The Medic's Guide to Work and Electives Around the World

The Medic's Guide to Work and Electives Around the World

Second edition

Mark Wilson BSc MBBChir MRCS MRCA Dip IMC

A member of the Hodder Headline Group
LONDON

First edition published in Great Britain in 2000.
Second edition published in 2004 by
Arnold, a member of the Hodder Headline Group,
338 Euston Road, London NW1 3BH

http://www.arnoldpublishers.com

Co-published in the United States of America by
Oxford University Press Inc.,
198 Madison Avenue, New York NY10016
Oxford is a registered trademark of Oxford University Press

British Library Cataloguing in Publication Data
A catalogue entry for this book is available from the British Library

Library of Congress Cataloging-in-Publication Data
A catalog record for this book is available from the Library of Congress

ISBN 0 340 810513

1 2 3 4 5 6 7 8 9 10

Commissioning Editor: Georgina Bentliff
Development Editor: Heather Smith
Project Editor: Anke Ueberberg
Production Controller: Lindsay Smith
Cover Design: Amina Dudhia, front cover pictures courtesy of Mark Wilson

Typeset in 9/9.5pt Times by Phoenix Photosetting, Chatham, Kent
Printed and bound in Malta.

What do you think about this book? Or any other Arnold title?
Please send your comments to feedback.arnold@hodder.co.uk

Contents

Foreword

Travel is one of life's gifts. Yet once the bug has bitten, the condition can be permanent. This book is incredible – how I wish it had been available when I started my own travelling career. Mark Wilson has clearly worked overtime to write it and has had tremendous enjoyment getting there.

As health services become ever more restrictive for the health professional or student, many look elsewhere for experience, teaching, greater personal responsibility and, let's be honest, fun. My own student elective, which took me from the comfort of London to Pakistan's remote and war-like North-West Frontier, started a process that continues to this day. India, Africa, the Middle East, the Far East, Central America, South America, Balkans . . . I could go on for pages. This year alone, I have been to a dozen distant lands: only last week, I was in Lapland talking to the Finns.

I look at those who do not travel and my heart goes out to them. They are missing so much and frequently do not realize it. Character building and med-ical training are not all about reading huge tomes and wafer-thin journals. I interview a lot these days, dozens of CVs passing across my desk for the handful of posts a teaching hospital can offer. Everyone – almost – is highly qualified, matching the specification like a glove. So how do I learn what the applicant is *really* like? Could I work with them? How will they react when under stress? I look for two things – personal interests and, wait for it, travel. They have never let me down. You only have to flick through these pages to feel a sense of excitement grow within your chest. What next? I want to be out there. I want to be everywhere. I want to journey to far-flung lands. Read this and I'll wager the travel bug will bite. Congratulations, Mark. You have done restless folk like me a gigantic service.

Richard Villar
Cambridge
Author of *Knife Edge – Life as a Special Forces Surgeon*

Preface to the second edition

'Medicine, as a doctor, nurse, physio or student, is your passport to the world.' That's how the first edition of this book started and it is still the best sentence to describe the wonderful and unique oppourtunities that we have. We have skills that are welcomed the world over. Most cultures have health as a central focal point and hence there is probably no other career that gets you involved in the heart of a community so easily.

Virtually all medical students and many nursing students get the opportunity during their training to spend some time overseas. This is a fantastic opportunity. While there is obviously the element of a holiday to such adventures, careful planning can make it very beneficial to both your training and future career. In addition, more and more of us are working overseas once qualified. The primary aim of this book is to offer an informal guide to what various hospitals are like all over the world. It also has information on other organizations for those that don't want to work in a hospital setting (flying doctors, forensic pathology, mountain rescue to name a few examples . . .).

This second edition has required a mammoth effort. In the last four years there have been massive changes – the principal one being the growth of the Internet. This now means that many more hospitals (even tiny ones) have websites. Where possible, all such adresses have now been included. The growth of medical schools has also occurred at a tremedous rate. For example, Nepal only had one medical school four years ago – now it has five! Many hospitals seem to have changed address and phone number; some have closed, new ones have opened. To top it all, half of Europe changed its currency! A few new countries have been included and, to make it all the more exciting, a new

Adventure Medicine section has been added.

The term 'Medic's' in the title of this book really does refer to all health professionals. The first edition of this book was primarily aimed at doctors planning work and medical students planning electives. Under most hospitals there is a section entitled 'Elective notes' and this contains jottings primarily from what medical students and doctors have reported. It may not therefore always be relevant directly to other health professionals, but it gives you a feel for what the hospital is like, both clinically and socially. Such information can be very difficult to come by as not all health schools keep elective reports from former students. As much information as possible has also been added regarding each country's regulatory bodies/professional organizations for nursing, physiotherapy, OT etc.

Here's the format of this second edition:

Section 1: Has up-to-date information on planning work and electives around the world. There is also a chapter on your health while overseas including vaccinations to think about getting and new information on HIV post-exposure prophylaxis.

Section 2: Provides details on healthcare systems, professional organizations, hospitals and what it's like to work in over 100 countries. Addresses (including website addresses) have all been updated. If you fancy some time in a warm environment, take a look at the Caribbean chapter. If 'hi-tech' is more your style, try the USA.

Section 3: This is a new adventure section covering expedition, diving, mountain, space and aviation medicine.

Section 4: The appendix has details on well over 100 non-governmental organizations. There's information on grants available to UK citizens and full listings of embassies in the UK, US and Australia.

As with the last edition, popular places and places people have enjoyed working in get the most coverage so apologies if 'your' big centre doesn't feature that highly. It's probably not visited that often – however, if you think you know a place that should be added or expanded upon, please do write and say. Remember that people move on, good hospitals go bad and bad hospitals sometimes improve (they rarely go bust!) . . . do let us know if you think somewhere has changed.

I have tried to make this book as up to date as possible, but the world seems to be changing at quite a pace. In the last few years there have been huge political changes especially with wars in the Middle East. Just because a country is not always in the news, it does not mean that it is necessarily safe. Please do get current advice before arranging an elective/work. A good website for this is run by the UK Foreign Office (www.fco.gov.uk)

As with the first edition, this book works hand in hand with the website www.medicstravel.org – here you will find updates to this book and useful tools such as a translation service, a jobs/CV database and information on locum/recruitment agencies/NGOs.

You have a wonderful opportunity to travel with your medical knowledge and skills. Plan well, you'll have a fantastic time. Please do let me know of your adventures! Good luck!

Mark Wilson
2004
E-mail: mark@medicstravel.org

Medicine, as a doctor, nurse, physio or student, is your passport to the world. We can turn up virtually anywhere around the globe, be welcomed and then be suddenly involved with the most important part of local people's lives, their health. There is probably no other profession that can offer this entrance into so many cultures. For this reason, if wanting to travel, doing it while working is a superb way of really experiencing life in another country.

All medical schools and many nursing schools have an 'elective' period offering a golden opportunity to undertake some training overseas. More and more qualified medics are taking time out of the normal career path to gain such experiences. However, whether studying or working, finding out about destinations can be difficult. You'll want to make sure you're going to the 'right' place for you. This book is designed to help.

Section 1 of this guide consists of three chapters giving advice on planning an elective, arranging work and organizing your own health requirements (both vaccinations and occupational) before departure.

Section 2 gives details about healthcare systems and hospitals in over 100 countries. If you know that you really want to work (play!) on a sunny tropical island, take a look at either the Caribbean or Pacific Island section. If you want developing world medicine, look in the Africa or Asia chapters. If it's hi-tech you're after, try the USA. Wherever possible, as much information about the hospital, its specialities and its social life and local activities (such as skiing or beaches) has been given. For elective students, there's some idea of accommodation costs. Medics can, of course, work in more than just hospitals. For the adventurers out there, other organizations, such as ski-patrols, NASA and the Royal Flying Doctor Service, are also listed at the end of their respective countries.

Section 3, 'The Appendix' is a valuable reference tool. If you want to work with an overseas organization rather than directly through a hospital, look under non-governmental organizations. This is a comprehensive list of agencies that provide aid overseas and require medics. A list of bursaries mainly for elective students in the UK is also given. Finally, details of embassies in Australia, the UK and the USA, as well as suggested vaccine requirements, are provided.

The countries that are popular and interesting have been the focus all along. In a similar fashion, interesting hospitals, even those with only 20 beds, may have more text than a hospital with 1000 beds. There is also more detail on countries where English is spoken or where translators are available.

The Medic's Guide is as up to date as possible at the time of writing, but of course hospitals and staff change. It has also sometimes had to rely on personal opinions. If you find things better, worse or in any way different, please let us know. Information on any hospitals not listed would also be greatly appreciated. There's a £200 prize, and you will of course get a mention in the next edition. Either fill in the coupon at the back of this book or e-mail us at updates@medicsworldwide.com.* Updates, lists of locum agencies and other information will also be provided on www.medicsworldwide.com*.

This information should give you some idea of where you would like to go and a taste of what medicine is like in that country. Everyone seems to benefit from time overseas. The patients benefit from some care they might otherwise not have had, and you benefit from what the experience teaches you. If you plan your trip well and choose a good destination, you will go a long way to insuring you have an interesting and enjoyable time. Remember, planning the trip is half the fun of it. Have a great time wherever your adventure takes you. If you do, please write and tell us.

MW
Whyalla, Australia
2000

*Now: updates@medicstravel.org
and www.medicstravel.org

Acknowledgements

There are many people who have helped to contribute to both the first and second editions of this book. The medical schools of the universities of Edinburgh and Cambridge, UCH and the Middlesex, and St Bartholomew's and the Royal London must be thanked for allowing me to look through their elective reports during preperation of the first edition. Those whose elective reports proved extremely useful and those whose signatures I could read are named below. Thank you for writing interesting and detailed reports. You've made it a great deal easier for others to find out about places. There are quite a few names I couldn't read: I'm really sorry I haven't been able to include you, but thank you just the same. Thanks also to the embassies and other medical schools in the UK that also supplied information. Much of the updated information came through medicstravel – I'm really grateful to all those who sent updates.

A number of other people have also helped with the project: Dr Dennis D'Auria, Alistar Wilson, Chris Oliver, Stephen Miles, Hugh Montgomery, Richard Villar, Richard Hanny, Paco (sorry mate … forgot your surname), Flynn Snell, Patrick Medd, Heather Le Cocq, Caphwin Laband, Mike Wells, Bip Nandi and Mr Paterson Brown for their enthusiasm. Dr Alan Hargens of NASA-Ames Research Center also has to be thanked for giving me such a great start.

The following have to be thanked for their help in my rather unusual career – Mr Mohammed Shibu, Mr Graham Moir and Mr Nigel Carver, and Drs Helen Cugnoni, Catherine Henderson, Fiona Lamb, Mr James Christie and Mr Chris Oliver.

Finally thanks to my family and Kelly for putting up with me whilst this was compiled. I'm sorry it took a bit longer than expected!

Grateful thanks to: Naa Annan, Dominic Hennessy, Lleona Lee Cam, Abigail Turner, Susan Dowling, C L Hardie, Helen Dormand, Sian Fiend, Simon Brown, K Gardiner, Stephen Kelly, Jennifer Kitson, Helen Briggs, Duncan Bew, Nicola Finneran, Lisa Clampitt, Marko Kerac, Hammon, H Law, Eric Yeung, Matthew Bur, S Lam, Amrit Ray, Bip Nandi, Sophie Coutouvidis, Mark Latimer, Gwyn Carney, Julia Relf, Madhumita Bhattacharyya, Anu Mitra, Katherine McGlone, Debi Ray, Sophie Dean, Diana Flemming, Julie Hutchison, Owen Anderson, H Sultan, G Sittampalam, Paul McGarry, Steven Epstein, Richard Edwards, Edward Hall, James Orr, Balsit Chander, Tara Bharucha, Anna Kirby, Mohini Varughese, Wanaratram Nasreen Jaffer, Emma Meikle, G Sittampalam, Sarah Gorman, Kate Janessy, S Cooper, Barnaby Major, Paul Albert, J Cheeseman, Joe Hall, Sonia Saha, Sheen Khanduri, Vicki Billing, Simon Calvert, Roger Patel, Ruth de Newtown, Neil McNamara, Gordon Peters, Stephen Wilson, Alan Clark, Freya Garbutt, Emma Nichols, Matthew Outram, R Henderson, Derek Kelly, S Bennett, Richard Bramble, James Porter, Catherine Theodorion, Rosie Davis, Kayode Adeniji, Lorna McCavat, Michael Chapman, Katherine Rank, Lisa Lewry, Paul Simons, Robin Johns, Catherine Scrutton, Brinda Murthsamy, Peter Williams, Geoffrey Corbett, A Morgan, T Thomas, Sarah Andersen, Giles Becker, Charlie Huins, Anna Bever, Vicky Johnson, Fraser, Georgia Page, Sally Ann Gibbs, Catherine Mackman, Angela Bell, Shareen China, S Teo, K Fong, Chumbi Chumbier, P Albert, Agarwala Godbolt, Lionel Tan, K M Nicol, Angela Bell, Susan Cook, Brinda Muthusamy, Alison Stewart, Lisa Andrews, Andrea MeKee, John

Woolmore, Judith Brown, C Lawthom, Helen Twydell, Priya Prasad, Sarah Wray, Roland Bunting, Lynn Brown, Mike Wallace, Stephen Kelly, Chris Butler, Kirsten Henderson, Sarah Hichens, Rebecca Underwood, Topun Austin, Hariet Fraser, G Hamlin, Emma Smith, Ed Fitzherbert, Baird, Maggie Ford, John LeMaitre, Eiva Tremaras, G Brynes, Simon Robinson, Emma Chan, R A Cadogan, W Mason, C Warwick, Katherine Oliver, Abigail Walker, Anne Baird, Heather Jack, Kerri Davidson, Kirstie Nicol, Joe McDowell, Dawn Alison, Kai Ren Ong, Alistair Brooks, M A Buchanan, K Graham, K Riddle, Andrew Fry, Angus Brown, Kirsty Friendly, Elspeth Macsween, Sam Cole, Eiva Trewavas, J McMillan, Berenice Oxford, R Reynolds, Sarah Sankey, Mark Craig, GR Dunn, Stephen Nicol, S Coutts, S Gulathakuta, E Doyle, Andrew Evans, K Connolly, Emma Davidson, Kryshani Fernando, Victoria Ferrar, Clare Byne, Ellen Rawlinson, Andrew Richardson, Sally Watkinson, A Sobaki, Sola Sobaki, Robert Carter, M Choudhry, Mohammed Belal, Leigh Crutchfield, Hilary Stephens, S Brown, Graham Collins, Chris Lambert, Kate Jarony, K Blight, Jennifer O'Brien, Annalisa Payton, Mathew Clark, Helen Twydell, Matthew Clark, Hevs Le Cocq, Richard Stumpfle, Jane Henderson, Thomas Martin, Emma Davidson, K Connolly, Jovina See, Li Wee, Choo Chin Hong, Charmaine Foo, Edwin Cooper, Stanley, James Crawford, Emeline Dean, Simon Butcher, David Porter, Nicholas Park, S Petrie, G Whitfield, Andrew McGin, C McAdam, Andrew Bracewell, James Henderson, Pete Wilde, Kay Seymour, Greenwood, Sinclair Gore, Chris Watts, Kamillar Porter, Sweeney, Nicola Marks, Jane Heraghty, Anne Chan, Jeremy Reynard, M Oddy, Thomas Bate, Sabastian Stur, Anton Bungay, Kim Williams, Simon Clint, Mark Wilson, Simon Matthews, Kate Washington, C McAdam, Tracey Sims, A Ransen, R Waller, James Myerson, Kate Williamson, Anya Wechsler, Ed Moran, Jennifer Anderson, Nicky Henderson, Laura Townsend, Kate Hodder, Stephen Ward, Nick Burfitt, Natalie Heaton, Deborah Wake, Hirst, K Gardiner, Alistair Brit, Elizabeth Davies, Richard Baxter, Nicola Smith, Tracey Smith, Alex Hart, C Efthymiou, Mike Wells, Z Christie, F Saunders, Neil Abeysinghe, Rachel Bullock, J Philips, Rosie Peet, Philip Hammond, Sarah Al-Termini, Charlotte Davies, Philip Davies, Julia Rebstien, Lara Tate, David Banks, Kate Chester, Choong-Sian Fong OCJ Thompson, Jasmin Hussein, Carolyn Cooke, Angharad Puw Davies, Sanjay Patel, Matthew Smith, Elizabeth Sapey, Ramani Moonesinghe, Michelle Lee, Rina Pancha, Stella Wong, Rachel Protheroe, Louise Tofts, Caroline Noakes, Eva Lew, Claire Plunkett, Vijai Ranawat, Mary Garthwaite, Adam Boyd, Hayley Barbet, Rosalind Tandy, Gareth Bashir, Russell Hawkins, Emily Watkinson, Helena Deeney, Anna Munday, Christina Thirlwell, Donna Gray, A Stanb, Ellis Hamilton, Mark Weatherall, Cathy Brice, Claire Mitchell, Baak Javid, Sarah Clark, Samantha Cole Haddon, Clare Cuckson, Eleanor Wood, Jonathan D'Souza, Stuart Benzie, Brain Chro-Kay, KT Porter, Sarah Lee, Claire G Harrison, Daniel Thurley, Lucy Meakin, Mark Braganza, Simon Harlin, Nick Haden, Charlotte Anderson, Paul Beirne, Paul Monks, Khan, Mohammed Ziaur Rahman, Samantha Stephen, Judith Littlejohns, Julia Maltby, Caroline H Costello, Hazel Wilkins, R Harisworth, Sarah Walmsley, Nicholas Conway, Suzanne O'Neill, Siobhan Whitley, Brian Lockey, Johanna Bell, Caphren Laband, Julian Harrold, Lawrence John, Clare McLaugh, Karen Julils, Elspeth Wise, Irene Chang, J Cheeseman, P Holmes, Andrew Douglas, Bryan Morland, Lindsey Smith, Lindsay Cosgrove, James Barry, B Choo-Kang, Jeanette Richard, C Harchie, Gordon Fetes, Jennifer Ketson, Karen Mitchell, Martin Chambers, Claire Neale, Stanley Chia, Yen-Ch'ing Chang Lee, Paul Kelland, Jonathan White, Rosie Davis, Kayode Adeniji,

Lorna McCavat, Michael Chapman, Katherine Rank, Lisa Lewry, Paul Simons, Robin Johns, Catherine Scrutton, Peter Williams, Roger Alcock, Fiona Collins, J Mills, M Guttikonda, Fiona Black, Kirsten Henderson, David Bacon, Jon Biro, Richard Griffiths, James Evans, Sarah Horn, Alison Stewart, Natasha Gilcrest, Sarah Gibson-Smith, Andrew Sykes, Roger Alcock, Marion Dimigen, Julie Baptie, Dominic Hennessy, Jeffrey Khoo, Peter Scholten, Amanda Clements, Julie Wood, Angela Luck, Patrick Fenny, Ruth Groves, Tim Caroe, Andy Curry, Helen Barker, Doug West, Georgia Libby, R Newell, Nick Green, Chin Whybrew, M Murray, Isabel Andrews, Beth Weatherley, Nicholas Brown, Tom Wright, P Crosbie, Lynsey McHugh, Edward Duncan, Kerry Gardner, Isabel Andrews, Emma Halliwell, Rachel Hoyles, Emma Wykes, Daniel Park, Jenny Dowler, Ambreen Kalhoro, Michael Hamblyn, Paul Barker, Bruce McManus, Joana Monjardine, Claire Neale, Monica Paris, Neil Abeysinghe, Ashlesha Dhairyawan, Anthony Cheesman, C A Mason, Zoe Astrouakis, KT Pother, Robert Henderson, M Sidery, Robin Johns, Morley, G Homill, M Cadamy, Jamie F Welch, Nicola Starritt, K Rice, Thereza Christopherson, Stephen Young, David Cairns, Amrit Ray, Stanley Chia, Andrew McDuff, Nilay Patel, Bobby Kumar, Maty Simpson, Serena K Ng, Paul Bishop, Bellemy, E Carling, Marcia Schofield, Sally Axelby, Adrian Cree, Jonathan Burns, Emma Spurrell, Andrew Sharp, Gavin Richard Speke, Megan Smith, Juliette Jackson, Mark Litchfield, Laurence Nunn, Kim Williams, Tom Konig, Natalie Morris, Luke Gompels, Mike Aratow, Sandy Green, Gita Murthy, Paul White, Ben Harrison, Catherine Walker, John Mathewson and Carrie Walker.

I am grateful to Irene Wells, Jane Fox, Ann Coney, Ann Cassey, Vicky Ibrahim, Shazia Jamal, Maria Brolley, Fiona Oaks, Heather Roberts, Diana Walton, Jane Zuckerman, Pratiba from UCL and all the other elective coordinators in the UK who have helped.

Others I would like to thank are Jenny Travis, Alistair Steel, Gavin Wooldridge, Riyaz Ahmed, Lorna Burn, Z Khan, Layla McCay, Ernesto Guiraldes, Toni Acton, Alexandra Clarke, David Morgan Griffith, Sujata Soni, Sarah Mackie, Andy Parrott (the God of MIU – or so he says!), Tom, Doro, Alex and Katie Gilkes.

I must also thank Glen Devich for his work on the New Zealand chapter, Rhona MacDonald of the *BMJ* for her fantastic support through the entire project and Dr Syed Ali, Dr Sarah Rafferty, Mr Christopher Oliver, Mr Lawrence Watkins and Ms Joan Grieve for their help with my career.

Finally I am hugely indebted to Penny Howes for her amazing hard work copy editing this book – thank you.

Abbreviations

ATLS	advanced trauma and life support
ALS	advanced life support
BNF	*British National Formulary*
CCST	Certificate of Completion of Specialist Training
CCU	coronary care unit
COPD	chronic obstructive pulmonary disease
CT	computed tomography
CV	curriculum vitae
CVA	cerebrovascular accident
DGH	district general hospital
ECG	electrocardiogram
ENT	ear nose and throat
ER	emergency room
EU	European Union
GDP	gross domestic product
GI	gastrointestinal
GMC	General Medical Council
GNP	gross national product
HIV	human immunodeficiency virus
IVF	*in vitro* fertilization
max-fax	maxillo-facial (surgery)
MCQ	multiple choice question
MDU	Medical Defence Union
MI	myocardial infarction
MPS	Medical Protection Society
MRC	Medical Research Council
MRI	magnetic resonance imaging
MRSA	methicillin-resistant *Staphylococcus aureus*
NGO	non-governmental organization
O&G	obstetrics and gynaecology
paeds	paediatrics
PET	positron emission tomography
SLE	systemic lupus erythematosus
STD	sexually transmitted disease
TB	tuberculosis
UN	United Nations
VSO	Voluntary Service Overseas
VT	vocational training

Section 1
Getting Ready

The period you have for your elective can be the best and most rewarding time of your student years. It's a time when you have complete autonomy to travel anywhere and do whatever you want. With that in mind, you'll want to make the most of the trip. Organized planning and having the right contacts are therefore vital. This book is designed to give you a few tips on how to plan your elective, but more importantly, it gives you the contacts that can otherwise be very hard to come by. For those who do not yet know where they want to go, the ideas generated from these places may spark further investigation. There are a whole host of factors that you should consider in choosing where to go.

DO I HAVE TO GO TO A HOSPITAL?

Do not immediately assume that you have to go to a hospital for an elective. Most sensible deans will see great potential if one of their students does, for example, research at NASA or forensic investigation in New York. You can push this further to diving medicine or joining a mountain rescue team (take a look at Section 3!). The world really is your oyster. Think about any hobbies or special interests you have ... can you squeeze them into your elective? If you're a nursing student who enjoys skiing, how about some work with an emergency ski patrol. You won't know if you don't ask!

HOME OR ABROAD?

For some people, financial or personal constraints (or exam re-sits) may mean that they have to do their elective at home. DO NOT DESPAIR. There are

still great opportunities to be had. If you're the academic type, there may be projects both at your home school and elsewhere. Think about what has really interested you. If you simply can't afford to go abroad, consider at least going somewhere different: if you're training in London, why not try a spell in Edinburgh or Dublin? Before you resign yourself to staying put, remember that there are plenty of travel awards for the taking. An award of only a few hundred pounds may well be enough to get you abroad and, if you pick a poorer area, the cost of living can be minimal. Whatever you do, do SOMETHING. It's never too late to organize an elective even if you have left it to the last minute or your original plans have fallen through.

DEVELOPED OR DEVELOPING WORLD HOSPITALS?

If you have decided on going to a hospital you need to consider what you want to get from your elective. Do you want space-age hi-tech investigations that you may not get at home? If so, one of the large university or private hospitals in the Western world (especially the USA, Canada or Australia) would be a wise choice. This may also give a different kind of cultural experience, showing how medicine can be with a big pot of money. Is it any better?

At the other extreme you can try the more destitute developing world scene. Although you will learn nothing about positron emission tomography, you will find out a great deal about common diseases and some that are rare back home. You will also be of more use to the hospital and more likely to be learning by experience than lectures. Medical students and nurses often find themselves behind a desk with (or without) a translator on their first day, being expected to run a clinic! There is no quicker way to learn than this. Many students find this incredibly frightening; the patient trusts you as they assume that you're a doctor. DON'T PANIC. Most hospitals of this sort have very limited resources therefore you'll only have access to a very limited weaponry with which to do harm. Make sure you have your Oxford Handbooks and the *BNF* to hand. Occasionally, things are very bad and students have found themselves the most-qualified (or least-unqualified) person around. In these situations, you tend to learn how not to do things. Whether patients benefit in these settings is debatable, but it may be all they can get. Working overseas to be allowed to do things you could not do back home poses some interesting ethical questions.

Think too about how much you need home comforts. If you're willing to rough it for a bit, the experience that developing communities offer can make it well worth your trouble. If you're on a tight budget, you may find you can live for next to nothing. If there is no way you can cope without a hairdryer or a McDonalds around the corner, try somewhere else. Along similar lines, consider whether you want urban or rural life. If you are stuck in a bush clinic, there may not be many clubs or bars at night. There may, however, be a great social life with other members of staff.

There is one other tip if you are going to a developing country. It is sometimes the case that government-run hospitals are underfunded, lack resources and have staff that may not be that interested in medical students. Missionary hospitals are also usually underfunded and lack resources, but usually they are more efficiently run, have staff that are trained overseas and they often have a better social life. This book has therefore occasionally concentrated on such hospitals in areas where the government hospitals are not recommended. Wherever possible, an idea of how 'Christian' they are is given so that you don't offend or feel awkward if it's not really your 'scene'.

In general, most missionary hospitals and organizations are happy if you just respect those with Christian beliefs; a few, however, require full participation.

As most medical/nursing schools provide 8–12 weeks for an elective, it may be worth trying both extremes of medicine.

ACTUALLY, I JUST WANTED A HOLIDAY:

Another very important consideration is what to do in your time off. If you are in a remote, isolated area, you may get incredibly bored unless the social life in the hospital is good. Under 'Elective notes' in the various sections hints on how the social life runs and what there is to do nearby are included. You can pick your hospital so that it is conveniently located next to a ski slope or beach. Remember that your elective is a big holiday as well. You may want to work for most of it and have a couple of weeks travelling. Alternatively, you may want to pop in the hospital for one day, get your forms signed then get out scuba-diving. Whatever, think about where you want to go and how good the transport links from your hospital are. Where possible, how much work consultants expect has also been included.

FINDING OUT ABOUT PLACES:

Well, you've begged, borrowed or stolen a copy of this book and it lists many places and gives ideas for electives outside hospitals. Maybe, however, you still want something else. There are a number of places you can look for more information.

The Internet:
The world-wide web is growing at a tremendous rate and is an excellent source of information, especially for the USA and Europe. Where available, web addresses have been included with hospitals listed in Section 2. Running in conjunction with this book is a website called Medics Travel (www.medicstravel.org). In

addition to supplying addresses and information on hospitals, it also has a discussion board and jobs noticeboard as well as updates for this book. So if you want to find someone to go on your elective with or need some idea of the cost of flights, this is the website for you. Another good website is Hospital Web, which has a full list of American hospitals and links to many 'Western' hospitals that are on the Internet (http://neuro-www.mgh.harvard.edu/hospitalweb.shtml). For medical schools, try the website of the Institue of International Medical Education: www.iime.org.

If what you're looking for isn't there, try a search engine such as Google (www.google.com) or AltaVista (www.altavista.com): you may be able to find the name of a specialist in the field you want to study. If you cannot find where the hospital is on a map, try www.multimap.com. Other useful sites are www.countrycallingcodes.com (for international dialling codes) and www.xe.com (to covert currency).

One big drawback of the Internet is that it doesn't supply information on small hospitals, for example in Africa and on Pacific or Caribbean islands. This book has therefore concentrated on such places. There are a number of websites giving information on missionary hospitals. One such is www.missionfinder.org – more are listed in Section 4.

Previous reports:
Students in the years above your own will be able to recommend or warn you off certain destinations. Their advice can be invaluable. Ask them and look at their elective reports.

Hospital staff:
Consultants and other senior staff tend to have buddies all over the world, especially in their field of interest. Ask if they can recommend people.

Medline:
If you want to work in a specialized field, type the keywords (e.g. 'surf board' and 'injuries') into Medline and see who is doing the latest research. This will give you an address that you can contact directly.

Organizations:
Many non-governmental organizations and missionary organizations (*see* Section 4) are happy to take students. That said, a few consider students to be a bit of a burden, so don't get upset if they don't rush to accept your 'help'. The **International Health Organization, Salvation Army, African Inland Mission** (and other Christian organizations) are examples of those which have been very helpful in the past.

There are also organizations specifically for medical students. The **International Federation of Medical Students' Associations** (IFMSA) (www.ifmsa.org) has previously helped with electives. They have a professional and research exchange programme.

Europe (excluding the UK) is not a popular elective destination, presumably because of language barriers. The **European Medical Student Association** (EMSA, c/o Standing Committee of European Doctors, Avenue de Cortenbergh 66/2, 1000 Brussels, Belgium. www.emsa-europe.org) has been set up to promote exchanges between European countries.

The **European Action Scheme for Mobility of University Students** (ERASMUS/SOCRATES Programme; UK Office, University of Canterbury, Kent CT2 7PD, UK. Tel: +44 1227 762712. Fax: +44 1227 762711. www.ukc.ac.uk/ERASMUS/erasmus/) organizes exchanges (for a minimum of 3 months) between European universities. It is open to all subjects and even helps with funding. Countries involved include Austria, Belgium, Cyprus, the Czech Republic, Denmark, Finland, France, Germany, Greece, Hungary, Iceland, Ireland, Italy, Liechtenstein, Luxembourg, Netherlands, Norway, Poland, Portugal, Slovakia, Spain, Sweden, Romania and the UK.

The World Health Organization has

published a directory of medical schools, although this really only gives addresses. University College London has an International Health and Medical Education Centre. They run a specific International Health Elective (www.ihmec.ucl.ac.uk).

The *Student BMJ* (www.student bmj.com) often has extremely good articles on electives in a number of countries, so keep an eye out there for more ideas.

CLIMATE:

You may have always had a burning desire to visit a particular country, but find out what the weather is like at the time of year that you can go. For example, the Himalayas are incredibly beautiful and relatively warm in October, but at other times of the year they are bitterly cold and dangerous. Some of the hospitals listed in Canada are always in snow, but certain times of the year are better than others. Ask at a student travel shop or look in the front of the Lonely Planet guide for that country. Also, remember that areas of large countries can vary tremendously. The coast of Australia is relatively cool compared with some of the deserts of its interior.

LANGUAGE:

It is obviously vital that you can converse with both the patients and the medical staff. Fortunately, English is often the language used to teach medicine even if it is not the local language. Also, because of their education, many doctors in non-English countries (e.g. many parts of Africa) speak English. It is, however, vital that you find out about this. In China and South America in particular, you may get very stuck if no one speaks English. Do not be put off if locals don't speak English as there will normally be nursing staff or translators available. Even if that is the case, try to learn some of the language, the pleasantries and a

few phrases such as 'Where does it hurt?' . You will often get out what you put in. Some people will love to chat to you to improve their English; if no one speaks it, you may get left by the wayside. Check the *BMJ* as courses in foreign languages are sometimes advertised (contact EMSA (*see* above) for more details). For an online web translation service that may be useful when writing letters, check www.medicstravel.org.

SAFETY AND SHOULD I GO ALONE OR WITH FRIENDS?

If you're lucky enough to have friends, you may well want to go with them. This has some great advantages and a few disadvantages. The most important consideration is whether you are going somewhere dangerous. Many places, especially in areas of South Africa, are really quite dodgy even for chaps travelling with a colleague. Seriously consider going with someone if you are planning to go as a lone female. On the subject of danger, try to avoid war zones. They may produce interesting stories but only if you're around to tell them.

The other big advantage of going with someone is that it gives you someone to talk to, to share your experiences with and generally have a good time with. Sharing travel costs (e.g. car hire) can also increase your spare cash. Problems may arise though if you fall out, if they want to go hiking while you would rather be on the beach or if you discover they've been sleeping with your boy/girlfriend etc. Make sure they are good buddies before you go. Remember that death (of patients) is common in developing countries. If on your own, this can be quite disturbing, especially if you have no one to talk to.

Something you may not notice is that with a companion you tend not get involved in the life of the local community as much as you otherwise would. You may not get quite the adventure or cultural experience you had hoped for.

Although every effort has been made to offer up-to-date advice at the time of printing, it is imperative that you establish the current situation before agreeing to work or study anywhere in the world. A good website is run by the British Foreign Office (www.fco.gov.uk). If going somewhere a little dicey, it is worth giving your home embassy in that country your details when you arrive so that if an emergency arises, they know where you are.

WHAT DISEASES WILL I SEE AND WHICH ONES CAN I CATCH?

Many Western countries have the diseases you are used to seeing at home. They also tend to be quite safe from the point of view of what you can catch. If you want to see the things that are rare at home then developing world countries are the places to go (see 'Your health whilst abroad' for more details). Think carefully. Countries differ greatly. Nepal, for example, has tuberculosis and rheumatic fever, but is low in trauma and HIV. Some areas of Africa have been swamped with the complications of HIV and in some Zulu townships the prevalence is approximately 50%. The population you see in a hospital setting therefore has an even higher prevalence. Although this means that you will see a wide variety of complications, you will see little being done about it. These hospitals can afford only basic care with antibiotics and no more. The other consideration is risk to yourself. The needle-stick transmission rate is around 0.3%, which is incredibly low. However, the prospect of tests hanging over you if you sustain one can ruin your elective. ALWAYS USE PRECAUTIONS, including goggles, and if you are going to a high-risk area, consider taking post-exposure prophylaxis. Some of these areas are very violent so there are plenty of minor operations and suturing. Great experience, just be careful.

OK, I'VE DECIDED WHERE TO GO. HOW DO I APPLY?

APPLY EARLY. If you know what you want, write as soon as possible. Chances are someone else wants to go there too. If you want to join the Royal Flying Doctors, for example, you should probably apply during your first or second year at college. Many associations will now only take Aussie students. Some Australian hospitals get booked up a year and a half in advance, as do some in the UK.

If you have left it until the year of your elective, don't panic. Apply anyway. People drop out and places may still be available. For hospitals in developing regions, it may not be so much of a problem, although slow postal services mean that you should still leave plenty of time.

How do you get in touch? This book lists addresses, phone and fax numbers and, where possible, websites. Unfortunately, names of individuals have not been included, primarily to stop them getting bombarded with mail, but also because people move on at an incredible rate. You don't want your letter to get put in the bin simply because the addressee doesn't work there any more. The best advice is to try to find out the name of the medical superintendent or equivalent; addressing your letter to a specific individual will increase the chances of getting a result. A visit to the hospital website or a quick phone call can do this. If this is too much effort, simply address the letter to the Medical Superintendent (for most developing country hospitals), the Chief Medical Officer (in Australia/New Zealand) or the Elective Coordinator or Admissions Organizer if applying via a university.

If the hospital is on the web, you may be able to find the name of someone in the speciality you're interested in. Write to that individual directly. He or she may say that they would be happy to have you shadow/assist them. You can then write to whoever is in charge saying that 'Dr X has kindly offered me an opportunity to follow his work for Y weeks . . .' and you are writing to enquire about accommodation, etc.

You may be wondering whether it's best to write, fax or e-mail: it really depends on where you are applying. If applying to do an established elective programme (e.g. in an Australian or US teaching hospital), then e-mailing the electives coordinator is fine. Small, remote developing world hospitals may, surprisingly, also have e-mail facilities, and many of these now prefer the speed and usually cheaper option of e-mail. However, there is something nice about recieving a formal letter with a crisp CV attached. This makes a letter far more difficult to ignore. If writing, do at least include your e-mail address so that you can get a speedy reply. If e-mailing, try to attach a copy of your CV, but bear in mind that developing hospitals may have very slow connections so make sure the file is not too large.

So you've sent your letter or e-mail but have heard nothing. For many areas, it can take weeks or months to get a reply. Try e-mailing again. If you receive a reply, you MUST write back and confirm acceptance or, if you have had other replies, politely say that you have already accepted another offer. Never just forget it. They may be making plans for you and you are also withholding someone else's elective place. By all means reply by fax or e-mail.

What if they don't speak English? Bear in mind that you're not going to get very far if you don't learn their language. If you want to write in, say, Spanish, either get a Spanish friend to do it for you or use the translation service on www.medicstravel.org. Type in your letter in English and it will be translated. It may not be 100% correct, but the recipient will be glad you tried. You can then translate their reply using the same service.

BUREAUCRACY:

Do you need a visa to study or work at a hospital? The official lines for the various countries have been included at the beginning of each chapter. If you're from outside the UK, you will have to enquire at the embassy in your country for more detail (*see* Section 4). Having said that, you will get into most countries as a tourist. Obtaining a tourist visa is usually not difficult. Most hospitals won't check (or care) what kind of visa you have. However, this can be a dangerous ploy as the last thing you want is for passport control not to let you in. This book is only allowed to give official advice, and therefore the official advice is to get a visa if required. If you're happy to take a bit of a risk and say that you're just on holiday as you walk through … good luck. For many countries (especially in the developing world), you'll probably be fine. Be very careful in the USA and Canada as they may well require a medical as well as a visa. Hospitals there may also be keener to check for security reasons. Most places have a limit to the length of time a tourist may stay so make sure that you're not going to exceed this. Landing cards often require an address for your stay in your destined country. Putting down a hospital is asking for questions. It is safer to get a visa.

FUNDING:

For most students, getting hold of some cash is vital for their elective. There are many organizations that can help you out. BE ORIGINAL. A list of commonly used bursaries is included in Section 4, but a very comprehensive database can be found on www.rdinfo.org.uk. Drug companies receive thousands of letters. Although a few of these may produce results, most drug companies have specific funds that require applicants to write an essay. It is still worth trying as this puts many people off. Other medically related companies (there are thousands, from nappy makers and baby food suppliers to those that make medical equipment) may well be worth approaching. If you can relate your elective to the company and state why they should sponsor YOU over anyone else, you immediately put yourself at an advantage. Canvass anyone and everyone. Offer a copy of your elective report on your return.

Your own institution may well have prizes and sponsor awards. If at Oxbridge, your college may be able to help a bit. If you went to a posh school, they too may have a bit of spare cash. Offer to give a talk about your trip when you get back.

Organizations such as Rotary Clubs and local churches are often keen to do a bit of fundraising for you. If taking money from Joe Public though, you really should be doing an elective where you are of use rather than funding a trip to Bondi Beach. Again, offer to give a talk on your return.

Local companies may also sponsor you. Apply to anyone you can link yourself with, from the local shops to the local brewery (after all, you have probably been funding THEM for the past five years). You could also try making a bit of money. Can you sublet your room while you're away? Can you rent out your bike or computer? Whatever you decide to do, apply to as many people as you can and try to be different from the thousands of other letters they receive.

Some books that list organizations include: *The Directory of Grant Making Trusts* (Charities Aid Foundation), *The Annual Register of Grant Support* (Macmillan Press) and the *Educational Grants Directory* (by French *et al.*).

If you haven't already got one, you can also apply for a student loan (which unfortunately has to be paid back, usually over a five-year period from the April after graduation). Contact the **Student Loans Company** (100 Bothwell Street, Glasgow G2 7JD, UK. Tel: +44 800 4050100. Fax: +44 141 306 2005).

When applying for funding, you should include a few items:
- A very nice (typed) letter introducing your application and reasons why it deserves funding
- A copy of your CV (*see* page 10)

```
                                    Bedside Manor
                                      St Cuthbert's
                                         London
                              justin@stcuthberts.ac.uk
Dr Nookie,
Medical Superintendent
The Tropical Island Hospital
Paradise
                                      20 April 2004
Dear Dr Nookie,
```

I am a final year student at St Cuthbert's Medical/Nursing/Veterinary School in London. During this year of my course I have the opportunity to spend X weeks abroad discovering how medical practice differs from here. I have heard impressive reports from those that have previously visited your hospital, and I am writing to ask if it would be possible for me to spend some time at the Tropical Island Hospital between X and Y 2004. I really would appreciate the chance to study in Paradise.

Please find enclosed a copy of my CV, and please do not hesitate to get in touch at the above address/e-mail/fax number if you have any questions.

Thank you for your time in reading this letter.

With best wishes

Yours sincerely

Sample covering letter

- A copy of your research proposal if appropriate (*see* page 10)
- Ideally, a letter from your dean confirming that you're not a fraud.

RESEARCH:

You may be using your elective purely as a holiday, but if you want financial help, are hoping to win a prize or are even trying to produce a paper, a project can be an excellent plan. It can be anything from estimating the prevalence of HIV in an African village to high-tech research for NASA. Whatever, plan early. Ethics committees often need to be consulted, and you'll want to work out a viable method for your investigation. Some organizations (*see* 'Elective and travel bursaries' in Section 4) will reward you handsomely for your efforts. The **Medical Research Council** (20 Park Crescent, London W1 4AL, UK. Tel:

Curriculum Vitae
Name: Justin Case
Date of Birth (Age): 1st April 1983 (20)
Address: Bedside Manor, St Cuthbert's, London e-mail justin@stcuthberts.ac.uk
Driving Licence: Full
Education: Dibelthwaite Comprehensive St Cuthbert's
Exam Results: GCSEs: 5 Grade A, 4 Grade B A levels: Home Economics A, Textiles B Media Studies N
Medical Exams: 1st MB 51% 2nd MB 52%
Intercalated BSc: Social Anthropology (2:2)
Publications: One hundred and one uses for a chocolate teapot. Case J and Bloggs J. *Home and Garden* 2002; 13: 110–111
Previous Employment: McDonalds Restaurant 1997–1999
Non-Academic Achievements: Blue Peter Badge 1997
Referees: Dr D.O. Little, Department of Social Studies, St Cuthbert's

+44 20 7636 5422. www.mrc.ac.uk) has contacts all over the world.

You will want to write a detailed but brief research proposal that you can submit when applying for funding. It should not really be more than one side of A4 paper. Some important tips are:

- Have a good clear title
- Start with an introduction or abstract that demonstrates you've done some background reading ('It has been found that …')
- State clearly and precisely the aim(s) of your project (but don't be over-ambitious)
- Outline your method, including the number of subjects you hope to use
- Outline how you will analyse your results
- Explain how what you may find will be of use in the future.

Setting a proposal out in this standard 'scientific' fashion looks much more impressive (and is hence more likely to get funding) than just stating a title in a letter.

YOUR CV:

By now, you have probably written many CVs, possibly for your house jobs. Everybody thinks their CV is the best. In case you've never written one before or want a few tips, an example is shown of how to set one out. Sticking (or cutting and pasting if you are really good on a computer) a photo in will also make your CV more appealing (unless of course the rear end of a camel is more attractive!).

WHAT SHOULD I TAKE?

Without wishing to state the obvious, don't forget your passport, tickets, clothes and a toothbrush. There are, however, items that you may not think of both for yourself and, if going to a remote area, for the hospital.

For the hospital and staff:

- British National Formularies. You've probably collected loads of these by now. Ever looked in one? You will need to now. If you are going to a developing country, take all the copies you have, no matter how out of date. You will make instant friends with the sister and clinic staff if you give them a new supply.
- Any slightly out-of-date textbooks that you're not going to use again will also go down well.
- Drugs/supplies. You may be asked to bring a few supplies out, and it's a very nice gesture to offer. If this is just a couple of boxes of gloves, it shouldn't be a problem. For medications, a bit more planning is necessary. Ask the hospital to send you a letter requesting exactly what they need. Keep this safe so you can produce it if any problems are encountered at customs. If they see a letter from their own country, customs officials will be more sympathetic

than if they see a scrap of paper signed by one of your mates.

Equipment for Charity Hospitals Overseas (ECHO; Ullswater Crescent, Coulsdon, Surrey CR5 2HR, UK. Tel: +44 20 8660 2220. Fax: +44 20 8668 0751. www.echohealth.org.uk. E-mail: cs@echohealth.org.uk) can give plenty of advice on what is legal/ illegal for you to take out.

• Sunday newspapers and magazines. If you know that there are missionaries or ex-pats where you are going who have been out of touch for years, you will guarantee friendships if you bring them news from home.

For yourself:
• If you're a medic, the (Cheese and Onion) *Oxford Handbook of Medicine*, the *Oxford Handbook of Specialties*, and probably also the mini Kumar and Clarke (*Clinical Medicine*, Saunders Pocket Essentials Series, by A.B. Ballinger and S. Patchett), are essential. If you are nursing in a developing country, consider getting these as well. Having your own *BNF* will save you having to search for their 1972 edition.
• A stethoscope (obviously).
• Gloves and goggles. Most hospitals, even the most primitive, have these, but some do not. If you are in any doubt, take your own. If you have allergies to any types of glove, take some you know you're ok with.
• A white coat. Some places may expect you to bring your own. In others, shorts and t-shirts are the dress. Take it just in case.

Other handy travellers' items can be:
• A padlock (and maybe a chain) to secure your bag to roofs of buses
• A thin plastic sheet for dirty hostel beds
• A Swiss Army knife
• A torch
• Sunscreen/lip balm
• An attack alarm for women
• A camera and a notebook or diary (especially if you have to write a report when you get back)

• An old passport. (Hand this one rather your real one over in hotels – they never check the date – and if you have to make a sharp exit, at least you can leave the country!)
• A first aid kit (*see* 'Your Health whilst Abroad').

TOP TIP: You may be worried about losing your passport, visas, etc. A cunning idea is to scan them into a PC and e-mail them to yourself as attachments. Then, if the worst does happen and all your bags go missing, you will still be able to get copies by walking into any Internet café.

INDEMNITY INSURANCE:

Once you've been offered an elective place, you'll need to think about medical indemnity insurance to cover any 'mistakes' you make. For many people, especially those going to developing countries, this isn't a major issue. However, it will be a problem in America, Canada and possibly Israel (which has the world's second-highest litigation rate). You should ask your destination whether cover is automatically provided or whether you can purchase cover through them. Ask your defence union too. The **Medical Defence Union**, **Medical and Dental Defence Union of Scotland** and the **Medical Protection Society** in the UK, for example, will cover nearly all destinations. If they can't cover you, they can recommend brokers who can. This area is obviously changing, and you must contact your union for advice. Further medico-legal matters are included in the entries for the relevant countries. Nurses are often covered by their UK provider, and in many developing countries this is not a problem anyway. Again, check with your institution and provider.

TRAVEL INSURANCE:

Most insurance policies appear pretty similar – they vary a bit on the number of millions they cover in medical expenses, but otherwise there is not much to choose between them. There are, however, a couple of points to consider. A number of insurance providers (e.g. **BMA Services**; www.bmas.co.uk) are now providing cover for canellation in case you fail your exams. Hopefully you won't need that. More importantly, cover for repatriation following needle-stick injury can now be provided. This may not seem like much, but it is a fantastic cover to have. You don't need to sero-convert or be unwell – if you've had a needle-stick injury and are scared to death (which you may well be), you can at least get home for some professional advice. Nurses should contact the **Royal College of Nursing** as they too often have affliated companies that can pro-vide good deals on insurance. And remember, if you're thinking of doing any barmy sports, make sure you're covered for hazardous pursuits!

TRAVEL ARRANGEMENTS AND COSTS:

This is the fun part. With everything confirmed, you can finally go and book your flights. Remember (as if you'd forget) that discounts are available for students.

You should now be ready to go. Before you leave, it may just be worth phoning or faxing your destination to make sure they are still expecting you. You've done all the hard work … now go and enjoy yourself.

More and more doctors, nurses and other health professionals are taking time out of their normal career path to work abroad. There are many reasons for this. An obvious one is to escape the pressures and strains of working back home, but this should by no means be a primary reason since, chances are, you'll have to come back one day. The vast majority of people want to travel to experience medicine in another culture. As 'medics', we are in a unique position. We can turn up virtually anywhere in the world, be welcomed and then suddenly be involved with the most important part of local people's lives, their health. There is probably no other profession that can offer this entrance into so many cultures.

Very early planning is extremely important in taking time out. Just going on a whim is asking for trouble. That said, if you want to work abroad and have found yourself without a job, there are a number of agencies that can arrange work in Australia and New Zealand with just a couple of months' notice. Reciprocally, locum work in the UK is usually abundant for visiting medics. You will get far better jobs though if you sit down and plan your trip.

If you are reading this, you are obviously at least toying with the idea or working abroad. There are, however, some questions you need to ask yourself.

SHOULD I TAKE TIME OUT FROM THE NORMAL CAREER PATH?

You will get plenty of advice from seniors in your field. This typically ranges from 'I wouldn't do that ... it's a competitive world you know' to 'Excellent idea – go for it'. Whose advice should you take? At the end of the day, both can be good or bad: it will depend on what you do and how well you sell yourself. You can guarantee that it will be a topic of conversation at any interview and will help them to remember you.

A very good piece of advice from a senior London A&E consultant was, 'Go down the pub with a pen and paper. Have four or five pints, not enough to get drunk, but enough to get merry and honest with yourself. Then write down the five things you MUST do in your life.' If travel is one of them ... read on.

Of note, the UK Department of Health has recently developed a website (www.doh.gov.uk/internationalhumanitarianandhealthwork) and 'Toolkit' with information to help all health professionals plan work overseas. It's well worth taking a look at this early on if you're thinking about doing voluntary or paid work abroad. It gives advice on career breaks, planning overseas work into your training and organizations that the NHS approves of.

WHERE SHOULD I GO AND DO I WANT PAID OR VOLUNTARY WORK?

WHERE and WHEN to go should be considered together. For your elective you probably knew whether you wanted a developed or a developing world setting. This time you have to consider the need for paid work. If you need pay, you are probably looking at going to a developed country. Remember though that developing countries are often extremely cheap to live in and, if you are going through an organization, living expenses are sometimes provided.

You should ask yourself what you want to get out of this trip. Most specialities have obvious advantages for either setting. What would you enjoy and benefit from most? If you want to do invasive cardiology, a trip to a high-tech speciality hospital may help your career more than listening to heart murmurs in Africa. If obstetrics is your forte, the frequency of complicated deliveries in a developing world setting may well be more use. If planning a trip that will last 6–12 months, there is no reason why you can't work in two or more places.

Nurses should consider their end career aims as well. The developing world setting, especially if the trip is arranged through a non-governmental organization (NGO), will probably have you diagnosing and treating more cases independently than you would back home. If you know that you want to be a nurse specialist in a specific field, ask your seniors at the hospital you currently work at whether they have any contacts.

WHEN SHOULD I GO?

This is a very important consideration. If you're currently without a job then now is probably as good a time as any, although even locum work abroad can take a couple of months to set up (because of visa and medical requirements).

If you're sensible and planning your trip carefully, bear the following points in mind. The earlier you go, the fewer ties you have (mortgages, partners, children, etc.) but the less experienced you are and hence the narrower the range of jobs available. The later you go, the more ties you'll have, and you may well get trapped in a job.

Doctors:

Once qualified, you could travel immediately. However, it is extremely difficult to get a clinical job anywhere if you haven't even registered in your own country. It really is probably a bad idea to travel in your pre-registration year (or in the first two years if working in a foundation post).

Many people go before their first SHO job. This is a good time as you're not on a rotation and, as said above, probably don't have much to sort out at home. You still have to ask yourself, 'How much use am I and where could I work?' Some agencies in Australia and New Zealand require a minimum of three years' postgraduate work (and in Canada they often want some obstetrics and gynaecology and/or paediatrics work). Do not let this put you off. If you plan things well, going at this point can be very much to your advantage. Some organizations are now offering work that can actually count back in the UK. This means that you can travel to Australia, do a six-month emergency department job and have it count towards, for example, the MRCP/MRCS qualification on your return. Make sure with the relevant Royal College that they will recognize it BEFORE you accept the post. If wanting to do developing world work while training as a GP, it is worth noting that the Royal College of General Practitioners now recognises programmes run by VSO and such work can actually count towards your training. Contact the college and VSO for more details.

You may, however, be looking for something a bit different. You would imagine that developing countries would be grateful for any help available and, indeed, individual hospitals usually are (hence writing directly will often give very positive results). NGOs and other agencies are often a little more picky however. They usually receive a number of applicants and will take those with the most experience. Overall though, with a decent plan, this is a reasonable time to travel. Try to get a job for your return before you go (see below).

After the first SHO job (usually in emergency medicine) is another common departure time. The added experience that just one SHO job gives makes you instantly more 'sellable', but remember that many agencies want those at the end of their house officer/foundation years. For example, ships' doctors are usually required to have a minimum of two years' experience as well as at least advanced life support or advanced trauma life support (posts being advertised in the *BMJ*). Apart from this, much of the advice is similar to that above.

In between house officer/foundation years and registrar posts is an excellent time to go, but waiting till then, remember that you may have ties. An irresistible job may also quash your ideas, and you may have to postpone travelling for some time. The experience you have at this stage (especially if you have some O&G, and paeds, under your belt) makes you valuable everywhere. Locum agencies in Australia and New Zealand will snap you up, as will NGOs and other organizations. This is currently a popular time for UK doctors to go as many people are waiting for training numbers, and travelling (as well as research) can obviously help. The only problem is continuing to apply for numbers and jobs whilst you're away. You will obviously have to keep in close contact with someone at home who can check your mail etc. Keep an eye on www.bmj.com.

As a registrar you can often take a year to work overseas and count it towards your training (at least on the CCST scheme in the UK). This opportunity varies from speciality to speciality and from country to country. You really do have to talk to your deanery and the college of the speciality you want to work in, both at home and in your desired country. There is not normally a problem if you want to work in a 'Western' hospital in somewhere like Australia. Arranging work in developing countries, while it may provide great experience, may not been seen so favourably. What you can get approved will very much depend on how well you can sell your idea. Alternatively, you can wait until you've completed your CCST.

As a consultant, you will have to tie in overseas work with your clinical commitments back home. Can you take a month off? Can you take time out as a sabbatical? Can you swap temporarily to part-time work? Can you job share? All this will very much depend on your speciality and the trust you work for.

Having the general skills (some medicine, O&G, and paeds) of a GP makes you very valuable to NGOs and remote hospitals. If you are in a practice, will your partners be happy for you to take time off? Could you get a job in a practice where everyone has a set time off on a rotating rota? Can you work as a GP locum? Could you 'job swap' (people often ask for swaps on www.medicstravel.org)? If a member of the BMA, you can access two useful resources on their website (www.bma.org.uk). One is entitled *The Members' Guide to Working Abroad*, the other *Opportunities for Doctors in Europe*.

Nurses and other health professionals:

Once registered, you have a valuable tool that enables you to travel at any time. The more experience you have, the more valuable you will be (especially if you have a broad range of experience and want to work in a developing country). However, as time passes, you may well develop restrictions such as a mortgage and a family.

How long do you want to go for? If for only a short period, would you be able to take a sabbatical? Many trusts (in the UK) allow you to take time out if you have been employed with them for a minimum period, and they keep your job to come back to. If you are going to a developed country such as Australia (from the UK) or the UK (from Australia), there is absolutely no reason why working overseas should halt your career progression. Once home, many people see great advantages in gaining experience in another health care system.

If you are a nurse specialist, do you want to do more specialist work overseas or have a period being more of a generalist again? Are you wanting to earn cash quickly? Take a look at the Middle East. Are you wanting to travel and just have a job to provide some funds while away? Try Australia. One important consideration is your ability to register with the relevant council/authority in your destination.

Where known, some details as to how much post-qualification experience is required is listed under each country.

Radiographers, theatre nurses, pharmacists, physiotherapists and occupational therapists all have careers that travel well. Are there any hospitals that might be of particular interest to you (e.g. physio – look under Rotorua, New Zealand)?

HOW DO I FIND OUT ABOUT AND APPLY TO PLACES?

This book has addresses and information on hospitals and other institutions as well as NGOs. You have a number of choices.

Applying directly to hospitals:

This is especially relevant if you want to go to a developing country, but many smaller hospitals, for example those in rural Canada and Australia, are desperate for people and will also welcome direct applications. This approach is ideal if you are looking for work of less than six months' duration. The main disadvantage is that you'll need to organize your own visa, registration, malpractice insurance and medical/nursing certification where appropriate. Check hospital websites as these are commonly used as a way of advertising jobs.

When writing to a specific hospital, try to address someone personally as this will give you a much better chance of a favourable reply. You can look on the web to find a suitable name, or ring and ask for the personnel department. For developing countries and small rural hospitals in Canada, Australia and New Zealand, you really want the name of the medical superintendent. As already said in 'Planning your elective', you should include a covering letter stating why you want to work there and a detailed copy of your CV. Write as early as possible, especially for work in developing countries, as the mail can take weeks. Try to include a fax number or e-mail address so they can respond quickly.

Let someone else do the work:

You can let an agency find you work. This can be either an NGO if you want to do voluntary work, or a locum-type agency if you need paid work. This approach may give you less choice about the precise destination and agencies will usually only arrange contracts for six months or longer.

Non-governmental organizations: There are many different agencies offering healthcare to those in need all over the world. Many are listed in section 4. Some are missionary based, but most are based on apolitical and secular principles and receive funds from charity donations. Some run permanent hospitals; some provide relief aid where and when it is needed. You will almost certainly find a charity that will be grateful for your services in the area you are wanting to go.

Be aware though that some NGOs can be quite choosey. If they have to go to the trouble of providing some preliminary training, organizing visas, accommodation, etc., they will probably ask for at least a minimum of six months' commitment, and many now ask for around two years. Do not be disappointed if they do not appear grateful if you offer to work for only a few weeks. For short-term work, it may be best to apply to a specific hospital. Note that Médecins du Monde (UK) and Voluntary Service Overseas (VSO) now take people for as little as three months. If it's disaster relief work you're after, an agency really is the only way. Although the work is usually voluntary, most agencies cover expenses and some also give a small allowance.

Medical employment agencies: Many agencies providing paid work advertise in the *BMJ*, *Nursing Times* and equivalent journals. For Australia, some can do virtually all the organizing (including flights). Remember though that they often only have places that Australians don't really want to work in. They are usually remote. This may be great if you want an outback experience, but be wary of committing a great deal of time if you don't know what the place is like.

If you can't find anything in this

book and you don't want to apply through an agency, look on the web. http://neuro-www.mgh.harvard.edu/hospitalweb.shtml is a very useful website that lists many hospitals around the world. Unfortunately, it does not help if you are looking for a hospital in a developing country that is not on the web. Asking colleagues in your hospital whether they have any contacts and looking through previous medical students' elective reports are other sources. The **International Health Exchange** (*see* Section 4) produces a magazine that advertises jobs around the world. Visit www.medicstravel.org and look under 'Planning your elective' for more ideas.

CONFIRMING A POST:

If you get an offer of work, either paid or voluntary, you must write back and accept or cancel it. If you have any concerns about a post, you can (if you are a member), discuss it with the BMA, although there is little that they can do to enforce 'working conditions', etc. since the post lies outside the UK. If you want a post to count towards your postgraduate exams, make sure you enquire with the appropriate Royal College before accepting it.

HOW WILL I JUSTIFY MY TRAVEL AT INTERVIEW AND WHAT ABOUT A JOB ON MY RETURN?

It's an excellent idea if you can get a job to return to before you go (hence the VERY early planning). Your potential employers will obviously want to know what your plans are. If you can't get a job, bear in mind that you will either have to come home early to try to get one, be able to apply from abroad or be willing to do locum work.

Whatever, at some point someone is going to ask you about your trip. They will want to know why you are going/why you went. 'I didn't like Great Yarmouth' and other negative reasons

should definitely not be mentioned. Emphasize the gains. Say that although you realize medicine is highly competitive, you are not wanting to race up the career path. State that you wanted to gain wider experience beforehand that you could then use in your later work. Remember that interviewers are usually not so bothered about academic qualifications at interview but rather the qualities of people they would enjoy working with – the kind of qualities that working abroad can enhance. Try to have some interesting stories from your time abroad or a good plan if you have not yet gone. As long as it is not obviously a huge holiday, most forward-thinking consultants see overseas work as a big plus.

FUNDING:

This may or may not be an important issue. If you have savings and a paid job to go to, there should be few problems. NGOs will often provide a small allowance. If you are doing something entirely voluntarily, your finances may be stretched. A fantastic website that lists numerous grants, for both travel and research, is www.rdinfo.org.uk. A number of grants are available (*see* 'Elective and travel bursaries' in Section 4), even for those who are qualified. Further details of other grant-making bodies can be found in *The Directory of Grant Making Trusts* (Charities Aid Foundation), *The Annual Register of Grant Support* (Macmillan Press) and *Educational Grants Directory* (by French *et al.*). You can also write to local companies, clubs, churches etc.

If you're not earning (e.g. you're working for an NGO or just volunteer work) and are a member of the BMA, you can save yourself the annual fee by telling the BMA that you are a 'medical missionary', thus getting free membership for a year. See the section on funding in 'Planning your elective' for more ideas on how to raise cash. Money can still be paid into a superannuation fund while you're away. Some NGOs now pay into these, and employers abroad may also be able to.

MEDICAL REQUIREMENTS:

Many countries require that an overseas doctor or nurse has a medical before practising. This is especially true of developed countries such as Canada and Australia. Details are given under the relevant country. A medical can usually be arranged through your GP, but you may be able to get the relative components carried out by hospital mates. A chest X-ray report, an HIV ($\pm$syphilis) test and a hepatitis B titre are sometimes required. *See* 'Your health whilst abroad' for information on how to organize this. Note that the UK now requires visiting medics (and medics who have been outside the UK for six months) who perform exposure-prone procedures to have HIV and hepatitis B and C tests.

INDEMNITY INSURANCE:

Your current provider may well cover you for work abroad in many countries (sometimes at no extra cost). A definite exception will be for those wanting to work in the USA or Canada. For both of these, the **Medical Defence Union** (MDU), **Medical Protection Society** (MPS) and **Medical and Dental Union of Scotland** (in the UK) can recommend insurance brokers (see the relevant country). If you are planning to work anywhere abroad, you must contact your provider to ensure that they cover you – and to get advice if they don't. If they do cover you, ask for a letter confirming this and take it with you as it may be required when you arrive. For example, the MPS and MDU have reciprocal arrangements with most government hospitals in Australia and New Zealand whereby you are automatically covered. This does not, however, include private or GP work.

TRAVEL INSURANCE:

At the time of press, no insurance company seems to be offering repatriation to medical staff who suffer a needle-stick injury, however as it has become possible for medical students to get this cover, things may change. Contact your insurer to see whether they can add it.

PROFESSIONAL REGISTRATION:

The requirements to register as a medical practitioner vary greatly. In the USA, for example, you have to sit a series of exams. In some developing countries, you probably don't even need to register. If you are going through a locum agency or NGO, your registration should be sorted out for you, but if going under your own steam, you will need to contact the appropriate medical council for that country. As much information as possible has been included under the respective countries in Section 2 (and visit www.medicstravel.org).

It is a similar story for nurses. Each country has an association or council that has a process to ensure that you are sufficiently up to standard. Where the information is available, these organizations are listed under each country and should be contacted directly for the latest advice.

A quick note about Europe. A qualification as a doctor from within the European Union is valid throughout Europe, and registration in the host country should be relatively straightforward. These countries include Austria, Belgium, Denmark, Finland, France, Germany, Greece, Iceland, Ireland, Italy, Luxembourg, the Netherlands, Norway, Portugal, Spain, Sweden and the UK. Graduates from Australia, New Zealand, South Africa, Hong Kong, Singapore and the West Indies also do not usually have any problems. Those who have qualifications from outside these countries may still be able to register, but contact the registration authority in the country concerned for more details.

YOUR PENSION:

If working in the UK, you are probably paying into the NHS pension scheme. If you have been working for the NHS for less than 2 years and then stop, the contribuitions you have paid are supposed to be returned to you and your pension scheme cancelled. You must therefore discuss your plans with the NHS agency BEFORE YOU GO and if necessary obtain written confirmation that you will be allowed to continue your pension on your return. This is normally not a problem if you plan to do medical work overseas. If you have been working in the NHS for more than two years, your pension is simply halted. You may wish to consider buying extra years on your return. For more information contact the **NHS Pensions Agency** (Hesketh House, 200/220 Broadway, Fleetwood, Lancashire FY7 8LG, UK. Tel: +44 1253 774774) or, if you are in Scotland, the **Scottish Public Pensions Agency** (St Margaret's House, 151 London Road, Edinburgh EH8 7TG, UK. Tel: +44 131 244 3292. Fax: +44 131 244 3336).

WHAT TO TAKE:

Apart from the obvious travel items for yourself, you might also want to consider taking the following.

For the hospital and staff:

- Spare *BNF*s
- Any unused textbooks
- Drugs/supplies (*see* 'Planning your elective' and contact ECHO, whose address can be found in Section 4)
- Newspapers and magazines.

For yourself:

- The *Oxford Handbook of Medicine*, *Oxford Handbook of Clinical Specialities* and any books relevant to what you will be doing (e.g. tropical medicine)
- Medical equipment (e.g. a stethoscope, ophthalmoscope, etc.)
- Gloves and goggles if there is a chance that they might not be provided. If you have an allergy to some types of glove, make sure that you take your own.

Other handy items include:

- A padlock (and chain) to secure your bag to bus roofs
- A thin plastic sheet for dirty hostel beds
- A Swiss Army knife
- A torch
- Sunscreen
- An attack alarm for women
- An old passport (hand it over in hotels rather than your real one – they never check the date, and if you have to make a sharp exit, at least you can leave the country!)
- A first aid kit (*see* 'Your health whilst abroad').

A top tip is to scan in your passport, visas and degree certificates and e-mail them to yourself before you go. That way, if all your bags are stolen, you can still get copies by walking into any Internet café.

Have a quick flick through the 'Planning your elective' section as quite a bit is still relevant for planning work. If everything is well organized, you should have few problems and you can start looking forward to a wonderful time ahead. The final job is to organize your flights (use an under-26 card if you can) and travel insurance. Give your destination a call before you leave to make sure they are still expecting you. Good luck!

Your health whilst abroad

The main reason for travelling as a medic (apart from the holiday) is to see things that you don't see at home. This can be anything from weird tropical diseases and herbal medicines to trauma. Under each country is a list of the common causes of death, but in this section an outline of infectious diseases and other conditions that can affect YOU is given. Although these conditions are rare in most of the Western world, some are common in developing countries. It's good to see them, but try not to catch them. Hence read through the diseases, and if you're going somewhere it is prevalent, get vaccinated.

This requires some planning a few months before you go as you can't always have all your jabs at once. It can also add quite a lot to your expenditure if you get them from a specialist travel clinic. The occupational health department of your hospital should be able to help and can usually get them for you free or at cost price. If you're friendly with your GP and he knows that you are a poor, underpaid junior doctor or nurse (or an unpaid student), you may also get them free.

For your own health, it is simplest to divide your needs into:
- What you need to do before you go
- What you need while you're away
- What you need to do when you get back.

Another occupational health issue is 'what will the host country require from you in order to work in one of their hospitals?' For most developing countries, no medical is needed. Where information is available, specific requirements have been included under the relevant country.

If you are planning to travel with medicine, either working or as a student, get some official documents sorted before you go. Ideally, the following test results/vaccinations should be drawn up and validated as a single document on official hospital or medical school notepaper. They should be signed and stamped by the college medical adviser or GP and preferably bear an official validating stamp. You may need to show:
- Hepatitis B status (indicating the titre level)
- A list of vaccinations you have had (with dates)
- A chest X-ray report from the last six months
- A statement of your good health.

A number of countries also require an HIV/hepatitis C test before you can work (this now includes the UK if you will be undertaking exposure-prone procedures). If you have all of the above, you should have little trouble with occupational health departments in most countries (but see Canada, which is an exception). Australian health organizations occasionally also ask for proof of MRSA screening – try to get this done before you go.

Most of the next section is written for those travelling from the UK, but requirements are similar no matter what your home country. Incidentally, the UK has a reciprocal arrangement with a number of countries. Seventeen of these are covered with the E111 system in Europe. A couple of other Commonwealth countries (e.g. Australia) also provide cover, but remember that you will not be covered for repatriation. See the Department of Health's booklet *Health Advice for Travellers* for more information (www.doh.gov.uk/traveladvice).

WHAT TO DO BEFORE YOU GO:

Your own health:
Once you've decided on your destination, the first thing to consider is 'Do I

have a condition that means I should not go there?' If you've had your spleen removed, it can be extremely dangerous to go to countries where pneumococcus or malaria are common. If you have asthma, is it well controlled? If you have a severe attack (possibly triggered by a strange environment) will your inhalers be enough, or can you get to a (decent) hospital? Are you epileptic and would having a seizure put you in danger? If you have any condition that may in some way be a problem, discuss it with your GP/occupational health department before you go. This is vital. It may well invalidate your travel insurance, and you may end up in a bad way and not able to get home.

It's also worth going to the dentist if you'll be away for a while or if you're planning to go diving (as the expansion of air bubbles in a tooth cavity on surfacing can be agony).

Try to find out, and make a note of, your blood group – write it in your passport.

If travelling from the UK, make sure you have adequate travel insurance or if going to a European Union country, get form E111 from the Post Office giving you free/reduced-cost emergency treatment.

Is the country safe?

Political situations are always changing and watching the news is simply not enough. It is obviously a good idea to avoid wars, but in some areas political struggles and fighting have been going on so long that they no longer attract any attention. **The Foreign Office** (www.fco.gov.uk) can give advice. Ask anyone you know who has recently been there or alternatively, ask the hospital you are going to.

Vaccinations:

About three months before your departure, you need to consider what vaccinations you might require. A brief list is given in Section 4, but it is vital that you get current information as the list is only a guide. A fantastic up-to-date reference

is provided free from the World Health Organization on www.who.int/ith/. This enables you to get the latest information on specific diseases and the latest recommendations country by country. There are a number of other up-to-date sources: *Doctor*, *Practice Nurse*, *MIMS* and *Pulse* magazines, your GP and your occupational health department. **The Medical Advisory Service for Travellers** (www.masta.org), a unit in the London School of Hygiene and Tropical Medicine (Keppel Street, London WC1E 7HT, UK. Tel: +44 20 7631 4408) can also give advice. They not only give vaccine requirements, but also a summary of the political stability of the country. Pre-recorded health advice is available from the **London Hospital for Tropical Diseases** (+44 898 345081) or **Liverpool School of Tropical Medicine** (+44 891 172111).

TROPICAL DISEASES THAT HAVE VACCINES:

Yellow fever:

Yellow fever is a viral disease transmitted by the mosquito in African and South American forests. The disease is usually confined to monkeys, but 'jungle' yellow fever occurs when an infected mosquito infects a human. Although this is bad news for the man, there is also a real danger that he can then act as a host and transmit to other mosquitoes that usually feed on humans. Once a cycle has been established in humans, 'urban' yellow fever is said to exist. Countries such as India (*see* Section 4) do not have yellow fever, but they do have a ready supply of mosquitoes to transmit it. It is for this reason that they require a certificate stating that you have been vaccinated if you are coming from a country that has it.

The vaccine is given only in yellow fever centres (ensuring that vaccine storage, administration and certification are correctly carried out) so that an internationally valid certificate is given. A list of centres is included in the Department of Health publication *Health Information for Overseas Travel*, but your friendly occupational health department or GP should be able to point you in the right direction. The vaccine is a single live attenuated vaccine, and the certificate is valid between ten days and ten years after it is given. Countries where yellow fever is currently a problem include: Angola, Benin, Burkina Faso, Congo, Gabon, Gambia, Ghana, Guinea, Liberia, Nigeria, Sierra Leone and Suda in Africa; and Bolivia, Brazil, Columbia, Ecuador, French Guiana and Peru in South America.

Typhoid fever:
Since typhoid is spread faeco-orally, the risk obviously increases as hygiene decreases. This varies within a country (from the top five-star hotel to the student flea-pit) as well as between individuals. In most areas of Europe, America, Canada and Australia, hygiene will be fine, but if you are going anywhere where there may be doubt, get vaccinated. (This is a single intramuscular/subcutaneous injection requiring a booster every three years.)

Hepatitis A:
Like typhoid, hepatitis A is transmitted faeco-orally and hence is more common where hygiene is poor. Two types of immunization are possible: the active vaccine (conferring immunity for 10–20 years after two doses given six months apart) and passive immunoglobulin (protecting for up to six months). These should be considered if you are visiting areas with reduced hygiene.

Hepatitis B:
Medics (including students), nurses and others who are at risk in the UK should already have been vaccinated and have had their antibody titre checked. It is vital to ensure that you are up to date on this. A booster is normally required after five years. Enquire with your occupational health department. Areas of extremely high risk include Africa, Malaysia, Thailand, the Pacific Rim and

Aboriginal and Maori clusters in Australia and New Zealand.

Meningococcus A and C:
Epidemics of meningococcal A infection are common in Africa between the Sahara and Egypt, and down to Malawi and Zambia. Areas of India, Nepal, Pakistan and Bhutan are also at risk. It's usually a problem in the first six months of the year. If staying there for any length of time, it is well worth getting vaccinated. It is mandatory if going to Saudi Arabia during the Haj. It's a single injection requiring a booster approximately every five years.

Rabies:
Rabies is still a major problem in many countries. Australia, New Zealand, the UK and the Antarctic are rabies-free. Epidemiologically, it is divided into 'urban rabies', transmitted by rabid dogs or cats, and wild rabies, in which a reservoir of disease is maintained in foxes, skunks, bats, etc. Once the clinical symptoms appear, death is inevitable. If you are travelling where rabies is a problem and immediate post-exposure treatment is not available, pre-exposure treatment should be considered. This consists of two injections four weeks apart. If a booster is then given a year later, up to three years' cover is gained. Note: If taking chloroquine, it may cause a problem as you get a reduced antibody response to the vaccine. If you are bitten, you still need treatment even if you have been vaccinated. Prophylaxis just buys you time and lowers the dose of treatment needed.

Japanese B encephalitis:
Endemic in Asia and the Pacific Islands, Japanese B encephalitis is spread by culicine mosquitoes that normally live on rice paddies. Monsoons can cause epidemics. The disease occurs between North-east India, throughout South-east Asia, and the Far East. Pigs and birds are the main hosts. High fever, headaches and meningism, with a 40% mortality rate, occur in humans. A two-dose

vaccine (one to four weeks apart) is available.

Tick-borne encephalitis:
This condition is transmitted by ticks in the forests of Scandinavia, central and eastern Europe. You are at risk if doing lots of walking/camping. You should wear long trousers and insect repellent. If bitten, a post-exposure immunoglobulin is available in high-risk areas (get it within four days). If contact with long grass is unavoidable, a two-component vaccine can be used.

Tuberculosis:
All tuberculin-negative school children should have a BCG by the age of 13. If unvaccinated and travelling to an area of increased risk (Asia, Africa, Central and South America and the Pacific Rim), immunization (if you are tuberculin negative) should be seriously considered.

Some diseases that have vaccines that are rarely given include the following.

Cholera:
The vaccine is very poor and now not available in the UK. Just watch what you drink in Africa, tropical Asia, South and Central America.

Plague:
This occurs mainly in India, some parts of Africa and South America. Vietnam has recently had quite a problem. However, unless contact with rodents is unavoidable, it is very unlikely that you will need vaccination.

VACCINES YOU MAY NEED BOOSTED:

Polio:
If not boosted in the past ten years.

Tetanus:
If not boosted in the past ten years.

Diphtheria:
Although this is part of the routine childhood immunization programme, some adults may not be immune. Diphtheria is common in overcrowded areas, especially Africa, Asia, eastern Europe, Russia and Central and South America. If working in such areas, vaccination or a booster (if not boosted within the past ten years) should be considered.

SOME DISEASES WITH NO VACCINES:

Malaria:
Around 12 UK travellers a year die from malaria. Up-to-date lists of the malaria status of different areas are available from the **Malaria Reference Laboratory** in London (+44 20 7636 8626), Glasgow (+44 141 946 7120) and Liverpool (+44 151 708 9393). Remember that the malaria status can change between different areas within a country.

There are three components to preventing malaria:
- Avoid being bitten by *Anopheles* mosquitoes
- Use the correct chemoprophylaxis (YOU MUST TAKE IT AS INSTRUCTED)
- Seek medical help as soon as possible if you develop a fever.

Avoiding bites: *Anopheles* mosquitoes tend to bite indoors and at night. Wear long sleeves and trousers where possible and use a good insect repellent. More than 15% but less than 30% Deet is recommended, but some people get a reaction to it (test a bit first). Mosquito nets impregnated with parmethrin and mosquito nets over windows are recommended. Using an insecticide around the room in the evening will help further.

Chemoprophylaxis: Countries (and areas within them) are divided into three categories with three different prophylactic regimens. In any category, start prophylactics (except mefloquine) a week before departure to ensure that there is no allergy to the medication, and continue it for four weeks after returning. Mefloquine needs to be started three weeks before departure to ensure that you don't go mad.

The advice in the table at the end of Section 4 is only a guide. You must check up-to-date information. Current regimens are as follows but do check for the latest information (try www.who.int/ith):

- *Regime A:* For areas where *Plasmodium falciparum* has not yet been found to be chloroquine resistant, a once weekly dose of chloroquine (500 mg salt, 300 mg base) alone is recommended. It is usually well tolerated, especially if taken with meals.
- *Regime B:* Where chloroquine-resistant *P. falciparum* exists, mefloquine (250 mg salt, 228 mg base) once a week is recommended. Those with a past history of seizures, psychiatric disorders or cardiac conduction defects should not take it.
- *Regime C:* Doxycycline (100 mg/day starting a couple of days before arrival) can also be used where there is chloroquine resistance. However, some people get gastrointestinal side-effects and/or thrush. It should also be noted that it reduces the effectiveness of the oral contraceptive pill.

Remember that even with prophylactics malaria is still possible, so seek medical attention if you develop a fever (which can be anything up to a year after your return). The fevers with malaria usually present with severe shaking and sweating. You feel quite well between them. If in doubt, assume that it's malaria and get to a hospital. In the meantime, take quinine (600 mg = two tablets) three times a day for three days and doxycycline (100 mg) daily for seven days at the same time. Fansidar (a single course of three tablets all at once) is an alternative but occasionally fails (especially in East Africa).

HIV AND POST-EXPOSURE PROPHYLAXIS:

HIV is probably the biggest concern for medics abroad. It has become a huge problem, reaching a prevalence of 60% or more in some areas of Africa. Avoiding transmission through sexual intercourse is hopefully fairly easy. For most, the real concern is from needle-stick injuries or receiving blood products if you become ill. It is important to remember that needle-stick transmission is rare – only 0.3% of injuries seroconvert. However, a needle-stick injury in an area of 60% prevalence with no one to talk to and no occupational health procedures can destroy your trip. (It is thought that one UK doctor has died from HIV that he probably contracted while on elective in Africa in the early 1980s.) A number of medical schools have now banned students going to places such as Africa for this reason. This is a shame, as a great deal can be learned from such places. Many people go to South Africa to see trauma. Unfortunately, this is probably the department where you are most likely to get a needle-stick injury. Think seriously before you go. Will you just act as an observer? When you arrive, you may be the only medical person around and have no choice but to get on with stitching someone up. Are you willing to take the risk?

The only advice possible is to ALWAYS USE UNIVERSAL PRECAUTIONS on everyone. Always wear gloves (double) and a mask; always wear goggles (splashes get around glasses); always wear a plastic apron under a gown in theatre (you'll never find a waterproof gown in an African hospital, and you won't be pleased when you undress to find blood, amniotic fluid, etc. soaked through to your skin); always take extra care with needles; and always keep your hands out of the way when assisting in theatre. Some things, such as goggles and gloves, should be provided, but often they are not. If in doubt take some with you.

Some medical schools and occupational health departments can now provide (usually for a small deposit) HIV post-exposure prophylaxis packs. These contain a seven-day starter combination pack of a zidovudine, lamivudine and nelfinavir or indinavir. Note that the protease inhibitors can be toxic, especially if you are dehydrated. If you are going to an area with a high prevalence of HIV, the

Department of Health strongly recommends you take one of these packs. If you sustain a needle-stick injury, you can always ring home, get the advice of an occupational health doctor or virologist and then take the medications as necessary. A significant exposure to HIV-infected or high-risk blood includes percutaneous injury (e.g. needle-stick, scalpel, bone/glass fragments), exposure to your own broken skin (cuts, etc.), penetrating bites and exposure to mucous membranes such as the eyes. You will obviously still need to discuss with an occupational health doctor how long you should take the prophyaxis for (a full course being four weeks) and the times of HIV testing post exposure. Of interest, there have been 300 cases of reported seroconversion from inoculation injuries and around ten failures of post-exposure prophylaxis packs.

It is very difficult to get accurate information on rates of HIV. A table of the average prevalance for each country (estimated in 1999) is given in Section 4. The rate varies widely within any particular country; it is often the small villages that have the high levels, whereas the average in the country may be low.

A NOTE ON INSURANCE:

For electives, consider taking out an insurance policy that covers your flights home in the event of a needle-stick injury (e.g. in the UK, from BMA Services). This is something unique about these policies that is to be highly praised. There is little worse than the desperate feeling of lonliness that you can get after being exposed to HIV in a remote area.

If you've done all the above and you are fit and vaccinated, the next thing you need to do is pack a medical kit. It should include most of the items you are likely to need for your own health while away. Components are listed in the next section.

WHILE YOU'RE AWAY:

While away, you should take precautions not to become ill and know what to do if you do.

Precautions to prevent illness:

All the advice below is common sense, but it can be so easy to forget.

Trauma: With all the concern about vaccines, you may think that you're safe once you have had them all. Sadly, you cannot be vaccinated against the common serious condition that travellers get: you are far more likely to be involved in some form of trauma than you are to catch dengue fever. Be constantly aware of this and try to protect yourself. Even if the local custom is not to wear a cycle helmet or seatbelt, it is still obviously safer to do so. If the bus has bald tyres, a smashed windscreen and a driver who is drinking, don't get in it. It's never worth it.

If a disaster does happen, try to avoid a blood transfusion unless a life-threatening blood loss demands it. For some areas of particularly high risk, you may wish to consider taking some cannulae, a giving set and plasma expander (*see* below).

Travellers' diarrhoea: Expect to get diarrhoea if you are going to India or somewhere hygiene is not perfect. There are a number of things you can do to avoid it:

- Try to eat only hot foods or fruit that you actually peel yourself
- Avoid salads, fish and meat unless you're entirely sure of their source
- It is best to boil water or use chlorine tablets or iodine drops in all the water you drink. Alternatively, use bottled water, but be careful if in any doubt of its authenticity. Famous (bottled) fizzy drinks are usually OK. (And say 'No' to ice cubes in drinks.)
- Avoid milk and its products
- Remember that foods such as coconut can provide a lot of fluid (for much less cost) that is safe. Maintain a high intake of fluids if it's hot or you have diarrhoea. (*See* 'Your medical kit' below for more details of oral rehydration therapy).

Swimming: While on the subject of water, make sure that any water you swim in is safe, both from drowning and schistosomiasis (which is common in Africa). Stick to either swimming pools or the sea.

Sunburn: As on any holiday, wear high-factor sunscreen and try to stay in the shade if you're the type that burns easily.

Sexually transmitted diseases: Try to avoid collecting venereal diseases! They are very common in tropical areas. The locals may also want to kill you for messing with their people. (This is actually an important point. In some parts of KwaZulu-Natal in South Africa, just looking at a girl – even if not in any kind of admiring sense – can cause great aggravation.) The risk of death in overseas travellers is ten times higher from HIV than malaria (*BMJ* 1990; 301: 984–5). It is patronizing to tell medics to be careful, and advising use of condoms should really not be necessary. Just remember that alcohol can make you forget.

Acute Mountain Sickness (AMS): AMS can occur in anyone at an altitude of over 2500 m. It is far more likely to occur if no time has been spent acclimatizing and you have flown in or climbed too quickly. It is thought to occur because the low oxygen tension at altitude causes electrolyte changes that favour fluid retention. This is evident as peripheral and, more worryingly, cerebral and pulmonary oedema. Over 50% of people get it if trekking above 4000 m.

Symptoms usually occur within the first 12 hours of arrival and disappear over a few days if you climb no further. Occasionally it develops over a few days and worsens. The symptoms are headache, nausea, vomiting, fatigue, dizziness, sleep disturbance and anorexia. All these can of course occur with the flu or if pissed. However, you should ALWAYS assume that it is AMS and not go any higher.

Some divide AMS into benign and malignant. The above symptoms are the benign part. It can then worsen as oedema accumulates further, causing breath-lessness, dry cough (becoming productive with pink frothy sputum), severe headache, vomiting, irritability, drowsiness and finally unconsciousness. Remember that AMS can and does kill even at 3000 m. For the benign symptoms, it is best just to wait at that altitude. If they worsen, or any of the malignant symptoms develop, get down as fast as possible and get urgent help. Drug treatments are always secondary. Preventative measures include:

- A slow, graded ascent. Each night above 3000 m should be no higher than 300 m above the last, with two rest nights every 1000 m. Sleep lower than the greatest height reached that day
- Drink plenty of fluids and avoid alcohol
- Do not use sedatives
- Prophylactic drugs that are sometimes recommended include acetazolamide 250 mg twice daily or dexamethasone (not as effective) 4 mg four times a day.

The *High Altitude Medicine Handbook* (*see* below) is vital reading for those working at high altitude.

YOUR MEDICAL KIT:

This is a list of items to obtain for your own medical kit and what they should be used for. As on the ads, 'always read the label' before using any of the following.

For gastrointestinal problems:

Loperamide (trade name Imodium): This is useful for diarrhoea, although the most important thing is to keep yourself hydrated. It is useful to relieve the pain if nothing else. Take two tablets with the first loose stool and then one for every subsequent one.

Dioralyte: Or other rehydrating mixture, especially if the diarrhoea is severe.

Antibiotics: If you note blood with the stool or develop a temperature, a short course of ciprofloxacin should do the trick. If the diarrhoea continues (especially if it may be an infection with amoeba or *Giardia*) with nausea, frothy stools and lots of wind, metronidazole is a wise choice.

Cyclizine or prochlorperazine: This may help if nausea and sickness are a major problem.

Oral rehydration therapy: Put one 5 ml teaspoon of salt with eight teaspoons of sugar in 1 litre of CLEAN DRINKING WATER and take one to two cups with each loose motion.

For allergies and insect bites:

Chlorpheniramine: Chlorpheniramine (e.g. Piriton) or promethazine is handy for most allergies, including those to insect bites. It also helps with motion sickness. It can make you drowsy, but this can be an advantage if the itchiness is keeping you awake.

Insect repellent: Repellent (and often a net) are essential (*see* 'Malaria'). If you are really prone to being bitten, 'afterbite'-type remedies are available.

For throat and skin infections:

Co-Amoxiclav: This (or doxycycline) is handy for a bad sore throat, most chest infections and skin that has become infected secondary to bites or sores. Combinations of amoxycillin and flucloxacillin can also be used.

For trauma and pain:

Analgesic: Aspirin or paracetamol, or a codeine/paracetamol combination. Note that the latter can make you drowsy and bung you up … handy for when you've finished the loperamide.

Bandages and plasters: These are useful for blisters.

Syringes and cannulae: These are for the adventurer who is going places you really don't want to be getting ill. Areas with high levels of HIV and hepatitis are not areas to have an accident. Although taking your own cannulae may protect you from contaminated needles, they won't help you much if they're being used to give you infected blood. If you really are going to take such risks, a bag of gelofusin or similar may be a good idea (although the chances are that if you need it, you're not going to be in a fit state to set it all up).

General items:

- Sunscreen
- Water purification tablets or iodine drops
- Scissors ± tweezers
- Antiseptic cream/Fucidin ointment.

Elective medical packs are available from **Trebova Medical Student and Junior Doctor Supplies** (7 Burton Close, Gustard Wood, Wheath Hampstead, Hertfordshire AL4 8LU, UK). These include some syringes, Sterets, cannulae, a suture kit, Steristrips, triangular bandages, pins and scissors. You may be able to obtain these from your school or occupational health department. To avoid any trouble with customs officials, you are well advised to carry a letter (get a qualified friend to sign it) stating that that you are a medical student or doctor carrying medical supplies.

WHEN YOU RETURN:

It's not over yet. If you are taking malaria tablets, continue them for another four weeks and keep an eye out for anything unusual. If you feel there is anything wrong, a persisting cough or occasional fever, go to your occupational health department as soon as possible. They can arrange a tropical screen.

FURTHER READING:

- *ABC of Healthy Travel* (E. Walker, F. Raeside, L. Calvert and G. Williams, BMJ Books, 1997)
- The infectious diseases chapters in *The Oxford Handbook of Medicine* (J.M. Longmore, M. Longmore, I. Wilkinson and E. Torok, Oxford University Press, 2001) and the *Oxford Handbook of Tropical Medicine* (M. Eddleston and S. Pierine, Oxford University Press, 1999)
- *The High Altitude Medicine Handbook* (A.J. Pollard and J.R. Murdoch, Radcliffe Medical Press, 2003)
- *International Travel and Health 2003* (World Health Organization, 2003).

Section 2
Destinations

AFRICA

Botswana

Population: 1.5 million
Language: English
Capital: Gaborone
Currency: Pula
Int Code: +267

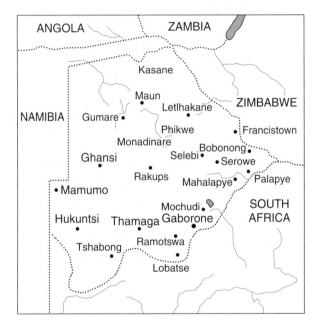

Botswana is a landlocked country just above South Africa. It gained independence in 1966 and has enjoyed relatively good econimic growth since then thanks to the discovery of diamonds. Botswana's population is mainly located in the eastern grasslands (where much of the diamond mining occurs). To the west lie the Kalahari Desert and the Okavango delta.

✛ Medicine:

Botswana is relatively fortunate in that poor nutrition and drought are no longer major detriments to health. Infectious diseases, especially HIV, are now of more concern. There is a 'Health for All' campaign that hopes to provide adequate healthcare to every citizen by the end of the decade. The doctor:patient ratio is 1:5150, which is actually pretty good for sub-Saharan Africa.

Botswana's public health system consists of different kinds of health facility: 23 district health teams, three referral hospitals (**Princess Marina, Nyangabgwe** and **Lobatse Psychiatric Hospital**), 12 district hospitals (of which six are operated by the government, three by missions and three by mining companies), 17 primary hospitals (at Bobonong, Ghansi, Gumare, Goodhope, Hukuntsi, Kasane, Letlhakane, Mmadinare, Palapye, Rakops, Sefhare, Thamaga, Tsabong and Tutume), 222 clinics, 330 health posts and 740 mobile stops.

The prevalence of HIV is very high (at 36%, probably the highest in the world), and this and other infectious diseases place a heavy burden on the health care system. Diarrhoeal diseases, measles, viral hepatitis, TB and, in the north, malaria are commonly seen.

In addition to the practice of Western medicine, there are a large number (possibly up to 2000) of traditional doctors such as herbalists, faith healers and diviners.

◎ Climate and crime:
The warmest times are November to March, but June and July have the lowest rainfall. The crime rate is generally low, diamond smuggling and robbery being the most prevalent crimes. The streets themselves are relatively safe.

⊃ Visas:
Visas are not required for most Commonwealth, Western European or US citizens who are 'visiting'. For official study or work, contact your local embassy.

USEFUL ADDRESSES:

Ministry of Health, Private Bag 0038, Gaborone. Tel: +267 352 000. Fax: +267 353 100. www.gov.bw/government/ministry_of_health.html.
Botswana Medical Council, Private Bag 0038, Gaborone.
Botswana Dental Association, Private Bag 00437, Garobone. Tel: +267 375 212.

MAJOR REFERRAL HOSPITALS:

Princess Marina Hospital
PO Box 258, Gaborone. Tel: +267 353 221.
The hospital: Princess Marina Hospital is the main government-run hospital in Botswana and therefore receives refer-

rals from many district hospitals. General medicine, surgery, O&G, paediatrics, ophthalmology and most major specialities are provided. Facilities include both CT and MRI. The staff are multinational and are often using Botswana as a stopping point on their way to somewhere else.

O Elective notes: They tend to be friendly, willing to teach and let you perform procedures. Most of the medical wards are filled with AIDS and TB patients. The paediatrics team is particularly keen to teach.

Nyangabgwe Hospital
Francistown, Botswana.
The hospital: This is Botswana's second major referral hospital. It has a range of specialities similar to that of the Princess Marina. It has a CT scanner but no MRI. It is also home to the Harvard HIV Institute laboratory.

Lobatse Mental Hospital
Lobatse, Botswana.
The hospital: Is Botswana's major psychiatric referral centre.

OTHER HOSPITALS:

District hospitals:
Lobatse Athlone Hospital, Box 20, Lobatse. Tel: +267 330 333.
Mahalapye Hospital, Bag 001, Mahalapye. Tel: +267 410 333.
Maun General Hospital, Box 12, Maun. Tel: +267 660 444.
Scottish Livingstone Hospital, Box 20, Molepolole. Tel: +267 320 333.
Sekgoma Memorial Hospital, Box 120, Serowe. Tel: +267 430 333.
Selebi Phikwe Hospital, Box 40, Selebi Phikwe. Tel: +267 810 333.

Primary hospitals:
Bobonong Primary Hospital, Box 7, Bobonong.
Ghansi Primary Hospital, Box 7, Ghansi.
Goodhope Primary Hospital, Box 175, Goodhope. Tel: +267 386 236.
Gumare Primary Hospital, Box 115, Gumare.
Hukuntsi Primary Hospital, Hukuntsi.
Kasane Primary Hospital, Box 3, Kasane.
Letlhakane Primary Hospital, Box 51, Letlhakane.
Mmadinare Primary Hospital, Box 72, Mmadinare.
Palapye Primary Hospital, Box 31, Palapye.
Rakops Primary Hospital, Box 12, Rakops.

Sefhare Primary Hospital, Box 23, Sefhare.
Thamaga Primary Hospital, P/Bag 4, Thamaga.
Tel: +267 399 250.
Tutume Primary Hospital, Box 36, Tutume.

Mission hospitals:
Bamalete Luthern Hospital, Box 6, Ramotswa.
(Very popular so apply early.)
Deborah Relief Memorial Hospital, Box 24,
Mochudi. (A medium-sized hospital about 70 km
from the city.)

**Seventh Adventist Hospital/Kanye Medical
Mission Hospital**, Box 11, Khanye. Tel: +267 340 333.

Mining hospitals:
BCL Mine Hospital, Box 3, Selebi Phikwe.
Jwaneng Mine Hospital, P/Bag 08, Jwaneng.
Orapa Mine Hospital, P/Bag 01, Orapa.

The country's private hospital:
Gabarone Private Hospital, Bag BR 130,
Gaborone. Tel: +267 301 999. Fax: +267 302 804.

The Gambia

Population: 1.1 million
Language: English
Capital: Banjul
Currency: Dalasi
Int Code: +220

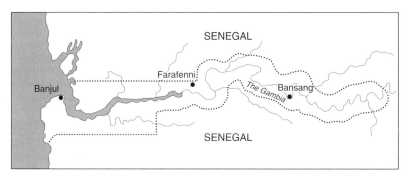

Gambia is a thin country – 48 km (30 miles) wide but 472 km (295 miles) long – situated on the west coast of Africa. It projects inland on both sides of the River Gambia and is totally surrounded by Senegal. From Banjul, it is possible to arrange trips to Senegal. It is not a popular elective destination, and most voluntary work has to be arranged through NGOs.

✪ Medicine:

Basic medical services are available to most of the population; however, neither medical care nor medicines are free. There is a vast shortage of doctors (only one for every 12 000 people), and a quarter of state doctors work in the main hospitals in the capital. Malaria, diarrhoea, malnutrition, TB, anaemia, snake bites, dysentery, pneumonia, burns and broken limbs are common, especially in the bush. The prevalance of HIV is around 2%. The three main hospitals in the Gambia are the Royal Victoria in the capital Banjul, the new facility in Farafenni and the Bansang Hospital in the remote area of Bansang.

➲ Visas and work permits:

Commonwealth nationals and those of countries who have abolished reciprocal visas do not need a Gambian visa for a stay of less than 90 days. Others must fill in the form (available from www.gambia.com) and send it to their embassy.

USEFUL ADDRESSES:

www.gambia.com, the official website of the republic of Gambia.
Ministry of Health, The Quadrangle, Banjul.
Tel: +220 227 300. Fax: +220 223 178.
Gambian Medical and Dental Council,
Kanifing (next to the Post Office), Kombo St Mary's Division.
Gambia Medical and Dental Association, PMB 430 SerreKunda. Tel: +220 495 934. Fax: 495 071.

MEDICAL SCHOOL:

University of the Gambia Medical School
Muammar Ghadaffi Avenue, Banjul.
Tel: +220 202 310.

THE HOSPITALS:

Royal Victoria Hospital
Independence Drive, Banjul.
Tel: +220 228 223. Fax: +220 225 832.
The hospital: This is one of the main hospitals in the capital, with a range of many unusual conditions. They also arrange field trips.

Bansang Hospital
Bansang. Tel: +220 674 222.
Fax: +220 674 425.
www.bansanghospitalappeal.com.
The hospital: Bansang Hospital is a 160-bed hospital deep in the African bush, 320 km (200 miles) east by road from the coast, and is responsible for the healthcare needs of around 600 000 Gambians. Patients are also accepted from Senegal, Mali, Guinea Bissau and Guinea Conakry, and refugees are seen from Sierra Leone. The hospital itself was built in 1938. Volunteers (from the UK) can apply through the hospital website.

Farafenni Hospital
Farafenni.
The hospital: This is the other main hospital, situated halfway along the River Gambia.

Ahmadiyya Hospital
Talinding, PO Box 708, Banjul.
Tel: +220 373 724. Fax: +220 390623.

MRC unit
Fajara, Atlantic Road, PO Box 273, Banjul.
Fax: 220 495 442/496 919.
The unit: The MRC unit is principally for research, although it does house a small 40-bed hospital.
O Elective notes: This is a great place if you want to do research (for funding help, *see* the Wellcome Trust information in Section 4), but there is little clinical exposure and you shadow on ward rounds. There is, however, good teaching. The beach is very close. You are better going to the Royal Victoria if you want procedures. Limited places available at the MRC and it is popular … apply early.

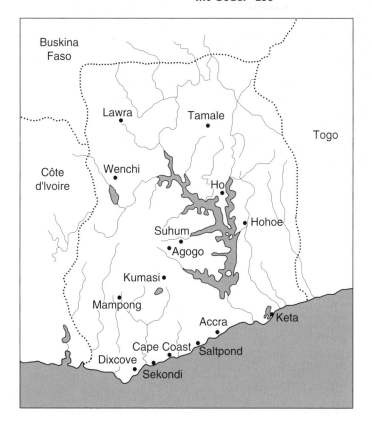

Ghana

Population: 18 million
Language: English
Capital: Accra
Currency: Cedi
Int Code: +233

Ghana is situated on the west coast of Africa. It gained independence from the UK in 1957 and subsequently came under intermittent military rule. In 1992, democratic elections were held. Although not a popular tourist destination, Ghana does have some beautiful beaches and coastal forts. The Ghanaian people are extremely polite and kind (although this can change if they want to sell you something!). Ghana is an excellent country to travel round in, being very safe and almost entirely unexposed to tourism (although this means that things like travellers cheques are difficult to deal with). It is politically stable now (unlike many of its neighbours), and there is no major tribal division. The people are curious about Westerners, and problems with police and officials are rare. The roads are, however, dreadful, and all forms of transportation are fairly erratic and uncomfortable. There are also supply problems for non-domestic products, although Ghanaian food and beer are good. In the North, the Mole Game Reserve has elephants, antelope and baboons. The Akosombo Dam, Lake Volta and the railway to Kumasi are all worth seeing. It is worth getting a multiple entry visa as this also allows you to visit the Côte d'Ivoire and Burkina Faso.

✪ Medicine:

Infectious diseases are very common, although public hygiene improvements have been of great benefit. Malaria, TB and gastroenteritis are regularly seen. Because of the economic situation, resources are universally scarce, and patients often have to pay for treatment (even bags of saline). The prevalence of HIV is around 3.5%.

USEFUL ADDRESSES:

Ministry of Health, PO Box M44, Accra. Tel: +233 21 662014. Fax: +233 21 666808.
Ghana Medical and Dental Council, PO Box 10586, Accra.
Ghana Medical Association, PO Box 1596, Accra. Tel: +233 21 670510. Fax: +233 21 670511.
Ghana Dental Association, University of Ghana Dental School, PO Box KB460, Korle-Bu, Accra. Tel: +233 21 662072.

MEDICAL SCHOOLS AND TEACHING HOSPITALS:

Ghana has two medical schools:

University of Ghana Medical School

PO Box 4236, Accra. Tel: +233 21 665101. Fax: +233 21 663062. www.ug.edu.gh.
This is the oldest and main medical school and is situated in the capital, which lies on the coast. One of its teaching hospitals includes:

Korle-Bu Hospital

Korle-Bu, Accra.
Tel: +233 21 665401/665481.
The hospital: Korle-Bu is the largest of the teaching hospitals in Ghana. As in most state hospitals, resources are limited. It is pretty run down, and hence some students have preferred Kumasi (see page 39).
○ **Elective notes:** Since this is a teaching hospital, there are well-organized tutorials and other students about. It is reasonably good for practical experience. You currently have to pay around $200 for an elective here.
Accommodation: Costs $50 a week.

University of Science and Technology

School of Medicine, University Post Office, Kumasi. Tel: +233 51 60303. Fax: +233 51 60302.
This is the only other Ghanaian medical school and is situated inland in Ghana's second biggest town. It uses:

Komfo Anokye Teaching Hospital

PO Box 1934, Bantama, Kumasi.
Tel: +233 51 208119.
The hospital: Komfo Anokye Hospital is a teaching hospital in Kumasi. All the specialities are here, but community health provides an excellent opportunity to see rural Ghana. Many of the diseases seen here are poverty or malnutrition related, and the expense and difficulty of getting to hospital make late presentation universal. There are a lot of strange tropical diseases.
○ **Elective notes:** The amount of support available on the ward is very limited, and you will see many postoperative problems rare to the West. There are a number of European doctors who give advice on everything, from where to change money to where to get football tickets. Kumasi itself is a beautiful city in the rainforest region of Ashanti, with wood-carving and weaving being commonplace. There are a number of hotels and bars. It is well sited for travelling to other parts of Ghana. Komfo Anokye is a very good choice of hospital since

Korle-Bu in Accra is very run down and the capital is pretty unattractive. Some of the district hospitals are incredibly isolated.

Accommodation: There are about 35 students in their sixth (final) year who all live in an excellent hostel (with elective students) built a few years ago, with security, laundry and meals provided. The hospital is within Kumasi town, but the rest of the university is on a large campus about 5 km (3 miles) outside town, with a supermarket, bars and a (very green) Olympic-sized swimming pool.

Mampong Herbal Clinic

Akwapim, Mampong. Tel: +233 872 22042/22103. Fax: +233 872 22087.

The hospital: This is a government-run hospital with a traditional medicine hospital and research centre.

OTHER HOSPITALS:

Kumasi, Ashanti Region:

Agogo Hospital

PO Box 27, Agogo. Tel: +233 51 20201/20202.

The hospital: This is a 200-bed hospital run by the Presbyterian Church of Ghana. It specializes in ophthalmology since many people here are affected by river blindness, carried by the filaria fly. This has increased since the Volta River Dam was built, providing an ideal breeding place for the fly. Ninety thousand people are seen as outpatients and 57 000 as inpatients annually. The hospital trains 120 nurses each year.

Radiant Medical and Dental Centre

Plot C. Blk 3 Ayigya, PO Box AS 399, Ayigya-Kumasi. Tel: +233 51 31451.

Western Region:

Nana Hima Dekyi Hospital

Dixcove, PO Box 5, Ahanta West, Western Region.

The hospital: Nana is a 50-bed hospital encompassing general medicine, surgery, paediatrics, O&G, and psychiatry. Ward rounds in the morning are followed by outpatients and surgery in the afternoon. There is a great deal of malaria, typhoid and other infectious diseases. Rural clinics are run from here. Again, there are severely limited resources, to the extent that running water is sometimes not available. Dixcove itself is a colourful fishing village, and the food is excellent.

O Elective notes: Your stay will be busy with quite a bit of responsibility, although there is always supervision.

Accommodation: There is a local hotel, but previous students have been able to stay with staff.

Effia Nkwanta

Box 229, Sekondi. Tel: +233 31 23151.

Afram Plains District:

Donkorkrom Presbyterian Hospital

Afram Plains.

The hospital: This 74-bed hospital is in a very remote area of Ghana surrounded by lakes, hence boats and ferries are required to get to it.

Central Region:
Ankaful Mental Hospital, PO Box 412, Ankaful, Cape Coast. Tel: +233 42 33686/33871.
Fynba Hospital, PO Box 131, Cape Coast. Tel: +233 42 33603.
Saltpond General Hospital, PO Box 29, Saltpond. Tel: +233 42 33850.

Volta Region:
Hohoe Government Hospital, PO Box 27, Hohoe. Tel: +233 935 2042/2031.
Keta Government Hospital (MOH), PO Box 82, Keta. Tel: +233 966 22309.
Ministry of Health Central Hospital, PO Box 49, Ho. Tel: +233 91 8209/8206.

Eastern Region:
Bawku Presbyterian Hospital, PO Box 45, Bawku. Tel: +233 743 22232/22246.
Suhum Government Hospital, PO Box 149, Suhum. Tel: +233 858 24380.

Northern Region:
Tamale Regional Hospital, PO Box 16, Tamale. Tel: +233 71 22454.

Brong Ahafo Region:
Emil Memorial Hospital, PO Box 96, Wenchi.
Tel: +233 652 22274.

Upper West:
Lawra Hospital, MOH, PO Box 19, Lawra. Tel:
+233 756 22809.

Kenya

Population: 29 million
Language: Swahili
Capital: Nairobi
Currency: Kenya shilling
Int Code: + 254

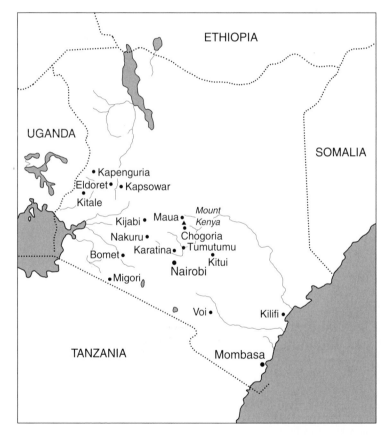

Kenya, situated in the east of Africa with the equator running through it, is probably best known for its game parks and coffee. Since its independence from the UK in 1963, tourism and agriculture (in the east) have become the country's mainstay. There has recently been trouble with political and tribal violence. There is plenty to do here: Climb Mount Kenya ($250 for porter, maps and meals over five days), visit Mombasa (the coast) and go on safari. Most people only speak Swahili (or a form of it), but English is *understood in the capital. At the time of writing, there is said to be a high threat from global terrorism. You should be vigilant in public places and tourist sites. Check* www.fco.gov.uk.

○ Medicine:

Both state and private healthcare institutions exist across Kenya. The state system has become very run down with limited resources, and, as the disparity in wealth between rich and poor grows, poverty-related diseases are on the increase. Some people who work have a minimal private insurance scheme through their employer. The private institutions are mainly charity- and mission-run hospitals. These tend to provide a better standard of care even though resources are as, if not more, restricted. In either, patients usually have to pay a small fee to be seen and/or the cost of medications. Most touring medics go to the mission/charity hospitals (even if they are not religious in any way) as they can get more involved, they are usually more hospitable, and there are usually other Westerners around. For these reasons, this chapter will tend to concentrate on these.

Infectious diseases such as malaria, chest infections and gastroenteritis are common. HIV has become a major problem, with an average prevalance of 14% (higher in the cities). There is only one doctor per 10 150 population.

Note that where stated, some hospitals are linked to the **African Inland Mission** (AIM, 2 Vorley Road, Archway, London, N19 5HE, UK. Tel: +44 20 7281 1184. Fax: +44 20 7281 4479). They run a number of hospitals across Kenya, and you can apply for electives/work places through them. They require you to complete a form confirming that you are a Christian. Take a look at www.aim-us.org (a more detailed site for the USA) or www.aim-eur.org (for Europe).

○ Visas and work permits:

Since the UK has introduced visas for former Commonwealth countries, Kenya

has reciprocated. You now need to get a visitor's visa costing £35.

Note: Be careful in Kenya if you are a female travelling alone … you are regarded as a second-class citizen. Always cover your legs, at least to the knees.

USEFUL ADDRESSES:

Public Health Office, Ministry of Health, Medical Officer of Health, PO Box 438, Nyambene. www.health.go.ke.
Kenya Medical Association, Chyulu Road, Upper Hill, PO Box 48502, Nairobi. Tel. +254 2 714991.
Kenya Dental Association, PO Box 20059, Nairobi. Tel: +254 2 544542.
Kenya Nurses Association, Tel: +254 2 229083.

MEDICAL SCHOOLS:

University of Nairobi, College of Health Sciences, PO Box 30197, Nairobi. Tel: +254 263 1638. Fax: +254 263 1102. www.uonbi.ac.ke. (The school, founded in 1967, is based in and uses the Kenyatta National Hospital in Narobi; see below.)
Moi University, Faculty of Health Sciences, Lumumba Avenue, PO Box 4606, Eldoret. Tel: +254 321 61562. Fax: +254 321 33041. www.moiuniversity.ac.ke.

THE HOSPITALS:

Nairobi

Kenyatta National Hospital
PO Box 20723, Nairobi.
Tel: +254 2 726300. Fax: +254 2 725272.
www.kenyattanationalhospital.org.
The hospital: A government-run teaching hospital providing care for the poor. Many patients are too poor to pay for their medications. It caters for most specialities (including cardiothoracic surgery) and has resources such as a CT scanner (even though it often does not work). Tropical medicine is big. HIV, malaria, TB and typhoid are common. The Wellcome Trust, in conjunction with Oxford University's Tropical Medicine Department, has a research centre here (and on the coast; *see* page 45). Their

address in Nairobi is the same as the hospital's above but the PO Box number is 43640 (Tel: +254 2 710672. Fax: +254 2 711673).

O **Elective notes:** As this is a teaching hospital, there are formal lectures and tutorials (in English). It is handy if you know Swahili. There are lots of procedures and signs. Taxis are expensive but safer than buses. Do not go around downtown at night.

Accommodation: Stay at the Nairobi Youth Hostel, which is basic but only a five-minute walk from the hospital.

Aga Khan Hospital
PO Box 30270, Nairobi.

The hospital: Built by charitable donations, it serves both insurance populations (the rich and the poor). It has departments of medicine, surgery, orthopaedics, neurology, paediatrics, O&G and an emergency department.

O **Elective notes:** It is well set up for elective students and can offer time in any of the above specialities.

Accommodation: There is none available to elective students. The YMCA offers cheap flats for £50–80 a month.

Note: There are a number of private hospitals (e.g. the Nairobi Hospital), which can easily be found on the Internet.

HOSPITALS OUTSIDE THE CAPITAL:

Bomet:

Tenwek Mission Hospital
PO Box 39, Bomet. Tel: +254 361 30086. Fax:+ 254 361 30165. www.tenwek.org.

The hospital: Originally founded in 1935, it has grown from a dispensary via a 35-bed cottage hospital to become a 300-bed referal centre. It is 240 km (150 miles) from Nariobi in Kenya's Rift Valley. It provides care for 600 000 Kipsigis within a 51 km radius and has general medicine, surgery, O&G, paediatrics and ophthalmology services. There

is a seven-bed ITU and good pathology department. There is also extensive training for doctors and nurses (the hosptial having its own nursing school).

Chogoria:

PCEA Chogoria Hospital
PO Box 35, Chogoria. Tel: +254 166 22620. Fax: +254 166 22122. E-mail: chogoria@africaonline.co.ke.

The hospital: Chogoria is a 250-bed mission hospital situated on the slopes of Mount Kenya, about five hours (200 km) north of Nairobi. It has two surgical, two medical, paediatrics and maternity wards as well as outpatient, ophthalmic, dental and community health departments. It is very well run by African standards, relying on patients' fees and charity. Drugs are always available. There are lots of tropical diseases – malaria, leprosy, TB, rheumatic heart disease, heart failure, nephrotic syndrome and HIV (its prevalence being approximately 10% in the surrounding area). There are usually six to eight doctors from all over the world as well as Africa. The nursing staff kindly translate.

O **Elective notes:** Elective students spend their first week with a doctor and are then set free, being first on call and prescribing. You do your own ward rounds, outpatient consultations, lumbar punctures, paracentesis, bloods (be careful) and catheterizations, and assist in theatre. There are lots of signs to see but few investigations. The doctors are all very relaxed and supportive, which all goes to make this a fantastic elective. Write to them very early as they only take two students at a time.

Accommodation: Great – a small cottage for two students with a cooker, fridge, bath and flushing loo. And there is a swimming pool on the staff compound.

Eldoret:

Eldoret District Hospital
PO Box 3, Eldoret. Tel: +254 32 133471.

Kapenguria:

West Pokot District Hospital
PO Box 63, Kapenguria.

Karatina:

PCEA Tomotomo Hospital
Private Bag, Karatina.
The hospital: This is a 180-bed government-run hospital 130 km (80 miles) north of Nairobi. Patients pay a small fee for treatment. There are usually approximately three doctors, and it is very busy – lots of TB, malaria, HIV and PV bleeding as a result of illegal abortion.
O Elective notes: It is busy, and medical students' help is greatly appreciated. There is a 1:3 rota for on call. There are plenty of practical procedures, and there is always someone to help. This comes highly recommended.

Presbyterian Mission Hospital
Tumu Tumu, PO Karatina.
E-mail tumutumu@africaonline.co.ke.

Kapsowar:

Kapsowar Hospital
PO Box 68, Kapsowar.
The hospital: A mission hospital (linked to AIM, and the cheapest for patients to attend) in the Rift Valley. It is very rural. There are three doctors with midwives and nurses from the West. O&G, paeds, medicine, surgery, an eye service and mobile clinics are provided.
O Elective notes: There is a 1:4 on-call rota for students. You can have as much responsibility as you are happy with, but back-up is always available. You are supposed to apply through AIM.
Accommodation: Accommodation is provided in a very nice house with mod cons.

Kijabi:

Kijabi Medical Centre
PO Box 20, Kijabe.
The hospital: Linked to AIM, this is a 208-bed general hospital in rural Kenya, 1 hour's drive from Nairobi. It is situated at 2286 m above sea level, overlooking the Great Rift Valley. The site also has a church, school (for 500 missionary children) and Bible college. Around 125 outpatients are seen each day and a mobile clinic offers women's and children's care to villages 12 times a month. There is an emergency department, O&G (1800 deliveries a year), paeds and general medical/surgical male and female wards. Student nurses are trained here to recognize common diseases and run rural dispensaries. A small fee is charged to patients for services. Trauma, HIV, malaria, TB, diabetes and hypertension are common.
O Elective notes: There are usually a couple of students from Nairobi University medical school, and this is a well-established elective destination. On call is every third night, and you are very well supported by staff. Note: This is a very Christian setting: Bible study in the mornings, lots of discussion with patients about God and literature given to them at the end of consultations. The language here is Kiku, and the nurses will translate for you.
Accommodation: Available with a cooker, fridge and washing machine (for 372 KES (US$5) a day).

Kijabi Dental Clinic
Same address as Medical Centre.
The clinic: This fully equipped dental unit sees around 30 patients a day.

Kikuyu:
Kikuyu, PO Box 45. Tel: +254 154 32412.
Fax: +254 154 32413.
E-mail pceagenhosp@maf.org.
The hospital: Has female, male and paediatrics wards, an orthopaedic clinic and an emergency department. Inpatients have to put a deposit of 5000 KES (£50) down to ensure that they pay for investigations at the end. Guards with clubs allegedly ensure they do not escape! HIV and TB are common. Most doctors are Kenyan or from the US.

O **Elective notes:** Students are on call two or three times a week with the on-call doctor.
Accommodation: Provided.

Kilifi

Kilifi District Hospital
PO Box 230, Bofa Road, Kilifi.
The hospital: Kilifi District Hospital is a medium-sized general hospital. It is also home to the Wellcome Trust's and the Kenyan Medical Research Instutute's (KEMRI's) unit, which carries out extensive research into malaria (especially in children) in East Africa (working in conjunction with Oxford University – www.jr2.ox.ac.uk/ndm/Tropical_Medicine/pages/kenya_unit.htm. Here you can do either a laboratory-based project and/or clinical work. In paediatrics at least, there is a great deal of interesting pathology. Most illness is related to malaria, gastroenteritis or malnutrition. There is less HIV than in other parts of Kenya. The Wellcome Trust runs an eight-bed paediatric intensive care unit equipped to Western standards. This contrasts markedly with the poor facilities in the rest of the hospital. The maternity unit has no running water and no obstetrician working there regularly. The British doctors doing research help out. Kilifi itself is a small seaside village situated 19 km north of Mombasa. It sits directly on the Indian Ocean and has a population of about 1000.
O **Elective notes:** The staff are friendly but do expect you to do a bit of work. There are a few procedures to do and patients to present at unit meetings. On the whole though, life is pretty relaxed. The beaches are spectacular, you can scuba dive or hop up to Watamu or down to Mombasa at weekends. Integrate yourself with the friendly locals or the VSO workers if you are looking for drinking buddies. The social life has very good reports. This elective is repeatedly thoroughly recommended.
Accommodation: There is a flat right in the middle of the village for approximately 178 KES (£1.50) a night.

Grants: Look for the Wellcome Trust under 'Elective and travel bursaries' in Section 4.

Kitui:

Mutomo Hospital
The Sisters of Mercy, PO Box 16, Mutomo, Kitui. Tel: Mutomo 16.
The hospital: Established by an order of Irish nuns in 1964, it now has 130 beds and a major and minor operating theatre. It is run by seven sisters and two doctors. This is in an extremely impoverished area 250 km south of Narobi. Malaria, AIDS (with a prevalence of 10% in blood donors) and leprosy are common.
Accommodation: Provided.

Maua:

Maua Methodist Hospital
PO Box 63, Maua, Nyambene. Tel: +254 167 21003/21107. Fax: +254 167 21121.
E-mail: linmaua@maf.org.
The hospital: Maua Methodist Hospital is a 150-bed hospital serving a large, widespread rural community in the eastern foothills of Mount Kenya at 1828 m above sea level. It has male, female, paediatrics and maternity wards. Like many mission hospitals, it is greatly overcrowded (especially with maternity cases and during dysentery season) and lacks funds. Patients pay 85 shillings (about £1, but one shilling buys a banana) to be seen. Malaria, dysentery, machete wounds, leprosy, HIV, rheumatic fever, malnutrition and parasitic worms are the order of the day. Maua is a relatively violent area, and there is a high incidence of serious trauma. Petrol permitting, there are rural clinics.
O **Elective notes:** This is a popular elective destination (taking 35 students a year). Medical students are integral to the running of the hospital, as the doctors are unable to cope with the workload. Some students have not found the nursing staff particularly helpful. However, the students from the nursing college and the other medical students are friendly. The medical experience is

great, as students are first on call at night and take outpatient clinics (a cross between an emergency department and a GP's surgery). There is little back up from the doctors. Although there is quite a bit of it, Maua is not a great place to study trauma as the HIV rate is high and nurses do all the suturing (they're better at it than you, and you are more useful diagnosing and prescribing). The night rota is an inaccurate 1:3. A couple of students have said that they felt they learned little and were taken for granted.

There are plans to make an elective here a minimum of eight weeks. If that is the case, think seriously before going as it can be hard work. The hospital would like students to play a part in the religious side of the hospital, but this is not compulsory. Smoking and alcohol are prohibited within the hospital grounds.

Accommodation: Provided with the other students for around $2 a night.

Migori:

Ojele Memorial Hospital
PO Box 355, Suna, Migori. Tel: +254 387 20346. www.omh2.org.
The hospital: This is a not-for-profit 96-bed private hospital in south-west Kenya. It has general medicine, surgery, paediatrics, ophthalmology and O&G services.

Mombasa:

St Luke's Hospital
PO Box 16, Kaloleni, Mombasa.
The hospital: A 150-bed missionary hospital run by one doctor, it is very busy, with limited facilities. Many beds are shared between two or three patients. Cholera epidemics, malaria, tetanus and HIV (with a prevalence of around 40% in some villages) are common. There is a great deal of interesting tropical medicine. Kaloleni is 50 km outside Mombasa. There are a few shops in the village.
O Elective notes: You will learn by doing and observing rather than direct teaching. It can get quite stressful.

Accommodation: Very basic (water collected from the rainwater tank). There's intermittent electricity and a gas cooker. It's clean and comfortable.

Mombasa Hospital
PO Box 90294, Mombasa. Tel: +254 11 312191/312099. Fax: +254 11 225086/229254.
www.mombasahospital.com.
The hospital: This is a not-for-profit private hospital with excellent facilities by Kenyan standards (air-conditioned rooms!). Most specialities are catered for, and there is a state-of-the-art ITU.

Nakuru:
Provincial General Hospital
PO Box 71, Nakuru.
The hospital: This is the referral centre for the Rift Valley province, with medical, surgical, paeds, O&G, TB and neonatal wards. There is a large outpatients and emergency department. They are very short of resources and staff here. Common diseases include malaria, TB and HIV (over half the inpatient population is HIV positive).
O Elective notes: Students are welcomed. The amount of 'hands on' experience is up to you. Most is observing. Students have no on-call duties.
Accommodation: Elective students need to stay at the Carnation Hotel in the centre of town. You can go and explore the Rift Valley, but it can get very lonely if you are on your own.

Nyans:

Nyans District General Hospital
Nyans.

Tumutumu:

Tumutumu Hospital
Tumutumu.
The hospital: A 203-bed mission hospital 130 km north of Narobi serving the largest tribe in Kenya (the Kikuyus). It trains around 100 nurses per year.

Kenya

Via Kitale:

Catholic Mission Hospital
Otrum, Via Kitale.

District Hospital
Kapenguria, PO Makutano, Via Kitale.

Voi:

Moi Hospital
PO Box 18, Voi. Tel: +254 147 2016.

Lesotho

Population: 2.1 million
Official Languages: English and Sesotho
Capital: Maseru
Currency: Loti
Int Code: +266

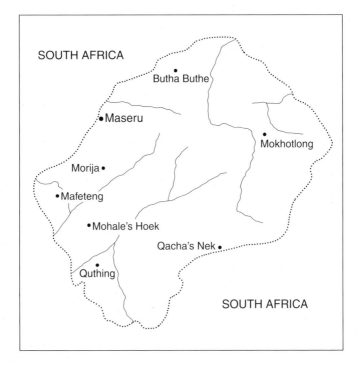

SOUTH AFRICA

• Butha Buthe

•Maseru

• Mokhotlong

Morija •

•Mafeteng

•Mohale's Hoek

Qacha's Nek •

Quthing

SOUTH AFRICA

Since Lesotho is entirely surrounded by South Africa, it is completely dependent on its neighbour for transport links to the rest of the world. It is a beautiful mountainous country, and the new highland water scheme aims to generate electricity for export. Its military rule ended in 1993, but it is still a very poor country, as its health statistics show. It is not a common elective destination. There are no medical schools.

✪ Medicine:

Health standards are generally poor, with low life expectancy and high infant mortality. Both private and government-run hospitals exist (*see* below). There is also a flying doctor service, but this does not cover the highlands adequately (only 13 300 people live in the capital, Maseru). The leading causes of mortality are TB, parasitic diseases and malnutrition. The prevalance of HIV is around 24%. The doctor:population ratio is a staggering 1:18 600.

➲ Visas and work permits:
Citizens of Australia, western Europe (including the UK) and most of the world do not need a visa to enter Lesotho. However, citizens of the USA, India, Pakistan, China and the Far East do. For them, a single entry visa (valid for three months) costs £5. For more information and information regarding work permits, write to the High Commission. To obtain a licence to practise, contact the **Lesotho Medical, Dental and Pharmacy Council**. You will need your diploma and a certificate of good practice from your previous employer.

USEFUL ADDRESSES:

Ministry of Health, Principal Secretary, PO Box 514, Maseru 100. Tel: +266 314404. Fax: +266 310467.
Lesotho Medical, Dental and Pharmacy Council, PO Box MS 726, Maseru 100. Tel/Fax: +266 322450.
Lesotho Medical Association, PO Box 588, Maseru 100.

GOVERNMENT HOSPITALS:

Botsabelo Hospital, Private Bag A149, Maseru 100. Tel: +266 312353.
Butha Buthe Hospital, PO Box 514, Maseru 100. Tel: +266 4602210.
Leribe Hospital, c/o PO Box 514, Maseru 100. Tel: +266 400305.
Machabeng Hospital, PO Box 8, Qacha's Nek 600. Tel: +266 950229.
Mafeteng Hospital, c/o PO Box 514, Maseru 100. Tel: +266 700208/700377.
Mohale's Hoek Hospital, PO Box 337, Mohale's Hoek 800. Tel: +266 785210/785292.
Mohlomi Mental Hospital, PO Box 540, Maseru 100. Tel: +266 313744.
Mokhotlong Hospital, PO Box Mokhotlong, Maseru 100. Tel: +266 920360.
Queen Elizabeth II Hospital, PO Box 122, Maseru 100. Tel: +266 312501. (This is Lesotho's main hospital.)
Quthing Hospital, PO Box 3, Quthing 700. Tel: +266 750213/750203.
Teyateyaneng Hospital, PO Box 514, Maseru 100. Tel: +266 500272.

MISSION/PRIVATE HOSPITALS:

St James' Mission Hospital
PO Box 3, Mantsonyane 150.
The hospital: This is a friendly, English-speaking, 70-bed mission hospital. They run a number of outreach clinics reached by 4×4. The hospital is a three-hour drive from the capital, Maseru, and the local village of Ha Toka is only ten minutes' walk away. Common problems are TB, HIV and obstetric complications

Scott Hospital
Hospital Road, Private Bag, Morija.
Tel: +266 360209.
The hospital: A 150-bed, four-doctor, acute care facility run by the Lesotho Evangelical Church that provides care for the surrounding 900 or so villages. It has grown tremendously since 1938 to include its own nursing school.

Maluti Seventh-Day Adventist Hospital
PO Box MG11, Mapoteng.
Tel: +266 540203. www.adventist.org.za.
The hospital: Maluti has become well known for its treatment of eye diseases.

St Joseph's Hospital
PO Roma 180, Roma. Tel: +266 340206.
The hospital: This is the largest non-governmental hospital in Lesotho.

Tebellong Hospital
Qacha's Nek.
The hospital: This is a small mountain hospital owned by the Lesotho Evangelical Church and built in 1965. It has 38 beds and is responsible for providing health services to about 52 000 people in the Tebellong Health Service Area in south-eastern Lesotho. It has many poor people, few development projects, no paved roads, many health problems and a very high infant mortality rate. The hospital is reached by Mission Aviation Fellowship planes, by rowing boat across the Orange (Senqu) River, or by horseback or foot. The hospital was built on the inaccessible side of the river, across from the main road,

since most of the people live on that side and the Basotho people do not like crossing the river in boats.

PRIVATE HOSPITALS:

Maluti Seventh Day Adventist Hospital, PO Box MG11, Mapoteng. Tel: +266 540203.
Maseru Private Hospital, Private Bag A58, Maseru 100. Tel: +266 313261/313260. Fax: +266 310142.

St Joseph's Hospital, PO Roma 180. Tel : +266 340206.
Scott Hospital, Hospital Road, Private Bag Morija. Tel: +266 360209.

DEFENCE HOSPITAL:

Makoanyane Military Hospital, Private Bag A166, Maseru 100.

Madagascar

Population: 15 million
Languages: Malagasy and French
Capital: Antananarivo
Currency: Malagasy franc
Int Code: +261

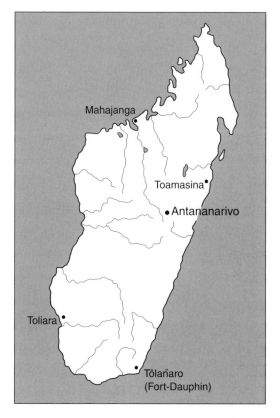

Madagascar is the third poorest country and fourth largest island in the world (being twice the size of the UK). The people are fantastically hospitable. Outside the hospitals, there are wonderful beaches (beware of sharks) and scenery. This can be a real adventure ... the odd cyclone and some amazing wildlife. The country now has a multiparty democracy. French is spoken widely and is the usual language of hospital work so a bit of knowledge is essential. Malagasy has 12 completely different dialects. Have a go!

Madagascar

○ **Medicine:**
A highly inefficient and underfunded state healthcare system can't cope, and private hospitals have now been set up for those with any money. Infectious diseases such as malaria are extremely common. There have been outbreaks of bubonic plague in recent years. It is thought that there is only one doctor per 8100 patients. HIV is not a major problem (affecting approximately 0.15% of the population); hence, if you are worried about needle-stick injuries, this is a good place for developing country medicine without the high risks. Only 3% of the population is aged over 65; therefore there is effectively no geriatrics. There are two medical schools.

Note: To arrange an elective here, it is best to write in French. Try to enclose an international pre-paid reply coupon as most hospitals are really strapped for cash.

◎ **Climate and crime:**
Madagascar has a tropical coast, temperate inland and near-desert south. Cyclones are pretty common. Crime is not a major problem but is rising.

⊃ **Visas and work permits:**
Enquire with the embassy as this is not a common elective destination and no clear information is available. At present, if you want to work, you need to register with the **Ordre de Médecins**.

USEFUL ADDRESSES:

Ministry of Health, BP 88, rue Jean Ralaemongo, Ambohidahy, Antananaviro 101. Tel: +261 2 23697.
Ordre de Médecins, Place Charles Renel, Antaninandro, Antananarivo 101.
Madagascar Dental Association, 9 Lalana Rabezavana, Antananarivo. Tel: +261 2 23818.

MEDICAL SCHOOLS AND TEACHING HOSPITALS:

Antananarivo

Université D'Antananarive
Faculté de Médecin, BP 566, Antananarivo 101. Tel: +261 20 22 24114.
www.refer.mg/madag ct/edu/minesup/anta nana/antanana.htm.

This is the principal medical school of Madagascar (founded in 1962). They can arrange electives in their main teaching hospital:

Befelatanana General Hospital (Hôpital Général Befelatanana)
PO Box 2097, 101 Antananarivo.
The hospital: Is the state-run, public, 1300-bed teaching hospital. It provides a free service and the patients are very poor. It has very restricted facilities. Drugs and even soap are in short supply. Rheumatic fever, TB, malaria and nephrotic syndrome (secondary to traditional drug use) are all common.

Mahajanga

Université de Mahajanga
Faculté de Médecine, Etablissement d'Enseignment supérieur des Sciences de la Santé, BP 652, Ambodrona, Mahajanga 401. Tel: +261 20 62 22724.
Fax: +261 20 62 23312.
www.refer.mg/madag ct/edu/minesup/mah ajang/mahajang.htm.
This is the only other medical school.

Hopitaly Loterana Antanimalandy
BP 653, Mahajanga 401.
The hospital: A Lutheran hospital about 8 km out of town. Owing to the very poor conditions, there is a great deal of pathology to be seen.
Accommodation: Difficult to arrange. Previous visitors have made friends with the local Lutheran missions and obtained accommodation through them.

Hopitaly Loterana Manambara
BP 108, Fort-Dauphin 614.
The hospital: Manambaro Lutheran Hospital is a small (50-bed) mission hospital with four doctors in a small fairly isolated village. Specialities include medicine, surgery, paediatrics and O&G. It can be a bit quiet, so do a bit of everything. Common illnesses include malaria, schistosomiasis, typhoid, diarrhoea and dehydration. Equipment is limited,

although there are ECHO, ECG and X-ray facilities. French is not spoken widely here; you will need a translator. Don't expect to improve your French at all.

O **Elective notes:** A normal day consists of ward rounds at 7.30 am, a couple of operations and outpatients in the afternoon. There is obviously not much to do in the local vicinity, but at weekends you can get out into the nearby town of Fort-Dauphin, which is beautiful.

Accommodation: Provided in a guest house (32 000 MGF (£3) a night) with a cook/housekeeper.

Toliara

Centre Hospitalier Regional (Hôpital Principal de Toliara)
Toliara, Southern Madagascar.

The hospital: Is a relatively attractive hospital with some new equipment and is fairly busy. Common conditions include typhoid, hepatitis, rheumatic fever, malaria, malnutrition and recently the plague.

O **Elective notes:** Electives have previously been difficult to arrange. All ward rounds are in French so some knowledge is ideal. Procedures can be done in the emergency department. There are some beautiful beaches close by.

Tamatave

Hôpital Principal de Toamasina
Toamasina.

The hospital: This is in Tamatave (the country's largest port, with a population of 100 000), a mile north of the town centre, right on the beach. It runs like a small district general hospital with X-ray and ECHO facilities. There are 400 beds and a two-tier system of care.

O **Elective notes:** You can do medicine, surgery, O&G, emergency medicine or radiology. There is a huge range of conditions to see: typhoid, malaria, TB and schistosomiasis are the bread and butter. Take any books you do not want and any copies of the *BNF* you can get your hands on. There is a sandy beach nearby but don't swim (because of sharks). Write to the Medécin-chef.

Malawi

Population: 11 million
Languages: Chewa and English
Capital: Lilongwe
Currency: Malawian kwacha
Int Code: +265

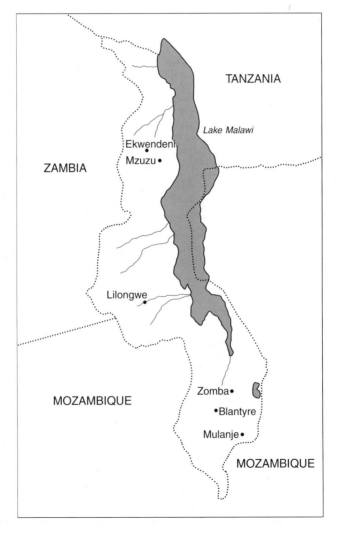

Until the early 1990s, Malawi was under the dictatorship of Dr Hastings Banda, a GP who practised in the UK and then went back to his own country and proclaimed himself president for life. It was a harsh time for the people: imprisonment without trial and other human rights abuses were common. Since 1994, however, democratic elections have been held. The country itself is beautiful. Its most prominent feature, Lake Malawi, supports a sizeable fishing industry.

✪ Medicine:

The country has a pretty poor record, with one of the lowest life expectancies (42 years) and highest infant mortalities. Over half of children under five are short for their age, but a massive vaccination campaign and combat malnutrition programme is beginning to work. Infectious diseases are common. The prevalence of HIV in some areas is thought to be over 30% (the population average being 16%). It has been estimated that there is only one doctor per 50 000 people. Prior to the change in government, there were no medical schools, but one has now been set up in Blantyre (*see* below).

The **Christian Health Association of Malawi** (CHAM, PO Box 30378, Lilongwe. Tel: +265 775 404. Fax: +265 776 492. E-mail: nympha@malawi.net) operates 20 hospitals in Malawi.

➲ Visas and work permits:

British passport holders do not require a visa to visit Malawi. If you are staying longer than three months or are from a country that does require a visa, a visitor's permit (approximately £25) is required. To get a temporary employment permit for working in a hospital or voluntary organization, contact the High Commission. It is usually quite easy to obtain one.

◎ Climate and crime:

The rainy season is in the winter (December–March). This is also when it is hottest. Malawi is a pretty safe country to travel in. Hitch-hiking is fine if there are a couple of you. Note for women: Showing your knees can make people think you're a bit of a slapper.

USEFUL ADDRESSES:

Ministry of Health, PO Box 30377, Capital City, Lilongwe. Tel: +265 783 044. Fax: +265 744 943.
Malawi Dental Association, Zomba C. Hospital, Box 21, Zomba. Tel: +265 523 266. Fax: +265 522 538.
National AIDS Control Programme, PO Box 30622, Lilongwe 3. Tel: +265 781 344.
Fax: +265 784 227.

Lilongwe

Lilongwe, the nation's capital, has recently set up a health sciences school and uses the Central Hospital.

Lilongwe Central Hospital, PO Box 149, Lilongwe. Tel: +265 721 555.
Lilongwe School for Health Sciences, PO Box 30368, Capital City, Lilongwe 3. Tel: +265 720 911.

Blantyre

University of Malawi College of Medicine
Private Bag 360, Chichiri, Blantyre 3.
Tel: +265 677 291. Fax +265 674 700.
www.unima.mw.
Founded in 1994, this uses:

Queen Elizabeth Central Hospital
PO Box 95, Blantyre.
The hospital: The main referral centre for southern Malawi and the largest hospital in the country, this is also the main teaching hospital for the College of Medicine (located in the university building opposite). Nurses, midwives and clinical officers are also taught here. It is very run down and desperately short of funds. There are six paediatric wards and there may be three or four children to a cot. At the time of writing, it had one of the two orthopaedic surgeons in the entire country. Many rare things are common here: malaria, TB, kwashiorkor and marasmus, HIV, typhoid, Burkitt's lymphoma, osteosarcoma, Kaposi's sarcoma, hippo and crocodile bites. The prevalence of HIV is nearly 100% on the TB wards and 50% on the general wards. HIV is also very common on the

Malawi

paediatric wards, although patients are often sent home to die.

O **Elective notes:** There is plenty to see and assist in. Teaching has been excellent but may vary depending on the consultants who are there now. It is a friendly hospital and highly recommended.

Another hospital in the region is:

Adventist Health Services
PO Box 951, Blantyre.

Ekwendeni

Ekwendeni Hospital
Ekwendeni.
The hospital: This is a 205-bed mission-run hospital in north Malawi, with most major specialities being catered for.

Embangweni

Embangweni Hospital
Embangweni.
The hospital: Is a 120-bed centre with general medical, surgical, paediatrics and maternity wards. There are 12 mobile outreach clinics to regions throughout northern Malawi. They have 1200 deliveries a year. It is currently run by two families.

Livingstonia

David Gordon Memorial Hospital
Livingstonia.
The hospital: This is a 65-bed hospital with a number of outreach posts.

Mulanje

Mulanje Mission Hospital
PO Box 45, Mulanje.
The hospital: A small hospital (set up in the early 1900s by Scottish ministers) in a Presbyterian mission at the foot of Mulanje Massif (3000 m above sea level). There are four doctors (recently all Dutch, but hospital work is carried out in English). Morning prayers and songs are in Chichewa.

There is a great deal of O&G, general medicine and surgery but not many opportunities for practical procedures. There are a total of 146 beds on female, male, maternity, paediatric, TB and private wards. There are also village clinics. Malaria, TB, pneumonia, malnutrition and AIDS are common. The prevalence of HIV around Mulanje is about 30%, which means that approximately three-quarters of hospital patients have AIDS-related illnesses.

O **Elective notes:** This place gets fairly booked up with elective students so apply well in advance. Mulanje has some VSO workers in it … go to the nightclub for a laugh. There is a sports club too. Some people have felt that a month is adequate here. Mulanje District Hospital is a lot more modern and bigger, but it is government run.

Accommodation: Very good (including a cook/cleaner) in a guest wing of the mission at a cost of £40 (2963 MWK) a month.

Mzuzu

St John's Hospital
PO Box 18, Mzuzu.
The hospital: A 216-bed mission hospital in northern Malawi. It is divided into male, female, paediatric, isolation and maternity wards, with a busy outpatient department. The hospital admits from all over north Malawi. It is a friendly hospital and well staffed by African standards.

O **Elective notes:** There's a great deal of responsibility and many procedures to do, but you are well supported. You can go to any department. At weekends, relax in town or on Lake Malawi. Try to go with someone as it can get a bit lonely in the evenings.

Accommodation: Accommodation for two is in a little flat for around £50 (3700 MWK) a month.

Nkhoma

Nkhoma Hospital
PO Bag 48, Nkhoma. Tel: +265 722 799.
Fax: +265 723 090. E-mail:
nkhoma@mlw.healthnet.org.

The hospital: Has 220 beds and is run
by four doctors. TB, HIV, malaria,
cholera, malnutrition and O&G complications are common. It is a very rural setting with limited investigations (the X-
ray machine is always broken); hence it
is a great place for clinical skills. It has a
fantastic eye surgery unit. Outreach clinics are also run.

O Elective notes: This hospital is well
organized and has friendly staff who
teach well. With lots of gross pathology
and procedures, it comes highly recommended. Apply early as it books up very
rapidly. It is quite isolated so take a good
book or a friend. It is a mission town but
not being religious is not a problem, just
no big swinging nights out. Access to
e-mail is available.

Accommodation: A lovely guesthouse
is provided for 40 MWK (50p) a day.
Bring a mosquito net.

Zomba

Zomba General Hospital
PO Box 21 Zomba. Tel: +265 523 195.

Mauritius

Population: I million
Language: English
Capital: Port Louis
Currency: Mauritian rupee
Int Code: +230

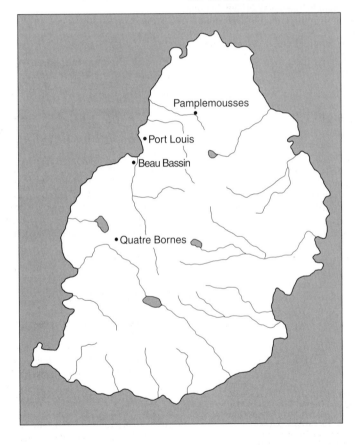

Pamplemousses

Port Louis

Beau Bassin

Quatre Bornes

Mauritius is a small and beautiful volcanic island in the Indian Ocean, hot with gorgeous white beaches and coral reefs. Unfortunately, it is terribly overpopulated, which has led to extreme social variation – the obscenely wealthy living very close to the very poor in slums and shanties. The population consists of Indian, Afro-Mauritian, Chinese and French Mauritian, each with their own culture, religion and cuisine. The economy is based on sugar, textiles and tourism. Since independence, the government has promised *a certain standard of (free) healthcare for all. The language is officially English, but in reality it is mainly Creole (based on French). Being able to speak French helps a lot. There are lots of watersports, including scuba-diving (especially on the west coast).*

✪ Medicine:

Mauritius has a healthcare system that is free to all. In the primary setting are 'dispensaries' (a cross between a chemist and a GP). There are also private doctors for the rich. Either of these can refer to hospitals. There are 13 government-run hospitals in Mauritius and one in Rodrigues (a small island about 560 km east of Mauritius); these provide 3505 beds. The three main hospitals on Mauritius are the **Sir Seewoosagur Ramgoolam National Hospital** (SSRN) in the northern district, the **Jetto** in the capital, Port Louis, and the **Victoria** in Quatres Bornes. The SSRN is the biggest. Many pathologies today are a result of the westernization of Mauritius. Big medical problems include hypertension, Type II diabetes, heart disease and alcoholism (and hence trauma). Rheumatic fever and diarrhoea and vomiting are also common conditions in paediatrics. The prevalence of HIV is very low, at 0.08%.

➲ Work permits:

Registration to work as a doctor or dentist can be obtained from the Medical and Dental Councils of Mauritius.

USEFUL ADDRESSES:

Ministry of Health, Emmanuel Anquetil Building, Port Louis. Tel: +230 201 1903. Fax: +230 201 3660.
Medical and Dental Councils of Mauritius, 6 Avenue des Jacinthes, Morc. St Jean, Quatre Bornes.
Mauritius Dental Association, 35 Labourdonnais Street, Port Louis.
Tel: +230 211 7206. Fax: +230 212 1502.

◉ Climate and crime:

The climate is subtropical, the warmest months being January and February. The crime rate is extremely low.

To do an elective in Mauritius, you are best to write to the elective coordinator at the Ministry of Health. They can sort the rest out. You may be asked to see the coordinator on arrival, in which case take some smart clothes. In addition, carry a letter from the coordinator with your passport as customs officials often do not understand why you are spending so long in Mauritius.

MEDICAL SCHOOL:

University of Mauritius Medical School
Reduit. Tel: +230 454 1041.
Fax: +230 454 9642. www.uom.ac.mu.

AG Jeetoo Hospital
Volcy Pougnet Street, Port Louis.
Tel: +230 212 3201.
The hospital: Is in the capital, very overcrowded, busy and not very well organized. The notes are in English (which the doctors speak), but the patients speak Mauritian Creole. There's plenty of rheumatic fever, alcohol-related problems and heart disease.
○ **Elective notes:** The staff are very friendly and translate in clinics (which can seem like a conveyer belt). It is not a complete holiday; you have to do a reasonable amount of work.

Pamplemousses

Sir Seewoosagur Ramgoolam National Hospital
Pamplemousses. Tel: +230 243 4661.
The hospital: The SSRN was built in 1968 as part of an independence agreement with the British. It is the largest hospital in Mauritius, with large, busy clinics and all major departments. The contrast between the rich and poor can be seen in the SSRN, where high-profile operations, such as heart and renal transplants, are carried out while patients may be two to a bed or lying on a mattress on the floor. The paeds unit, for example, has previously had only one peak-flow meter. Birds and dogs are free to roam the wards.

Mauritius

O **Elective notes:** Most of the consultants are British- or French-trained and keen to teach. There are lots of patients to see and as much 'hands-on' activity as you like. There is plenty of time off to do as you wish. This is probably a better elective if you really want a holiday.

Accommodation: A list of apartments is provided; however, the north west is the 'happening area', and apparently renting a flat in Grand Baie is better. Try to book in advance as entering Mauritius without a booking can be difficult.

Quatre Bornes

Victoria Hospital

Candos, Quartre Bornes. Tel +230 425 3031.
The hospital: Is a very busy, govern-ment-run converted army barracks but it is a major hospital for the region. It is understaffed but has a wide range of facilities. It also contains the Princess Margaret Orthopaedic Centre.

O **Elective notes:** You can see some great clinical signs, but as it is so busy, it can be difficult keeping up on ward rounds. There's a great deal of type II diabetes and hypertension. The staff are very friendly, and the teaching is good.

Accommodation: Not provided.

OTHER HOSPITALS:

Brown Sequard Hospital, Pope Henessy Street, Beau Bassin. Tel: +230 454 2071.
Medical and Surgical Centre Ltd, Georges Guibert Street, Floreal. Tel: +230 686 1477.
Moka Hospital, Moka. Tel: +230 433 4015.

Namibia

Population: 1.5 million
Language: English
Capital: Windhoek
Currency: Namibian dollar
Int Code: +264

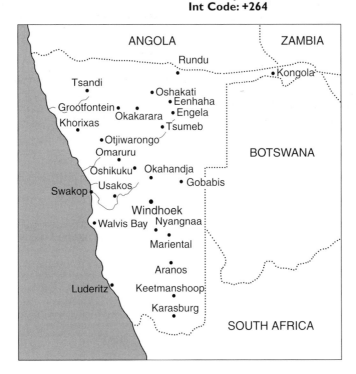

Namibia is a land of amazing contrast, from desert on the coast and in the east to green farmland in the north, mountain ranges in the centre and Fish River canyon in the south. There is also a great diversity in culture, with influence from the original San Bushmen and the European and South African colonial invasion. There are many local dialects (e.g. Ovambo, Nama and Damara), but the nurses in each area are fluent in these and translate.

✪ Medicine:

Namibia is a vast country, making health provision awkward. All major areas have hospitals. To be seen in a government hospital, patients pay N$9 (about £1), which entitles them to any care they require. Family practitioners in cities are inaccessible for most of the population. In remote rural areas, there are clinics, as it may take days to walk to the nearest hospital. Most of the doctors are

Namibians who have trained abroad or South Africans. Windhoek is the referral centre for the whole of Namibia. If the service cannot be provided there, the patient either has to be transferred to South Africa or wait until the specialist does his annual visit. Basic hygiene is still a big issue, many areas not having safe water. Infectious diseases are very common. HIV has become a major problem across the country (with an average prevalence around 20%).

➲ Visas and work permits:

For stays of up to three months, British citizens do not require a visa. If officially studying or working, you will need to get a letter of acceptance/employment from the institution you are visiting, and the High Commission will then issue the appropriate permit.

Note: At the beginning of 1998, the Namibian Ministry of Health said that foreign medical students would only be allowed in the capital, Windhoek. Contact the High Commission as things are changing.

USEFUL ADDRESS:

Ministry of Health, Old State Hospital, Harvey Street, Private Bag 13198, Windhoek. Tel: +264 61 2039111. Fax: +264 61 227607.

HOSPITALS:

There are literally hundreds of small hospitals and clinics, too many to list here. Up-to-date information on all of them, with contact details of the doctors in charge, can be found on www.medicstravel.org.

Katatura State Hospital

Harvey Street, Private Bag 13198, Windhoek. Tel: +264 61 203911/ 2032589. Fax: +264 51 221332/ 222706.

The hospital: Is part of the Windhoek Medical Complex, including the Windhoek Central Hospital (which admits some private patients; same address but Tel: +264 61 2033037), a TB hospital and a psychiatric hospital.

Katatura (entirely state run) has 16 wards for medicine, surgery, paeds, trauma and O&G. There is also an outpatients/emergency department. In the emergency department, a triage nurse refers directly to the relevant speciality. TB, malaria, HIV and malnutrition are common. It has been estimated that between 20% and 30% of babies born in Namibia are HIV positive. As this hospital is the referral centre for the entire country, many unusual conditions are also seen.

Accommodation: Provided free in the doctors' residence at the central hospital. There is also a large swimming pool and barbecue on site. It is very sociable. The lively town centre (with shops, cinema and restaurants) is about a mile away.

MISSION HOSPITAL IN THE CAPITAL:

Rhino Catholic Hospital, 92 Stubel Street, PO Box 157, Windhoek. Tel: +264 61 237237. Fax: +264 61 236416.

GOVERNMENT-RUN HOSPITALS:

These all have many associated clinics:
Omaruru District Hospital, P/Bag 2021, Omaruru, Erongo. Tel: +264 64 570717. Fax: +264 64 570602.
Swakop District Hospital, P/Bag 5004, Swakop, Erongo. Tel: +264 64 412400. Fax: +264 64 400946.
Usakos District Hospital, P/Bag 1003, Usakos, Erongo. Tel: +264 64 530067. Fax: +264 64 530293.
Walvis Bay District Hospital, P/Bag 5010, Walvis Bay, Erongo. Tel: +264 64 203441. Fax: +264 64 202086.
Aranos District Hospital, P/Bag 2001, Aranos, Hardap. Tel: +264 63 272027/70. Fax: +264 63 272122.
Mariental District Hospital, P/Bag 2014, Mariental, Hardap. Tel: +264 63 242092. Fax: +264 63 240765.
Karasburg District Hospital, P/Bag 2001, Karasburg, Karas. Tel: +264 63 270167. Fax: +264 63 270407.
Keetmanshoop District Hospital, P/Bag 2101, Keetmanshoop, Karas. Tel: +264 63 223388. Fax: +264 63 223781.
Luderitz District Hospital, P/Bag 2002, Luderitz, Karas. Tel: +264 63 202446. Fax: +264 63 203602.
Andara District Hospital, P/Bag 2072, Nyangana, Kavango. Tel: +264 66 259311. Fax: +264 66 255184.

Nyangana District Hospital, P/Bag 2074, Nyangara, Kavango. Tel: +264 66 258266. Fax: +264 66 255184.

Rundu Intermediate Referral Hospital, P/Bag 2094, Rundu, Kavango. Tel: +264 66 255025. Fax: +264 66 255371.

Khorixas District Hospital, P/Bag 2010, Khorixas, Kunene. Tel: +264 67 331064. Fax: +264 67 331398.

Opuwo District Hospital, P/Bag 3003, Opuwo, Kunene. Tel: +264 65 273026. Fax: +264 65 273022.

Outjo District Hospital, P/Bag 2567, Outjo, Kuene. Tel: +264 67 313044. Fax: +264 67 313271.

Eenhana District Hospital, P/Bag 2006, Eenhaha, Ohangwena. Tel: +264 65 263023/5. Fax: +264 65 263024.

Engela District Hospital, P/Bag 502, Engela, Ohangwena. Tel: +264 65 266600. Fax: +264 65 2266678.

Kongo District Hospital, P/Bag 2038, Kongo, Ohangwena. Tel: +264 65 695003. Fax: +264 65 695002.

Gobabis District Hospital, P/Bag 2099, Gobabis, Ohangwena. Tel: +264 62 563720. Fax: +264 62 563489.

Oshikuku District Hospital, P/Bag 5567, Oshikuku, Oshakati. Tel: +264 65 254550.

Tsumeb District Hospital, P/Bag 2004, Tsumeb. Tel: +264 67 221082. Fax: +264 67 221370.

Outapi District Hospital, P/Bag 504, Outapi. Tel: +264 65 250318. Fax: +264 65 251020.

Tsandi District Hospital, P/Bag 502, Uukwaluudhi. Tel: +264 65 258121. Fax: +264 65 258121.

Oshakati Intermediate District Hospital, P/Bag 5538, Oshakati, Oshana. Tel: +264 65 2233143. Fax: +264 65 221390.

Onandjokwe District Hospital, P/Bag 2016, Ondangwa. Tel: +264 65 240111. Fax: +264 65 240688.

Grootfontein District Hospital, P/Bag 2052, Grootfontein, Otjozondjupa. Tel: +264 67 242141. Fax: +264 67 242141.

Okahandja District Hospital, P/Bag 2026, Okahandja, Otjozondjupa. Tel: +264 62 503039. Fax: +264 62 501731.

Okakarara District Hospital, P/Bag 2102, Okakarara, Otjozondjupa. Tel: +264 67 317028. Fax: +264 67 317448.

Otjiwarongo District Hospital, P/Bag 2516, Otjiwarongo, Otjozondjupa. Tel: +264 67 300900. Fax: +264 67 304963.

Tsandi District Hospital, P/Bag 502, Uukwaluudhi. Tel: +264 65 258121. Fax: +264 65 258121.

Nigeria

Population: 126 million
Language: English
Capital: Abuja
Currency: Naira
Int Code: +234

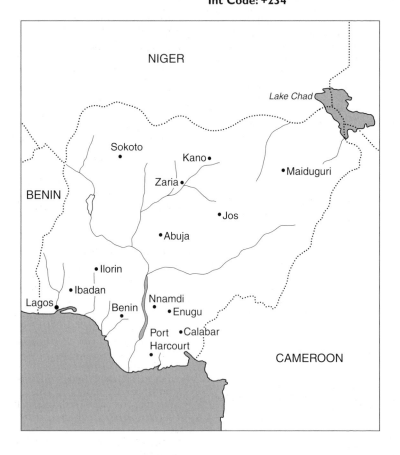

Nigeria gained independence from the UK in 1960. Since then it has had a number of military governments which has had dire consequences for what was one of Africa's most productive countries. There is now a great deal of poverty. The country itself has desert in the north and dense rainforest in the south.

✪ Medicine:

Healthcare is very poor and really only available to those living near cities. As a result, infectious diseases, including yellow fever, malaria, yaws and trachoma, are commonly seen. The prevalence of HIV is relatively low, averaging 5%.

⊃ Visas and work permits:

To do an elective in Nigeria, you will need a visitor's visa. This requires a passport (valid for at least six months), a completed visa application form (IMM 22), a letter of invitation from Nigeria addressed to the visa section, Nigeria High Commission, accepting full immigration/evidence of sustaining yourself while you are in Nigeria, a return ticket and a fee if appropriate. Allow at least five working days for your visa to be processed.

To work as a medical practitioner, you have to register with the **Nigeria Medical Council**. You will need a work permit and may be asked to sit the Nigeria Medical Council Assessment Examination.

USEFUL ADDRESSES:

Federal Ministry of Health, Block 4A, (301–99) Third Floor, New Federal Secretariat Complex, Shehu Shagari Way, PMB 83, Garki Post Office, Abuja. Tel: +254 9 523 4590.
Nigeria Medical Council, PMB 12611, Plot PC 13, Idowa-Taylor Street, Victoria Island, Lagos.
Nigerian Medical Association, 74 Adeniyi Jones Avenue, Ikeja, PO Box 1108, Marina, Lagos. Tel: +234 1 497 7292 Fax: +234 1 583 1027.
Nigerian Dental Association, Department of Oral Pathology and Biology, College of Medicine, University of Lagos, PO Box 3971 Marina, Lagos. Tel: +234 1 545 3760.

SOME OF THE MAIN MEDICAL SCHOOLS:

Abia State University, College of Medicine and Health Sciences, PMB 2000, Uturu, Abia State. Tel: +234 88 220 785.
Ahmadu Bello University, Faculty of Medicine, PMB 1008, Zaria, Kaduna. Tel: +234 88 220 785.
Bayero University, Faculty of Medicine, PMB 3011, Kano. Tel: +234 69 32 688.
Danfodiyo University, College of Health Sciences, Sultan Abubakar Road, PMB 2370, Sokoto 02254, Sokoto State. Tel: +234 60 233 012. Fax: +234 60 230 709.
Nnamdi Azikiwe University, College of Health Sciences, Nnewi Campus, PMB 5001, Nnewi, Anambra State. Tel: +234 46 463 663. Fax: +234 46 460 124.

Ogun State University, Obafemi Awolowo College of Health Sciences, PMB 2002, Ago-Iwoye, Ogun State.
University of Benin, College of Medical Sciences, PMB 1154, Benin City, Bendel. Tel: +234 52 600 547. Fax: +234 52 600 273. www.uniben.edu.
University of Calabar, College of Medical Sciences, PMB 1115, Calabar, Cross River State. Tel: +234 87 222 855. Fax: +234 87 221 766.
University of Ibadan, College of Medicine, Queen Elizabeth Road, PMB 5017, Ibadan, Oyo. Tel: +234 2 241 3922. Fax: +234 2 241 1768. www.ui.edu.ng.
University of Ilorin, Faculty of Health Sciences, PMB 1515, Ilorin, Kwara State.
Tel: +234 31 221 844. www.unilorin.edu.ng.
University of Jos, Faculty of Medical Sciences, PMB 2084, Jos, Plateau.
www.uiowa.edu/intlinet/unijos.
University of Lagos, College of Medicine, PMB 12003, Idi-Araba, Lagos Tel: +234 1 832 049. Fax: +234 1 837 630.
University of Maiduguri, College of Medical Sciences, PMB 1069, Maiduguri, Borno. Tel: +234 076 232 537.
University of Nigeria, College of Medicine, PMB 01229, Enugu, Anambra.
University of Port Harcourt, College of Health Sciences, East West Road, PMB 1, Choba, Port Harcourt, Rivers State.

At the time of writing, most of the above do not have websites, but www.widernet.org/nigeriaconsult/ gives a great deal of information on them.

ECWA-Evangel Hospital

PMB 2009, Jos, Plateau State.
The hospital: Is a 160-bed mission hospital and teaching hospital for GP residents (with many lectures). The staff are very welcoming, and medicine, surgery, O&G, and paeds can be practised. There is also a busy outpatients' department. This is a good place to see Christian Medical Evangelism in action. Most of the trainees are from the **Jos University Teaching Hospital**, but the seniors are missionaries from all over the globe. It is one of a number of fistula centres in Nigeria.
Accommodation: A comfortable house is provided.

Vom Christian Hospital

PMB 06, Vom, Via Jos, Plateau State.
The hospital: This is another mission hospital in the same area.

Seychelles

Population: 80 000
Language: Creole
Capital: Victoria
Currency: Seychelles rupee
Int Code: +248

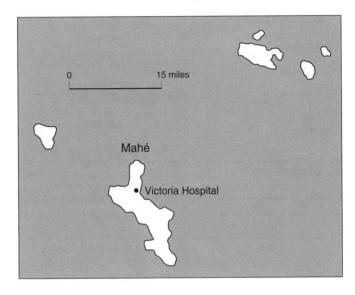

0   15 miles

Mahé

● Victoria Hospital

Fancy medicine in paradise? The Seychelles is a group of 115 islands in the Indian Ocean. Formerly a British colony, it has had democracy since 1993. There are beautiful beaches, excellent diving sites (including diving with whale sharks in June–August) and a very relaxed lifestyle. Be warned though, the main economy is tourism, and this is an incredibly expensive place to visit (it costs £4 for a drink).

✪ Medicine:

The government provides a free state healthcare system employing mainly a few ex-pat doctors and local nurses. Western diseases (cardiovascular, heart and cancers) are the common pathologies. There are many small private hospitals that can be easily found on the web. Small rural hospitals are usually affiliated with the Victoria Hospital.

◎ Climate:

Hot (not surprisingly). It rains quite a bit between November and February.

USEFUL ADDRESS:

Ministry of Health, PO Box 52, Victoria Hospital, Victoria, Mahé. Tel: +248 388 000.
Fax: +248 224 792.

Victoria Hospital

PO Box Mont Fleuri Road, Victoria, Mahé.
Tel: +248 224 400.
The hospital: This is the main hospital

and has 300 beds, including an eight-bed ITU. Reports say that, despite the good funding, the relaxed lifestyle leaves something to be desired with regard to efficiency. There are good surgical, medical and radiographic departments.

O **Elective notes:** If it's 'hands on' experience and teaching you want, it's best to look elsewhere. The anaesthetic department is, however, keen. If you want a very relaxed time with sunny beaches, then this is the place. Community medicine (with a local GP) has received very good reports (this can be arranged through the Ministry of Health).

Accommodation: Has previously been provided by the Ministry of Health.

South Africa

Population: 43 million
Languages: English, Afrikaans and
nine separate African languages
Capitals: Pretoria, Cape Town and
Bloemfontein
Currency: Rand
Int Code: +27

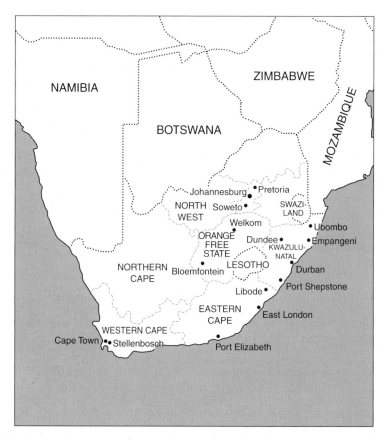

In 1994, the 80 years of apartheid and white minority rule ended, giving a new-found freedom to so many of the natural population. It has, however, meant that many whites have decided to leave the country. It will be a test of the government to see whether it can maintain the country's economy during this change. The land itself

has many natural resources (diamond and gold mining) and some beautiful countryside, the Drakensberg Mountains and the Garden Route for example. Many students go here as it is renowned for violence and trauma, and hence can offer great experience in emergency departments. You might think that the place would be becoming more peaceful with the change in politics, but the opposite is true. Many poor and unskilled people now have just enough money to buy a gun (available for a few pounds), and these have replaced traditional fighting weapons.

✪ Medicine:

It is often described as Third World medicine in a First World setting. Until 1990, medical care in South Africa could be segregated into that for whites (good, very high-quality Western-style care) and that for blacks (much more of a developing country situation). Indeed, the incidence of diseases still reflects this divide. Infectious diseases (especially HIV and TB) are extremely common in Zulus. Out of every 1000 children, 200 die before the age of five. Western diseases of ageing lie in the domain of the white people. There has been a huge push to try to improve the health of rural folk. This has involved plans from basic sanitary care to immunizations and the building of new hospitals.

Two points have to be stressed about South African medicine. Trauma and violence are common. This is great if it's your speciality; it's not great if you happen to be actually experiencing it. Many people who have been there will say that stressing this point is just scaremongering as they never saw any trouble. Indeed, most tourist areas are pretty safe. Chances are though that if you're going to a hospital, it's not in a tourist area. In years gone by, the worst that could happen was a threat with a knife or *nob keri*. You could run away. You can't run away from a gun. For this reason, it is not illegal to jump red lights at night. Try not to look too much like a tourist – rip the map out of the Lonely Planet guide rather than carrying it open. Road traffic accidents (especially among Zulu taxi dri-

vers, who also have taxi wars) are common. These problems are really only confined to certain areas, mainly in KwaZulu-Natal, Johannesburg and townships near Cape Town. Speak with someone who has been there recently.

HIV also has to be mentioned. A number of UK medical schools have now banned students from going to South Africa unless they sign a disclaimer. This is a real shame as it is a wonderful place to see a great deal of medicine. The concern surrounds the risk of getting a needle-stick injury. Again, this depends on location. Some areas have an HIV rate below 10%, others as high as 50%, the average being 20%. There are a number of options. You can refuse to do any exposure-prone procedure, although this may be difficult if they have taken you on to help them out. You should (as you would anywhere) always use universal precautions (*see* 'Your health whilst abroad'). Remember that the seroconversion rate from needle-stick injuries is very low (<1%), but the prospect of tests on your return will absolutely destroy your elective.

Note: South African students have their summer holiday during November–December. This means that there are only elective students on the wards … can be fun, can be lonely.

➲ Visas, registration and work permits:

○ Electives: Some universities (e.g University of Witwatersrand) say that if you are doing an elective in a teaching hospital, you have to (by law) apply to the **Health Professions Council of South Africa** (HPCSA). This costs US$20 and can take around 12 weeks. The forms are usually available from the host institution.

Most European Union, US, Australian and New Zealand citizens do not require a visa to 'visit' South Africa for up to 90 days. The official line for elective students from the European Union and US is, however, that they require a *study permit*, for which a letter from the host institution and proof of acceptance from the HPCSA is needed. The visa costs R500 (£90). Many students going to rural areas do not bother with it and say they are going on holiday (which indeed many of them are). In recent years, however, the law has been enforced more rigorously. If you are going to a university hospital, you will definitely need a study permit. If you don't want to risk having your elective ruined, it is best to follow the bureaucracy. Obtaining a work permit for paid employment will also cost £90.

Work: Regulations have started to change in this area. Until recently, UK qualifications were automatically recognized. Now you have to submit your details to the HPCSA, who then assess you for registration. The process varies depending on whether you wish to do general practice (public or private), academic or specialist work. If wishing to work privately, you will have to do one year of public work (as all South African graduates do). Contact the HPCSA for more details.

USEFUL ADDRESSES:

Department of Health, Hallmark Building, Proes St, Pretoria 0002. Tel: +27 12 312 0000.
Health Professions Council of South Africa, PO Box 205, Pretoria 0001. Tel: +27 12 338 9300. Fax: +27 12 325 2074. www.hpcsa.co.za.
South African Medical and Dental Council, PO Box 205, Pretoria 0001. Tel: +27 12 328 6680. Fax: +27 12 328 5120.
South African Medical Association, PO Box 74789, Lynnwood Ridge 0040, Castle Walk Office Park, Block F, Nossob Street, Erasmuskloof Ext 3, Pretoria 0153. Tel: +27 12 481 2000.
Fax: +27 12 481 2100. www.samedical.org.
South African Nursing Association, PO Box 1280, Pretoria 0001. Tel: +27 12 343 2315. Fax: +27 12 344 0750.
South African Nursing Council, PO Box 1123, Pretoria 0001. Tel: +27 12 343 0121. Fax: +27 12 343 5400.
South African Dental Association, 31 Princess of Wales Terrace, Parktown, Gautang.
Tel: +27 11 484 5288. Fax: +27 11 642 5718. www.sadanet.co.za.
South African Society of Physiotherapists, PO Box 92125, Norwood 2117.
Tel: +27 11 485 1467. Fax: +27 11 485 1613.
South African Occupational Therapy Association, 946 Shoeman Street, Arcadia 0083. www.linx.za.occther.

⊚ Climate and crime:

It can get very hot (over 35°C) in January and February and quite cold in winter (June–August). With regard to crime, *see* above. Avoid townships and heed local advice.

Western Cape

The Western Cape has two universities – Cape Town and Stellenbosch – the latter being more Afrikaans. There is also the Faculty of Dentistry and Allied Medical Disciplines in Bellville (Private Bag X17, Bellville, Cape 7535. Tel: + 27 21 959 2911. Fax: +27 21 951 3627).

CAPE TOWN:

An amazing city with lots to do, including Table Mountain, beautiful beaches, diving, surfing, climbing, penguins at Balder's Bay, Stellenbosch (winery), Cape Point, sky-diving, great restaurants and clubs. Hire a car (£20 a day) if you're over 23 and go down the Garden Route. It is relatively cheap to eat out (£7 for a three-course meal and a couple of beers).

University of Cape Town

Faculty of Medicine, Anzio Road, Observatory, Cape Town 7925. Tel: +27 21 650 9111. Fax: +27 21 478 955.
www.uct.ac.za.

For electives, apply to all the University of Cape Town (UCT) hospitals via the university, but note that most elective places are filled up to a year in advance. The processing of applications can take several months. You may well be best writing to your destination first and saying, 'Dr X has said I can work with him …'. If organized through the university, there is a fee for administration. This costs 600R (£100, and has been increasing), and then you have to pay to register with the **South African Medical and Dental Council** (SAMDC), giving you permission to practise in the country and covering you for malpractice. Write to the elective coordinator at

Medfac@medicine.uct.ac.za or the above address for a form. Note: The UCT also runs a **Student Health and Welfare Community Organization** (SHAWCO). This consists of UCT students and a doctor going out into townships to run clinics. Previous elective students have found it an excellent experience and it may be worth enquiring about.

Hospitals associated with the University of Cape Town:

Groote Schuur Hospital
Anzio Road, Observatory 7925, Cape Town. www.gsh.co.za.

The hospital: This is a huge hospital serving a large segment of Cape Town and the townships. All specialities are here. It has a level one trauma unit, which is busy seeing 35 000 cases a year, half deliberate acts and half penetrating trauma. This is mainly gunshots, stabbings and car accidents (the latter making up only 20% of the total). There is an acute arm – admitting and stabilizing trauma patients – and a surgical arm – performing acute and subacute procedures on them. Common trauma includes thoracic cases such as stabbed hearts, neck trauma, abdominal and vascular injury. The hospital spends R1 000 000 a year on security to stop gangs coming in to finish the job. There is a high incidence of HIV (15%). There is also an excellent neurology and cardiothoracic department.

O **Elective notes:** Apply at least a year in advance if you want to do trauma. It is popular with Australian, German, Dutch and British students (because of the excellent social life). It's good for trauma, with many practical procedures (chest drains and central lines), and there is a good lecture programme (an optional two hours day). There are, however, lots of UCT students who have preferential treatment. Reports say that the head of department is VERY strict … you do not manage any patients without senior consultation, and you must be present (to work) when you are supposed to. Medical pathology includes TB, AIDS

and rheumatic fever. Cardiothoracic surgery is good as the students have a rota system giving plenty of time off, but ward rounds start at 7 am. There are 22 languages used in the area, not a problem unless you are doing psychiatry, where it really does limit you to being an observer.

Accommodation: The Lodge (36 Milton Road, Observatory, Cape Town. Tel: +27 21 448 6536) is a good place to stay (£3 a night). It seems as if all the medical students stay here (and some people have left because of this and questions of security). Nelly (the owner) is friendly and handy if you are going to Namibia or Zimbabwe. They can also arrange cheap car hire. The Green Elephant Hostel (a two-minute walk from the hospital) is also good. Some people have preferred Sunflower Stop (Main Road, Greenpoint. Tel: +27 21 434 6535. Fax: +27 21 434 6801), which is nearer the beaches and waterfront.

Victoria Hospital
Private Bag x2, Wynberg, Plumstead 7800, Cape Town.

The hospital: A small (160-bed) state hospital in a leafy suburb of Cape Town (20 minutes by car from the centre). It has medical, surgical, O&G, and paeds wards as well as a fairly busy trauma department. It has repeatedly been described as very friendly.

O **Elective notes:** UCT students are attached here, although not to the emergency department. There are quite a lot of gunshot cases, but most major trauma is seen at the Groote Schuur. Groote Schuur, however, has a very large number of students … and here there are only elective students. Many people have said that this is a better place for practical experience, as you get taken on as an important member of the team.

Red Cross Children's Hospital
Klipfontein Road, Rondebosch 7700, Cape Town. www.kidshospital.co.za.

The hospital: Is the largest paediatric hospital in South Africa and has a huge range of conditions, spanning those of the developing to the developed world. Common conditions include HIV, TB, malnutrition, asthma and meningitis. It sees the acute paediatric emergencies in Cape Town, who can then be referred on for supportive care. It has very specialized departments, from paediatric cardiology to surgery.

O **Elective notes:** Working for the Red Cross requires quite a bit of dedication and responsibility. When working, a full day's work is expected. It makes you very confident in your clinical skills. Thoroughly recommended.

Accommodation: Stay at Nelly's (*see* Groote Schuur Hospital).

Somerset Hospital

Private Bag, Green Point 8051, Cape Town. E-mail: somhosp@ilink.nis.29.

The hospital: A medium-sized public hospital, this is located by the V and A waterfront, an area with excellent night-life. The hospital is lacking in facilities, and trauma (stabbings and gunshots) makes up a large part of the surgical workload. There are medical, surgical, paeds and O&G departments. Malnutrition, TB, meningitis, gastroenteritis and HIV-related disease are common in paeds. There are three busy wards, although acute paeds is seen at the Red Cross Hospital rather than here.

O **Elective notes:** The teaching on ward rounds (at 8 am) is excellent, and there is a relaxed attitude towards how much you put in. An administration charge of R30 is requested. This is a highly recommended elective.

Accommodation: In the nurses' home, costs about R360 a month (£13 a week) and is basic (there are no catering facilities).

GF Jooste Hospital

Manenberg Road, Manenberg 7767, Cape Town. Tel: +27 21 691 7962. Fax: +27 21 691 7962.

The hospital: Is in the Cape Town townships in the area of the Cape Flats (20 minutes' drive from Cape Town). It is a secondary referral centre and has a trauma unit, male, female, high-dependency and surgical wards, totalling 180 beds. A great deal of penetrating trauma is seen in the emergency department. The HIV rate in patients is thought to be 50%. This is a dangerous area (the security guard is behind bulletproof glass, and you have to go though a metal detector in reception). There is incredible poverty in the townships.

O **Elective notes:** You will need transport as public transport is not safe. Some of the junior doctors don't want to be here. The consultants are, however, excellent, and there are plenty of opportunities for practical procedures such as chest drains. Go with friends to spread the cost of car hire and for safety.

Princess Alice Orthopaedic Hospital

White Road, Retreat 7945, Private Bag X13, Tokai 7966, Cape Town.

The hospital: A relatively small hospital with six wards of a dozen beds. It carries out all the elective orthopaedic surgery for the Cape in two theatres. It also has a large rheumatology department.

Stellenbosch University

Private Bag X1, Matieland 7602. Tel: +27 21 808 9111. Fax: +27 21 931 7810. www.sun.ac.za.

This is very much the Afrikaans' university. Many German elective students go here. Surgery is popular with them as it involves less work than in Germany and, once done, they don't have to do it at home. The university is quite a way out of Cape Town (30 minutes on the train … don't do it after dark). Write to the elective student officer at the above address.

Accommodation: Usually provided in the elective student residence.

Tygerberg Hospital

Private Bag x3, Tygerberg 7505. Fax: +27 21 931 1451.

The hospital: Part of the University of Stellenbosch but is some way from it and also some way from Cape Town. It is a very Afrikaans hospital, which can cause language problems. The violence here is incredible, stabbings, gunshot wounds and accidents being the run of the mill.

O **Elective notes:** The trauma unit is incredibly busy, and there is loads of assisting in theatre. The ward rounds are sometimes in English, sometimes in Afrikaans, and there is not that much to do in the local area. You need to get into Cape Town.

Johannesburg and Pretoria

Some people will say this is overstated but Johannesburg is VERY DANGEROUS. Elective students get mugged here. If you can live in fear, you will learn loads and the opportunities are immense. Once inside the hospitals, everything is fine, but be careful if going out alone. Try to make friends with a local who can show you the sites. Despite all this, Johannesburg is a good base for getting up to Kruger National Park and Pretoria. Pretoria, on the other hand, is the base of the government, safer and much more pleasant. There is one medical school in Johannesburg (Witwatersrand) and two in Pretoria (Medunsa and Universiteit van Pretoria).

Johannesburg:

University of the Witwatersrand Medical School
7 York Road, Parktown 2193, Johannesburg. Tel: +27 11 6447 1111. Fax: +27 11 643 4318.
E-mail: elective@chiron.wits.ac.za.
www.wits.ac.za.
The university: The University of Witwatersrand has plenty of information on electives on its website (www.wits.ac.za/fac/med/elective/index.html) – it can seem extremely off-putting though. It all sounds very strict, saying that you have to apply through the university to get a place in any of their hospitals (marked on page 79 with a *). This is basically a money-making scheme for

the university since they then charge you US$200 a month for the privilege. They warn you that your elective will not be recognized if you apply directly. If you plan to work in one of their teaching hospitals, you will have little choice but to follow the rules. However, many medical schools around the world have had links with rural hospitals going back decades, and students still apply directly, usually without any problems (just get the medical superintendent to sign your forms). As is suggested throughout this book, a donation to the local hospital would be far better than funding the university.

Johannesburg General Hospital
Jubille Road, Parktown, Johannesburg.
The hospital: Is huge (1800 beds, but not as big as the Bara), with the medical school next door. It has a very busy trauma department with a helicopter service. The transplantation unit and cardiothoracic unit serve the entire community of greater Johannesburg.

O **Elective notes:** Students become very much part of the emergency room team, and there are plenty of opportunities for procedures. The South African students have a two-week trauma attachment and elective students can attend their lectures. This offers great experience for plastic surgery and there are plenty of opportunities for 'hands on' work.

Accommodation: Available at the Johannesburg College of Education residences for about R40 (£6) a day. There's a large outdoor swimming pool.

Chris Hani Baragwanath Hospital
PO Bertsham 2013, Soweto, Johannesburg. Tel: +27 11 647 1111. Fax: + 27 11 643 4318.
www.chrishanibaragwanathhospital.co.za.
The hospital: Is part of the University of the Witwatersrand and is massive. It has 4000 beds serving the 3–4 million people in Soweto. It is like no other hospital. The surgical pit in the emergency department is world renowned for the amount of trauma seen. It is like working in a

war zone. The prevalence of HIV is thought to be around 15%.

O Elective notes: This is a very, very dangerous area. Once inside the guarded hospital you are safe. The medicine seen is very impressive. The final-year students (and yourself) basically do the job of a house officer. You must try to spend some time in the surgical pit. There are many local and elective students. Say hello to everyone and you'll get loads out of it. Students get to do many procedures while the big boys remove the bullets. Fifty per cent of patients have stab or gunshot wounds. It is very popular with German students. An elective here comes extremely highly recommended if you are interested in a trauma career.

Accommodation: Can be arranged through the university, which supplies a list of private houses and hostels. Account for around £5 a day.

Coronation Hospital, which opened in 1944, is 10 km west of the university and has 350 beds. It offers a full range of services and is the largest centre for the treatment of thalassaemia in the province.

Helen Joseph (JG Strijdom) Hospital is located 7 km west of the medical school and has 450 beds.

Pretoria:

Medical University of South Africa (MEDUNSA), PO Box 210, Pretoria 0204. Tel: +27 12 529 4321/521 4111. Fax: +27 12 529 5811/560 0086. www.medunsa.ac.za.
University of Pretoria (Universiteit Van Pretoria), Dr Savage Weg, Riviera, PO Box 667, Pretoria 0001, Gauteng. Tel: +27 12 319 2541/420 4111. Fax: +27 12 329 1351/362 5190. www.up.ac.za.

Pretoria Academical Hospital
Private Bag 169, Pretoria 0001.
The hospital: Is the main government hospital in Pretoria and has a good quality of medicine. It is situated next to the medical faculty. The main conditions are TB, malnutrition and HIV. The staff are friendly and, although it tends to be an Afrikaans area, everyone speaks English.

O Elective notes: Elective fees are around R1300 (£125), half payable in advance. It's busy and you'll see loads here. The local students are friendly and will help you out. Paeds ward rounds start at 7 am. There are plenty of opportunities for procedures. Pretoria is nicer and safer than Johannesburg but still don't walk around alone, especially at night.

Accommodation: This is good quality, close to the university and costs about £150 (R1564) a month.

KwaZulu-Natal

KwaZulu-Natal is, as its name implies, a predominately Zulu area of South Africa. It has a great deal to offer: the Drakensberg Mountains, a number of National Parks, St Lucia wetlands, Cape Vidal, some excellent diving and water sports, as well as the City of Durban. Beware though as some areas are pretty dodgy.

DURBAN:

This is a multicultural city that is not (yet) as dangerous as Johannesburg. There is a pleasant coastal area to the city, however there are areas that are dangerous. Take local advice seriously and drive with your car doors locked at night.

University of Natal
Faculty of Medicine, Student Affairs, Box 17039, Congella 4013. Tel: +27 31 260 4248/260 4377. Fax: +27 31 260 4410. www.nu.ac.za.
They can arrange electives in Durban and in Natal, but most people write direct to the hospital. Other adresses are:

Durban Campus, University of Natal, Durban 4041. Tel: +27 31 260 1111. Fax: +27 31 260 2214.
Pietermaritzburg Campus, University of Natal, P Bag X01, Scottsville 4013, Tel: +27 331 260 5111. Fax: +27 331 260 5599.

King Edward VII Hospital

PO Box Congella, Durban, KwaZulu-Natal.

The hospital: This is main teaching hospital in Durban. Before the end of apartheid it was a blacks-only hospital with Indian medical students. Today, the vast majority of patients are still Zulu.

O **Elective notes:** This is a superb place to study trauma. Often both emergency trauma theatres are running throughout the day with little or no elective surgery. Gunshots, stabbings and car accidents are the common conditions. You will get lots of practical experience.

Addington Hospital

Durban, KwaZulu-Natal.

The hospital: It has a big trauma and orthopaedics department.

O **Elective notes:** This elective is highly recommended if you're into orthopaedics/trauma.

McCord Zulu Hospital

28 McCord Road, Overport 4065, Durban 4001. Tel: +27 268 5700.

The hospital: This is a Christian mission hospital serving the African and Asian communities of Durban. It has 278 beds and an extremely busy outpatient department. Despite this, the staff are friendly and there is a relaxed atmosphere. Over half the patients on the wards are HIV positive.

O **Elective notes:** Elective students can do whatever speciality they feel like when they get up in the morning. There are no formal academic teaching sessions, but much can be gained from practical experience. In surgery, they'll teach you to perform circumcisions and lumbar punctures, insert chest drains, drain liver abscesses and suture. Do as much or as little as you wish. You can get out to do clinics at rural hospitals in Natal. McCord is now charging R3000 (£350) for the privilege of doing an elective here.

Accommodation: Accommodation and food are cheap and provided by the hospital.

RURAL KWAZULU-NATAL

For details on all hospitals, including e-mail addresses and the names of the current medical superintendents, check out the KwaZulu-Natal government's own health website www.kznhealth.gov.za.

Ngwelezana Hospital

Private Bag X20021, Empangeni, 3880, KwaZulu-Natal. Tel: +27 35 901 7000. Fax: +27 35 794 1684.

The hospital: Ngwelezana is a township approximately 7 km from Empangeni (300 km from Durban) and the hospital serves this township. The population is Zulu; very few speak English. It has 800 beds with about 40 beds per ward. There is a great deal of trauma in this violent, eye-opening area. If doing orthopaedics, you will get a wide range of experience, a couple of days a week in theatre, a couple of days on the wards and a day in outpatients. The prevalence of HIV is thought to be 14% in the general population and 25% in the inpatients. The obstetrics experience is superb (200 deliveries a week, no privacy and no analgesia), but there is obviously a lot of blood contact. Be very careful.

O **Elective notes:** You can choose to do what you want when you get there depending on what other students are doing. Empangeni itself is beautiful, and there is a free commonwealth pool for you to use opposite the hospital. There is also a cinema and several restaurants. The doctors are friendly and regularly arrange weekends away and barbecues. However, some have not found this to be their cup of tea as you are very isolated if you do not have a car.

Accommodation: Was in flats nearby where the doctors live but is now often in a house on the opposite side of town. Expect to pay R600 (£90) a month.

Mseleni Hospital

PO Sibhayi 3967, KwaZulu-Natal. Tel: +27 35 574 1004 Fax: +27 35 5741 0126.

The hospital: Mseleni is a mission hospital (established in 1908, although it was

1959 before the first doctors came) situated in the bush in KwaZulu-Natal approximately 80 km from Empangeni. The hospital has 120 beds and up to 200 patients, covering general medicine, surgery, infectious diseases and orthopaedics. The nursing staff are predominantly Zulu. Ward rounds are in English and Zulu nurses translate for non-Zulu-speaking doctors. As well as the six wards there is a busy outpatient department (seeing 100 people a day; patients pay R4 (60p)), two operating theatres, a maternity block and facilities for X-ray, ultrasound, haematology, microbiology and biochemistry. Specialized clinics visit the hospital, and mobile clinics from the hospital go out into the bush.

HIV is endemic, and TB and bilharzia are common. Malaria, worm infections, malnutrition and gastroenteritis are other common pathologies. Mseleni joint disease is a form of osteoarthritis confined to the local area and associated with a genetic collagen defect. Hip and knee replacements are required at an early age, and to this end an orthopaedic surgeon visits once or twice a month. Clinics (by plane) are also carried out from here.

O **Elective notes:** This is a good opportunity for responsibility and practical procedures in a lovely setting with very friendly doctors. Lake Sibhayi (with crocodiles and hippos) is close by, and there is a good sports complex. It is quite remote (11.5 hours from the nearest tarmac road). Take a mosquito net. Repeatedly highly recommended. It still has a mission hospital feel to it. This hospital is linked to the **Africa Evangelical Fellowship** (6 Station Approach, Borough Green, Sevenoaks, Kent TN15 8AD, UK).
Accommodation: Is free, as is the (somewhat predictable) canteen food.

Benedictine Hospital
Private Bag X5007, Nongoma 3950, KwaZulu-Natal. Tel: +27 35 831 0221.
The hospital: A rural hospital with around 750 beds. The wards consist of

male and female medical and surgical, O&G, paeds, TB, psychiatry and ITU.
O **Elective notes:** Some have had a fantastic time here. There is a large paeds department (burns and gastroenteritis) and community clinics to be reached in a 4×4. There's a great deal of orthopaedics and Caesarean sections. Nearby hospitals include **Empangeni** (Ngwelezana Hospital) and **Hlabisa**.
Accommodation: A real problem. Because of this, it may be better to apply to another hospital.

Charles Johnson Memorial Hospital
Private Bag X5503, Nqutu, KwaZulu-Natal 3135.
Tel: +27 34 271 1900. Fax: +27 34 271 0234.
http://charlesjohnsonmem.tripod.com/main.html.
The hospital: Has approximately 400 beds. It is in an entirely Zulu area. It has male and female medical and surgical wards, obstetrics and a large paediatric department. Currently, the doctors (very friendly) are mostly Cuban, although the superintendent is from Mozambique. Common conditions include malnutrition, TB and HIV. It is estimated that there may be an HIV prevalence of up to 45%.
O **Elective notes:** There is a responsibility to do rounds and outpatient clinics, but there is always good support. There are rumours that the area around the hospital is VERY dangerous. (The hospital has barbed wire fencing all around it and gun checks on the gates.) Going to the market is safe, but check before you go. This elective is highly recommended but it is advisable to go with someone.
Accommodation: A good bungalow and food are provided free.

Bethesda Hospital*
Private Bag X602, Ubombo 3970, KwaZulu-Natal. Tel: +27 35 595 1004.
Fax: +27 35 595 1007.
The hospital: Ubombo is a settlement in the Lebombo mountains, Maputoland, about 320 km east of Durban. Methodist

missionaries started the hospital in the 1930s. The Provincial Department of Health now operates it, although there are usually Western doctors here. It has 245 beds serving 100 000 people.

Ubombo is 15 km on a dirt track up a hill from the larger town of Mkuze (on the main road from Durban). It is high and malaria is not a problem here, unlike the valley below. It has a post office and general store. The doctors do not really specialize (although there are male, female, isolation, paeds and maternity wards) but there is usually a surgeon. Patients pay R4 (60p) to visit the busy outpatient department. Most of the population are Zulus. The prevalence of HIV is around 30% in some areas. Malaria, schistosomiasis, TB and STDs are also common. Tuesday is flying day, when small villages are reached by light aircraft.

O **Elective notes:** Responsibilities include doing rounds and clinics. The flying involves flights over Mkuze Game Park and is beautiful. This is an excellent elective as it gives some responsibility and an opportunity to see many conditions. Some have found it difficult to get to. It is best to go with a companion.

Accommodation: About R20 (£2) a day.

Mosvold Hospital
PO Box X2211, Ingwavuma, 3968 KwaZulu-Natal. Tel: +27 35 591 9122. Fax: +27 35 591 9133.

The hospital: Is a rural hospital with the basic specialities and friendly staff. The HIV rate is very high (over 60% on the wards). Medicine, surgery, paeds, O&G and anaesthetics can be undertaken. TB and malaria are common. There is a busy outpatient department and rural clinics (reached by car/plane). The actual hospital is on top of a mountain so there is no malaria. The locals speak only Zulu, but the nurses translate. The nearest big town is Mkuzi.

O **Elective notes:** You're only limited by how much you want to get involved. There's responsibility with good support and opportunities in theatre. The staff are friendly and will see sites with you. You

really need a car. This elective repeatedly comes highly recommended. There are excellent game parks nearby (Mkuzi/Hluhluwe) and in Mozambique. Go to Sodwana bay for diving.

Accommodation: And food are provided free although a donation should be made. It's advisable to bring a mosquito net. The local market stocks basic foods.

Edendale Hospital
Postbag X509, Plessislaer 4500, KwaZulu-Natal. Tel: +27 33 195 4370.

The hospital: Serves the local township and is busy with a large amount of trauma, TB and HIV. Medicine, surgery, paeds, O&G, and anaesthetics are the specialities.

O **Elective notes:** There's plenty of pathology, and doctors are keen for students to get procedures done. It's also very sociable, but a car is essential to get out.

Accommodation: And food are both basic but free.

St Mary's Catholic Mission Hospital
Private Bag X16, Ashwood 3605, KwaZulu-Natal. Tel: +27 31 717 1000.
www.stmarys.co.za.

The hospital: Is a small rural hospital about 20 km from Durban. Its 300 beds provide paeds, O&G, medicine and surgery services. The doctors are not specialists but can work on any ward. A great deal of trauma (road traffic accidents and violence) is seen here. Very serious trauma gets referred to Durban.

O **Elective notes:** An elective here offers plenty of opportunity for procedures. It is an isolated town so a car is ideal. There are usually no other students so going with a friend is advised.

Emmaus Hospital
Private Bag X16, Winterton 3340, KwaZulu-Natal. Tel: +27 36 488 1570.
Fax: +27 36 488 1156.

The hospital: Has 150 beds with five wards (male, female, maternity, paeds and TB) and is situated in the

Drakensberg Mountains. The outpatients functions as a GP/emergency department. There are rural clinics and surgery is carried out one morning a week. The patients are all Zulu. It is not wildly busy so not the best if you are wanting stabbings and gunshot wounds.

O **Elective notes:** There is a friendly group of eight doctors from Europe and South Africa. English is the common language. You can choose what you want to do. It is isolated so a car is advisable.

Accommodation: Free in the new nurses' home. Meals cost £1 (R10) a day.

Dundee Municipal Hospital
Dundee, KwaZulu-Natal.

The hospital: Dundee (population 150 000) is a small, mainly middle-class town close to the Drakensberg Mountains. The hospital has private (which still means mainly white) and government wards. The private wards are as good as, if not better than, those in the West. There are 250 beds in the government part. Most medical, surgical and obstetric procedures can be carried out by one of the four doctors working there, but serious cases are transferred to Peitermaritzberg. The doctors also run the town's GP service.

O **Elective notes:** There is a great deal of freedom to do what you want.

Accommodation: Normally available.

Murchison Hospital
Private Bag 701, Port Shepstone 4240, KwaZulu-Natal.

The hospital: This rural mission hospital with 250 beds is in a very poor area of KwaZulu-Natal. It lies 120 km north of Durban and 15 km from Port Shepstone. It has a small emergency department, two paeds, a maternity and two combined medical and surgical wards. There is a small operating theatre. HIV is a major problem. It is estimated that 40% of the hospital population is infected, 27% in the community. TB is also rife. A hospice team visits the terminally ill (mainly AIDS-related) in their homes. There are peripheral clinics.

O **Elective notes:** They are very welcoming to students and you are free to rotate round and do what you want. The staff are friendly, encourage you to do practical procedures and often invite you round for dinner. The surrounding countryside is beautiful and there are great beaches in Port Shepstone. The staff offer lifts but having your own transport is ideal.

Accommodation: And meals are provided free in the nurses' home (make sure you like rice).

Provincial Hospital
Private Bag X5706, Port Shepstone 4240, KwaZulu-Natal.

The hospital: The main hospital for the area south of Durban.

O **Elective notes:** It has no students of its own and does not receive many elective students. Because of this, there is not the 'student fatigue' that you get at teaching hospitals. The staff are friendly and will let you do as much or as little as you wish. There is no library, but there is a fully stocked, reasonably priced bar. It is situated half a kilometre from the coast in an area packed with surfing/fishing beaches, golf courses, tennis courts and rugby fields. This elective will not suit those wanting city life and may not be pleasant for those who object to spending lots of time with white conservative South Africans.

Accommodation: Cheap and basic but wonderful. The rooms have a balcony and overlook the Indian Ocean.

Manguzi Hospital
Private Bag 301, Kwangwanase 3973, KwaZulu-Natal.

The hospital: Manguzi is a rural hospital, miles from the nearest city. The population is entirely black South Africans, and there is plenty of TB, HIV, bilharzia, worms, malaria and marasmus. By South African standards, the trauma load is very small. Travelling outside the town is difficult without a bike or car. There are many game reserves close by and the beach is about 16 km away, but there is no road. Mozambique is 16 km away.

Accommodation: Is in the hospital with the other doctors. They form a tight-knit, family group, but it can get a bit lonely.

Other rural hospitals in KwaZulu-Natal:
Ceza Hospital*, Private Bag X200, Ceza 3866, KwaZulu-Natal. Tel: +27 358 320001/320002. Fax: +27 358 20027.
Church of Scotland Hospital*, Private Bag X502, Tugela Ferry 3504, KwaZulu-Natal. Tel: +27 33 493 0004/0023/0038. Fax: +27 33 493 0073.
Donald Fraser Hospital*, Private Bag X1172, Vhufuli, Northern Province 0971, KwaZulu-Natal. Tel: +27 15 963 1778. Fax: +27 15 963 1796.
Elim Hospital*, PO Box 12, Elim, Northern Province 0960, KwaZulu-Natal. Tel: +27 15 556 3201/3204. Fax: +27 15 556 3160.
Embhuleni Hospital*, Private Bag X1001, Elukwatini, Mpumalanga 1192, KwaZulu-Natal. Tel: +27 17 883 0093. Fax: +27 17 883 0044.
Manguzi Hospital*, Private Bag X301, KwaNgwanase 3973, KwaZulu-Natal. Tel: +27 35 592 0150/0151/0152/0153/0154/0155.
Mosvold Hospital*, Private Bag X2211, Ingwavuma 3968, KwaZulu-Natal. Tel: +27 35 591 0122. Fax: +27 35 591 0148.
St Apollinaris Hospital*, Private Bag 206, Creighton 3263, KwaZulu-Natal. Tel: +27 33 833 1045. Fax: +27 39 833 1062.
Shongwe Hospital*, Private Bag X301, Shongwe Mission, Mpumalanga 1331, KwaZulu-Natal. Tel: +27 13 781 0219. Fax: +27 13 781 0219, ext. 2015.
Themba Hospital*, Private Bag X1002, Kabokweni, Mpumalanga 1245, KwaZulu-Natal. Tel: +27 13 796 0201. Fax: +27 13 796 0339.
Tintswalo Hospital, Private Bag X407, Acornhoek, Mpumalanga 1360, KwaZulu-Natal. Tel: +27 13 797 0000/0076. Fax: +27 13 797 0082.
Tshilidzini Hospital*, Private Bag X924, Shayandima, Northern Province 0945, KwaZulu-Natal, Tel: +27 15 964 1061/1068. Fax: +27 15 964 1492.

*You should really apply through the University of Witwatersrand to do an elective in these hospitals (see page 73).

Eastern Cape

EAST LONDON:

East London is a city on the south coast between Cape Town and Durban. It is close to some lovely beaches (if you have a car) and is small enough to be very friendly. There are some nice pubs and clubs and diving is popular.

There is only one medical university in the Eastern Cape:

University of the Transkei
Faculty of Medicine and Health Sciences, 2 East London Road, Private Bag 11, Umtata 5100, Eastern Cape. Tel: +27 47 130 2 233. Fax: 471 302 235. www.utr.ac.za.

Frere Hospital
Private Bag x9047, East London 5200.
The hospital: Is pretty busy and the patients reflect the conditions outside. Every night there are stabbings and RTAs. Diseases tend to be almost Third World, HIV being a major problem. Translators translate Xhosa to English.
O Elective notes: Try to go with someone or go out with Frere students as it can be a bit dangerous at night.

Cecilia Makiwane Hospital
Mdantsane, Private Bag X13003, Cambridge, East London 5207, Eastern Cape. Tel: +27 403 618 2134. Fax: +27 40 361 1158.
The hospital: A fairly run-down general hospital 25 km from East London in Mdantsane (South Africa's second largest black township). Major specialities are catered for. TB, HIV, malnutrition, diabetes mellitis and poverty problems (including trauma) are commonly seen.
O Elective notes: This is very much 'have a go' medicine in a supportive environment.
Accommodation: Usually available somewhere.

PORT ELIZABETH:

Port Elizabeth is a pretty town on the South Coast of South Africa. It is a pleasant drive through the Garden Route to Cape Town. See www.pe.org.za/info.html for more details.

Dora Nginza Hospital
Private Bag X11951, Algoa Park, Port Elizabeth 6005, Eastern Cape. Tel: +27 41 406 4201. Fax: +27 41 644683.
The hospital: Dora is an impressive new

hospital with the major specialities (medicine, surgery, paeds and O&G). It is in the heart of a township where poverty and crime are major problems. Common conditions include HIV (lots of it), TB, pneumonia and trauma.

O **Elective notes:** The hospital is pretty short on facilities and hence some students have found that although they have seen a fair bit, procedures and drug treatments might not be that appropriate at home.

Accommodation: On-site you can get fairly lonely. King's Beach Backpackers (about R210–270 (£30) a week) is in Port Elizabeth and near the beach.

St Barnabas Hospital

PO Box 15, Libode 5160, Eastern Cape. Tel: +27 47 555 1010.

The hospital: St Barnabas is a small (approximately 200-bed) rural hospital in the heart of the Transkei (a former 'independent' black homeland created during apartheid). There are normally around six doctors and six wards: male, female, maternity, paeds, TB and outpatients/emergency. The doctors rotate through these. TB, HIV and malnutrition are commonplace.

O **Elective notes:** You can go anywhere you want and visit rural clinics. The doctors are friendly but it can get a bit lonely if you are on your own.

Accommodation: There is free accommodation in a singles quarter in the hospital grounds.

Kiriman Hospital

Main Road, Private Bag 910, Kiriman 8460, Eastern Cape.

The hospital: Is a busy, government-funded rural hospital with one medical and one surgical ward. Clinics occur daily from 11 am to 5 pm. TB, AIDS, hypertension and diabetes are very common. The nurses are happy to translate.

O **Elective notes:** Recently the two doctors have been Cuban and keen to teach and encourage practical procedures.

Accommodation: Available at the Moffat Mission.

Orange Free State:

There is only one medical school in Orange Free State:

University of Orange Free State

PO Box 339, Bloemfontein 9300, Orange Free State. Tel: +27 51 401 2847. Fax: +27 51 444 3101. www.oovs.ac.za.

SOMETHING DIFFERENT:

Ernest Ppenheimer Hospital Welkom

Part of the Anglo-American Corporation of South Africa Ltd, PO Box 61587, Marshaltown 2107, Eastern Cape.

The hospital: Deals with the acute medical and surgical problems of the 100 000 employees of this big gold and diamond conglomerate. It is in Welkom, a purpose-built gold mining town. There are many admissions due to industrial accidents. The life here is very Afrikaans, but the miners speak Sootoo.

Phelophepa Mobile Health Care Train

Transnet Park, 8 Hillside Road, Parktown 2193, PO Box 72501, Eastern Cape. www.mhc.org.za.

The train: This is a train that travels around the country at weekends and then sets up a clinic for the following week. It has 12 carriages, each with a different role. There is a health clinic, eye care clinic, dentist, pharmacy and X-ray carriages as well as living quarters. It is run by nursing, dentistry and ophthalmology students under the supervision of their tutors. There is a minimal fee for treatment but it is very busy and serves a very worthwhile purpose in the communities it visits.

O **Elective notes:** Write to the senior manager at the above address. They may only be able to take you for a week while they are stationary. Note: The train only runs between January and September.

Swaziland

Population: 900 000
Languages: Siswati and English
Capital: Mbabane
Currency: Lilangeni
Int Code: +268

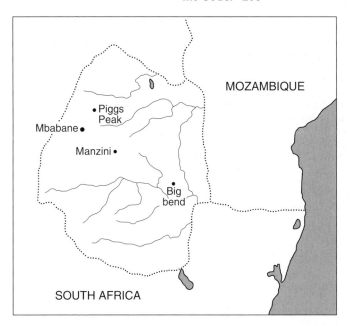

Swaziland is a very small country populated by friendly people with strong cultural and traditional beliefs (including witch doctors). It has a powerful monarchy led by King Mswati III. The dry season is from May to October (20–25°C) getting cooler at night but there are no mosquitoes. In the summer the place buzzes with them. To get around, you will need to hire a car or use the 'kombi' vans. It is easy to get to Mozambique and South Africa.

✛ Medicine:

There is no health service and there are no medical schools. Healthcare therefore relies on a few mission- and a few government-run hospitals (*see* Section 4 for organizations that run these). Infectious diseases, AIDS/HIV, TB, STDs, malnutrition and diarrhoea are all very common. The prevalence of HIV in adults averaged 25% at the turn of the millenium – so be careful...

USEFUL ADDRESSES:

Ministry of Health, PO Box 5, Mbabane. Tel: +268 42431. Fax: +268 42092.
Swaziland Dental Association, PO Box 1291, Matsapha.

Mbabane

Mbabane is the capital and the main hospital is:

Mbabane Government Hospital
PO Box 8, Mbabane. Tel: +268 42111.

Manzini

Manzini is the industrial hub of Swaziland … not exactly pretty. There is a small cinema and a few restaurants, although it's best not to go out late at night if you don't want to get stabbed, robbed, etc. Hire a car and get out into the bush.

Raleigh Fitkin Memorial Hospital
PO Box 14, Manzini. Tel: +268 52211.
The hospital: The hospital is very busy, with 60 paediatric beds and 70 for general medicine. The obstetrics ward has around 20 deliveries a day. The outpatient clinic runs throughout the day. The hospital has strong Nazarene church connections so no smoking, drinking or 'cohabitation'. Females in trousers and wild jewellery are also completely unacceptable. Apart from these rules, it is very friendly.

O Elective notes: You will be consulting alone, but the other doctors are close at hand. You will also need a Swazi person to translate. Students are expected to be first on call on a 1:3 rota. You are given a great deal of responsibility and practical experience. This is great if you swim rather than sink.

OTHER HOSPITALS:

Piggs Peak Clinic, PO Box 260, Piggs Peak. Tel: +268 71176.
Ubombo Ranches Hospital, PO Box 131, Ubombo Ranches, Lot 311, Big Bend. Tel: +268 36332.

Tanzania

Population: 29.7 million
Languages: English and Swahili
Capital: Dodoma
Currency: Tanzanian shilling
Int Code: +255

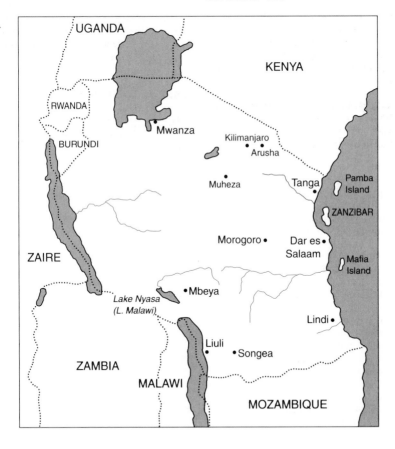

On the East African coast, Tanzania comprises the mainland and a number of small islands such as Zanzibar and Tanganyika. There is a great variety of scenery, from the coastal lowlands to the volcanic highlands and the Great Rift Valley.

The highlands are home to Mount Kilimanjaro, Africa's highest peak. Tanzania is famed for its wildlife. Herds of wildebeest, zebras, lions, cheetah and hyenas are in abundance. The beaches are beautiful and the cities friendly. If you want an exotic island *break, visit Pemba or Mafia. These are not yet overrun by tourists. Tanzania has a long history. One of the oldest human remains (1.75 million years old) was recently found here. The various African tribes (mainly Masai from Kenya) intermarried with trading Arabs 2000 years ago, forming a new people with their own language, Swahili. Tanzania later became a German territory but was surrendered to the British after World War I. Tanzania then became independent in the 1960s. After you have climbed Mount Kilimanjaro, head to the north for Ngorongoro Crater (the largest unbroken caldera in the world), Olduvai Gorge, Serengeti, Arusha, Tarangire and Lake Manyara National Parks. Then go south to Selous Game Reserve, Mikumi, Ruaha and Udzungwa Mountains National Parks. Other places to visit are Katavi, Gombe, Rubondo Island and Mahale Mountains National Parks, Lake Victoria and Tanganyika. Don't forget Zanzibar!*

◎ Medicine:

Basic medical care is state funded, although there are also a number of Christian missions. There are four major referal hospitals (the **Muhimbili National Hospital**, which caters for the eastern zone; **Kilimanjaro Christian Medical Centre**, which caters for the northern zone; **Bugando Hospital**, which caters for the western zone; and **Mbeya Hospital**, which serves the southern highlands), then 17 regional and 55 district government-run hospitals. In addition, there are around 56 mission hospitals. Despite relatively good medical care, diarrhoea, respiratory diseases and malaria are still big killers. HIV is increasing and has a prevalance of around 20% in rural regions (the national average being 8%). Most hospital work (e.g. ward rounds and notes) is done in English; however, the majority of patients only speak Swahili. A detailed background to the healthcare structure in Tanzania can be found at www.tanzania.go.tz/health.

◎ Climate and crime:

The coastal areas are hot and humid, with an average daytime temperature of 30°C. The central plateau has hot days and cool nights. The hills below the northern highlands are pleasant between January and September, with temperatures of around 20°C. The area around Mount Kilimanjaro is warmest between December and March (22°C). For the whole country, October to February is the hottest and March to May the wettest. The crime level is low, although theft is rising in Dar es Salaam.

⊃ Visas and work permits:

A visa is needed. For up-to-date information visit www.tanzania-online.gov.uk. Alternatively, contact the embassy.

USEFUL ADDRESS:

Ministry of Health, PO Box 9083, Dar es Salaam. Tel: +255 51 20261. Fax: +255 51 39951.

MEDICAL SCHOOLS:

Muhimbili University College of Health Sciences

Office of the Principal, PO Box 65001, Dar es Salaam. Tel: +255 22 215 3026. Fax: +255 22 215 1586. www.muchs.ac.tz (university website: www.udsm.ac.tz).
They can organize electives, for example in **Mbeya Consultant Hospital**. Only around 50 Tanzanian students enrol a year, and there is a high drop-out rate. This makes Tanzania very short of doctors. It uses:

Muhimbili Medical Centre

PO Box 65000, Dar es Salaam. Tel: +255 51 150939/1500816.

Kilimanjaro Christian Medical College

Moshi Towa, Kilimanjaro. Tel: +255 55 543 77. Fax: +255 55 543 81. www.kcmc.ac.tz. The college is situated in the foothills of the snow-capped Mount Kilimanjaro and was opened as a government referal hospital in 1971. It is huge, with over 450 beds. It is a Christian hospital and since 1997 has had its own medical and nursing school. It uses:

Kilimanjaro Christian Medical Centre

PO Box 3010, Moshi. Tel: +255 57 54263/52291. Fax: +255 55 54381. www.kcmc.ac.tz.

Two new medical schools are:

Faculty of Medicine, Hubert Kairuki Memorial University, 322 Regent Estate, PO Box 65300, Dar es Salaam. Tel: +255 22 270 0021. Fax: +255 22 277 5591.
Faculty of Medicine, Vignan's International Medical and Technological University, PO Box 77594, Saruji Complex, New Bagamayo Road, Dar es Salaam. Tel: +255 51 647 257. Fax: +255 51 647 038. www.imtu.edu.

GOVERNMENT HOSPITALS:

Bugando Hospital

PO Box 1370, Mwanza. Tel: +255 68 40610. www.bugando.org.
The hospital: The University College of Health Sciences at Bugando Medical Center is established as a Catholic college, having four schools: medicine, nursing, pharmacotherapy and dentistry. The hospital has 800 beds, providing for a population of 8 million in north-west Tanzania.

Mbeya Referral Hospital

PO Box 419, Mbeya. Tel: +255 65 3576.
The hospital: Is a large (by Tanzanian standards) referral hospital in south-west Tanzania. It is a teaching centre for clinical assistants (who do a similar job to junior doctors). Common pathologies are malaria, pneumonia, meningitis, malnutrition and sickle cell disease. HIV is also very common.
O Elective notes: They do not often get students so it is up to you what and how much you do. If you stay around, you can end up running wards. There is good support. Lake Nyasa (Malawi) is only a couple of hours away by car. Mbeya itself is a busy town at the bottom of Mbeya Mountain. It has a small ex-pat community of coffee-buyers, NGO workers and missionaries.

Mnazi Mmoja Hospital

PO Box 338, Zanzibar. Tel: +255 54 31071.
The hospital: Zanzibar is a beautiful place … sun, sea, sand, palm trees. The hospital, however, is a bit disorganized. It is government run and underfunded so most of the doctors spend their time in private practice. Despite this, the staff are very friendly and helpful and there are interesting clinics to attend.
O Elective notes: A surgical elective is especially recommended here (the main surgeon is very efficient and helpful). There's also acupuncture and the chance to go on outreach clinics.

OTHER GOVERNMENT-RUN HOSPITALS USED FOR ELECTIVES:

Hindu Mandal Hospital

PO Box 581, Dar es Salaam.
Tel: +255 51 110237/110428.

Agha Khan Hospital

PO Box 2289, Dar es Salaam.
Tel: +255 51 114096.

Nachingwea District General Hospital

Nachingwea, Lindi.
The hospital: With 179 beds, this hospital was built in 1952 principally as a TB centre. It is government run (with two doctors), and resources are scarce. Malaria, anaemia, pneumonia, meningitis and diarrhoea are the common causes of death. Mortality is high for infants (124 per 1000) and the under-fives (209 per 1000). There is a busy outpatients/ emergency department, a theatre, an X-ray machine and very basic laboratory facilities. There is an AIDS department.
O Elective notes: The hospital has long-standing links with St Andrews Church, Stapleford, Cambridge, and hence a lot of Cambridge students. There is plenty to see and do.
Accommodation: And food are provided in the teacher training college.

Teule District Designated Hospital
Muheza, Tanga Region.

The hospital: This was recently designated a district hospital. It is currently run by an amazing British doctor. Its 260 beds are usually at 150% capacitance, catering for its catchment population of 250 000. Muheza itself has a population of 30 000 and lies 35 km from Tanga and 350 km from Dar es Salaam. The local language is Kiswahili.

The hospital is partly government funded but still receives overseas aid. It was originally an Anglican Mission hospital (in a Muslim area) and still receives help from the church. The hospital has nine wards: two medical, two surgical, two paediatric, one maternity, one isolation and one diarrhoea. There is a theatre, ITU, X-ray and delivery suite. There is also a mobile clinic. There are a couple of doctors, a surgeon and a number of assistants. There is a nursing and midwifery school of 120 students. Malaria is the biggest problem, along with TB, typhoid, dysentery and meningitis. The prevalence of HIV is around 17%. Patients pay 2000 shillings (about £2) for a week in hospital – a week's income. This covers food and medicine but X-rays, etc. are extra.

O Elective notes: You are very much needed here. From day one you may well find yourself doing ward rounds alone. There are opportunities to go to rural dispensaries. It can get lonely … try to go in pairs. There are daily prayer meetings. Try to learn a little Swahili. It comes highly recommended.

Accommodation: This is basic but costs only £2 (2500 TZS) a month.

MISSION HOSPITALS:

Berega Mission Hospital
Berega, Morogoro.

The hospital: This is a 120-bed mission hospital established in the 1890s. It is often described by Paul White in the 'Jungle Doctor' series. Most of the locals are subsistence farmers. Berega has a population of only a few hundred, but the hospital covers a vast population of 200 000 (some of whom have to walk for two days to get there). There are male and female, paeds and O&G wards, and recently community health services. Most diseases are infectious: malaria, pneumonia, gastroenteritis, skin infections and worm infestations. Common paediatric conditions include measles, malnutrition, burns and fractures. The community health team is trying to immunize the population. There are a lot of complicated deliveries (the normal ones do not come in).

Conditions in the hospital (run by a Tanzanian, a couple of Australians and a British doctor at the time of writing) are very poor. Patients often have to share beds, families live under them and provide nursing care and food (there are only 15 nurses in the hospital). There is a bucket of water in the corner for washing. The flying surgeon occasionally visits. The electricity generator is switched on if the theatre is needed. Some laboratory facilities (including HIV testing) are available. The HIV rate in those donating for blood transfusion is 13%. The nearest phone box is 80 km away, and post relies on a weekly visit to Morogoro (135 km south).

O Elective notes: An excellent if somewhat isolated elective.

St Anne's Hospital
PO Box 2, Liuli (via Songea).

The hospital: Liuli is a small village on the Tanzanian side of the banks of Lake Malawi with the Livingstone Mountains behind it. It is very remote: when the road is washed away in the wet season, the only way to it is by boat. The hospital, connected with the charity USPG, is an Anglican mission hospital established in 1906, rebuilt in the 1970s but still very shabby. There are 100 beds (20 female, 20 male, 20 paeds, 23 maternity and 17 isolation) but many more patients. It serves a population of 100 000 with very limited resources. Common rare diseases include malaria (especially with the lake), TB, HIV, typhoid and meningitis. Schistosomiasis occurs but not that commonly as there are no reeds in this area of Lake Malawi.

○ **Elective notes:** Your help is very much appreciated, for example in taking clinics. There are plenty of procedures in theatre.

Accommodation: Available in a guest-house. A cook costs 25 500 TZS (£20) a month.

St Francis Hospital
Kwo Mkono, Handeni District.
The hospital: Another Anglican 70-bed general mission hospital offering a range of health programmes. The maternity and child health clinic undertakes child monitoring and immunization. Rural clinics are also perfomed.

SOMETHING DIFFERENT:

Tanzania's Flying Doctor service is based in Arusha (Tel: +255 2548578); *see* the new and exciting 'Adventure Medicine' section for more details.

Uganda

Population: 22 million
Language: English
Capital: Kampala
Currency: New Uganda shilling
Int Code: +256

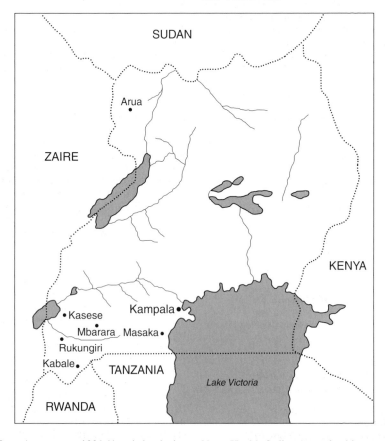

Since democracy in 1986, Uganda has had good economic growth. However, some areas are still very poor and, especially in the north, rebel attacks and ambushes still occur. Uganda is a former British colony and 80% Christian. The official language is English, but it's really only used in cities.

Note: Health Online (www.health.go.ug) is a fantastic site with full lists of hospitals and other health facilities and information on AIDS, child health programmes, public health programmes and disease surveillance in Uganda.

✪ Medicine:

Fifty per cent of healthcare in Uganda is provided by NGOs. Uganda has 104 hospitals, 57 of which are run by the government, 44 by NGOs and three by private organizations. In addition, there are 250 health centres. The mission hospitals rely on charity, small donations from the government and small contributions from patients. Government hospitals provide free care. By the end of 2000, 55 000 cases of AIDS had been reported, with an estimated 1.5 million HIV positive. It is thought that 30% of the urban and 15% of the rural population are positive. Be VERY careful if doing procedures. Other infectious diseases, especially malaria, measles and gastroenteritis, are also very common. The national health research organization in Uganda oversees research units specializing in viruses, cancer, TB, public health, trypanosomiasis and cardiology (*see* www.health.go.ug).

USEFUL ADDRESSES:

Ministry of Health, PO Box 8, Entebbe.
Tel: +256 42 20201.
Uganda Medical Council, PO Box 16115,
Wandegeya, Kampala.
Uganda Medical Association, Plot 8, Katonga Road, PO Box 2243, Kampala.
Tel. +256 41 236 539. Fax. +256 41 532 591.

MEDICAL SCHOOLS:

Uganda has three medical schools:

Kigezi International School of Medicine

Kabale Hospital, PO Box 7, Kabale.
Tel: +256 24 822 006. www.kigezi.edu.

Makerere University Medical School

Faculty of Medicine, PO Box 7072,
Kampala. Tel: +256 41 530 020.
Fax: +256 41 531 091. www.makerere.ac.ug.

Mbarara University of Science and Technology

Faculty of Medicine, PO Box 1410, Mbarara.
Tel: +256 48 520 782 Fax: +256 48 521 373.

NATIONAL REFERRAL HOSPITALS (BOTH GOVERNMENT RUN):

Mulago Hospital

PO Box 7051, Kampala. Tel: +256 41 541 250/533 560. Fax: +256 41 532 591.
This has 1500 beds.

Butabika Hospital

PO Box 7017, Kampala
With 850 beds.

There are also regional referral hospitals with specialist fields (Arua, Gulu, Hoima, Jinja, Kabarole, Masaka, Mbale, Mbarara and Soroti). These also act as teaching hospitals.

MISSION HOSPITALS:

Some of the hospitals run by NGOs also have specialists (Nsambya, Rubaga, Mengo (Kampla district), Lacor and Matany (Moroto district)). Addresses for all these hospitals can be found on www.medicstravel.org under Uganda, or on Uganda Health Online (www.health.go.ug). Some mission hospitals that come highly recommended for electives include the following:

Kisiizi Hospital

PO Box 109, Kabale. Tel: 00 871 761 587 164. Fax: 00 871 761 587 166
(both satellite phone and very expensive).
www.kisiizi.supanet.com.
The hospital: Is a medium-sized (200-bed plus floor space) rural mission hospital (founded in 1958) over an hour from the main road through south-west Uganda. It is usually run by around four British and Ugandan doctors and has maternity (900 deliveries a year), surgical, medical, paediatric, SCBU and isolation wards and two operating theatres. The emergency/outpatient department commonly sees malaria (occasional epidemics), HIV medicine, pneumonia, rheumatic fever, malnutrition, diabetes, meningitis, STDs, trauma and alcohol-related disease. The hospital has basic

laboratory facilities, X-ray and ultra-sound. There are community visits to local villages and a newly developed AIDS programme (including an AIDS orphans programme). Patients have to pay for care here, but a scheme of community health insurance is being set up. A nursing school has just opened.

O **Elective notes:** While here, be pre-pared to work fairly hard and have a fair bit of responsibility, although it is quite flexible when you want to go. You will have clinics and ward rounds to do. The staff (mainly Western doctors, currently a British surgeon and a GP) are keen to teach and support during practical proce-dures. There are medical students (elec-tive and Ugandan) most of the year. Kisiizi is very Christian (chapel is at 8 am every morning) but no one holds anything against non-Christians as long as they are sympathetic to their beliefs. There are beautiful walks in the nearby hills and a hospital football team. Alcohol is frowned upon.

Kabale, the nearest town, is over two hours (48 km (30 miles)) away. There's plenty to do nearby: Lake Bunyonyi, Kisoro (Mgahinga National Park with gorillas), Queen Elizabeth National Park. It has been described as a great experience and very friendly. It is a very popular elective destination. Take Angel Delight (NOT banana flavour!) and the Sunday newspapers to make friends.

Accommodation: Provided for students in a guesthouse for £10 (24 000 UGX) a week.

Note: This elective can be arranged through the **Mid-Africa Ministry** (157 Waterloo Road, London SE1 8UU, UK. Tel: +44 207 261 1370. Fax: +44 207 401 2910). They will send a lot more information about the place.

Kagando Hospital

Private Bag, Kasese. Tel: +256 41 267 462 (the Mission Aviation Fellowship in Kampala … they can radio a message to Kagando, as there is no phone there). Fax: +256 41 241 413 (the Uganda Protestant Medical Bureau, which can also radio the hospital).
www.aim-uganda.org/ministries/kagando.htm.

The hospital: A missionary hospital of 220 beds with some government fund-ing. It is very much part of the commu-nity of Kagando and situated near Kasese and the Rwenzan Mountains ('mountains of the moon') in western Uganda. It serves a population of 380 000 and is run by three or four physicians, two surgeons and two anaes-thetists. There are also Ugandan house officers. There is a wide variety of pathologies. Cholera, TB and malaria are common. There are also major prob-lems with a rebel versus government war, with families being displaced and children even being burned. This puts great restrictions on travel outside the hospital. It has also caused more malnu-trition and surgically there are many casualties from gunshots, burns and mines. Dental and ophthalmic services are also provided.

O **Elective notes:** It is a Christian hos-pital and accordingly there is a prayer service at 8 am. You can see patients on your own in outpatients but there is always support. There is much to see and the area is very beautiful with mountains and woodland. Overall, this elective is recommended, but enquire about safety regarding rebel activity before you go.

Accommodation: This is very good (approximately 10 000 UGX (£4) a day, including a cleaner and cook … this money helps to fund Ugandan medical students).

Nyakibale Hospital

PO Box 31, Rukungiri.

The hospital: An ex-mission hospital with about 300 beds and a large materni-ty wing. It is in south-west Uganda close to the Zaire border and about 400 km from Kampala. It is a 20 minute walk to the small town of Rukungiri. About four Ugandan doctors (±Westerners), who are very welcoming, usually run it. The hospital provides medical, surgical, orthopaedic, paeds and O&G services. There is a large outpatients and primary healthcare programme. Common dis-eases include malaria, HIV, typhoid and meningitis. Despite an HIV prevalence of approximately 15%, malaria still causes twice as many deaths.

O **Elective notes:** The surrounding countryside is beautiful.

Kuluva Church of Uganda Hospital
PO Box 28, Arua.
www.aim-uganda.org/ministries/kuluva.htm.
The hospital: A rural hospital. Malaria, malnutrition, with gastroenteritis, TB, HIV, pneumonia and meningitis are on the menu.

O **Elective notes:** Students normally do a 1:3 rota and have a great deal more responsibility than in Western hospitals. It can be organized through AIM in London (*see* website given above).

Masaka Hospital
PO Box 18, Masaka. Fax (in local post office) +256 48 120 514.
The hospital: Has the basic specialities (medicine, surgery, paeds, O&G). It is basic healthcare in a friendly hospital.

O **Elective notes:** It is up to you how much you do. A car is ideal so you can get out to national parks.

Zambia

Population: 9.8 million
Languages: English, Bemba and Nyanja
Capital: Lusaka
Currency: Zambian kwacha
Int Code: +260

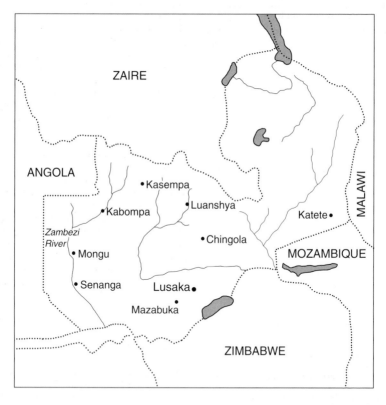

Zambia is a large, landlocked country. It gained independence from the UK in 1964 and has since been one of Africa's poorest nations. The situation's not improving. The country previously had a large copper industry, but since prices dropped this has been drastically cut back. The largest bank note is 500 kwacha (worth about 30p).

People live in small villages in mud huts and the economy is now based on subsistence farming. With all that said, it is a beautiful country with very friendly people. There is a police system but corruption is rife. There are half a dozen languages with many dialects but the official language is English and staff in hospitals usually translate.

✪ Medicine:

Healthcare is based on a government-run scheme like the British NHS. This was fine when the copper industry was booming, but since it collapsed, healthcare has fallen apart. The government is currently trying to give more money to local areas so that they can decide their own priorities. In the Western Province the Dutch have stepped in to try to provide primary healthcare.

Rarities that are common here include malaria, TB, schistosomiasis (be careful if you go swimming), syphilis, Burkitt's lymphoma, sickle cell anaemia, osteomyelitis, meningitis and trauma. HIV is rife with an estimated prevalence of between 30% and 60% depending on location (the average being 20%). Like much of Africa, culture states that the more partners a man has, the higher his position in society. This, combined with the fact that traditional healers commonly treat with escarification, increases transmission.

Zambia has 11 300 people per doctor, and the University of Zambia trains only around 100 per year. They are, however, training clinical officers. They have three to four years' basic medical training and do the jobs of junior doctors. A number of mission hospitals are listed below. For more information, contact the Christian Missionary Association of Zambia (PO Box 8085, Woodlands, Lusaka).

USEFUL ADDRESSES:

Medical Council of Zambia, Dental Training School Premises, PO Box 32554, Thornpak, 10101, Lusaka.
Zambia Medical Association, PO Box 50903, Lusaka.
Zambia Dental Association, PO Box 50363, Lusaka 15101. Tel: +260 1 221 257. Fax: +260 1 263 401.

MEDICAL SCHOOL:

School of Medicine at Zambia University
PO Box 50110, Lusaka. Tel: +260 1 252 641. Fax: +260 1 250 753. www.unza.zm.

They can recommend places and help with electives. The main teaching hospital is:

University Teaching Hospital
PO Box 50110, Lusaka.
The hospital: This is the main hospital in Zambia and has all major specialities. The staff (and patients) are incredibly friendly; morale is, however, low as resources have been limited for so long. There is a great deal of HIV, malnutrition, tropical and infectious diseases (malaria and TB).
✪ Elective notes: English is widely spoken, although it is handy to know a little Nyanja. Some teachers have been excellent, and there is a great deal of pathology. You are made to feel useful.
Accommodation: That provided by the university (HS$1 a day) is pretty appalling. You may be able to arrange something when you get there.

St Francis' Mission Hospital
Private Bag 11, Katete.
E-mail: stfrhosp@zamnet.zm.
The hospital: Is situated 500 km northeast of Lusaka, although it is actually another 5 km from the town of Katete (population 10 000). It is a district general hospital serving 165 000 people from a wide area. It has 365 beds forming male, female, surgical, paeds, maternity and TB wards as well as an outpatients, SCBU and isolation units. It is a very busy hospital run by six doctors who specialize in everything from ophthalmology to surgery. There are three operating theatres, ultrasound and X-ray facilities and an AIDS department. By Zambian standards the hospital has good facilities but they are very low on many drugs and do not stock expensive ones. Rural outreach clinics are often held.

It has a very good reputation (John Cairns, author of *Primary Surgery*, worked here for years) and people come from the university to study for the FRCS.
✪ Elective notes: There is a great deal of pathology to see and you get a good

deal of opportunity to run clinics with help whenever needed. Nurses take blood so the only exposure-prone procedures are in theatre (goggles being provided). Although this is a Christian (Catholic and Anglican) mission, there is no pressure to get involved. There is a football team to try to join.

Note: They are very keen that you spend your entire elective (at least 45 days) with them. You work every weekday and Saturday mornings. Lake Malawi is three hours away, and there is also a game park. It is advisable to go with someone so as not to get lonely.

Accommodation: Provided for around £5 (23 316 ZMK) per night, including full board and laundry. Katete has a Barclays Bank.

Mpanshya Mission Hospital
PO Box 32789, Lusaka.

The hospital: A 100-bed general hospital 200 km from Lusaka that serves 600 000 people over a very wide area. Three Polish nuns (of the order of St Charles Borromeo) run it. There is some funding from the Zambian government (£380 a month), the rest coming from charity. Facilities are very basic. There is no mains electricity, no telephone and only a limited range of drugs. It has a male, two female, a paediatric and maternity ward, an isolation unit and outpatient department. There is one doctor and his clinical officer. Big problems are malaria, TB, HIV, pneumonia, malnutrition and gunshot wounds. Satellite clinics are also run. The local culture has a very high pain threshold. Women give birth in silence.

O Elective notes: Medical students are very welcome as it gives the doctor (and his clinical officer) a bit of a break as you can see patients at night. If the doctor is ill, you have to see the patients. It can be hard work but the staff are very friendly and appreciative, and make sure you are OK. This elective is popular with students from Poland, New Zealand and Ireland.

Accommodation: Provided in a guesthouse.

Chikankata Hospital
Private Bag S-2, Mazabuka.

The hospital: A Salvation Army mission hospital with 250 beds, Chikankata lies 130 km south of Lusaka (the local language being Tonga). The nearest town, Mazabuka, is 60 km away. Five doctors, mostly Western volunteers, work at the hospital. Basic investigations and X-ray are available. There are general medical and surgical wards, male and female, TB, paeds, labour, gynaecology, and mother and baby wards. There are also an ITU and a ward for terminally ill patients with HIV. It has two operating theatres. Facilities are not bad but drugs are in short supply. HIV, leprosy, malnutrition and malaria are the order of the day. There are also outreach clinics to attend. Consultations cost about 6p.

O Elective notes: Lots to see and do, and well recommended.

Accommodation: Accommodation is available (previously at around £100 (470 000 ZMK)).

Murkinje Mission Hospital
Mailing address: PO Box 31981, Lusaka.
Local address: PO Box 120092, Kasempa.
E-mail: mukhosp@zamnet.zm.
www.webmissions.org/mukinge.

The hospital: A busy, 180-bed mission hospital with separate ward buildings (connected by a covered sidewalk) for general medical/surgical (male and female), maternity (1000 deliveries a year), paeds, isolation, TB and rehabilitation. Operating room facilities include two theatres with a reasonable range of instruments (including an operating microscope) for general, orthopaedic and eye surgery. The laboratory is run by a medical technician with two assistants and is capable of doing haematology, culture and sensitivities, serology for HIV, electrolytes and the usual run of low-tech lab tests. There is a dedicated HIV team and around 350 outpatients are seen each day. There is also a nursing school. It works with Mission Flight Zambia which provides air transport for medical staff, patients and supplies.

Senanga District Hospital

Senanga, Western Province.
Tel: +260 7 230 022.

The hospital: The largest and busiest district hospital in Senanga (one of the largest districts in the western province). It is on the Zambezi River about an hour south of Mongu and ten hours west of Lusaka. South, a dirt road leads to Namibia, Botswana and Victoria Falls. Within the district, 23 rural health centres provide basic care, Senanga being the referral centre. Senanga itself (population 10000) has a few shops, a post office and the hospital. The hospital is well run and very busy. The basic specialities are catered for.

O Elective notes: Students get to take responsibility for one or two wards and help with on call. There are opportunities in outpatients and theatre as well as any projects they are interested in. It's a lot of work, but the Dutch doctors are very friendly and there are plenty of trips to sites such as game parks, Victoria Falls and Botswana. The town has running water, electricity, a phone line, bus service and e-mail. Do not send heavy things to them as they have to pay postage at the other end. Fax and e-mail are the best ways to get in touch.

Accommodation: Provided.

A couple of other hospitals are:

Kabompo Rural District General Hospital, PO Box 140046, Kabompo.
Mpongwe Mission Hospital, PO Box 90096, Zambia.

SOMETHING DIFFERENT:

Zambia Consolidated Copper Mines Ltd

Nchanga Division, South Hospital, PO Box 10063, Chingola.

The hospital: ZCCM Ltd is a mining company that funds the North and South hospitals in Chingola. It is free for employees although there is a private facility as well. Medicine, surgery, paeds and O&G are all available.

O Elective notes: This elective is popular with Belfast students as one of the consultants is from Belfast.

Accommodation: Available in the nurses' home.

Zimbabwe

Population: 11.3 million
Language: English
Capital: Harare
Currency: Zimbabwe dollar
Int Code: +263

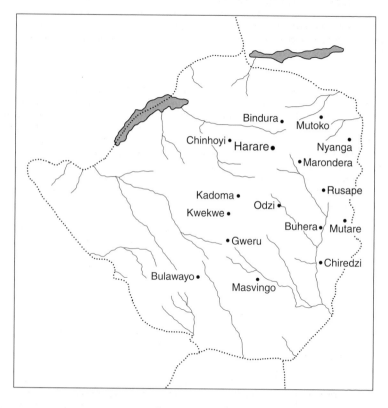

Zimbabwe borders Botswana, Mozambique, South Africa and Zambia and is famed for possessing the Zambezi River which goes on to form the Victoria Falls. Zimbabwe is currently going through a period of great unrest, with popular uprisings against the leader, Robert Mugabe. This is causing a geat deal of violence and disruption. You MUST consult the Foreign Office or equivalent before planning to work here. Since Zimbabwe's independence from the UK in 1980, clashes between the two ethnic groups – the Ndebele (known as the Matabele, making up 15% of the population) in the south and the Shona (known as the Mashona, comprising 80%) in the north – have been a problem. It reached a peak in the mid-1980s and riots and clashes have

become a serious problem in the new millenium. Tourism is growing as there are a number of attractions: safaris in the many national parks, the Victoria Falls, the Kariba Dam, the Great Zimbabwe ruins near Masvingo and World's View in the Matopo Hills. In recent years, action/adventure trips, such as white water rafting, bungee jumping and climbing, have become more popular. Public transport is pretty poor and buses always break down. Food is, however, cheap. There's widespread use of English, but Shona and Ndebele are used among locals. A note for girls going to rural areas: do not wear trousers (wear below-knee skirts instead) – it is not the local custom as 'prostitutes wear trousers'. In the cities it's OK.

✆ Medicine:

Health services are free for those who earn less than Z$400 (about £26) a month, but the quality is poor owing to the lack of staff and resources. Most districts in Zimbabwe have government-run hospitals and a mission hospital. Since independence from the UK, there has been a high priority on developing primary healthcare, especially in rural areas although the government has a pretty poor track record, especially on its slow reaction to AIDS. There is a severe shortage of doctors and the newly qualified ones often leave the country.

Despite HIV, the population is still growing at 3.5% per annum. In adults aged less than 45, the seroprevalance of HIV is thought to be around 60%, with 80–90% of the hospital population being infected. (Government statistics say that the general prevalence is 30%, but it is thought by doctors to be much higher.) The rate of antenatal HIV in Gwanda district has risen from 17% to 33% over the past five years. There is a real taboo about AIDS, and the health services are nowhere near tackling the problem. There is so much denial that it even has another name – 'New Serology (NS) positive'. It is particularly bad in rural areas as husbands go to the cities to get work, use prostitutes and then return to their wives. Zimbabweans come to hospital late after visiting a traditional

healer (the *Nyanga*). They encourage sex with a virgin as a cure for AIDS and also perform escarification, which probably transmits it. Malaria and TB are also very common.

◎ Climate and crime:

Owing to the high altitude, Zimbabwe is actually cooler than you might expect for a tropical country. It is wettest between November and March, but drought is also common. October to April are the warmest months. Crime is mainly a problem of urban areas. The murder rate is 17 per 100 000, and drug-related crime is increasingly problematic. It is a very safe area to visit for tourists.

➲ Visas and work permits:

British passport holders do not require a visa to visit Zimbabwe (for less than three months), but they do require permits to do official study or work. Applications for student permits should be forwarded to the Chief Immigration Officer, Department of Immigration (P Bag 7717, Causeway, Harare, Zimbabwe). They will require:
● A statutory fee of US$80 or the equivalent in any foreign currency
● A letter from the institution of affiliation
● A certified photocopy of your birth certificate
● Documentary proof of accommodation
● Two passport-sized photos
● Radiological certificate if the duration of stay is in excess of six months.

The university and the immigration department state that you need a student permit to do an elective. Most medical students not going through the university get away with saying that they are visitors. Even many of those going via the university still do not bother. If doing this make sure that you state that the purpose of your visit is tourism. If you are going to work in Zimbabwe, your prospective employer will apply for a work permit on your behalf.

Note: Some students have been told that you need to register with the university wherever you are doing your elective, the fee being US$200. If going to a rural hospital the money stays at the university and the hospital sees none. Instead, make a donation when you are actually there. You may have to pay it if you are going to a hospital in Harare or the Mipilo in Bulawayo.

USEFUL ADDRESSES:

Health Professions Council, PO Box A 480, Avondale, Harare.
Zimbabwe Medical Association, PO Box 3671, Harare. Tel: +263 4 735401. Fax: +263 4 720731.

Harare

Harare is the capital and a convenient base to tour the Eastern Highlands.

MEDICAL SCHOOL:

University of Zimbabwe Clinical School

Parirenyatwa Hospital, PO Box A 178, Avondale, Harare. Tel: +263 4 791631. Fax: +263 4 724912.

Write to the electives secretary, electives office at this address. Some students have had no problems but others have not been impressed by their organization. They can arrange electives in Harare and country hospitals but charge US$200 for the privilege. There have also been reports of students who have arranged electives with peripheral hospitals only to arrive there (with letters of confirmation) and be told that they weren't expected. This has even led to students having to go home. If you do organize your elective through them, get letters of confirmation and ring your destination to ensure they are expecting you. To add insult to all this, some people have been asked to get a chest X-ray to make sure that they do not have TB (chances are you will have by the time you get back!).

GOVERNMENT HOSPITALS:

Parirenyatwa Hospital
Box CY 198, Causeway, Harare.

The hospital: Is a government-run teaching hospital. It was initially the 'white' hospital, whereas the Central was the 'black', but there is no division now. It is big with lots of up-to-date equipment, including a CT scanner (although a lack of funds may mean things don't work). Most specialities (medicine, surgery, emergency medicine, neurology/surgery and plastic surgery to name but a few) are catered for. Practical experience is limited. Some medicine is very similar to typical Western medicine. Malaria and HIV (up to 50% prevalence) are common. Ward rounds are in English.

O **Elective notes:** Apply through the university (*see* address above). By applying through them you join their own student groups. This can mean that you do not get to see or do much. Students are expected to attend ward rounds, outpatients and tutorials. Plastic surgery is recommended as there are no other students. There's no shortage of gloves (remember to double-glove for everything). You may be able to get out to Rusape and do some minor surgery. Socially, if you find a few friendly local students, it's pretty good.

Accommodation: Available in the medical residency opposite the main entrance to the hospital, but space is limited so apply early. The cost is Z$31 (£1.20) a night. There are many local and elective students so the place is quite lively. A backpackers' place around the corner (Possum Lodge) costs Z$50 (less than £2) a night. Harare has many good places for eating and drinking, but get out to the rest of the country.

Central Harare Hospital
Lobengula Road, ST 14 Southerton, Harare. Tel: +263 4 664695/664690.

The hospital: Originally the 'black' hospital, it now has no division. It is in the more industrial part of town. It does have fewer facilities than the Parirenyatwa but has nearly all the same specialities (including an emergency department). It is the other teaching hospital. The conditions seen are very similar to those at the Parirenyatwa and are often AIDS related.

O Elective notes: A number of students have said that the Central offers a better elective experience with a wider range of pathologies; however, the clinical school and students are based in the Parirenyatwa.

Avenues Clinic, PO Box 4880, Harare.
Harare Hospital, Lobengula Road, ST 14 Southerton, Harare. Tel: +263 4 664695/664690.
Montague Clinic, 135 J. Chinamano Avenue, 5th Street, Harare.
Secretary for Health and Child Welfare, Box CY 1122, Causeway, Harare. Tel: +263 4 730011.
Sekuru Kaguvi Hospital, Milton Avenue, Box CY, Causeway, Harare. Tel: +263 4 726121.

Bulawayo

This is the country's second-largest city but seems to be stuck somewhere in the 1950s. Old buildings and old cars line the streets. The language here is Ndebele, and the people are very friendly.

Bulawayo has three main hospitals: the Mpilo, United Bulawayo Hospital (the central) and Mater Dei (a private hospital).

Mpilo Central Hospital
Vera Road, Box 2096, Bulawayo
Tel: +263 9 72011/72019.
The hospital: Large and very busy. It is understaffed, overcrowded and commonly runs out of drugs, but by African standards it is quite well run. The care given is very good. Most major specialities are provided. HIV is common, up to 90% of patients admitted being (according to recent reports) HIV positive.
O Elective notes: Time is spent on the wards, in outpatients and visiting outlying hospitals. They occasionally have to visit Victoria Falls Hospital (a short plane trip), which has 200 beds and is run entirely by nurses and one doctor. On call is twice a week. People have found this a very enjoyable elective. There's currently a British consultant who is an excellent teacher. Take gloves as they are not always available on the wards.

Bulawayo Central Hospital
United Bulawayo Hospitals, PO Box 958, Bulawayo.
The hospital: Is an urban, state-run hospital. The diseases seen are typical of Zimbabwe and possibly a bit more complicated as it is a referral centre. Unlike more rural hospitals, there is no drug shortage and it is well equipped. The United Bulawayo has an emergency department, medical and surgical wards (including orthopaedics and paeds), operating theatres, radiology and outpatients. There is also an infectious diseases unit. Outpatients is very busy.
O Elective notes: Reports say that it has been pretty disorganized in the past. It has a modern ITU and CT scanner, but sometimes items like glucometers cannot be found. You can get involved in lots of procedures in the emergency department and assist in theatre. Surgery is recommended. There are opportunities to fly to rural clinics.
Accommodation: Usually, someone puts you up. If not, there are youth hostels in town.

Ingutsheni Hospital, 23rd Avenue, Belmont East, Box 8363, Belmont, Bulawayo. Tel: +263 9 66463/72420.
Lady Rodwell Maternity Hospital, PO Box 958, Bulawayo. Tel 09-72111.
Ministry of Health and Child Welfare, Box 441, Bulawayo. Tel:+263 9 62914. Fax: +263 9 79891.
Nervous Disorders Hospitals, Box 949, Bulawayo. Tel: +263 9 60021/62328.
Richard Morris Hospital
Robbie Gibson Hospital
St Francis, Box 8256, Bulawayo, Tel: +263 9 63411.

GWERU

Birchenough Maternity Hospital, Box 59, Gweru. Tel: +263 54 2399.
General Hospital, Box 135, Gweru. Tel: +263 54 21301/51301. Fax: +263 54 2406.

Mutare

This is Zimbabwe's fourth largest city and is situated in a valley surrounded by mountains.

Zimbabwe

Mutare Provincial Hospital

PO Box 30, Mutare. Tel: +263 20 64321.

The hospital: Mutare is a 250-bed hospital on the outskirts of town and is the referral centre for the whole of the eastern highlands. Common conditions include malaria, TB, AIDS, kwashiorkor, schistosomiasis, STDs, rheumatic fever and congestive cardiac failure. Presentations are usually late due to ignorance and the fact that seeing a doctor costs a whole week's wages.

O **Elective notes:** There are lots of practical procedures and rare diseases.

Accommodation: This is free, in the nurses' home. The town centre is 15 minutes away for food.

Marange Rural Hospital, PO Odzi.
Sakubva District Hospital, Box 3039, Paulington, Mutare. Tel: +263 20 64204.

OTHER HOSPITALS:

Kwekwe:
Kwekwe General Hospital, Box 39, Kwekwe. Tel: +263 55 2333/2337.

Masvingo:
Masvingo General Hospital, Box 114, Masvingo.
Ngomahuru Hospital, P Bag 9028, Masvingo.

Rusape:
Rusape General Hospital, PO Box 10, Rusape.

Marondera:
Chiota Rural Hospital, Box 20, Marondera.
Marondera General Hospital, Box 20, Marondera.

Chinhoyi:
Chinhoyi General Hospital, PO Box 17, Chinhoyi.

Bindura:
Bindura Provincial Hospital, PO Box 260, Bindura.

MISSION HOSPITALS:

Mtshabezi Mission Hospital

P Bag M 5212, Bulawayo.

The hospital: Lies 120 km south-east of Bulawayo in the Gwanda district and was founded in 1951 by the American Evangelical church Brethren in Christ. Funding comes from the Ministry of Health, although it receives four or five times less than government-run state hospitals. One doctor runs 110 beds, including male, female, paeds, TB, antenatal, surgical, labour wards and outpatients. There are 17 nurses and 11 nurse aids. A surgeon from United Bulawayo Hospital visits once a month. The hospital's catchment area covers an 80–100 km radius and 17 000 patients, but many come from outside this area too. AIDS has become a severe problem and has greatly increased the number of patients. It is the most common cause of failure to thrive in paediatrics. The outpatient department is very busy. An extensive system of rural clinics is also visited from here. These provide immunizations, women and children services and advice to small, nurse-run hospitals.

O **Elective notes:** There is an open-air chapel service in the morning (attendance is not expected but is appreciated) followed by ward rounds (which you gradually do yourself) and then outpatients. There's loads of 'hands-on' experience in outpatients (plastering, incision and drainage experience) and theatre. The countryside around the hospital is beautiful although there's not much to do.

Accommodation: This should be available somewhere in the hospital.

Bonda Mission Hospital

Box T7903, Mutare.

The hospital: This is a small, very friendly hospital in the beautiful eastern highlands. It is a well-run though overcrowded mission hospital in a rural area. Malaria, TB, abscesses and HIV are common.

O **Elective notes:** This is a very pretty area and comes highly recommended.

Note: They only take two students at a time so book in advance. It is also best to book with a friend.

Murambinda Mission Hospital

PO Box 20, Buhera. Mobile
Tel: +263 11 423122. www.vanstam.net.

The hospital: Buhera is the second poorest district in Zimbabwe. The hospital was established in 1968 by a group of Catholic nuns, the Little Sisters of Mary. It's about a three-hour drive south-east of Harare. It is both a mission hospital and government run. There are 120 beds (and floor space). One wing is for O&G; the other wing caters for everything else. There are usually three doctors here (often two from the UK). In addition, they visit rural clinics. The hospital has X-ray facilities and a midwifery school (with 2000 deliveries a year). TB, malaria, malnutrition, gastroenteritis and AIDS are commonly seen. It is thought that approximately 40% of antenatal patients and up to 70% of inpatients are HIV positive. A home-based care programme has been established with the role of educating people and caring for HIV patients. There is a busy (220 patients a day) outpatient department (the nurses translating). Drug shortages are a major problem.

O Elective notes: There are usually a maximum of two elective students, but the University of Zimbabwe also uses it. You can tag onto anything you like. Lots of 'hands on' experience in theatre (most operations being carried out under local anaesthetic, although there is a nurse trained in general anaesthesia). It is very friendly and the elective comes highly recommended.

Accommodation: A two-bed bungalow is provided (for approximately Zim$100 a week). Murambinda is a medium-sized town but has no banks (Mutare, two hours away, is the nearest).

Mutambara Mission Hospital
PO Box 90, Nhedziwa, Manicaland.

The hospital: Mutambara is a small Methodist mission 80 km south of Mutare with 1500 people. There is a hospital and a school on site. The hospital has 120 beds (although 200 patients) and family (who may have the same disease) sleep on the floor. It has very limited resources, and equipment for investigations such as X-rays is often broken. Drug shortages are another major prob-

lem. The prevalence of HIV in patients is thought to be around 60%.

O Elective notes: This is a very close-knit community which is very friendly and welcoming. The staff are very stretched so you will have your own clinic. There are plenty of practical procedures as well. Take gloves. There is a morning chapel service you are welcome to attend. This is highly recommended.

Accommodation: Students have previously have stayed with local families.

Tshelanyemba Mission Hospital
P Bag, Maphisa 5703, South Matabeleland.

The hospital: Tshelenyemba is a Salvation Army mission complex 150 km south of Bulawayo, with schools, a midwifery training centre and (no surprises) a chapel. It serves around 30 000 between Tshelenyemba and the Botswana border. The hospital has about 100 general and 20 maternity beds. There is also a shelter for women more than 37 weeks pregnant. One doctor runs everything – the wards, outpatients, surgery – and is on call 24 hours a day, seven days a week. The nurses, however, are very experienced and admit patients and run clinics. Common diseases include malaria, TB, STDs and AIDS (the prevalence of HIV being around 70% in adults and 30% in children). Rural clinics are also conducted within a 30 km radius.

O Elective notes: If it's procedures you want, you should be following the role of the nurse rather than the doctor! When the doctor is away, students find themselves running the show and are often the anaesthetist in operations. There is a chapel service everyday at 7.30 am. There are also prayers before meals and before operations (while the patient is awake!). You do not have to be in any way Christian to go here. This elective is recommended but not if you are going alone as there is not much to do outside the hospital. You may not learn a great deal about treatments, but you will see a great number of unusual conditions.

Accommodation: Provided in a hut, which is in good condition with an (occasionally) flushing loo.

Luisa Guidotti Hospital

PO Box 201, Mutoko.

The hospital: A Catholic mission hospital owned by the Archdiocese of Harare and partly aided by the Zimbabwe government. It was founded in 1966 by Luisa Guidotti. She was accused of helping terrorists and was gunned down by the Rhodesian Guard Force. The hospital has 160 beds for a population of 130 000 in the Mutoko district. Wards include male (acute cases and HIV), female, maternity, paeds and two TB isolation wards. There is also an outpatients and an emergency department. A number of small rural clinics refer to here. The hospital is run by one doctor. There are many cases of AIDS, and the hospital does its best to care for them.

Elim Mission Hospital

PO Box 2007, Nyanga. Tel: +263 29 8516.

The hospital: Has 75 beds and lies 90 km north of Nyanga, forming part of a mission compound. It is in the tribal highlands of north-east Zimbabwe. Staff and drug shortages are common. Conditions are similar to those seen everywhere else in Zimbabwe: TB, HIV, rheumatic fever, meningitis, snake bites and burns.

O Elective notes: There are excellent signs and teaching here. However, it is very isolated (do not go alone). Although it's a mission hospital, the doctor there at the time of writing is not Christian so don't worry if that's not your thing. After a couple of weeks settling in, you do your own clinics and ward rounds. There's no electricity.

Songati Baptist Hospital

P Bag 735, Kadoma.

The hospital: Is a busy but friendly mission hospital. HIV is the major problem.

O Elective notes: Great, but expect to work very hard. There's quite a bit of responsibility. The prevalence of HIV is very high (think hard as you can't really go and then not help out with procedures). The doctors are friendly and can

be asked at any time. It is a mission hospital and therefore they prefer Christians, but this is not vital.

Rusitu Mission Hospital is another popular mission hospital in the Eastern Highlands of Zimbabwe. It has links with the Christian Medical Fellowship. To do an elective here, you need to get in touch with the Fellowship (*see* Section 4); they may interview you, and then you have to sign to confirm that you are a Christian.

SOMETHING DIFFERENT:

Hippo Valley Health Centre

PO Box 1, Chiredzi.

The hospital: Is in an unusual situation. In the 1930s, a project was undertaken to dam tributaries of the Save and Runde rivers. This has provided agricultural land and now the Hippo Valley Company (a large Anglo-American corporation) has set up in Chiredzi (450 km from Harare). It farms sugar cane and employs 40 000 people. The area has supermarkets, schools and hospitals. The hospital serves the workers through the company insurance scheme. Despite its corporate backing, it is still a busy hospital, run by only five doctors. HIV is estimated to be prevalent in 30% of the workforce. Education is the main weapon being used against it. Malaria, TB, Kaposi's sarcoma, rheumatic fever, meningitis, malnutrition and syphilis are also common. Sector and peripheral clinics run by nurses (which the doctors visit) refer here. The hospital has male (16 beds), female (5 beds) and paediatric wards as well as an outpatient department.

O Elective notes: You are encouraged to see your own outpatients with a translator. It is excellent if you want a well set up hospital in a developing world rural setting. There is no need to take gloves with you but take spare *BNF*s. White coats are not used.

Accommodation: This can be arranged at the Hippo Valley Country Club. It

costs around £7 a night, including breakfast for two sharing but is very comfortable with a golf course, pool, bar and
tennis and squash courts.

Flying Doctor service
Check out Section 4 for details of the
Flying Doctor service in Africa.

ASIA

Bangladesh

Population: 134 million
Language: Bengali
Capital: Dhaka
Currency: Taka
Int Code: +880

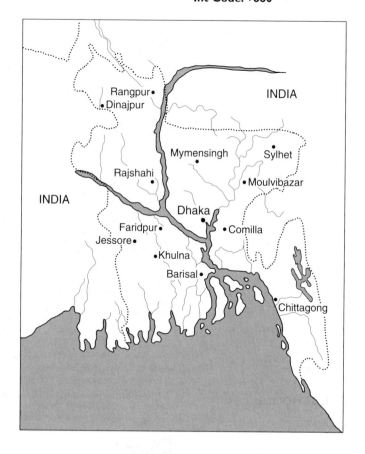

Bangladesh borders India and Burma, and to the south has the coastline of the Bay of Bengal. Although most of the country consists of fertile alluvial plains, the north is mountainous. Bangladesh has had a troubled past, both politically and from natural disasters. Knowing some Bengali will obviously be an advantage, although many in the hospitals speak English. It is not a particularly common elective or work destination.

✪ Medicine:

Bangladesh has severe health problems. There are many reasons for this, but staff and resource shortages and the repeated demand caused by natural disasters are the main ones. Over the past decade, rural health and birth control have taken priority. This has reduced the population growth rate from 23% 15 years ago to less than 3%. Diseases such as cholera and dengue fever are relatively common.

◎ Climate and crime:

Up to two-thirds of the country can become flooded in the monsoon season (March–October). During this time, the water level can rise to 6 m above sea level. As well as the heavy rain, the melting snow of the Himalayas causes the Ganges, Meghna and Jamuna rivers to swell and flood the delta where they converge. Cyclones can build in the Bay of Bengal and can be particularly devastating (killing 140 000 in 1991). Crime has been rising, but severe penalties are curbing it.

➲ Visas and work permits:

A visa is required to visit Bangladesh, as is a work permit if you are intending to do more than voluntary work. Contact the embassy.

Notes for the visitor: Friday is the day off … they work all the others.

USEFUL ADDRESSES:

Ministry of Health, Bangladesh Secretariat, Building 2, Dhaka 100. Tel +880 2 865 063.
Bangladesh Medical Association, BIRDEM Hospital, Shahbag, Dhaka 1000. Tel: +880 2 861 1734. Fax: +880 2 861 3004.

MEDICAL SCHOOLS:

Each has its own associated hospitals:

Dhaka:
Bangabandhu Sheikh Mujib Medical University, Dhaka. Tel: +880 2 861 2550. www.bsmmu.edu.
Bangladesh Medical College (which has the Bangladesh Medical Studies and Research Institute), House No 35, Road 14/A, Dhanmondi Residential Area, Dhaka 1209, Tel: +880 2 816 699. Fax: +880 2 912 5655. www.du.bangla.net.

Dhaka Medical College, 100 Ramna, Dhaka 1000. Tel: +880 2 500 698. It uses: **Dhaka Medical College Hospital**. Tel: +880 2 318 202.
Jahurul Islam Medical College, Dhaka University, Bhagalpur, Bajitpur, Kishoreganj. Tel: +880 2 966 1900. Fax: +880 2 861 5583.
Medical College for Women, Road 8, Sector 1, Uttara, Dhaka 1230. Tel: +880 2 893 939. Fax: +880 2 893 939.
National Medical College, 53 Johnson Road, Dhaka 1100. Tel: +880 2 233 469.
Sir Salimullah Medical College, Midford, Dhaka. Tel +880 2 236 486.
Zainul Haque Sikder Women's Medical College, Monika State, West Dhanmondi, Dhaka 1209. Tel: +880 2 815 951. Fax: +880 2 815 965.

Outside Dhaka:
Barisal Medical College, Barisal. Tel: +880 431 52151.
Chittagong Medical College, KB Fazul Kader Road, Chittagong 4203. Tel: +880 18 637 071. It uses: Chittagong Medical College Hospital. Tel: +880 312 12155.
Comilla Medical College, Comilla. Tel: +880 818 583.
Dinajpur Medical College, Rajshahi Division, Dinajpur.
Faridpur Medical College, Faridpur 7800. Tel: +880 631 64911.
Jessore Medical College, Jessory. Tel: +880 421 5509.
Khulna Medical College, Jessore Road, Khulna.
Mymensingh Medical College, Mymensingh. Tel: +880 915 5601.
North Bengal Medical College and Hospital, Campus, Sushratanagar, Siliguri, Darjeeling District.
Rajshahi Medical College, Rajshahi 6000. Tel: +880 741 772 150. It uses: **Rajshahi Medical College Hospital**. Tel: +880 721 5051.
Rangpur Medical College, Rangpur 5400. Tel: +880 10 521 2288.
Sher-E-Bangla Medical College, Band Road, Barisal. Tel: +880 43 152 151.
Sylhet MAG Osmani Medical College, Sylhet 3100. Tel: +880 821 714 368. It uses: Sylhet MAG Osmani Medical College Hospital. Tel: +880 821 4613.

The language of instruction in most institutions is English. You can write to one of these to ask for an elective in its teaching hospital, but most people write directly to a hospital.

Dhaka

Dhaka, the capital, is becoming a rapidly developing, heaving metropolis with lots to see and do (e.g. the old forts from the British Raj and many shops). Many of the foreign embassies have small cinemas and social clubs for you to meet fellow travellers. The weather is best around Christmas. Only some of the hospitals listed provide accommodation, but hotels in Dhaka cost around £6 a day. Try to make friends with some Americans as the American Embassy supposedly has some good facilities.

International Centre for Diarrhoeal Diseases Research, Bangladesh (ICDDR, B)

Mohakhali, Dhaka. Tel: +880 2 881 1751.
The centre: The ICDDR, B was established by the Bangladesh government in 1981 as a successor to the former Cholera Research Laboratory. It is the world centre for diarrhoea research. It receives some funding from the Bangladesh government, but most comes from foreign governments. It's a place to see every type of diarrhoea: acute watery diarrhoea … persistent diarrhoea … invasive diarrhoea. Lots of pooh, lots of causes.
O Elective notes: The hospital itself is (surprisingly!) clean, and there is good teaching. This elective has been highly recommended a number of times.
Accommodation: Has been available before.

Institute of Postgraduate Medicine and Research

Dhaka, Bangladesh. Tel: +880 2 865 010.
The hospital: Is very large, with all faculties of medicine and surgery. It mainly caters for training postgraduates. It is claimed that it has some of the best departments in Bangladesh. Despite this, owing to the economic situation, some investigations that would be routine in the West are not done. There's much more emphasis on clinical skills.
O Elective notes: Presentations are in English, but ideally you should speak Bengali.
Accommodation: Not provided.

Bangladesh Institute of Research and Rehabilitation in Diabetes, Endocrine and Metabolic Disorders

Ibrahim Memorial Diabetes Centre,
122 Kazi Nazrul Islam Avenue, Dhaka 100.
Tel: +880 861 664 150.

The hospital: Is unique in treating almost exclusively diabetic patients. It houses all departments and manages diabetics who develop illnesses either as a result of diabetes or otherwise. It is a centre for research and a WHO Collaborating Centre for diabetes. As well as the common type I and type II diabetes that we see in the West, there is the tropical form of diabetes called malnutrition-related diabetes mellitus.
O Elective notes: The people and doctors are very friendly. They are busy but make time to teach.
Accommodation: And living are cheap: the total cost (for food and accommodation) should no be more than 8061 BDT (£100) a month.

Dhaka Shishu Hospital

Shar-e-Bangla Nagar, Dhaka-1207.
The hospital: The main children's hospital in Dhaka.
O Elective notes: It's interesting, but there isn't much in the way of practical skills or responsibility.

Centre for Rehabilitation of the Paralysed

PO CRP, Chapain, Savar, Dhaka.
The hospital: Has both an inpatient (mainly orthopaedics and plastic surgery) and an outpatient department specializing in spinal cord injuries. It is well organized, but there is a lack of equipment.
Accommodation: Previously available in the hospital grounds.

A few other specialist hospitals in Dhaka:

Aysha Memorial Specialized Hospital, Mohakhali, Dhaka. Tel +880 912 268 990.
Bari-Ilizarov Orthopedic Centre, Dhanmondi, Dhaka. Tel: +880 912 0309.
Central Hospital, Dhanmondi, Dhaka.
Tel +880 966 001 519.
Christian Medical Hospital, Gulshan, Dhaka. Tel: +880 2 988 6298.
City Dental College and Hospital, Malibagh, Dhaka. Tel +880 934 16624.
Dhaka Ear, Nose, and Throat Hospital, Dhanmondi, Dhaka. Tel: +880 861 3936.
Holy Family Red Crescent Hospital, Eskaton, Dhaka. Tel +880 831 172 125.
National Institute of Cardiac Vascular Disease, Ser-e-Banglanagar, Dhaka.
Tel +880 912 2560.

SPECIALIST HOSPITALS OUTSIDE DHAKA:

Chittagong Diabetic Hospital, Batali Road, Chittagong. Tel: +880 031 617 495.
Holy Crescent Hospital, Zakir Hossain Road, Chittagong. Tel: +088 031 616 001 4.
Institute of Community Opthalmology, Pahartoly, Chittagong. Tel: +880 031 654 051.

Heed Bangladesh Kamalganj Project

Keramatnagar (near Srimangal), Moulvibazar. Contact the Leprosy Mission (TLM, Goldhay Way, Orton Goldhay, Peterborough PE2 5GZ, UK. Tel: +44 1733 370505.)

The project: Is responsible for TB and leprosy control in the whole Sylhet division of Bangladesh. They have a TB/leprosy hospital and many field clinics.

O **Elective notes:** The staff are friendly and speak good English, and the tea gardens and jungle nearby are beautiful. It is excellent if you want to be a leprosy expert. The area, however, is pretty isolated.

Accommodation: In the project guest-house, costs around £3 a day.

Bangladesh

China

Population: 1.3 billion
Language: Mandarin
Capital: Beijing
Currency: Yuan (CNY)
Int Code: +86

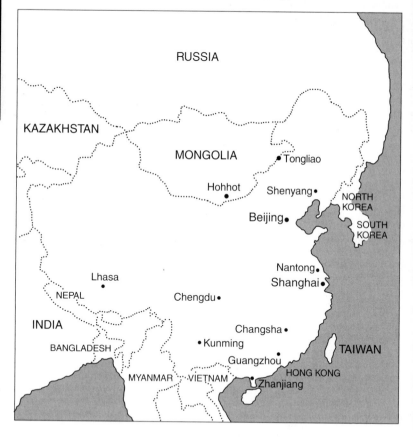

China is a huge country with mountains bordering the north (the Tien Shan Mountains) and south-west (the Tibetan plateau). Two-thirds of China's vast population lives in the low-lying eastern region of the country. Ninety-three per cent of the population are Han Chinese. Of the remaining 92 million, many are of minorities, such as Tibetans, Mongolians and Muslim Uygurs. They inhabit disputed border areas. These small groups do not face the one-child policy that the Han Chinese do, as otherwise *they would soon become extinct. Tourism has increased over the past decade with the relaxation of immigration control. The Great Wall, the Terracotta Army and the Forbidden City are popular tourist attractions. It is very difficult to get an elective or do medical work in Tibet as the Chinese do not want you to see what they are doing to the people.*

✪ Medicine:

Traditional Chinese medical treatments are still very widely used, and a number of medical schools specialize in these. Western medicine has, however, also become accepted and a number of institutions practise both. With communism, all have had access to a relatively high standard of medical care. However, in recent years an economic gap has started to form a split between public and private practice. Attempts to curb families to one child only have had limited success. City hospitals tend to be extremely busy and some are very large, commonly having more than 1000 beds. China is not a common destination for the Western medic, probably because of language and political reasons. The major centres and places of interest are given below.

In some of the central teaching hospitals, there will be doctors who can speak some English, but very few patients will be able to. Further out, there is a high chance that no one will speak any English at all, so a little knowledge of Mandarin or the appropriate language is highly advisable.

◎ Climate:

Being a vast country, there is a great range of weather. In general, the north around Beijing is fairly arid, the south being warmer but wetter.

➲ Visas and work permits:

For all types of Chinese visa, you will require one completed application form, a passport photo and a passport with blank pages. Then you need the following. For a **tourist visa**, you need travel information, including a return airline ticket and itinerary. For a **student visa** (where necessary), you should present the application form for international students (JW-201 or 202 form) issued by the Ministry of Education of China, and a letter of admission from a Chinese university or college. A work visa requires a letter and an employment permit from the Ministry of Labour or the State of Foreign Experts of China.

Note: British passport holders enjoy six-month, visa-free treatment for Hong Kong only for the purposes of tourism or short-term business. Other nationalities should ask the Visa Officer or phone +44 20 7436 1248. Allow three days for visas to be processed.

For travel to Tibet: contact the **Tourist Bureau of Tibet** (Fax: +891 6334632) to obtain approval before applying for a Chinese visa. They will send an itinerary of where you are allowed to go and charge you for this 'tour'. (*See* Section 4 for embassy addresses or visit the website www.chinese-embassy.org.uk).

USEFUL ADDRESSES:

Ministry of Health, 44 Houhaibeiyan, Xicheng Qu, Beijing 100725. Tel: +86 10 403 4433.
Chinese Medical Association, 42 Dongsi Xidajie, Beijing 100710, Tel: +86 10 6513 4885, Fax: +86 10 6512 3754. www.chinamed.org.cn provides extensive details about health care in China and how to organize an exchange.

MEDICAL SCHOOLS:

There are about 130 medical schools – not all can be listed here. For more information, check www.iime.org or www.medicstravel.org.

Beijing

Formerly Peking, China's capital has a huge population (19 million) and is a busy centre for commerce and industry.

Peking Union Medical College Hospital

Chinese Academy of Medical Sciences, Dong Dan, San Tiao, Beijing 100730. Tel: +86 10 201 7620. www.pumch.ac.cn.

China

The hospital: The Peking Union Medical College and its hospital lie in the heart of Beijing. It stands as one of the foremost medical institutions in China, with 900 beds catering for every speciality. Over 3000 outpatients are seen a day. The department of internal medicine, especially the specialities of endocrinology and rheumatology, is considered to be the best in China. The hospital was established in 1921 by the Rockfeller Foundation, USA, and it continues to retain an American tradition in its organization. The standards of clinical practice are very high, with MRI, angioplasty and transplant procedures being performed. These all depend, however, on patients' financial abilities.

O **Elective notes:** The amount of clinical material to be seen is exceptional as it acts as a tertiary referral centre, and even if a disease has an incidence of only 0.0001%, there will be plenty of it in China.

Accommodation: Not provided by the hospital. Hotels are costly and hostels basic. It's best if you have friends you can stay with. Transport around the city is cheap and easy by bus and taxi.

Beijing Medical University
38 Xue Yuan Road, Beijing, Post: 100083. Tel: +86 10 201 7620. Fax: +86 20 201 5681. www.bjmu.edu.cn.
Founded in 1912, the BMU is a comprehensive and leading medical university in China, situated in the north-west suburb of Beijing. It is huge (1500 professors) and affiliated with eight teaching hospitals. Three hospitals are incorporated as colleges of clinical medicine.

The **First Affiliated Hospital (the First College of Clinical Medicine):** Originally founded in 1915, the hospital has very up-to-date facilities and 42 wards providing 1136 beds and an outpatient department seeing 5000 patients per day. It is a centre of excellence for both clinical care and research. As well as being a tertiary referral centre, it runs a special primary care office for local people. It is renowned for its excellence in renal, cardiovascular and oncological dis-

eases. It has an outpatient acupuncture department treating sciatica, headaches, tinnitus, etc. There are also six very active research institutes. It's quite a way out of Beijing and a slog to get to.

The **Peoples' Hospital at Beijing Medical University:** Is effectively the second affiliated hospital. It too has a number of specialities.

The **Third Affiliated Hospital:** Was founded in 1958 as a general hospital, and in 1987 the Beijing Medical University decided to set up its third college of clinical medicine there. It has 945 beds and all major medical and surgical specialities. Some interesting departments include the department of traditional Chinese medicine and the central sterilization room. It has the national departments of sports medicine. There are four research centres, including sports medicine, laser medicine and plastic surgery.

There are a number of other affiliated hospitals (the sixth being concerned with mental health); contact the university for more details.

O **Elective notes:** Write to the **Foreign Students Office** (Beijing Medical University, Beijing 100083). You need to fill in forms four months in advance, and there is a cost of US$400 a month. Although many doctors speak some English, you will not be able to clerk patients if you cannot speak Mandarin. Electives here come recommended.

Accommodation: Provided in the foreign students' building at a very cheap rate. Food is also cheap.

A centre for traditional Chinese medicine:

Beijing University of Chinese Medicine
11 Bei San Huan Dong Lu, Chaoyang District, Beijing 100029, Tel: +86 10 642 13841. Fax: +86 10 642 13817. www.bjucmp.edu.cn.
Was founded in 1956 and has 700 beds. It uses both Western and traditional medicines, with obvious emphasis on the latter.

Guangdong

In the south-east of China, Guangdong Province is becoming a centre for foreign investment, hence industry is growing.

Guangdong Medical College
2 Wenming Dong Donglu, Xiashan District, Zhanjiang, Guangdong Province 524023. Tel: +86 759 228 1544. Fax: +86 759 228 4104. www.gdmc.edu.cn.

Guangzhou College of Traditional Chinese Medicine
San Yuan Li, Guangzhou, Guangdong Province.
The hospital: Combines traditional Chinese medicine with Western medicine. It is one of only two hospitals like this that are centrally funded.

Hunan

This area of China is mainly agricultural.

Hunan Medical University
22 Bei Zhan Road, PO Box 46, Changsha 410078. Tel: +86 731 447 2685. Fax: +86 731 447 1339.
The medical school uses the three main hospitals. The **Xiang Ya Hospital**, one of the oldest hospitals of Western medicine in China (founded in 1906), now has 1085 beds and sees 2000 outpatients a day. It has many areas of speciality, including organ transplantation. The **Second Affiliated Hospital of Hunan Medical University** (Remin Road, Changsha) was founded in 1958 and has 1200 beds. Both of these hospitals pride themselves on their strict, hard-working reputation. There is also a third affiliated hospital.

Inner Mongolia

Inner Mongolia College of Medical Sciences
5 Xinhua Street, Hohhot, Inner Mongolia Autonomous Region 010059. Tel: +86 471 696 3300. Fax: +86 471 696 5120.

Inner Mongolia College of Traditional Mongolian Medicine
16 Cui Lin He Street, Tongliao Inner Mongolia Autonomous Region 028041. Tel: +86 475 696 7406.

Liaoning

Most of the north-east of China is sparsely populated, Liaoning being the exception. It is a booming city receiving a great deal of investment.

China Medical University
92 North Road, Heping District, Shenyang, Liaoning, PR 110001. Tel: +86 24 386 3731. Fax: +86 24 387 5539. www.cmu.edu.cn.
Initially, a mobile medical school (founded in 1931) following the Red Army, it settled in its present place in 1948. It has all major departments, including stomatological, nursing and a very large forensic department. Three teaching hospitals and eight general hospitals are associated, providing 6000 beds. It has a number of research centres, including brain, cancer and paediatrics. Instruction is in English and Chinese.

Jiangsu

Jiangsu is a state just north of Shanghai.

Nantong Medical College
19 Qixiu Road, Nantong, Jiangsu 226001. Tel: +86 513 551 7191. Fax: +86 513 551 7359. www.ntmc.edu.cn.
This medical college, at the end of the Yangtze River, uses 34 teaching hospitals and is associated with a nursing school (in the First Affiliated Hospital).

Shanghai

Shanghai is very overcrowded (population 12.5 million). It previously had an important role in the formation of the Communist Party but now, like much of China, it to is gearing up as a manufacturing city.

Shanghai Second Medical University
280 South Chong Qing Road, Shanghai 200025. Tel: +86 21 632 008 79. Fax: +86 21 632 029 16. www.shsmu.edu.cn.

One of the hospitals it uses is:

Rui Jin Hospital
Shanghai Second Medical College, 197 Rui Jin ER Road, Shanghai.

The hospital: Rui Jin hospital is surprisingly well equipped. The wards are crowded and there is a great opportunity to see traditional Chinese medicine combined with Western practice. There is a great deal of pathology to be seen.

O **Elective notes:** There are acupuncture and herbal clinics for you to attend if you wish. The staff are very friendly and visiting students have been treated very well. Most doctors speak English and all the medical students are expected to learn either English or French. A number of ward rounds and teaching sessions are conducted in English. Try the street food markets and the Jade Buddha temple and visit the areas around Shanghai.

Accommodation: Basic, and hygiene standards are Chinese rather than Western. There are rats and cockroaches to keep you company and no electrical appliances (e.g. no fridge). The shower can only manage a dribble. It is, however, very liveable owing to the large number of friendly visiting medical students (mainly from Taiwan, Malaysia and other parts of south-east Asia and Africa). They know where the parties are.

Sichuan

Chengdu in west China is a busy town and the gateway to China for people who travel via Tibet.

West China University of Medical Science
17 Section 3, South Ren Min Road, Chengdu, Sichuan 610044. Tel: +86 28 550 100. Fax: +86 28 558 3252.

The university/hospital: The university is central in Chengdu and is reported to be the third-largest medical school in China. The university hospital has most specialities, and knowledge is similar to Western standards. However, facilities are limited.

O **Elective notes:** Fees are charged to do an elective here – at least $400 a month. However, accommodation is provided and it's a very cheap place for food and travel (you can survive on less than £20 a week). English classes are part of the medical school curriculum so students can speak it (although may be shy). Rent a bike from the Traffic Hotel (CNY 10 a day) to get around. The students are very friendly. You can organize electives through the WaiBan (Office for International Co-operation) at the above address.

Accommodation: This is provided in a foreign guesthouse within the university (luxury ... your own bathroom, TV and telephone).

Tibet Autonomous Region

Yanwangshan School of Traditional Tibetan Medicine
6 Bai Ta Road, Lhasa 850003.
This is the Chinese replacement for the Tibetan Medical School that used to be here. If you want to see uninfluenced practice then go to Dharamsala, North India.

The main Western hospital in Lhasa is:

Tibet No 1 People's Hospital
Tel: +86 891 633 2462.
Fax: +86 891 633 3478.

Yunnan

Kunming City is the capital of Yunnan Province which is the most south-western province in China, bordering Burma, Laos and Vietnam. In China, it is known as the 'city of

*eternal spring' because of the pleasant
weather all year round.*

Kunming Medical College

84 Western Ren Min Road, Kunming,
Yunnan 650031. Tel: +86 871 531 6570.
Fax: +86 871 531 1542.
www.kmmc.edu.cn.

The hospitals: Kunming uses a number
of hospitals. Conditions are fairly poor in
all of them. Relatives stay day and night,
and hence provide for many of the
patients' needs. The second Affiliated
Hospital (Kunming Medical College,
Kunming, Yunnan 65010) has a specialist hepatobiliary and pancreatology
department.

O Elective notes: It seems a bit odd.
Nurses take blood and give intravenous
drugs while medical students change
dressings. That said, there is plenty to do
in theatre and outpatients.

Accommodation: Provided by the medical college. It has good facilities but
also cockroaches. (The doors are locked
at 11 pm so make sure you are back!)
Food is cheap. A reasonable meal should
cost about Y1.20 (10p).

East Timor

Population: 800 000
Languages: Indonesian, Tetum and Portuguese
Capital: Dili
Currency: US dollars
Int Code: +670

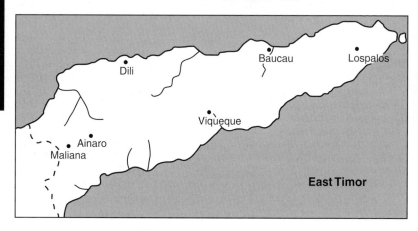

East Timor

After the atrocities with Indonesia, the Democratic Republic of Timor-Leste (or East Timor or Timor-Lorosae) became fully independent in May 2002. The violence resulted in 60% of doctors fleeing the country and the theft of much medical equipment. For a country that already had horrific health problems, the war made things even worse. The situation is, however, improving. Obviously, with the formation of a new government, changes are rapid. Up-to-date information can be found on the government of East Timor's website (www.gov.east-timor.org). You must discuss the possibility of doing an elective in East Timor with your occupational health department and seek the latest advice from the Foreign Office. The country is becoming a common destination for Australian students, but details for other students are sketchy. An elective here would, however, be a fascinating experience. A few people have gone to work here both through aid agencies and the Bairo Pite Clinic. In addition to the medicine, local attractions include Atauro Island (an ecotourism destination run by Oxfam) and trips to Suai and Mount Ramelau.

SAFETY:

The UK Foreign Office (www.fco.gov.uk) currently advises against all holiday and non-essential travel to East Timor. Anti-governmental violence occasionally still erupts. In addition, Westerners in South East Asia are under a general threat from terrorism (some extremist Muslims having condemned the separation of East Timor from Indonesia). If you decide to go on an elective or work in East Timor, register with the British (or your own) embassy as soon as you arrive. If you have a second passport, take it with you because replacements are not possible. Make sure you have proper insurance, medical cover (including evacuation) and secure accommodation provided. Do not go out of town after dark, and drive slowly as the streets are the main gathering place for children and livestock (insurance is not available and crashes can result in nasty arguments). The mobile phone network is good; take your mobile and buy a SIM card there. Flights to Dili are usually via either Bali or Darwin. Check with the Foreign Office before booking your route.

○ Medicine:
TB is still the main cause of death. Malaria, dengue fever, Japanese encephalitis, diarrhoea, pneumonia and skin infections are some of the other common pathologies. *Chikungunya* (Swahili for 'contorts' or 'bends up') is another viral infection transmitted by mosquitoes. The average life expectancy is 46 years for men and 48 for women. Malnutrition is a serious problem, especially in children.

○ Visas:
So far, most electives to East Timor have been by Australian students. Since Australia was so heavily involved in the conflict, they have much closer arrangements. A charge of $25 (£15) is payable for a 30-day visit. Thirty-day extensions cost $30. There is an exit fee of $50 and a $10 departure tax. Contact the embassy in Dili or your destination clinic for fully up-to-date information on visas as this is constantly changing.

The British Embassy in East Timor (Avenida de Portugal, Dili; postal address PO Box 194, The Post Office, Dili. Tel: 390 723 1606. Fax: 390 312 652. E-mail: dili.fco@gtnet.gov.uk) does not offer consular and visa services (such as replacing passports) and has only limited facilities to help in an emergency. For such problems, contact the British Embassy in Jakarta, Indonesia.

HOSPITALS:

The East Timor Interim Health Authority (www.gov.east-timor.org/old/social/health/iha.php) currently coordinates all non-governmental organizations and would be a good starting point for finding out about current projects.

Before independence, East Timor had 10 government-run hospitals and around 20 Catholic-run clinics. There were also 67 *puskesmas* (health dispensaries). The **National Hospital** (formely run by the Red Cross) is situated in Dili (Tel: +670 311 022). Other civilian hospitals can be found in Baucau, Maliama, Viqueque, Ainaro, Oecussi, and Los Palos. The **United Nations Military Hospital** is near the Obrigado barracks and has a continuing education programme every Tuesday evening, which students can attend, but electives cannot currently be arranged here. Another hospital run by the United Nations is in Suai.

Bairo Pite Clinic
PO Box 259, Dili.
www.bairopiteclinic.tripod.com.
The Bairo Pite is a fantastically run primary care clinic in Dili. A number of students and doctors have gone to work here. Their website tells of the experiences encountered.
Accommodation: Accommodation for students working here has previously been provided by the local car rental franchise. A nun in Parunas (Sister Lourdes) can also provide accommodation a little closer. Local families may also offer.

Hong Kong

Population: 6.5 million
Languages: English and Cantonese
Capital: Victoria
Currency: Hong Kong dollar
Int Code: +852

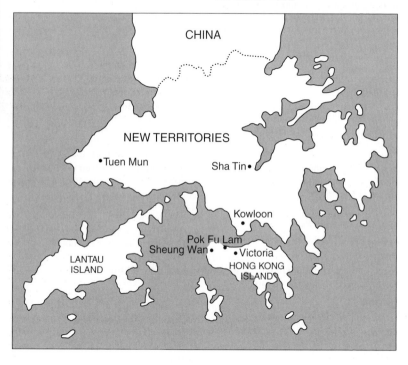

Since the hand-back in 1997, Hong Kong has become a 'Special Administrative Region' of China. The area itself comprises Hong Kong Island, Kowloon and the New Territories. It is a financial and trade centre and, despite its hand-back, this should not change. What may change over the coming years are the (currently British) names of hospitals and places. Hong Kong is a multicultural society, and there is plenty to do and buy (you can shop 24 hours a day!). There are even night markets that open at 10 pm.

All lectures and meetings in hospitals are currently in English. However, the local language is Cantonese so having some knowledge of this is essential for getting the most out of contact with local patients.

✪ Medicine:
The state provides subsidies for medical care so patients only have to pay a fraction of the cost of hospital treatment. Emergency and maternity/paediatric care

is given entirely free. There is no public GP service, although private hospitals and private GPs are popular. Since this is a highly Westernized part of Asia, Western diseases (cardiovascular and cancers) are common causes of mortality.

○ Visas and work permits:

This is currently changing. British, Commonwealth, US and most European citizens are allowed to enter Hong Kong without a Chinese visa, although a permit may soon be required. Elective students are now required to get a student visa. You will also require a visa if you are intending to work. Other nationalities should contact their local Chinese embassy.

USEFUL ADDRESSES:

Hong Kong Medical Association, Duke of Windsor Building, 5th Floor, 15 Hennessy Road, Wanchai. Tel: +852 2527 8452 Fax: +852 2865 0943. www.hkma.com.hk.
Hong Kong Nurses College, 221 Gloucester Road, 12th Floor, Hyde Centre, Wanchai. Tel: +852 2572 9255. Fax: +852 2838 6280. www.fmshk.com.hk.
Hong Kong Dental Association, Duke of Windsor Building, 5th Floor, 15 Hennessy Road, Wanchai. Tel: +852 2528 5327. Fax: +852 2529 0755. www.hkda.org.
Hong Kong Physiotherapy Association, PO Box 10139. Tel: +852 2336 0172. Fax: +852 2338 0252. www.hongkongpa.com.hk.
Hong Kong Occupational Therapy Association, PO Box 98241, Tsim Sha Tsui Post Office.

Full Internet links to all of Hong Kong's hospitals can be found at the **Hong Kong Polytechnic University School of Nursing** website http://nhs.polyu.edu.hk/nhs/

UNIVERSITIES AND ASSOCIATED HOSPITALS:

University of Hong Kong

Faculty of Medicine, 7 Sassoon Road, Pok Fu Lam. Tel: +852 2819 9214. Fax: +852 2855 9742. www.hku.hk/facmed/index.html (this website is excellent and tells you all you need to know for planning an elective in Hong Kong).

Hong Kong University Medical School

is in the western part of Hong Kong, and the **Queen Mary Teaching Hospital** is across the road. It was founded in 1911. This is a large medical school admitting 170 students a year. Apply to the electives supervisor here to do an elective in one (or more) of its affiliated hospitals. You will probably find yourself attached to some Hong Kong students and may have to move around hospitals with them. It is all well organized. They require a letter from your dean saying that he or she approves your proposal. You can then select one of the following options: medicine, surgery, paeds, obstetrics, gynaecology, orthopaedics, psychiatry, radiology or general practice (although you must speak fluent Cantonese for the latter). You can apply to one or more for a total of no more than eight weeks. Some departments will not accept elective students during their elective periods and exams:

- Medicine: December, January, February and May
- Paediatrics: January, February and mid-July to mid-August.

No fee is charged. It is not the university's responsibility to find accommodation (which is possible at hostels or the YMCA, but note that Hong Kong is expensive – it is best to see if you have any relatives or friends there). You can occasionally find accommodation in the Madam SH Ho Residence for Medical Students (6C Sassoon Road; write directly if you are desperate). If accommodation cannot be organized, they may not take you. Bring a white coat.

Chaps need to wear a tie and chapesses need to wear a dress. Jeans and t-shirts are a definite no-no. APPLY AT LEAST 12 MONTHS IN ADVANCE.

Queen Mary Hospital

102 Pok Fu Lam Road.
The hospital: A large, acute, modern teaching hospital for the University of Hong Kong. Established in 1937, it provides most specialities.

○ **Elective notes:** If you select surgery you can choose between a number of specialities: ENT, upper gastrointestinal, vascular, etc. However, you isolate yourself from most other students if doing this so you are better off going for medicine, where most of the other students are. Ward rounds start at 7 am and there is another at 5 pm. During the day there is theatre to visit (all operations are filmed and shown on overhead monitors for you to see) and clinics to attend. In medicine there are ward rounds and teaching in the morning and in the afternoon you go out to peripheral hospitals ... the other students make sure you get there. There may be up to 15 students in one clinic with just one patient. It is not the best way to learn. Paeds has some interesting cases: Kawasaki disease, for example, is much more common.

Accommodation: When available, it has been universally described as poor, but it is right opposite the hospital. Do anything to avoid it. Stay with family or friends if you have them.

Princess Margaret Hospital
Lai Chi Kok, Kowloon, Hong Kong.
The hospital: A district general hospital in eastern New Territory serving approximately one million people in the western part of the Kowloon Peninsula. It is a busy, crowded (45 beds per ward, 1000 in total) hospital and, although ward rounds and meetings are in English, the local population speaks only Cantonese. It has the only infectious diseases centre in Hong Kong.

Other hospitals associated with the University of Hong Kong are:

Grantham Hospital (near Ocean Park), where the first heart–lung transplant in Hong Kong was carried out: a big place for cardiology
Queen Elizabeth Hospital, the largest in Hong Kong with 2500 beds serving the entire population of the Kowloon Peninsula. It is a general hospital
Ruttonjee Hospital, good for respiratory medicine
Duchess of Kent Hospital (12 Sandy Bay Road, Pok Fu Lam. Tel: +852 2817 7111. Fax: ++852 0684. www.ha.org.hk/hospserv/hospital/ dkch.htm), on the western part of Hong Kong is a paediatric hospital for the mentally handicapped. It's in a very picturesque setting.

Chinese University of Hong Kong
Faculty of Medicine, Faculty Office, G03 Choh-Ming Li Building, Sha Tin, New Territories. Tel: +852 2609 6870. Fax: +852 2603 6958. www.cuhk.edu.hk/med/.
The main hospital used is the **Prince of Wales**. Apply to the above for the application forms. Specialities you can choose include general medicine and surgery, O&G, paeds, emergency medicine, orthopaedics and psychiatry. They make it their policy NOT to provide accommodation and the cheapest hotels are around £20 a night. You really do need friends or relatives to go here. Alternatively, if in a crowd, you can try to share a hotel room (e.g. the Regal Riverside). It's not cheap (£290 a month each if sharing with two others) so HAGGLE!

Prince of Wales Hospital
30–32 Ngan Shing Street, Sha Tin, New Territories. Tel: +852 2632 2211.
www.ha.org.hk/pwh/greeting.html.
The hospital: Is one of the two major teaching hospitals for the Chinese University of Hong Kong and the regional hospital for the eastern New Territories. It is large (1400 beds) and has a new children's cancer centre which receives paediatric oncology patients from most of Hong Kong. There is a busy emergency department.
O Elective notes: You blend in with the local students attending their tutorials. You can do what you want. Local students will translate when talking to patients. But teaching is in English.

OTHER HOSPITALS IN HONG KONG:

Castle Peak Hospital
15 Tsing Chung Koon Road, Tuen Mun, New Territories. Tel: +852 2456 6289. Fax: +852 2455 9330. www.ha.org.hk.
The hospital: Opened in 1961, this is a massive 1741 bed psychiatric hospital. Every branch of psychiatry imaginable is here: child, adolescent, psychogeriatrics and forensic to name but a few. It has close links with community units.

St Teresa's Hospital

327 Prince Edward Road, Kowloon. Tel: +852 27119111. Fax: +852 27119779.

Tuen Mun Hospital

Tsing Chung Koon Road, Tuen Mun, New Territories. Tel: +852 2568 5111. Fax: +852 2455 1911. www.ha.org.hk/tmh/.

The hospital: Completed in 1990 and has 1606 beds. It is an acute hospital serving the north-west region of the New Territories.

Tun Wah Group of Hospitals

12 Po Yan Street, Sheung Wan. Tel: +852 2859 7500.

The hospitals: Tun Wah is a charity (which receives government funding) established in 1870. It has set up a number of hospitals to care for the poor and needy throughout Hong Kong.

Hong Kong

India

Population: 1.03 billion
Official Languages: Hindi and English
Capital: New Delhi
Currency: Rupee
Int Code: +91

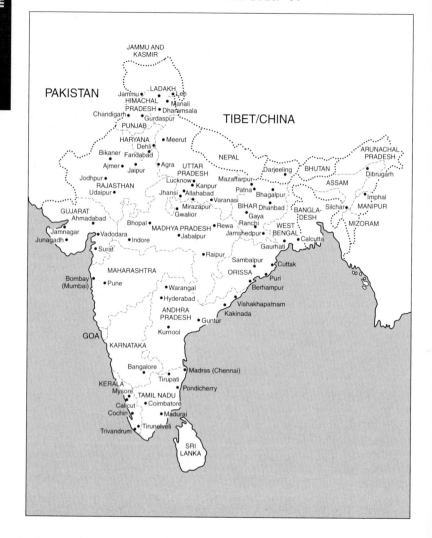

India is huge. It also is a land of great diversity. The landscapes and lifestyles in India contrast considerably from the highly polluted bustle of Delhi to the tranquil and spectacular Himalayas. It is also the second most populous country after China with a great deal of poverty and this is reflected in the medicine seen. There is a subtle division between the south (more vegetarian) and north (more omnivore), which stems back to 1000BC when the original Indian civilization was pushed south by invaders from central Asia. There are 18 official languages in India and, as a result of this, English is still commonly used, especially in politics and bureaucracy (as well as by most doctors). Hindi is the main other language but varies tremendously in different regions, again keeping English in use, especially in Tamil Nadu and Himachal Pradesh.

A number of organized missions and charities run projects and hospitals in India. Some are listed in the information on NGOs in Section 4. The Emmanuel Hospital Association (808/92, Nehru Place, New Delhi 110019, India) runs a number of missionary hospitals across India, as do the Salvation Army. Contact their HQ in your home country (in the UK, 101 Queen Victoria Street, London EC4P 4EP).

✪ Medicine:

The government does provide a health service, but this only stretches to one doctor and two healthcare workers per 2000 population and is very restricted in resources. Malnutrition is still common and contributes to an infant mortality of 80 per 1000. Infectious diseases, especially respiratory, diarrhoeal and malaria, are also big killers. Oral cancers (owing to the habit of chewing betel quids) are much more common. Because of the difficulty accessing healthcare in some regions, many diseases present at a very late stage. Rheumatic fever affects 1% now but many more in the past; therefore, there are lots of heart murmurs. Multidrug-resistant TB is a growing problem, mainly due to patients wanting to avoid the social stigma of TB by stop-ping treatment as soon as their symptoms cease. Because of this stigma, it is often referred to as 'Koch's disease'. To tackle this, the WHO now makes anti-TB drugs freely available to anyone with AFB-positive sputum. In addition, to ensure compliance, a directly observed therapy regime is employed in which patients return to the clinic three times a week to be observed swallowing their medication.

The population is still rising rapidly despite desperate attempts to curb it with policies such as forced sterilization and a campaign of giving away transistor radios in exchange for sterilization. What is really needed is education. Literacy is around 50% but varies dramatically between different castes (an Indian form of class system). The castes consist of *Brahmins* (priests) at the top, with *Kshatriyas* (soldiers and administrators) and *Vaisyas* (artists and business types) below. The *Sudras* are the lowest of the low ... the peasants and toilet-cleaners. Between these four castes, the average wage turns out to be Rs 12 000 a year (about 70p a day).

To Western eyes, India can seem a very unfair society. As well as the caste system (which has rituals to keep them all separate), women get a particularly rough deal. Fifty per cent have had their marriages arranged for them by the age of 20, and with that the bride's parents have to pay a sizeable dowry (e.g. if marrying a doctor they can expect to pay around £15 000). This involves loans and families are plunged into poverty for years as they try to pay it off. Because of this, female infanticide is not uncommon. In some areas, the population average age has reached 45% female and 55% males so 'sex determination' units have been banned. Abortions, however, still occur after illegal ultrasound clinics. Women who get married become very much the underdog in the relationship. Many are subjected to physical and mental abuse and bride-burning continues.

The government-run hospitals tend to be overcrowded and inefficient. There are Christian and charity-based hospitals which are also overcrowded but run much better. These are probably the better places to go for experience on electives (and, if you become ill, better places to be treated). There are a number of private hospitals. Only a few are listed here as they are on the web and aren't used much for electives or temporary work. You may think that in India they would be grateful for all the help they could get ('see a couple of appendectomies and then start doing them' sort of thing). This is generally not the case as India has many of its own juniors. You will, however, get much more stitching and assisting experience than normal in a Western teaching hospital.

Not surprisingly, India has thousands of hospitals and over 100 medical schools. A comprehensive list is not possible here. The main institutions are listed and examples from each region given.

◉ Climate and crime:

The climate varies tremendously from north (hot, but occasionally cool, especially in the Himalayas) to south (very hot). Beware of going in May (as the heat may kill you) or after September in the monsoon season (when malaria probably will).

➲ Visas and work permits:

A three-month visitors' visa is available from the High Commission. A work permit is required for anything more than voluntary work.

Note: If planning an elective, you are advised to organize things early (at least 6–12 months in advance) as post is slow and India is renowned for unnecessary bureaucracy. The vast majority of students get in with just a visitor's visa, but some (on a pretty random basis) have found that they required permission from the government and Ministry of Health of India, which can itself take six months. Hospitals have occasionally found that before they can confirm a place, they have to apply to the Indian government for permission to have a student visitor observer. Once that hurdle has been negotiated, they then have to

get specific permission to have an elective student! Another example of the paperwork is the need to have your passport to buy a train ticket.

USEFUL ADDRESSES:

Ministry of Health, Nirman Bhavan, New Delhi 110 011. Tel: +91 11 301 8863. Fax: +91 11 301 4252. www.mohfw.nic.in.
Medical Council of India, Temple Lane, Lotla Road, New Delhi.
Indian Medical Association, IMA house, I.P. Marg, New Delhi 110002. Tel: +91 11 331 8819. Fax: +91 11 331 6270. (There are branches in every state with their own websites – do a Google search.)
Indian Dental Association, 20A Dewan Bahadur Road, R.S. Puram, Coimbatore 641 002, Tamilnadu. (Again, each area has its own website.)

Delhi

Delhi consists principally of Old and New Delhi. The smaller Old Delhi contains much of the Islamic heritage and is separated from the larger New Delhi in the south by Connaught Place, an area of offices, banks and government buildings as well as some cheap accommodation. New Delhi was set up by the English and was completed in 1911. Overall, Delhi is a busy, heavily polluted city with a great deal of history. Some love it ... others can't wait to get out. Some of the many things to do include train rides to Corbett National Park, the Taj Mahal and Jaipur.

MEDICAL SCHOOLS AND TEACHING HOSPITALS:

All-India Insitute of Medical Sciences (AIIMS)

Ansari Nagar, New Delhi 110029. Tel: +91 11 661123/11 686 45851. Fax: +91 11 686 26630. www.aiims.ac.in.
The hospital: AIIMS, located in the capital (30 minutes' bus ride from the centre), is India's premier teaching hospital and medical research institution. It is a tertiary referral centre and is where Indira Gandhi was brought after her assassination. Even if a disease has a

prevalence of 0.01%, India will have 10 000 cases of it, many of which will be seen at the AIIMS. It is not government run but does receive some funding from the government. Patients (not in the emergency department) pay a registration fee of Rs 10 (approximately 20p), after which all consultation and staff fees are free, although medications and equipment have to be paid for. The hospital is well equipped by Indian standards with its own (working) X-ray machine. The emergency department is busy with four teams doing a four-day rotating cycle.

O **Elective notes:** The doctors are friendly, speak good English and are happy to teach. The patients, however, speak only Hindi so a good grasp of the language is necessary to be able to take a history. You'll get plenty of experience, for example trauma, TB, meningitis, cardiac arrests and drug-induced psychoses. You set your own timetable so (if you have any sense) there's plenty of time to explore Delhi and the surrounding areas. Departments that are quieter than the emergency department may be better if you do not speak Hindi as the doctors will have more time to explain things (although some students have found them very hierarchical). Between January and June, rural placements are offered.

Accommodation: If you want to be where it's happening with a lot of foreign travellers, the central youth hostel is a good bet but not at all cheap at Rs 694 (£10) a night. However, it's clean, has good facilities and one bus takes you straight to AIIMS in 25 minutes. AIIMS will send you a list of local guest houses/B&Bs, claiming to cost about Rs 1400 (£20) a week. Most are considerably more expensive or really a challenge to live in.

The Upkar Guest House has been highly recommended. It is cheap – Rs 210 (£3) a night single, (Rs 280 (£4) a night double – and clean, and has good toilets and showers. As you come out of the main entrance of AIIMS, cross the busy main road, walk left for about 400 m into the shopping area, and there

is a small alley on the right before the Indian Oil House (on the left). It is in Yousef Surrai near the post office. The canteens in the student hostels provide good Indian and Chinese food at bargain prices.

OTHER MEDICAL SCHOOLS:

College of Medical Sciences, University of Delhi, Ring Road, New Delhi 110029.
Government Medical College, Maharishi Dayanand University, Rohtak 124001.
Lady Hardinge Medical College, University of Delhi, Connaught Place, New Delhi 110001. Tel: +91 11 334 3984.
www.mohfw.nic.in/kk/95/ib/95ib0i01.htm.
Maulana Azad Medical College, University of Delhi, Bahadur Shah Zafar Marg, New Delhi 110000. Tel: +91 11-323 1478. Fax: +91 11 372 5574.

OTHER HOSPITALS:

St Stephen's Hospital
Tis Hazari, Old Delhi.
The hospital: St Stephen's is a large general hospital founded by British missionaries to provide subsidized healthcare for working-class Indians in north Delhi. Funding initially came from churches in the UK but it is now predominantly funded by cross-subsidy from private practice and money from the Overseas Development Agency. The hospital employs guards armed with large sticks (called *Latti's*) to marshal the endless patients into outpatients. The patients are usually very poor and there is a lot of noise and bustle. Wards are much the same as clinics except that the patients are better behaved.
O **Elective notes:** There are good reports of theatre work. All the doctors speak English, and they're a pretty jovial bunch. Language barriers can be a bit of a problem.

All India Blind Relief Society, f2 Lajpat Nagar, New Delhi 110024; Willingdon Hospital, New Delhi 110001.
Amar Heart Centre, S357 Pnch Shl Park, New Delhi 110017.
Batra Hospital and Medical Research Centre, 1 Tughlakabad Institution Area, Mehraula Bbd Road, New Delhi 110062.

Deen Dayal Upahdyay Hospital, Harinagar, New Delhi 110064.
Delhi Child Health Centre AIIMS Fountain View, B. Ram Road, 24 Darya Ganj, New Delhi 110002.
Dr Ram Manohar Lohia Hospital and Nursing Home, New Delhi. Tel: +91 336 5525. (This has a bed strength of 937 and is spread over an area of 25 acres, as well as having 4 acres of land that house the nurses' hostel.)
Escorts Heart Institute and Research Centre, Okhla Road, New Delhi 110025.
Hamdard Research Clinic and Nursing Home, 2/3a Ali Road, New Delhi 110001.
Kasturba Hospital, Near Jama Masjid , New Delhi 110002.
Lady Hardinge Medical College and Hospital, P. Kuin Road, New Delhi 110001.
Lajpat Nagar Hospital, Laj Nagar, New Delhi 110024.
Lala Ram Sarum Hospital, Sri Aurobindo Marg, New Delhi 110030.
Lok Nayak Jai Parkash Narain Hospital, Jawarhal Nehru Marg, New Delhi 110002.
National Chest Institute, Sitaram Jiwarajka Hospital, Gautam Nagar, New Delhi 110049.
Nature Cure Hospital, Jawahar Nagar, New Delhi 110007.
New Delhi Tuberculosis Centre, Jawarhal Nehru Marg, New Delhi 110002.
Orthopaedic and Trauma Accident Clinic, 71 Ring Road, Laj Nagar III, New Delhi 110024.
Roshan Lal Bajaj Memorial Hospital and Medical Research Institute, 1C/D Guru Gs Marg, New Delhi 110005.
Safdarjang Hospital, Safdarjang, New Delhi 110016.
Sri Moolchand Khairati Ram Hospital and Ayurvedic Research Institute, Laj Nagar III, New Delhi 1100024.
St Luke's Clinic, 70 Vasant Marg, Vasant Vihar, New Delhi 110057.
University College of Medical Sciences and GTB Hospital, Sgagdara, Delhi 110095. Tel: +91 11 228 0208.

Punjab and Haryana

This area was originally just the Punjab and was severely affected by the great divide when the border with Pakistan was formed. Political unrest has persisted and only in recent years has it become safe to visit. Amritsar was the capital, but it's a bit too close to Pakistan for comfort. Apart from the Golden Temple, there's not a lot to do in the city itself. Chandigarh has been built to be the new capital. Haryana was formed during another split in 1966. You have to go through it to get north from Dehli.

MEDICAL SCHOOLS AND TEACHING HOSPITALS:

Christian Medical College and Hospital
Punjab University, Brown Road, Ludhiana 141008, Chandigarh, Punjab. Tel: +91 161 665 950. Fax: +91 161 609 958.
http://education.vsnl.com/cmcl/.
The hospital: A 600-bed joint mission- and government-run hospital with its own medical school. It is linked to the British Medical Fellowship.

Postgraduate Institute of Medical Education and Research
Sector 10, Chandigarh (VT), Haryana.
The hospital: The PGI is a 1000-bed tertiary referral hospital serving Chandigarh and areas of Himachal Pradesh, Punjab and Haryana. It has a reputation as a centre of excellence and is advanced by Indian standards. Patients pay Rs 10 (20p) for a consultation and a similar fee per day in hospital. They also have to supply or pay for their medications, needles and dressings. Relatives do most nursing duties. It is busy with many different pathologies.

OTHER MEDICAL SCHOOLS:

Dayanand Medical College and Hospital, Punjab University, Tagore Nagar, Civil Lines, Ludhiana 141001. Tel: +91 161 471 500. Fax: +91 161 472 620. www.dmchonline.com.
Government Medical College, Punjab University, Sector 32, Chandigarh, Punjab. Tel: +91 665 253 259. www.gmch.nic.in .
Guru Govind Singh Medical College, Punjab University, Faridkot 151203, Punjab. Tel: +91 163 951 111. www.universitypunjabi.org.
Guru Nanak Dev University Medical College, Magitha Road, Amritsar 143001. Tel: +91 183 220 618.

OTHER HOSPITALS:

Macrobert Hospital
Chariwai District, Gurdaspur, Punjab.
The hospital: Run by the Salvation Army and has 110 beds providing for general medical and surgical needs. Outreach eye clinics are also run. There is a small nursing school.

Escorts Hospital and Research Centre

Neelam Bata Road, Faridabad 121 001, Haryana.

The hospital: Escorts is a very well-equipped (e.g. having a CT scanner) private hospital 30 km south of Delhi. It has all major specialities, including neurosurgery and intensive care. Tropical diseases (TB, malaria, typhoid and meningitis) are all pretty common. It's third world medicine, but this hospital has the facilities to do something.

O Elective notes: Lots to see, but few patients or nurses speak English, and students do not have much responsibility. Great if you speak Hindi.

Accommodation: A guesthouse is nearby Rs 210 (£3) a night, but hospital accommodation may be available.

Ajit Prasad Jain Civil Hospital, Rajpura, Patiala, Punjab.
Christian Medical College and Hospital, Ludhiana, Punjab.
ESI Hospital, Ludhiana, Punjab.
Guru Nanak Mission Hospital, Jalandhar, Punjab.
Kdirhna Charitable Hospital, Model Town, Ludhiana, Punjab.
St Joseph's Hospital, Rani Col Camp, Hoshiapur, Punjab.

Maharashtra (including Mumbai (Bombay))

Mumbai is the financial centre of India with a large manufacturing industry and the world-famous 'Bollywood'. Its prosperity, however, also attracts migrants hopeful of a richer life. This has meant that the slum areas have grown. The result is a diverse, vibrant city with an odd mixture of rich and poor in an unusual Victorian setting.
Maharashtra itself is a large and prosperous state. The coast has plenty of beaches and small fishing villages. In the north are many buddhist caves such as the Ajanta and Ellora caves.

MEDICAL SCHOOLS AND HOSPITALS:

ADLI:Armed Forces Medical College, University of Pune, Sholapur Road, Pune 411040, Maharashtra. Tel: +91 212 606 009, Fax: +91 212 674 759. www.unipune.ernet.in.
BJ Medical College, University of Pune, Sassoon Road, Pune 411001, Maharashtra. Tel: +91 212 626 010. Fax: +91 212 626 868. www.unipune.ernet.in.
Dr Vaishampayan Memorial Medical College, Shivaji University, Golibar Maidan, Sholapur 413003.
Government Medical College, Marathwada University, Ghati, Aurangabad 431001, Maharashtra. Tel: +91 240 331 298. Fax: +91 240 334 418.
Grant Medical College, Mumbai University, Sir J.J. Hospital Compound, Byculla, Mumbai 400008, Maharashtra. Tel: +91 22 373 1144. Fax: +91 22 373 5599. www.mu.ac.in.
Indira Gandhi Medical College, Nagpur University, Central Avenue Road, Nagpur 440018. Tel: +91 712 726 126. Fax: +91 712 728 028.
Lokmanya Tilak Municipal Medical College, Mumbai University, Sion, Bombay 400022. Tel: +91 22 407 6381. Fax: +91 22 407 6100.
Mahatma Gandhi Institute of Medical Sciences, Nagpur University, Pune–Mumbai Highway, Sector 18, Kamothi Navi Mumbai 400209, Maharashtra. Tel: +91 22 742 1723. Fax: +91 22 757 1162. www.mu.ac.in.
Medical College Nagpur University, General Hospital, Nagpur 440001. www.gmcnagpur.net.
Miraj Medical College, Shivaji University, Miraj 416410.
Rajiv Gandhi Medical College, Chhtrapati Shivaji Maharaj Hospital, Kalwa, Thane 400605, Maharashtra. Tel: +91 22 538790. www.mu.ac.in.
Seth GS Medical College, Mumbai University, Acharya Donde Marg, Parel Bombay 400012. Tel: +91 22 413 6051. Fax: +91 22 414 3435. www.kem.edu.
SRTR Medical College, Marathwada University, Ambajogai 431517.
Topiwala National Medical College, Mumbai University, Dr A.L. Nair Road, Byculla, Bombay 400008. www.mu.ac.in.

Sion Hospital

Bombay.

The hospital: One of four large government-funded hospitals in Bombay serving the population of 14 million. It is very busy and situated next to Dharvi, the largest shanty town, with many hundreds of thousands of people. (Dharvi itself has its own WHO-funded primary care hospital.) Even as a shanty town, it is expensive. A house can cost £20 000 so many can't even afford to live here and are forced onto the streets. There is no sewage system so faeco-oral infections are common. Illiteracy and malnutrition are also highly prevalent. Sion Hospital is very large, with most specialities. It provides a basic service free, but if patients can 'afford' it, they get better investigations and the drugs they really need.

P.D. Hinduja National Hospital

Veer Savarkar Marg, Mahim, Mumbai. Tel: +91 445 1515.

The hospital: A large hospital with most specialities including cardiology, nephrology and ITU. As with much of India, there is a great deal of TB and malaria.

O Elective notes: There are no other students. Staff are friendly and provide good teaching.

OTHER HOSPITALS IN MAHARASHTRA:

Jamkhed Hospital

Jamkhed, Ahmed Najar District, Maharashtra.

The hospital: There are 40 beds over three wards (one obstetrics and gynaecology, and two general). The outpatient department sees around 100 patients a day. It is very rural and outreach clinics are run in local villages. Minor operations (there is no general anaesthesia unless a surgeon visits) can be carried out. Rare conditions commonly seen here include TB, malaria, snakebites (lots of them), trauma and dowry-burning. Asthma is also quite a problem. There are plenty of doctors so students are not given much responsibility. Currently there's not a high incidence of HIV here.

Richardson Leprosy Hospital

Miraj 416410, Sangl District, Maharashtra. **The hospital:** Is run by Leprosy Mission International and is a tertiary referral centre covering a population of 330 000 with reconstructive surgery, ophthalmology and dermatology. It has 120 beds and a very busy outpatients. It is the headquarters of the government leprosy survey. It can, however, get a bit special-

ized but they have links with nearby general medical hospitals. It is a friendly place and a good base in India.

Mure Memorial Hospital

Nagpur 440001, Maharashtra.

The hospital: This is a 120-bed mission hospital providing general and maternity services.

O Elective notes: Work is pretty hard here, but there is plenty to see.

N.M. Wadia Hospital

283 Shukrawar Peth, Pune 41102.

The hospital: This 200 bed missionary hospital provides all general medical, surgical, maternity and ophthalmological services.

Catherine Booth Hospital

Ahmedangar, Maharashtra, India.

The hospital: A 350-bed, Salvation Army-run hospital providing all basic medical, surgical, obstetrics and orthopaedic needs.

Acworth Leprosy Hospital, Wadala, Bombay 400031, Maharashtra.
B. Nanavati Hospital, Swami Vivekanand Road, Vile Parle, Bombay 500056, Maharashtra.
B.A.I. Jerbai Wadia Hospital for Children, Acharya Donde Marg, Bombay 400012, Maharashtra.
B.C.J. Santa Cruz General Hospital, Swami Vivekanand Road, Bombay 500054, Maharashtra.
Bhatia General Hospital, Chikalwadi, J. Dadajee Road, Bombay 400017, Maharashtra.
Bombay Trust Hospita l, Antop Hill Road, Bombay 400031, Maharashtra.
Breach Candy Hospital (and Nursing Home), 60 Bhulabhai Desai Road, Cumbella Hill, Bombay 400026, Maharashtra. Tel: +91 22 363 2657.
B.Y.L. Nair Hospital, near Bombay Central Railway Station, Bombay 400008, Maharashtra.
Cama and Albess Hospital, Mahapalika Marg, Bombay 400001, Maharashtra.
Chinchpada Christian Hospital, Chinchpada, Maharastra. A mission hospital linked to the Emmanuel Hospital Association (see Introduction).
Kasturba Hospital, Sane Guruji Marg, Bombay 400011, Maharashtra.
KB Bhabha Hospital, Bandra, Bombay 400050, Maharashtra.
King Edward Memorial Hospital, King Edward Road, Bombay 400012, Mahahashtra.
Lokmanya Tilak Municipal General Hospital, Sion, Bombay 400022, Maharashtra.
Mansadevi Tulsiram Municipal General Hospital, Mulund, Bombay 400080, Maharashtra.

Mental Hospital, Thane, Bombay 400064, Maharashtra.
Municipal Eye Hospital, Kamathipura, Bombay 400008, Maharashtra.
Municipal General Hospital, Rajawadi, Ghatkopar, Bombay 400077, Maharashtra.
New Hospital for Women, M. Permanand Marg, Bombay 400004, Maharashtra.
Nowrojee Wadia Maternity Hospital, King Edward Road, Bombay 400012, Maharashtra.
Osteopathic Clinic, Dunkeld, J.M. Mehta Road, Bombay 400006, Maharashtra.
Petit Bomanjse Dinshaw Parsee General Hospital, B. Desai Road, Bombay 400026, Maharashtra.
Raonibai Watumull Sanatorium, 120 Savarkar Marg, Bombay 400016, Maharashtra.
Ram Kunvar Charitable X-ray Institute, Dnayaneshwar Mandir Road, Bombay 400002, Maharashtra.
Saifee Hospital, 15 Karve Road, Bombay 400001, Maharashtra.
Sk Patil Arogya Dham, Daftary Road, Bombay 400064, Maharashtra.
St George's Hospital, P. D'Mello Road, Bombay 400001, Maharashtra.
Seth A.J. Bankerbihari Mun, ENT Hospital, Napier Road, Bombay 400001, Maharashtra.
Sir Hurkisondas Nurrotumdas Hospital, Prathnasamaj, Bombay 400001, Maharashtra.
Wanless Hospital, Miraj, Maharashtra.

West Bengal (including Calcutta)

Calcutta, once the Indian capital, conjures thoughts of Mother Teresa and desolate slums. Initially, a town that prospered from jute production, it was plunged into poverty with Partition which divided the mines from the refineries. Since then it has suffered a number of influxes of refugees. It is an amazing city that attacks the senses and can be quite trying. Within India it is known as a centre for arts and culture as well as being a thriving metropolis (the noble laureate Rabindranath Tagore and the film director Satyajit Ray came from these parts). To turn back the clock it is trying to change its name back to its original, Kalikata. Calcutta is a huge experience. Most hospitals won't provide accommodation; try Sudder Street in central Calcutta, which is where all the foreign travellers head. The northern end of West Bengal is another extreme, with quiet serenity in the tea plantations of Darjeeling and the Himalayan foothills.

MEDICAL SCHOOLS AND TEACHING HOSPITALS:

Nilratan Sicar Medical College and Hospital
138 Acharya J.C. Bose Road, Calcutta 700014. Tel: +91 33 244 3213.
The hospital: One of the largest in India and a government-run teaching hospital. It provides care for the very poor and is very overcrowded with poor facilities. Cats and goats roam freely around and there is no limit to the number of patients that can be squeezed in. Lots of tropical diseases. The staff are, however, very knowledgeable and have excellent clinical skills.
O **Elective notes:** There is good teaching with the local students. Being able to speak Bengali is a BIG plus. Very few patients speak English and the staff are too busy to translate. Try to go to a private hospital in Calcutta to see the difference.

Ramakrishna Seva Pratishtan Hospital
99 Sarat Bose Road, Calcutta 700026. Tel: +91 33 475 3636/3637/3638/3639. Fax: +91 33 475 4351.
The hospital: This is a charitable hospital but is also recognized as a postgraduate training institute by the University of Calcutta. It has an educational unit with a reasonable library and some organized seminars/lectures. Patients have to pay for their own drugs, venflons, pacemakers, etc., which prevents the poorest being treated here. Surgery is a luxury beyond the means of most people.
O **Elective notes:** Some of the surgeons can give excellent teaching. Being able to speak Bengali is an obvious advantage. Again, as is common in India because of the hierachical system, do not expect any more responsibility than in a Western hospital.
Accommodation: The hospital has a list of local accommodation.

Institute of Ophthalmology
Calcutta Medical College, Calcutta.
The hospital: State run and busy. Only the very poor come here. The beds are

very close to each other with no curtains. There are only two or three nurses to cover several wards. Each operating theatre has two or three tables. Many of Calcutta's own students study here.

Accommodation: Not provided.

North Bengal Medical College

PO Sushruta Nagar, Darjeeling Pin: 734432, West Bengal. Tel: +91 35 375 201. Fax: +91 35 345 0285.

The hospital: This is a large busy teaching hospital, with most specialities and lots of unusual pathologies. The hospital is pretty dirty and crowded. Villagers come from miles to get to here.

O **Elective notes:** Highly recommended for surgery, but it is hard work.

Accommodation: Provided on campus for Rs 10 (8p) a week, with food around Rs 100 (£1.50) a week.

North Bengal Poly Clinic

Nivedita Road, Pradhan Nagar, Siliguri, 734403 West Bengal. Tel: +91 353 433120.

The hospital: Fairly large with all major specialities.

O **Elective notes:** Good teaching from friendly staff. The patients all speak Bengali.

Advanced Medicare and Research Institute

Calcutta, West Bengal.

The hospital: Privately run and some patients here speak English. The contrast to government hospitals is incredible; it is like a Western hospital. Patients have to pay £5 a night here, but that can only be afforded by the well-off.

OTHER MEDICAL SCHOOLS:

BS Medical College, University of Calcutta, Bankura 711303, West Bengal. Tel: +91 32 425 1324.

Calcutta National Medical College, University of Calcutta, 32 Gorachand Road, Calcutta 700014, West Bengal. Tel: +91 33 244 4834. Fax: +91 33 350 0639.

Medical College, Burdwan University, Burdwan 713101, West Bengal.

Medical College, University of Calcutta, 244 Acharyya Jagadish Chandra Bose Road, Calcutta 700020, West Bengal Tel: +91 33 241 4901. (This is the oldest and largest medical college in Calcutta.)

R.G. Kar Medical College, University of Calcutta, 1 Khudiram Bose Sarani, Calcutta 700004, West Bengal.

OTHER HOSPITALS:

Belle Vue Clinic, 9 Loudon Street, Calcutta 700016, West Bengal.

Calcutta Nursing Home, 231/1 Lower Circular Road, Calcutta 700020, West Bengal.

Kumup Sankar Ray TB Hospital, Jadavpur, Calcutta 700032, West Bengal.

Marwari Relief Society Hospital, 392 U. Chitpur Road, Calcutta 700007, West Bengal.

Matri Mangal Pratisthan, 51 U. Chitpur Road, Calcutta 700007, West Bengal.

M.N. Chatterjee Memorial Eye Hospital, 295/1 Acharya P. Chander Road, Calcutta 700009, West Bengal.

North Howrah Hospital, 22 Guha Road, Ghusuri, Howrah, West Bengal.

Park Nursing Home, 4 Victoria Terrace, Calcutta 700017, West Bengal.

Paschim Banga Samaj Seva Samity, Baranagar Hospital, 282 Madjid Bari Lane, Calcutta 700055, West Bengal.

Woodlands Nursing Home, Alipore, Calcutta 700027, West Bengal.

Karnataka

Previously known as Mysore, Karnataka has historic temples, ruins and natural beauty (especially the beaches). It is a major producer of silk, coffee and spices, and its capital, Bangalore, is growing at an incredible rate with its high-tech industries. It is now the fifth-largest city in India and extremely 'Westward' for India, with an almost 'pub culture'. Hampi, a 500-year-old deserted city, is eight hours by train, 12 hours by bus and one hour by plane (for £67). The main language is Kanada and the predominant religion Hinduism.

MEDICAL SCHOOLS AND TEACHING HOSPITALS:

St John's Memorial College Hospital/St John's Medical College

Sarjapur Road, Bangalore 560034. Tel: +91 80 553 0724. Fax: +91 80 553 1786. www.kar.nic.in/rguhs.

The hospital: St John's is a large (900-bed), private, Catholic teaching hospital and tertiary referral centre situated in the south of the city. Both the outpatient department and the inpatient wards are incredibly busy. Guards man the wards to ensure that no outsiders climb into a bed to be fed. Many patients have to leave hospital mid-treatment as their finances run out. Overall, it is all fairly disorganized. By Indian standards, however, it is well equipped and does excellent research. There are facilities for cardiac catheterization and CT scanning, and they recently carried out their first heart transplant.

O **Elective notes:** It is a popular choice for elective students. You are encouraged to rotate around as many departments as possible but are really given free rein over what you want to do. The doctors are friendly and helpful. There are trips into the surrounding villages with the community outreach health team, giving a great insight into village and slum life. Many of the students there are Catholic sisters who train specifically for a life dedicated to working in the slums. There is no real integration with the Indian students, but there are usually a few (10–15) elective students there at any one time. As Bangalore has become more Western, so have the diseases – myocardial infarctions, diabetes and asthma. HIV is increasing (about five cases a day). There are many opportunities for minor procedures. Most people speak English, and it's pretty easy to get around and away from. You have to pay £70 to work here. Overall, this is a good gentle introduction to India and a good place to explore from, although not a good place to see *Indian* medicine.

Accommodation: Cheap (Rs 50 (£1–£3) a night) and adequate (with en-suite toilet and basin), and the food is not bad. The are usually other British/ American elective students there so the social life is pretty good. There are many restaurants (KFC, Pizza Hut, Wimpey) up to five-star hotels. An evening out (posh) with food and drinks costs Rs 150–700. There's a café on Brigade Road with e-mail and Internet access.

Kasturba Medical College/Hospital

Mangalore University, Light House Hill Road, PO Box 53, Mangalore 575001, Karnataka. Tel: +91 824 26482. Fax: +91 824 28183.

The hospital: One of the largest teaching hospitals in Karnataka with many services. A wide range of pathology is seen. Electives here have been well recommended.

Accommodation: Has previously been available.

Cheluvamba Hospital for Women and Children (Krishna Rao Hospital)

Mysore 570001, Karnataka.

The hospital: A government hospital that treats very poor patients from Mysore. It is a teaching hospital for the state-run medical school, with 600 beds and most specialities (e.g. plastic surgery). Although the staff are very good, they perform this service with a shortage of drugs and in poor conditions. There is only one nurse per ward. Malnutrition, gastroenteritis, rheumatic fever and TB are all common. There is a busy outpatient department and busy paeds ward.

Manipal Academy of Higher Education

Manipal, Karnataka 576119.

The hospital: A large teaching hospital, with all major specialities. Manipal itself is a university town on a hill. The location is beautiful and there are plenty of sporting activities. Highly recommended for students.

Accommodation: The school has supplied rooms for Rs 100 a day.

Al-Ameen Medical College, Athani Road, Bijapur 586108, Karnataka. Tel: +91 83 527 0045. www.alameenmedical.edu.

Bangalore Medical College, Bangalore University, Bangalore 560001, Karnataka. Tel: +91 80 611 3342 Fax: +91 80 661 3342. www.kar.nic.in/rguhs.

Gandi Health University, Bangalore and Karnataka University. Dharwad. (It has 100 students a year.)

Government Medical College, Gulbarga University, Bellary 583101, Karnataka.

Jadadguru Jayadeva Murugarajendra Medical
College, Mysore University, Davangere 577004,
Karnataka. Tel: +91 81 923 1388. Fax: +91 81 923
1201. www.jjmmc.bizland.com.
J.L.N. Medical College, Karnataka University,
Poona Bangalore Road, Nehri Nagar, Belgaum
590010, Karnataka.
Karnataka Medical College, Karnataka
University, Hubli 580020, Karnataka.
Mahadevappa Pampure Medical College,
Gulbarga University, Gulbarga 585105, Karnataka.
Mysore Medical College, Mysore University,
Mysore 570001, Karnataka. (This is the oldest in
Mysore.)

OTHER HOSPITALS IN KARNATAKA:

Church of South India Hospital
2 Col Hill Road, Chikballapur 562101,
Karnataka. Tel: +91 8156 72269.
The hospital: An overcrowded, self-
funded, 175-bed hospital in Chikballapur, a small town 60 km north of
Bangalore. It gives a wide range of
experiences with good general medical,
surgical, O&G, and paeds cases daily.
Five consultants and a few juniors run
the show. Rural clinics are run three
times a week. Presenting pathology
includes malaria, leprosy, typhoid fever,
burns, cardiac failure, liver failure,
snake bites, bull gores and many normal
and complicated deliveries. Diagnostic
aids and medication are, unsurprisingly,
lacking. Few of the patients speak
English, however all the doctors and
nurses do.
O Elective notes: It is currently run by
a Scottish-trained surgeon who will turn
his hand to anything. His surgery starts at
6.30 am so take an alarm clock. There are
three weekly trips to treat patients in the
community. Chikballapur (population
40 000) is a very quiet and peaceful
place, with Bangalore just 1½ hours
away by bus. From there, the rest of
India can be explored.
Accommodation: Previously available
for about Rs 70 (£1) a day.

Holdsworth Memorial Hospital
Mysore City, Mysore, Karnataka.
The hospital: A 300-bed mission hospital with basic specialities and a heavy
maternity load.

Jaya Vijayam Tribal Hospital
Virekananda Ginjana Kalyana Kenda, BR
Hills 571441, Mysore District, Karnataka.
The hospital: This hospital was set up
for the local tribes who, until 15 years
ago, moved through the forests of the
wildlife sanctuary. It has attempted to
provide good medical care while pre-
serving the traditional plant medicine
knowledge that the locals have. There
is a very high incidence of sickle cell
disease, TB and obstetric complications.

Manipal Hospital
98 Ruston Bagh, Airport Road, Bangalore,
Karnataka. Tel: +91 80 526 6646. Fax: +91
80 526 6757.
The hospital: A large private hospital
with excellent facilities and plenty of
pathology to be seen.
O Elective notes: This is a very friendly place, and electives here have been
recommended.
Accommodation: Can be arranged.

Anath Ayurvedic Centre
3/89 Bull Temple Road, Bangalore 560019,
Karnataka.
The hospital: Practises ayurvedic medicine, a 4000-year-old traditional medical
culture based on the holy scriptures of
Hindu texts. It has specialities such as
surgery, paeds and O&G, but its diagnoses and treatments are very different,
using herbs, oils and powders. It is very
popular. Visit herb gardens and see it
used in general practice.

A.B. Shetti Hospital, Mangalore, Karnataka.
Baptist Mission Hospital, Bebal, Bangalore,
Karnataka.
Bowring and Lady Curzon Hospital, Shivaji
Nagar, Bangalore, Karnataka.
ESI Hospital, Indiranagar, Bangalore, Karnataka.
ETCM Hospital, PO Box 4, Kolar, Karnataka
563101. (This is a mission hospital run by the
Emmanuel Hospital Association.)
**National Institute of Mental Health and
Neuro Sciences**, PO Box 2979, Hosur Road,
Bangalore 560029, Karnataka.
St Martha's Hospital, Nrupathunga Road,
Bangalore, Karnataka.
Victoria Hospital, K.R. Market, Bangalore,
Karnataka.

Tamil Nadu (including Madras (Chennai))

Chennai (formerly Madras) is a large city and, compared with other Indian cities, is clean and quiet. A large business and manufacturing industry contributes to its wealth, although as a tourist destination it does not have many 'sites'. Tamil Nadu State as a whole is the area of India least influenced by outsiders. The Muslims didn't get very far into it, and the British haven't left much of a mark either. As a result, it is predominantly vegetarian and in some areas alcohol can be difficult to obtain. Pondicherry is the exception as it has had a strong French influence since the 18th century.

MEDICAL SCHOOLS AND TEACHING HOSPITALS:

Christian Medical College and Hospital Vellore

University of Madras, Ida Scudder Road, Post Box 3, Vellore 632004, Tamil Nadu. Tel: +91 416 22603. www.cmch-vellore.edu.

The hospital: A missionary hospital with a medical school. It is the biggest hospital in south India, with 1700 beds and specialities such as cardiothoracic medicine and plastic surgery. People come from all over India to be seen here. It is very highly regarded. It was founded by an American lady, Dr Ida Scudder, and trains male and female doctors and nurses. It offers care regardless of income, race or religion. Malnutrition is common (but it is mainly male children who are brought to see the doctor).

O Elective notes: The staff are friendly and you can do rounds or clinics or join in the student teaching. It is not great for 'hands on' experience, but you will learn a lot as the teaching is excellent. Owing to the language problem (Tamil and Hindi), the doctors take the history and then point out things to you. Language barriers can restrict what you get out of it. They don't like you wandering off during the week, but weekends are free. This is Third World medicine in an almost First World hospital. There is a small charge for electives here. The Community Health and Development Department (CMC Vellore, Tamil Nadu) is excellent for getting to study paediatrics and experience India's culture.

Accommodation: The college provides a list of hostels that you must write to directly. Some students have had basic accommodation in the hospital (less than £1 a day). You will be expected to share in that. New accommodation has recently been built.

Sri Ramachandra Medical College and Research Institute

1 Ramachandra Nagar, Porur, Madras/Chennai 600116, Tamij Nadu. Tel: +91 482 8027 29. Fax: +91 44 482 7008. www.srmc.edu.

The medical school is deemed a university and uses the Sri Ramachandra Hospital.

The hospital: A non-profit-making organization with 1050 beds in the suburbs of Madras. It caters for city and rural folk. Many advanced specialities, such as neurosurgery and cardiothoracic surgery, transplantation and advanced trauma services are provided. Approximately 2000 outpatients are seen each day and given free consultations, investigations and prescriptions. Rates for inpatients range from Rs 1 to Rs 150. It has CT and MRI facilities. A great deal of tropical medicine is seen in rural patients.

O Elective notes: It is very friendly and you will see more pathology than you thought possible. The hospital itself is partly private (300 beds) so there is not much 'hands on' experience, but the teaching is superb. Surgery has been highly recommended. A special 'tropical medicine' elective programme has been set up. Full details and an application form are on their website. Unfortunately, they charge $500 for the privilege.

Accommodation: Free, but you'll have to confirm this in advance.

Chingleput (or Chengalpattu) Medical College, University of Madras, Chingleput 603001, Tamil Nadu. Tel: +91 915 26 566. www.tnmmu.ac.in/medical.htm.
Coimbatore Medical College, University of Madras, Avinashi Road, Aerodrome Post Office Coimbatore 641014, Tamil Nadu. Tel: +91 422 574375. www.tnmmu.ac.in/medical.htm.
Jawaharlal Institute of Postgraduate Medical Education and Research, University of Madras, Dhanvantari Nagar 605006, Pondicherry, Tamil Nadu. Tel: +91 413 372066. Fax: +91 413 372067. www.jipmer.edu. (This is a large institute that comes recommended.)
Kilpauk Medical College, University of Madras, E.V.R. Salai, Chennai 600010, Tamil Nadu. Tel: +91 44 641 2979. Fax: +91 44 641 2979.
Madras Medical College, University of Madras, Periyar E.V.R. Salai, Park Town, Chennai 600003, Tamil Nadu. Tel: +91 44 536 3001. Fax: +91 44 536 3008. www.mmcindia.edu.
Medical College, Madurai University, Madurai 625020, Tamil Nadu. Tel: +91 452 533 230.
Stanley Medical College, University of Madras, Madras 600001, Tamil Nadu. Tel: +91 445 13311.
Thanjavur Medical College, University of Madras, Thanjavur 613001, Tamil Nadu. Tel: +91 4362 40854. www.tnmmu.ac.in/medical.htm.
Tirunelvelu Medical College, Madurai University, Tirunelveli 627002, Tamil Nadu.

OTHER HOSPITALS:

Christian Fellowship Hospital

Oddanchatram, Anna District, Tamil Nadu 624619. www.cfc-ambilikkai.org .
The hospital: A mission hospital (with nursing school) in rural Tamil Nadu. It is very popular for electives and voluntary work, hence the detail below. It is subsidized and attracts patients from miles around: they come to queue in their hundreds at the outpatient clinics. Very few laboratory tests are available. This results in clinicians with excellent clinical skills. Oddanchatram is a semirural area about 120 km from Madurai, the south Indian city most famous for its huge Meenakshi temple, silk and cotton.

It has an interesting history. In the late 1940s, a group of Christian medical students from Miraj decided to venture into the poverty-stricken village. In 1955, one doctor, one nurse and one paramedic came to work here permanently, setting up in a bamboo hut. Many patients came, and it quickly grew to become a 40-bed hospital. In 1958, the hospital moved to new premises when a patient offered five acres of land and a builder offered his services for free. The hospital now has 270 beds and an average of 800–1000 outpatients a day.

The hospital is entirely self-sufficient, accepting no outside funds from mission societies or other organizations. Patients have to pay for all tests and treatments, but it is entirely at the doctor's discretion to allow concessions for those who are genuinely financially restrained. Despite this, poverty is still a problem. Many diabetic patients can't afford their insulin so complications become a problem. A number of open-air clinics are performed in surrounding villages. They tackle education, housing, water and nutrition as well as starting cottage industries such as basket-weaving.

Common conditions include gastroenteritis and malnutrition in children, treated with the WHO strategy of basic oral rehydration. Following that successful campaign, they are starting another for lower respiratory tract infections. Primary healthcare workers in villages are trained to count a child's respiratory rate using an hour glass and act accordingly. It is taking off and effective. TB is also very common, often diagnosed on clinical grounds. Compliance with treatment is a common problem. Women are encouraged to be sterilized immediately after the birth of their second child in an attempt to reduce the population growth.
O Elective notes: Students are expected to see and treat patients on their own, an excellent way to learn medicine. There is also good teaching within the hospital itself, especially in ITU. The staff are very friendly and involve you in their postgraduate programme. However, because it is a rural hospital, there is very little to do in the evenings. The hospital is well served by buses, and it's a great place from which to explore the south of India. Overall, it is an excellent place to learn, but take some good books. Once you have learnt a bit of Tamil you can examine patients very quickly. All the doctors speak English.

Accommodation: Provided, but very basic.

Government General Hospital
Indiragandi Nagar Road, Madras 60002, Tamil Nadu.
The hospital: This is the major general hospital in Madras.

Institute of Thoracic Medicine
Chetput, Chennai 600031, Tamil Nadu.
The hospital: Good for chest disease and infectious/tropical medicine.

CSI Rainy Hospital
Royapuram, Madras 60021, Tamil Nadu.
The hospital: A 170-bed mission hospital with all the basic specialities.

Catherine Booth Hospital
Nagercoil 629001, Tamil Nadu.
The hospital: This is a 350-bed Salvation Army hospital situated on the tip of India, providing all general medical and surgical needs.

MV Diabetes Specialties Centre
35 Conran Smith Road, Chennai 600086, Tamil Nadu. Tel: +91 826 3038/828 2657.
The hospital: This is a specialist centre for diabetes.
Accommodation: Provided free.

Arignar Anna Government Hospital of Indigenous Medicine, Arumbakkam, Madras 600029, Tamil Nadu.
ESI Hospital, 37 Madhavakkam Tank Road, Madras 600023, Tamil Nadu.
Government Chest Institute and TB Training Centre, Spur Tank Road, Madras 800031, Tamil Nadu.
Government Kasturba Gandhi Hospital for Women and Children, Madras 600005, Tamil Nadu.
Government Kilpauk Medical College and Hospital, PH Road, Madras 600010, Tamil Nadu.
Government Ophthalmic Hospital, Egmore, Madras 600008, Tamil Nadu.
Government Royapettah Hospital, Madras 600014, Tamil Nadu.
Government TB Sanatorium, Tambaram, Madras 400047, Tamil Nadu.
Government Thiruvoteswarar TB Hospital, Konnur High Road, Otteri, Madras 600012, Tamil Nadu.
Gremaltes Hospital, Shannoy Nagar, Chennai. (Excellent for leprosy and skin diseases. They also run rural clinics.)

Institute of Child Health and Hospital for Children, Halls Road, Madras 600008, Tamil Nadu.
Raja Sir Ramaswamy Mudaliar's Lying-in Hospital, Kamraj Road, Madras 600013, Tamil Nadu.
Stanley Hospital, Old Jail Street, Madras 600001, Tamil Nadu.
Tuberculosis and Chemotherapy Centre, Spur Tank Road, Madras 600031, Tamil Nadu.

Kerala

Kerala is a beautiful narrow strip in the south-west corner of India that is separated from the rest of the country by dense forest. This has protected it from land invasion and enhanced its use of the sea. It has a large maritime as well as agricultural industry. International influence has created an area of well-educated (nearly 100% literacy) and relatively well-off Indians.

MEDICAL SCHOOLS AND TEACHING HOSPITALS:

Kottayam Medical College, University of Kerala, Gandhi Nagar, Kottayam 686008, Kerala. Tel: +91 481 597 311. Fax: +91 481 597 284.
Medical College, Calicut University, Calicut 673008, Kerala. (This is the largest medical school, with over 2000 beds.)
TD Medical College, University of Kerala, Aleppey 688005, Kerala.
Trivandrum Medical College, University of Kerala, Pattom Palace PO, Trivandrum 695011, Kerala. www.mctrivandrum.com. (This is the oldest.)

OTHER HOSPITALS:

Lal Memorial Hospital
Asan Nagar, Maddayikonam Irinjalakuda, Trichur Kerala.
The hospital: Lal Memorial Hospital is in a small town about two hours' drive from the nearest big city (Trivandrum). It is a small general hospital with departments of medicine, surgery, O&G, paeds, ENT and ophthalmology. It is run by a charity and is very basic, but there are plenty of opportunities to learn. They never have local students so the doctors are very keen to teach and help.
Accommodation: This is provided free in the hospital grounds where most of the doctors and nurses live. This is very

sociable ... you won't have a minute to yourself. The surrounding area is magnificent and typically rural India. There is an elephant next door in the local timber yard!

Mar Kurilose Mission Hospital
Anjoor, PO Thozhiyur 680520, Trissur Dt, Kerala.

The hospital: Built in 1976 by the Malabar Independent Syrian Church. It is three minutes' walk from the St George Cathedral (the church's headquarters) in Thozhiyur, a small town near the west coast of south India. It is financed completely by the church. It has 25 beds and employs one consultant and two junior doctors. Most of the medical consultations are for hypertension and diabetes. Heart disease is therefore a major problem. TB, typhoid and malaria are also seen. Women in Kerala are well-informed about the risks of childbirth so most want hospital births. Perinatal and maternal mortality rates are low (comparable to Western rates) and the Caesarean section rate is 10–20%. Education about family size is rigorous (sterilization being offered after second child). Psychiatric complaints are very common, especially among the young women – their husbands commonly go off to work in the Gulf, leaving them with the family. Depression is treated with simple antidepressants. Any psychosis is still managed by the church, the priest removing the demons.

Holy Cross Hospital, Cheriakadau, Cochin, Kerala.
Iruvella Medical Mission, Tirunelveli, Kerala. Tel: +91 473 630144.
Josgiri Hospital, Tellicherry, Cannanore, Kerala.
Sree Chitra Tirunal Institute for Medical Sciences and Technology, Trivandrum 695011, Kerala.
St Mary's Hospital, Kattakada, Trivandrum, Kerala.

Goa

Unlike the rest of India, the Portuguese influence is still very evident here. Roman Catholicism is still a major religion and there are more churches than temples. It is famed

for its idyllic beaches, although this has made it a bit of a tourist trap. This has in turn made it a rich area with relatively good healthcare and education. It is also a much fairer society towards women.

MEDICAL SCHOOL:

Goa Medical College and Ribandar Hospital, Mumbai University
Ribandar, Panaji 403001 (or Bambolim 402202). Tel: +91 832 226 288. Fax: +91 832 226 288.
www.goacom.com/unigoa/medi.
The hospital: A very busy teaching hospital with many students about. It was founded in 1963 and has 700 beds.
O Elective notes: The teaching is very didactic and there is not much in the way of 'hands on' experience. Students translate though.

OTHER HOSPITALS:

Asilo Hospital Mapusa, Rajvedda, Mapusa, Goa.
Dr Fernando Menezes Hospital, Rai Salcete, Goa.
Goa Dental College & Hospital, PO Bambolim, Goa.
Rebello Hospital, Madel, Margao, Goa.
Salgonkar Medical Research Centre, Vasco da Gama, Goa. Tel: +91 834 512 524.
Shri Kamaxi Nursing Home, Shiroda 403103, Goa.
Sirsat Hospital, Tiska, Ponda 403401, Goa.
Usganonkar Hospital, Sadar, Ponda 403401.

Gujarat

On the west coast, Gujarat has ancient temples and tribal villages and is home to the Asiatic lion. There are also some beautiful beaches at Diu and Mandvi.

MEDICAL SCHOOLS:

Baroda Medical College, Sayiji Gunj, Vadodara, Baroda 390001, Gujarat. Tel: +91 265 421 594. www.msub.edu.
BJ Medical College, Gujarat University, Ahmadabad 380016, Gujarat. Tel: +91 272 376 074. www.gujaratuniversity.org.in.

India

Government Medical College, South Gujarat University, Surat 395001, Gujarat. Tel: +91 261 41596.
MP Shah Medical College, Sauashtra University, Jamnagar 361001, Gujarat. www.saurashtrauniversity.edu.
NHL Municipal Medical College, Gujarat University, Ellisbridge, Ahmadabad 380006, Gujarat. Tel: +91 79 657 5388. Fax: +91 79 657 9282.

OTHER HOSPITALS:

Sheth Vadilal Sarabhai General Hospital and Sheth Chinas Maternity Hospital
Ellisbridge, Ahmadabad, Gujarat 380006.
The hospital: The VS Hospital is a fairly large hospital seeing the poorer communities of Ahmadabad. Most facilities are available, but the conditions are poor, with wards holding 80 patients plus relatives and pigeons. Some equipment, including gloves and needles, are recycled. The language can be a problem: although the notes and teaching sessions are in English, the signs are in (and most people only speak) Gujarati.
O Elective notes: The staff are friendly and you'll get to perform procedures on your own. The VS receives very few elective students, but they are fairly well set up for them. You are encouraged to go to theatre; however, you may be behind six other heads. Ahmadabad ('the Manchester of the east') is a friendly, safe place, but there is little to do, alcohol being prohibited (although it is available for tourists).

Note: Between April and August it can get very hot (47°C). Also, if you're Caucasian, prepare to be stared at a lot.
Accommodation: Cannot be provided, and it can be difficult to arrange.

Emery Hospital
Anand 388001, Gujarat.
The hospital: This is a 200-bed mission hospital with all basic specialities.
Accommodation: Has previously been provided for students.

Bhagat Nursing Home, Valsad, Gujarat.
Dr D.M. Gandhi's Hospital, Bardoli, Surat, Gujarat.
Dr J.K. Patel's Hospital, Vadodara, Gujarat.

Dr Johar Thakkar's Hospital, Veraval, Junagadh, Gujarat.
Dr K.M. Shah Hospital, Laldarwaja, Ahmadabad, Gujarat.
Dr N.G. Savsani's Hospital, Junagadh, Gujarat.
Dr Sakaruta Neducak and Surgical Hospital, Saraspur, Ahmadabad, Gujarat.
ESI General Hospital, Surat, Gujarat.
M.V. Rajda Charitable Hospital, Jamkhambhalia, Jamnagar, Gujarat.
St Mary General Hospital, Gomtipur, Ahmadabad, Gujarat.

Himachal Pradesh

This beautiful area extends from the foothills of the Himalayas high up to the Tibetan plateau. It differs greatly from the rest of India in its climate, altitude and religion. Tibetan Buddhism is the mainstay here. This is reflected in the practice of Tibetan as well as Western medicine. Shimla in the south is a very pleasant town with great colonial influence. Dharamsala is an old British Hill station but now better known as the home of the Tibetan government in exile and the Dalai Lama. It is in the Himalayan foothills and has beautiful views. Many Tibetan monks are here, giving it a very unusual feel for India. It is a pleasant and popular place for electives and volunteers, and these both a Tibetan and Western institute are listed below. To the north are yet more impressive landscapes. Manali in the Kullu Valley is not so attractive since it has been overrun by tourism, especially honeymooning couples. (It does, however, grow some of the finest marijuana in the world apparently.)

MEDICAL SCHOOLS:

Himachal Pradesh/Indira Gandhi Medical College
Himachal Pradesh University, Simla 171001, Himachal Pradesh. Tel: +91 177 204 251. Fax: 177 230 775. www.hpuniv.nic.in/med.

Tibetan Delek Hospital
Gangchen Kyishong, Dharamsala 176215, Dist. Kangra, Himachal Pradesh. www.tibet.net/eng/delekhospital.
The hospital: Run by the Tibetan community but serves the needs of the

Tibetans, Indian people and Westerners living in the area. Although it is Tibetan run, the doctors are mainly unpaid Western volunteers. There is a long-stay TB ward, and much of the outreach work also focuses on TB treatment. There are about 20 inpatient beds for adults and children and daily or twice-daily outpatient clinics, including a weekly antenatal clinic. The medicine practised here is Western style. There is also a torture victims unit on site (for new refugees from Tibet).

O **Elective notes:** There is a real sense of community at the Delek. Everyone cooks and eats together on the roof of the doctors' accommodation. There is plenty of medicine to get involved in and procedures such as draining abscesses and ascitic taps to do. The hospital, and the two listed below, are up in the mountains. Many travellers come via here to see the Dalai Lama or to learn Buddhism. This elective gives an excellent insight into developing world medicine as well as the plight of the Tibetan people, their religion and culture.

Men-Tsee-Khang

Tibetan Medical and Astrological Institute of HH the Dalai Lama, Gangchen Kyishong, Dharamsala 176215, Dist. Kangra, Himachal Pradesh.
www.mentseekhang.org.

The hospital: This is the institute for the preservation of and further investigation into Tibetan medicine. It has a number of clinics all over India (and now throughout the world) that continue to practise Tibetan medicine. It has a clinic on site and also one just up the road in Macleod Gange. The staff are incredibly friendly and if you fancy tasting medicine from a very different culture, this is highly recommended. Most of the time is spent in outpatients clinics. There are no beds here, although the Delek Hospital (for Western medicine) is right opposite.

Accommodation: Occasionally provided, but there are plenty of cheap guesthouses.

Medical Dispensary

Geden Choeling, Nunnery, PO Macleod Gange 176219, Dharamsala, Dist. Kangra, Himachal Pradesh. (Run by Association un Dispensaire pour Dharamsala, Angigonda, 5 Bordeaux St Augustin 33035, Bordeaux, France.)

The clinic: This is a drop-in clinic seeing relatively minor complaints in the local community.

O **Elective notes:** Excellent teaching and plenty of opportunities to do minor procedures and, if it is busy, see patients independently. An elective here has been highly recommended.

Accommodation: There are plenty of guesthouses, but accommodation has previously been provided.

Lady Wellington Hospital

Manali, Kullu, Himachal Pradesh 17131.

The hospital: This is a mission hospital in the foothills of the Himalayas with 40 beds and a busy outpatient department run by about four doctors. Manali itself is a nice, but touristy town.

O **Elective notes:** It's busy and there are plenty of minor procedures. Lots of superb trekking up to Lahaul or Ladalch. There are usually two medical students here. It can be hard work (on call three nights a week); hence some people have not enjoyed it, whereas others have got stuck in and loved it. There are outlying clinics. You don't have to be Christian, but do respect it.

Accommodation: Pretty squalid and dirty.

Bihar

Although Bihar is a holy area for Buddhists, Hindus and Jains, it also seems to be cursed. It suffers great floods and its inhabitants are among the poorest and most illiterate in India. Violence and crime are also commonplace compared with the rest of India. Watch your belongings if you are travelling through.

MEDICAL SCHOOLS AND TEACHING HOSPITALS:

Anugrah Narain Magadh Medical College, Magadh University, Bodhgaya, Gaya 823001, Bihar. Tel: +91 631 420 339.

Darbhanga Medical College, L.N. Mithila University, Laheriasarai 846001, Bihar. Tel: +91 627 233 093.

Mahatma Gandhi Memorial Medical College, Ranchi University, PO Mango, Dimna Road, Jamshedpur 831001, Bihar. Tel: +91 657 462 108. Fax: +91 657 462108.

Medical College, Bhagalpur University, Bhagalpur 812001, Bihar Tel: +91 641 401 078.

Nalanda Medical College, Magad University, Bodhgaya, Patna 800001, Bihar. Tel: +91 612 354 871. Fax: +91 612 354 821.

Patliputra Medical College, Ranchi Uinversity, Dhanbad 826001, Bihar. Tel: +91 326 204 165. Fax: +91 326 204 165.

Patna Medical College, Patna University, Patna 800004, Bihar. Tel: +91 612 653 343.

Rajendra Medical College, Ranchi University, Ranchi 834001, Bihar. Tel: +91 651 301 533.

Sri Krishna Medical College, Bihar University, PO Umanager, Muzaffarpur 842001, Bihar. Tel: +91 621 261 366.

OTHER HOSPITALS:

St Luke's Hospital

PO Hiranpur, District Sahebganj, Bihar 816104. Tel: +91 643 58262.

The hospital: St Luke's is a mission hospital in north-east India. It is the largest hospital in the area and serves one of India's poorest and most backward areas. It has 100 beds and deals with general medicine and surgery, orthopaedics, obstetrics and ophthalmology.

O Elective notes: A typical day consists of a ward round, outpatient clinic and theatre. There's plenty of pathology and tropical diseases to see – TB, malaria and kala-azar. Normally there are about three doctors, all of whom speak and conduct ward rounds in English. However, few patients speak English and this can be a problem. There is some good teaching and there is often the opportunity to assist in theatre and perform minor procedures. You can do any speciality you like. Village clinics are also run.

Note: It is important to consider which season you will be visiting in. In the monsoon season (June–September), most people stay working on the paddy fields despite their illness. The hospital is happy to give you time off to travel. There is not much to do in the evenings, but it is easy to visit Darjeeling (ten hours away), Calcutta (six hours), Nepal and to travel around India from the hospital. This elective has repeatedly been highly recommended; apply early.

Accommodation: Provided in the hospital for around £3 a day.

Duncan Hospital

Raxaul, Champaran District, Bihar.

The hospital: A 200-bed mission hospital with general medial, surgical and obstetric specialities.

Nav Jiwan Hospital

Satbarwa, Bihar, India.

The hospital: A mission hospital run by the Emmanuel Hospital Association.

Uttar Pradesh

In the north Uttar Pradesh has the foothills of the Himalayas, whereas the south has vast plains that often flood forming the basin of the Ganges. Hinduism is the religion and there are many holy places, especially Varanasi on the banks of the river Ganges. There's Agra, home of the Taj Mahal. For wildlife, there is the Corbett Tiger Reserve. Uttar Pradesh is the most populated region of India.

The Director General for the region is at Medical and Health Services, Lucknow, Uttar Pradesh.

MEDICAL SCHOOLS:

Baba Raghav Das Medical College, Gorakhpur University, Gorakhpur 273013, Uttar Pradesh. Tel: +91 551 311 736. Fax: +91 551 311 736.

GSVM Medical College, Kanpur University, G.T. Road, Kanpur 208001, Uttar Pradesh. Tel: +91 512 214 145. Fax: +91 512 570 006. www.kanpuruniversity.org.

Institute of Medical Sciences, Banaras Hindu University, Varanasi 221005, Uttar Pradesh. Tel: +91 542 367 501. Fax: +91 542 316 068. www.bhu.ac.in/.

JLN Medical College, Aligarh Muslim University, Aligarh 202002, Uttar Pradesh. Tel: +91 571 400 603. Fax: +91 571 400 392. www.amu.nic.in.

KG Medical College, University of Lucknow, Lucknow 226001, Uttar Pradesh. Tel: +91 522 257 540. Fax: +91 522 257 539. www.kgmcindia.edu/.

LLRM Medical College, Meerut University, Meerut 250001, Uttar Pradesh. Tel: +91 121 760.888. Fax: +91 121 760 577.

MLB Medical College, Kanpur/Bundelkhand University, Khansi (Jhansi) 284128, Uttar Pradesh. Tel: +91 517 440 858. Fax: +91 517 440 858.

MLN Medical College, University of Allahabad, Lowther Road, Allahabad 211001, Uttar Pradesh. Tel: +91 532 601 983.

SN Medical College, Agra University, Agra 282002, Uttar Pradesh. Tel: +91 562 562.

OTHER HOSPITALS:

Mahanagar Civil Hospital

Lucknow, Uttar Pradesh.

The hospital: In Lucknow (population 5 million), this was originally a small dispensary set up by two doctors. It now has 35 doctors, 30 inpatient beds, four GP clinics, an outpatient department, O&G, respiratory medicine, paeds, orthopaedics and family planning. Facilities are very limited. Patients pay Rs 2 (4p) on arrival in the hospital. TB, malaria, typhoid, leprosy, tropical pulmonary eosinophilia and asthma are common. No one knows the extent of HIV.

Mahila Women's Hospital

Mirazapur, Uttar Pradesh.

The hospital: In a small town east of Lucknow. It has 62 beds in two obstetric and two gynaecology wards. It caters for a large rural population of Hindu and Muslim women. There are 3000 deliveries a year and the wards are often crowded. Abortion here is legal up to 20 weeks. This hospital does not do ultrasound scans. Some, however, go to private hospitals (Rs300 (£3) for a scan), find out the sex of the fetus and then ask for an abortion if it is a girl.

Kachhwa Christian Hospital

Kachhaw, Uttar Pradesh
and

Landour Community Hospital

Mussoorie, Uttar Pradesh.

These are mission hospitals run by the Emmanuel Hospital Association.

St Mary's Hospital

Patna, Uttar Pradesh.

The hospital: A 360-bed, privately funded hospital, located in the small town of Patna. As it is private, you can see and examine patients, but you will not be allowed to do any procedures. However, the staff are keen to teach. There is a wide range of conditions, infectious diseases being the most common.

Asopa Hospital

Gailana Road, Agra, Uttar Pradesh.

The hospital: This is a general hospital, with plenty of tropical diseases. The patients don't speak English. Agra is a pretty ugly place but it does have the Taj Mahal.

Accommodation: A hostel near the hospital costs Rs 300 (£3) a night.

Madhya Pradesh

Lying in the centre of India, this huge state is mainly dry desert. It has mainly Hindi tribal people, most of the tourist attractions being in the north near Delhi. It has numerous Hindi temples and in the centre there is the forested Kanha National Park where Kipling's The Jungle Book was set.

MEDICAL SCHOOLS:

Gajra Raja Medical College, Pune University, Gwalior 474003, Madhya Pradesh. Tel: +91 751 321 400. www.unipune.ernet.in/.

Gandhi Medical College, Bhopal University, Bhopal 462021, Madhya Pradesh. Tel: +91 755 541 376.

JLN Medical College, Ravi Shankar University, Raipur 492001, Madhya Pradesh. Tel: +91 771 523 919.

Medical College, Jabalpur University, Jabalpur 482001, Madhya Pradesh. Tel: +91 761 422 851. Fax: +91 761 422 851.

MGM Medical College, Indore University, AB Road, Indore 452001, Madhya Pradesh. Tel: +91 731 527 383. Fax: +91 731 534 628. www.mgmmc.edu.

SS Medical College, A.P. Singh University, Rewa 486001, Madhya Pradesh. Tel: +91 866 241 655. Fax: +91 766 251 167.

OTHER HOSPITALS:

Padhar Hospital

PO Padhar, Dist. Betul, Madhya Pradesh 460005.

The hospital: Padhar is a small village (population about 300 people) in southern Madhya Pradesh (about 180 km south of Bhopal). The nearest town (with a phone) is Betul, 20 km away, with a population of 30 000. The hospital was founded in 1939 by Reverend Moss, an English missionary who was not a doctor at the time. He spent several years there using a medical textbook to diagnose and treat patients before he was persuaded to go to medical school (in India) and become a doctor.

Since then, the hospital has grown and now has about 250 beds and a busy outpatient department. It serves an area of 300 km diameter. It employs 15 doctors covering general medicine, surgery, O&G, ophthalmology and radiotherapy. It also runs outreach clinics. It is run by the Evangelical Lutheran Church, which also has several other projects based in Padhar, working with the people in the local villages. Although this means that most (but not all) of the staff are Christian, the vast majority of the patients are Hindus and Muslims from the surrounding villages, and religion does not play a part in the day-to-day work apart from 'morning devotion', which is at 8 am each day. Despite donations from the Evangelical Lutheran Church making the hospital well equipped with facilities such as endoscopy and ultrasound, the hospital expects patients to pay for at least part of their treatment. About 60% of the general medical work involves TB, but hypertension, angina and diabetes are also common.

O Elective notes: The doctors are trained in and speak good English. The patients, however, speak Hindi, and this is the language of consultations. The doctors are willing to translate. This is highly recommended as a very Indian, unspoilt elective.

Accommodation: In the 'Big Bungalow', a guesthouse run by the hospital for foreign visitors. It's very comfortable, with hot showers, electricity, all meals cooked for you and even a guard at night. The cost is about Rs 300 (£3) a night. Hire of the jeep and a driver to Betul costs £3.

Chhatapur Christian Hospital

Chhatapur, Madhya Pradesh.
and
Lakhnadon Christian Hospital

Lakhnadon, Madhya Pradesh.
These are missionary hospitals run by the Emmanuel Hospital Association.

Rajasthan

Rajasthan is a beautiful area in north-west India, full of colour and immense history. It is famed for its Rajiput warriors and there are numerous forts and museums.

MEDICAL SCHOOLS:

Birla Institute of Technology and Science, Pilani 333031, Rajasthan.
Dr S.N. Medical College, University of Rajasthan, Jodhpur 342003, Rajasthan. Tel: +91 291 31987.
Jawaharlal Nehru Medical College, University of Rajasthan, Ajmer 305001, Rajasthan. Tel: +91 145 22842.
RNT Medical College, University of Rajasthan, Udaipur 313001, Rajasthan. Tel: +91 294 23613.
Sardar Patel Medical College, University of Rajasthan, Bikaner 334003, Rajasthan. Tel: 151 23443.
Sawai Man Singh (SMS) Medical College, University of Rajasthan, Jaipur 302003, Rajasthan. (This is the largest and oldest medical school in the area.)

Jammu and Kashmir

This area is highly dangerous because of the Pakistan conflict. Don't go there.

MEDICAL SCHOOLS:

Government Medical College, Jammu University, Bakshi Nagar, Jammu 180001. Tel: +91 191 46824. Fax: +91 191 547 647.

Government Medical College, University of Kashmir, Karan Nagar, Srinagar 190010, Jammu and Kashmir. Tel: +91 194 453 314. Fax: 194 453 115. www.gmcsrinagar.net.

Andhra Pradesh

This east coast state, high on the Deccan plateau, is one of the poorest and most underdeveloped areas in India. It has a strong Muslim influence and attractions such as the Golconda Fort and Qutb Shahi tombs. Like all proper poor areas, it gets more than its fair share of tropical storms and floods.

MEDICAL SCHOOLS:

Andhra Medical College, Andhra University, Vishakhapatnam 530001, Andhra Pradesh.
Tel: +91 891 563 413. Fax: +91 891 495 538.
Gandhi Medical College, Osmania University, Basheerbagh, Hyderabad 500001, Andhra Pradesh.
Tel: +91 40 232 452.
Guntur Medical College, Nargarjuna University, Guntur 522001, Andhra Pradesh.
Kakatiya Medical College, Osmania University, Warangal 506002, Andhra Pradesh.
Tel: +91 871 225 971. www.kuwarangal.com/.
Kurnool Medical College, Sri Venkatesvara University, Kurnool 518001, Andhra Pradesh. Tel: +91 851 820 150.
Medical College, Sri Venkatesvara University, Tirupati 517501, Andhra Pradesh.
Osmania Medical College, Osmania University, Hyderabad 500001, Andhra Pradesh.
Tel: +91 404 651 936.
Rangarya Medical College, Andhra University, East Godavary District, Kakinada 533003, Andhra Pradesh.

OTHER HOSPITALS:

CSI Campbell Hospital
Jammalamadugu, Cuddapah District, Andhra Pradesh. Tel: +91 8560 70218.
The hospital: A 320-bed mission hospital. Most pathology is infectious disease, such as TB and leprosy, but O&G, and orthopaedics are also catered for.

Assam

Assam, in the north-east, grows much of India's tea, produces oil and has the rare horned rhinoceros, but be careful if going there. There is a great deal of strife between

the United Liberation Front wanting Assam's independence, and the Indians. The Bodo community is also getting in on the violence.

MEDICAL SCHOOLS:

Assam Medical College and Hospital, Dibrugarh University, Dibrugarh 786002, Assam.
Tel: +91 373 300 080.
Gauhati Medical College, Gauhati University, Gauhati 781001, Assam. Tel: +91 361 261 323.
www.gmchassam.nic.in.
Silchar Medical College and Hospital, Gauhati University, Ghungoor, Silchar 788001, Assam. Tel: +91 384 233 832.

Manipur

Manipur also high in the north-east, has a craft and agriculture industry. Violent struggles are also commonplace so this is another area to avoid.

MEDICAL SCHOOL:

Regional Institute of Medical Sciences, Manipur University, Lamphelpat, Imphal 795001, Manipur. Tel: +91 385 222 2234, Fax: +91 385 231 0625.

Orissa

Orissa is a predominantly rural area with poor but friendly people. There is usually the odd cyclone, flood or drought to make sure they stay poor. For the visitor, there are temples in Bhubaneswar and a beautiful beech in Puri.

MEDICAL SCHOOLS:

Maharaja Krishna Chandra Gajapati Medical College, Berhampur University, Ganjan District, Berhampur 760004, Orissa. Tel: +91 6812 200 746.
Fax: +91 6812 200 720.
SCB Medical College, Utkal University, Cuttak 752001, Orissa. Tel: +91 671 614 355. Fax: +91 671 614 147. www.utkaluniversity.org.
VSS Medical College, Sambalpur University, PO Sambalpur, Burla 768017, Orissa. Tel: +91 663 430 768. Fax: +91 663 430 933.

Ladakh and Zaskar

If remote is what you want, this is it. The main town, Leh (which is of medium size with its own polo ground), is at 3505 m and right at the tip of northern India. There are many festivals, approximately one a month, at the nearby Gompas. Acute mountain sickness is not uncommon. If you fly in you may well get it yourself.

MEDICAL SCHOOL:

Sonam Narbu Memorial Hospital, Leh, Ladakh, India. Tel: +91 198 252 014.

Private hospitals in India

There are a number of private hospital groups, the largest is the Apollo which has a number of centres. Some have previously taken elective students.

Apollo Hospitals Group

www.apollohospitals.com.

The hospitals: The Apollo Hospitals is a group of private hospitals throughout India, set up in 1983 by Dr P Reddy to try to bring international healthcare standards within the reach of every individual. They are major referral centres and centres of excellence providing high-tech specialities such as cardiac surgery. Although much of the medicine seen is Western, topical medicine is still common. From an educational point of view, it can be argued that you learn more by seeing diseases and how to treat them here than you do seeing diseases and then not having the facilities or drugs to treat them in government hospitals. You may feel, however, that you didn't go to India to see the well-off in an air-conditioned hospital (although they do have schemes for the 'economically weaker'). The group has a number of hospitals in a number of states:

Apollo Speciality Hospitals, 320 Anna Salai, Nandanam, Chennai 600 035, Tamil Nadu. Tel: +91 44 433 1741. Fax: +91 44 434 3996. (This 200 bed hospital specializes in neurology/surgery and cancer.)
Chennai (Madras): Apollo Hospitals, 121 Greams Lane, off Greams Road, Chennai 600 006, Tamil Nadu. Tel: +91 44 829 3333. Fax: +91 44 823 4429. (This is a superspeciality and the first Apollo hospital.)
Hyderabad: Apollo Hospitals, Jubilee Hills, Hyderabad 500 034, Andhra Pradesh. Tel: +91 40 360 7777. Fax: +91 40 360 8050. (A 400 bed, high-tech speciality hospital (especially cardiac) and the Apollo Cancer Centre.)
Madurai: Apollo Hospitals, Lake View Road, KK Nagar, Madurai 625 020. Tel: +91 452 650 892. Fax: +91 452 650 199. (It has 135 beds.)
Mumbai (Bombay): Apollo Cliniq, Bogilal Hargovind Das Building, 18/20, K. Dubash Marg, Mumbai 400001, Maharashtra. (This provides a clinic service to Bombay.)
New Delhi: Indraprastha Apollo Hospitals Delhi, Mathura Road, New Dehli 110044, Uttar Pradesh. Tel: +91 11 683 0861. Fax: +91 11 682 3629. (A 700 bed superspeciality hospital, it is the largest private hospital outside the USA. The ITU has an incredible 92 beds. Multiorgan transplants, non-invasive neurosurgery, trauma … they do it all.)
Ranchi: Abdur Razzaque Ansari Memorial Weavers Hospital, PO Irba, Ranchi, Bihar. Tel: +91 651 535 717. Fax: +91 651 535 786. (This is the first rural Apollo hospital.)

India

Japan

Population: 125 million
Language: Japanese
Capital: Tokyo
Currency: Yen
Int Code: +81

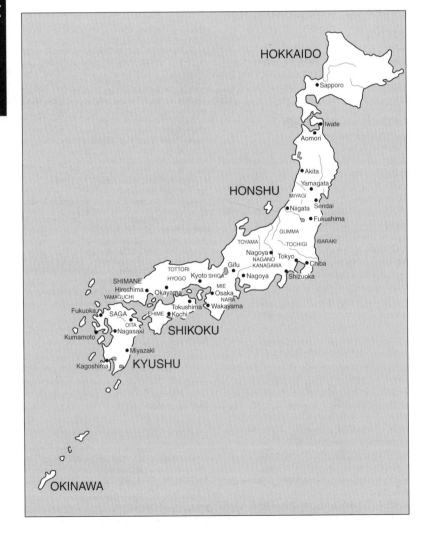

Japan, in the north Pacific, is made up of four islands with most cities being situated near the coast. It is well known for its powerful economy and hard-working people. It is not a common elective or work destination, presumably owing to language barriers. The schools are in general, however, very willing to offer exchanges. If you can understand Japanese, the world-wide web is a good place to start looking, although many schools are difficult to find. For this reason, all the medical schools and their main teaching hospitals are listed below.

✪ Medicine:

Japan has a first-class health system in which most people pay into an insurance scheme related to their pay (*see* below). The poorest receive free treatment. Japan has some of the highest longevity and lowest infant mortality figures in the world. The common causes of death are heart and cardiovascular diseases, cancer (especially gastric) and TB. The ageing population will present a major problem to healthcare, but intermediary health-care services for the elderly are already being set up. There are 9400 hospitals in Japan, of which 80% are privately owned but run on a not-for-profit basis (they can make a profit but they cannot give it to shareholders). The remaining 20% of hospitals are publicly owned; they account for 34% of beds.

Nearly all Japanese citizens participate in a medical care insurance programme. The current system consists of four different insurance groups depending on the size of the organization you work for, and an elderly health-providing group. Although there are variations, patients may under all schemes visit medical clinics and hospitals, and be hospitalized when necessary. They personally pay deductibles and co-payments. People of low income are eligible for medical assistance. They do not need to pay deductibles or co-payments.

✪ Working and advanced training in Japan:

Japan's Medical Practitioners' Law strictly prohibits diagnosis and medical treatment by those without the requisite medical licence. This therefore applies to foreign nationals. Technically, without a Japanese licence you are not allowed to do anything except observe. In 1987, The Law on Exceptions to the Medical Practitioners' Law, Article 17 was passed, which allows advanced clinical training. With a permit for advanced clinical training, you are able to carry out all medical and surgical procedures (in a specified speciality) but only:

- Under guidance of a practitioner certified in advanced clinical training
- At a hospital permitted to give advanced clinical training (*see* below)
- If you can provide documents listed below.

You are not allowed to write prescriptions and all notes must be countersigned by your supervisor.

To apply for a permit you need:

- A medical practitioner's licence from your country
- A certificate of clinical experience (at least three years after qualification)
- Documents to prove you will return to your own country upon completion
- A certificate of language proficiency in Japanese or English
- Proof that you have not been 'struck off' in your country
- A certificate of your own medical health
- Insurance for any injury to patients
- Proof that you have no criminal record
- An application form (and 11 000 yen)
- Passport and photos.

All this will give you a permit for up to two years in a specific field of surgery or medicine at a specific hospital. Write to the **Office of National Examinations and Licences** (*see* below).

USEFUL ADDRESSES:

Japan International Educational Association, 4-5-29, Komaba, Meguro-ku, Tokyo 153. Tel: +81 3 467 3521.

Ministry of Education, Kasumigaseki, Chiyoda-ku, Tokyo 100. Tel: +81 3 581 4211.

Ministry of Foreign Affairs, 2-2-1, Kasumigaseki, Chiyoda-ku, Tokyo 100. Tel: +81 3 580 3311.

Ministry of Health and Welfare, 1-2-2, Kasumigaseki, Chiyoda-ku, Tokyo 100.
Tel: +81 3 503 1711. Fax: +81 3 501 4853.
Office of National Examinations and Licences, Medical Professions Division, Health Policy Bureau, Ministry of Health and Welfare, 1-2-2 Kasumigaseki, Chiyoda-ku, Tokyo 100-45.
Tel: +81 3 503 1711.
Japanese Medical Association, 2-28-16 Honkomagome, Bunkyo-ku, Tokyo 113.
Tel: +81 3 3946. 2121. Fax: +81 3 3946 6295.
www.med.or.jp.
Japanese Nursing Association, 8-2, 5 Chome, Jingumae, Shibuya-ku, Tokyo 150-0001. Tel: +81 3 400 8331. Fax: +81 3 400 8336. www.nurse.or.jp.
Japanese Dental Association, 4-1-20 Kudan-kita, Chiyoda-ku, Tokyo 102-0073.
Tel: +81 3 3262 9213. Fax: +81 3 3262 9885.
www.jda.or.jp.
Japanese Physical Therapy Association, Health Department, School of Medicine, Hiroshima University, 1-1-89, Higashisends, Naka-ku, Hiroshima. Tel: +81 82 241 1221. Fax: +81 82 241 0508. www.ne.jp/asahi/jpta/international.
Japanese Occupational Therapy Association, 2-2-8 Nishi-Waseda, Shinjuku-ku, Tokyo 162.
Tel: +81 3 3203 1286.

SOME SPECIALIST HOSPITALS:

Cancer: Cancer National Cancer Center, 5-1-1, Tsukiji, Chuo-ku, Tokyo 104. Tel: +81 3 542 2511.
Cardiovascular disorders: National Cardiovascular Center, 5-7-1, Fujishiro-dai, Suita-shi, Osaka 565. Tel +81 6 833 5012.
Forensic medicine: Tohoku University School of Medicine, 2-1 Seiryo-machi Aoba-ku, Sendai 980-8575. Tel: +81 22 717 8110. Fax: +81 22 717 8112. www.med.tohoku.ac.jp/index-e.html. (The forensic medicine department has been recommended by elective students.)
Gene therapy: Hospital of Nagoya University, 65, Maizuru-cho, Showa-ku, Nagoya-shi, Aichi 466-8550.
Tel: +81 52 741 2111. Fax: +81 52 744 2428.
www.nagoya-u.ac.jp. (Founded in 1871, the hospital is huge with 1035 beds and a new gene therapy centre.)
Neurology and psychiatry: Konodai Hospital, National Center of Neurology and Psychiatry, 1-7-1, Kono-dai, Ichikawa-shi, Chiba 272.
Tel +81 47 372 0141.
Paediatrics: National Children's Hospital, 3-35-31, Taishido, Setagaya-ku, Tokyo 154.
Tel +81 3 414 8121.

HOSPITALS OF UNIVERSITIES AND MEDICAL COLLEGES:

There are around 80 medical and nursing schools in Japan. As it is not a common destination for most Western health professionals, details are spared. All the schools now have websites, and the addresses for these are included below where available.

Aoto Hospital of the Jikei University, 6-41-2 Aoto, Katsushika-ku, Tokyo 125. Tel: +81 3 603 2111.
Branch Hospital of Nagoya University, 1-1-20 Daiko-minami, Higashi-ku, Nagoya-shi, Aichi 461.
Tel: +81 52 723 1111.
Branch Hospital of Tokyo University, 3-28-6 Mejiro-dai, Bunkyo-ku, Tokyo 112.
Tel: +81 3 942 1151.
First Hospital of Nihon Medical School, 3-5-5 Iidabashi, Chiyoda-ku, Tokyo 102.
Tel: +81 3 3972 8111.
Fujigaoka Hospital of Showa University, 1-30 Fujigaoka, Midori-ku, Yokohama-shi, Kanagawa 227. Tel: +81 45 971 1151.
General Medical Centre of Saitama Medical School, 1981 Aza-Tsujido-machi, Ooaza-Kamoda, Kawaboe-shi, Saitama 359. Tel: +81 49 225 7811.
Hachioji Medical Center of Tokyo Medical College, 1163 Tate-machi, Hachioji, Tokyo 193.
Tel: +81 42 665 5611.
Higashi Hospital of Kitazato University, 863-1, Asamizo-da, Sagamihara-shi, Kanagawa 228.
Tel: +81 42 748 9111.
Hospital of Aichi Medical Universtiy, 21 Aza-Karimata, Ooaza-Iwasaku, Nagakude-cho, Aichi-gun, Aichi 480-11. Tel: +81 56 162 3311. Fax: +81 561 62 4866. www.aichi-med-u.ac.jp. (Established in 1971, Aichi has 100 students a year and all major departments.)
Hospital of Akita University, 1-1-1, Hon-michi, Akita-shi, Akita 010. Tel: +81 188 34 1111.
www.jazz.akita-u.ac.jp.
Hospital of Asahikawa Medical College, 5-3-11, 4-sen, Nishi-Kagura, Shikawa-shi, Hokkaido 078.
Tel: +81 166 65 2111. www.asahikawa-med.ac.jp/.
Hospital of Cancer Research Institute, Kanazawa University, 4-86 Yoneizumi-cho, Kanazawa-shi, Ishikawa 921. Tel: +81 762 41 8245.
Hospital of Chest Disease Research Institute, Kyoto University, 53 Kawahara-cho, Shougo-in, Sakyo-ku, Kyotot-in, Kyoto 606.
Tel: +81 75 751 3802.
Hospital of Chiba University, 1-8-1 Inohana, Chiba-shi, Chiba 280. Tel: +81 472 22 7171.
www.m.chiba-u.ac.jp.
Hospital of Dokkyo University, 880 Ooaza-Kita-Kobayashi, Mibu-cho, Shimo-tsuga-gun, Tochigi 321-02. Tel: +81 282 86 1111.
www.dokkyomed.ac.jp.
Hospital of Ehime University, Ooaza-Shizugawa, Shienobu-cho, Onsen-gun Ehime 791-02.
Tel: +81 899 64 5111. www.m.ehime-u.ac.jp.
Hospital of Fujita Gakuen Health University, 1-98 Dengakugakubo, Kutsukake-cho, Toyoake-shi, Aichi 470-1. Tel: +81 562 93 2000.
www.pathy.fujita-hu.ac.jp.
Hospital of Fukui Medical School, 23 Shmo-Aizuki, Matsuoka-cho, Yoshida-gun, Fukui 910-11.
Tel: +81 776 61 3111. www.fukui-med.ac.jp.
Hospital of Fukuoka University, 7-45-1 Nanakuma, Jonan-ku, Fukuoka-shi, Fukuoka 814-01.
Tel: +81 92 801 1011. www.fukuoka-u.ac.jp.

Hospital of Fukushima Prefectural University, I Hikarigaoka, Fukushima-shi, Fukushima 960-21. Tel: +81 245 48 2111. www.fmu.ac.jp.

Hospital of Gifu University, 40 Tsukasa-machi, Gifu-shi, Gifu 500. Tel: +81 582 65 1241. www.gifu-u.ac.jp.

Hospital of Gunma University, 3-39-15 Showa-machi, Maebashi-shi, Gunma 371. Tel: +81 272 31 7221. www.sb.gunma-u.ac.jp.

Hospital of Hamamatsu University, 3600 Handa-cho, Hamamatsu-shi, Shizuoka 431-31. Tel: +81 534 35 2111. www.hama-med.ac.jp.

Hospital of Hirosaki University, 53 Hon-machi, Hirosaki-shi, Aomori 036. Tel: +81 172 33 5111. www.hirosaki-u.ac.jp.

Hospital of Hiroshima University, 23 Kasumi 1-Chome, Minami-Ku, Hiroshima 734-8551. Tel: +81 82 25 7555. www.med.hiroshima-u.ac.jp.

Hospital of Hokkaido University, 5-chome, Nishi-Juushijo, Kita-ku, Sapporo-shi, Hokkaido 060. Tel: +81 11 716 1161. www.med.hokudai.ac.jp.

Hospital of Hyogo College of Medicine, 1-1 Mukogawa-cho, Nishinomiya-shi, Hyogo 663. Tel: +81 798 45 6111. www.hyo-med.ac.jp.

Hospital of Institute of Medical Science, Tokyo University, 4-6-1, Shiroganedai, Minato-ku, Tokyo 108. Tel: +81 3 443 8111.

Hospital of Iwate Medical University, 19-1 Uchimaru, Morioka-shi, Iwate 020. Tel: +81 196 51 5111.

Hospital of Jichi Medical School, 3311-1 Yakushiji, Minamikawachi-machi, Tochigi-ken 329-0498. Tel: +81 285 44 2111. www.jichi.ac.jp.

Hospital of the Jikei University, 3-19-18 Nishi-Shinbashi, Minato-ku, Tokyo 105. Tel: +81 3 433 1111.

Hospital of Juntendo University, 3-1-3 Hongo, Bunkyo-ku, Tokyo 113. Tel: +81 3 813 3111. www.med.juntendo.ac.jp.

Hospital of Kagawa Medical School, 1750-1 Ooaza-Ikenobe, Miki-cho, Kida-gun, Kagawa 761-07. Tel: +81 878 98 5111. www.kms.ac.jp.

Hospital of Kagoshima University, 1208-1 Ushiki-cho, Kagoshima-shi, Kagoshima 890. Tel: +81 992 64 2211. www.kufm.kagoshima-u.ac.jp.

Hospital of Kanazawa Medical University, 1-1 Daigaku, Uchinada-machi, Kawakita-gun, Ishikawa 920-02. Tel: +81 762 86 3511. www.kanazawa-med.ac.jp.

Hospital of Kanazawa University, 13-1, Takara-machi, Kanazawa-shi, Ishikawa 920. Tel: +81 762 62 8151. www.kanazawa-med.ac.jp.

Hospital of Kansai Medical University, I Fumizono-cho, Moriguchi-shi, Osaka 570. Tel: +81 6 992 1001. www.kmu.ac.jp.

Hospital of Keio University, 35 Shinano-machi, Shinjuku-ku, Tokyo 160. Tel: +81 3 353 1211. www.med.keio.ac.jp.

Hospital of Kitazato University, 1-15-1 Kitazato, Sagamihara-shi, Kanagawa 228. Tel: +81 427 78 8111. www.kitasato-u.ac.jp.

Hospital of Kobe University, 7-5-2 Kusunoki-machi, Chuo-ku, Kobe-shi, Hyogo 650. Tel: +81 78 341 7451. www.med.kobe-u.ac.jp.

Hospital of Kochi Medical School, Kohasu, Okatoyo-machi, Nangoku-shi, Kochi 781-51. Tel: +81 888 66 5811. www.kochi-ms.ac.jp.

Hospital of Kumamoto University, 1-1-1 Honjo, Kumamoto-shi, Kumamoto 860. Tel: +81 96 344 2111. www.cms.kumamoto-u.ac.jp.

Hospital of Kurume University, 67 Asahi-machi, Kurume-shi, Fukuoka 830. Tel: +81 942 35 3311. www.kurume-u.ac.jp.

Hospital of Kyorin University, 6-20-2 Shinkawa, Mitaka-shi, Tokyo 181. Tel: +81 422 47 5511. www.kyorin-u.ac.jp.

Hospital of Kyoto Prefectural University of Medicine, 465 Kajii-cho, Noboru, Hirokoji, Kawarachodori, Kamigyo-ku, Kyoto-shi, Kyoto 602. Tel: +81 75 251 5111. www.kpu-m.ac.jp.

Hospital of Kyoto University, 54 Kawahara-cho, Shougo-in, Sakyo-ku, Kyoto-shi, Kyoto 606. Tel: +81 75 751 3111. www.med.kyoto-u.ac.jp.

Hospital of Kyushu University, 3-1-1 Umaide, Higashi-ku, Fukuoka-shi, Fukuoka 812. Tel: +81 92 641 1151. www.med.kyushu-u.ac.jp.

Hospital of Medical Institute of Bioregulation, Kyushu University, 4546 Tsurumihara, Beppu-shi, Oita 874. Tel: +81 977 24 5301.

Hospital of Mie University, 2-174 Edobashi, Tsu-shi, Mie 514. Tel: +81 592 2 1111. www.medic.mie-u.ac.jp.

Hospital of Miyazaki Medical College, 5200 Kihara, Kiyoyake-cho, Miyazaki-gun, Miyazaki 889-16. Tel: +81 985 85 1510. www.miyazaki-med.ac.jp.

Hospital of Nagasaki University, Sakamoto-cho, Nagasaki-shi, Nagasaki 852. Tel: +81 958 47 2111. www.med.nagasaki-u.ac.jp.

Hospital of Nagoya University, 65 Maizuru-cho, Showa-ku, Nagoya-shi, Aichi 466-8550. Tel: +81 52 741 2111. Fax: +81 52 744 2428. www.med.nagoya-cu.ac.jp.

Hospital of Nihon Medical School, 1-1-5 Sendagi, Bunkyo-ku, Tokyo 113. Tel: +81 3 822 2131. www.med.nihon-u.ac.jp.

Hospital of Niigata University, 754 Ichiban-cho, Asahi-machi-dori, Niigata-shi, Niigata 951. Tel: +81 25 223 6161. www.med.niigata-u.ac.jp.

Hospital of Oita Medical College, 1-1506 Idaigaoka, Hazama-machi, Oita-gun, Iota 879-56. Tel: +81 975 49 4411. www.oita-med.ac.jp.

Hospital of Okayama University, 2-5-1 Shikata-cho, Okayama-shi, Okayama 700. Tel: +81 862 23 7151. www.okayama-u.ac.jp.

Hospital of Osaka Medical College, 2-7 Daigaku-machi, Takatsuki-shi, Osaka 569. Tel: +81 726 83 1221. www.osaka-cu.ac.jp.

Hospital of Osaka University, 1-1-50 Fukushima, Fukushima-ku, Osaka-shi, Osaka 553. www.osaka-u.ac.jp. (This hospital has previously been highly recommended for electives, but note that language can be difficult. There are also only limited procedures for medical students.)

Hospital of Research Institute for Microbial Diseases, Osaka University, 3-1 Yamadagaoka, Suita-shi, Osaka 565. Tel: +81 6 877 5121.

Hospital of Saga Medical School, Sanbonsugi, Ooaza-Nabeshiima, Nabeshima-cho, Saga-shi, Saga 840-01. www.saga-med.ac.jp.

Hospital of St Marianna University, 2-16-1 Sugao Miyamae-ku, Kawasaki-shi, Kanagawa 213. Tel: +81 44 977 8111. www.marianna-u.ac.jp.

Hospital of Saitama Medical School,
38 Morohongo, Moroyama-machi, Iruma-gun,
Saitama 350-04. Tel: +81 429 95 1111.
www.saitama-med.ac.jp.
Hospital of Sapporo Medical College, 16-chome,
Nishi-Minami-Ichijo, Chuo-ku, Sapporo-shi, Hokkaido
060. Tel: +81 11 611 2111. www.sapmed.ac.jp.
**Hospital of Shiga University of Medical
Science**, Tukinowa-cho, Seta, Otsu-shi, Shiga 520-
21. Tel: +81 775 48 2111. www.shiga-med.ac.jp.
Hospital of Shimane Medical University, 89-1
Shioji-cho, Izumo-shi, Shimane 693. Tel: +81 853 23
2111. www.shimane-med.ac.jp.
Hospital of Shinshu University, 3-1-1 Asahi,
Matsumoto-shi, Nagano 390. Tel: +81 263 35 4600.
www.med.shinshu-u.ac.jp.
Hospital of Showa University, 1-5-8 Hatanodai,
Shinagawa-ku, Tokyo 142. Tel: +81 3 784 8000.
www.showa-u.ac.jp.
Hospital of Teikyo University, 2-11-1 Kaga,
Itabashi-ku, Tokyo 173. Tel: +81 3 964 1211.
www.teikyo-u.ac.jp.
Hospital of Tohoku University, 2-1, Seiryo-cho,
Sendai-shi, Miyagi 980. Tel: +81 22 274 1111.
www.med.tohoku.ac.jp.
Hospital of Tokai University, 143 Shimokasuya,
Isehara-shi, Kanagawa 259-11. Tel: +81 463 93 1121.
www.pr.tokai.ac.jp.
Hospital of Tokushima University, 2-50-1
Kuramoto-cho, Tokushima-shi, Tokushima 770.
Tel: +81 886 31 3111. www.tokushima-u.ac.jp.
Hospital of Tokyo Medical College, 6-7-1
Nishi-Shinjuku, Shinjku-ku, Tokyo 160. Tel: +81 3
342 6111. www.jikei.ac.jp.
**Hospital of Tokyo Medical and Dental
University**, 1-5-45 Yushima, Bunkyo-ku, Tokyo 113.
Tel: +81 3 813 6111. www.tmd.ac.jp.
Hospital of Tokyo Women's Medical College,
8-1 Kawada-cho, Shinjuku-ku, Tokyo 162.
Tel: +81 3 353 8111. www.twmu.ac.jp.
Hospital of Tokyo University, 7-3-1, Hongo,
Bunkyo-ku, Tokyo 113. Tel: +81 3 815 5411.
www.m.u-tokyo.ac.jp.
Hospital of Tottori University, 36-1 Nishi-
machi, Yonago-shi, Tottori 683. Tel: +81 859 33
1111. www.tottori-u.ac.jp.
**Hospital of Toyama Medical and
Pharmaceutical University**, 2630 Sugitani,
Toyama-shi, Toyama 930-01. Tel: +81 764 34 228.
www.toyama-mpu.ac.jp.
Hospital of Tsukuba Univerity, 2-1-1 Amakubo,
Sakura-mura, Shinji-gun, Ibaragi 305. Tel: +81 298 53
3900. www.md.tsukuba.ac.jp.
**Hospital of University of Occupational and
Environmental Health**, 1-1 Ibugaoka, Yahatanishi-
ku, Kitakyushu-shi, Fukuoka 807. Tel: +81 93 603
1611. www.uoeh-u.ac.jp.
Hospital of University of the Ryukyus, 207
Aza-Uehara, Nishihara-machi, Nakagami-gun,
Okinawa 903-01. Tel: +81 9889 5 3331. www.ie.u-
ryukyu.ac.jp.
Hospital of Wakayama Medical College, 1
Nanaban-cho, Wakayama-shi, Wakayama 640. Tel:
+81 734 31 2151. www.wakayama-med.ac.jp.
Hospital of Yamagata University, Aza-
Nishinomae, Iida, Zao, Yamagata-shi, Yamagata 990-
23. Tel: +81 236 33 1122. www.id.yamagata-u.ac.jp.

Hospital of Yamaguchi University, 1-2-3
Kasumi, Minami-ku, Hiroshima-shi, Hiroshima 734.
Tel: +81 82 251 1111. www.yamaguchi-u.ac.jp.
Hospital of Yamanashi Medical College, 1110
Shimo-Kawahigashi, Tamaho-cho, Nakakoma-gun,
Yamanashi 409-38. Tel: +81 552 73 1111.
www.yamanashi-med.ac.jp.
Hospital of Yokohama City University, 3-46
Urabune-cho, Minami-ku, Yokohama-shi, Kanagawa
232. Tel: +81 45 261 5656.
Ise Keio Hospital of Keio University, 2-7-28
Tokiwa, Ise-shi, Mie 516. Tel: +81 596 22 1155.
www.yokohama-cu.ac.jp.
Itabashi Hospital of Nihon University, 30-1
Kami-machi, Ooyaguchi, Itabashi-ku, Tokyo 173.
Tel: +81 3 972 8111. www.med.nihon-u.ac.jp.
Kashiwa Hospital of the Jikei University,
163-1, Kashiwa-shita, Kashiwa-shi, Chiba 277.
Tel: +81 471 64 1111.
**Kasumigaura Hospital of Tokyo Medical
College**, 3-20-1 Chuo, Amimachi, Inajiki-gun,
Ibaragi 300-03. Tel: +81 298 87 1161.
Koshigaya Hospital of Dokkyo University,
2-1-500 Minami-Koshigaya, Koshigaya-shi, Saitama
343. Tel: +81 489 65 1111.
**Misasa Branch Hospital of Okayama
University**, 827 Yamada, Misasa-cho, Tohaku-gun,
Tottori 682-02. Tel: +81 858 43 1211.
Naruko Branch, Hospital of Tohoku University,
67-1, Aza-Shin-Yashiki, Naruko-machi, Tamatsukuri-
gun, Miyagi 989-68. Tel: +81 229 82 2531.
Oohashi Hospital of Toho University,
2-17-6, Oohashi, Meguro-ku, Tokyo 153.
Tel: +81 3 468 1251.
Ooiso Hospital of Tokai University, 21-1
Tsukikyo, Oiso-machi, Naka-gun, Kanagawa 259-01.
Tel: +81 463 72 3211.
Oomori Hospital of Toho University,
6-11-1 Oomori-nishi, Oota-ku, Tokyo 143.
Tel: +81 3 762 4151.
**Rakusei New-Town Hospital of Kansai
Medical University**, 3-6, Ooeda-Higashi-shinrin-
cho, Nishigyo-ku, Kyoto-shi, Kyoto 610-11.
Tel: +81 75 332 0123.
Second Hospital of Nihon Medical School,
1-396 Kosugi-machi, Nbakahara-ku, Kawasaki-shi,
Kanagawa 211. Tel: +81 44 733 5181.
**Second Hospital of Tokyo Women's Medical
College**, 2-1-10 Nishi-Oku, Arakawa-ku, Tokyo
116. Tel: +81 3 810 1111.
Surugadai Hospital of Nihon University,
1-8-13 Kandasuruga-dai, Chiyoda-ku, Tokyo 101.
Tel: +81 3 293 1711.
Third Hospital of Jikei University,
4-11-1 Izumihon-machi, Komae-shi, Tokyo, 201.
Tel: +81 3 480 1151.
Tokyo Hospital of Tokai University, 1-2-5
Yoyogi, Shibuya-ku, Tokyo 151. Tel: +81 3 370 2321.
Toyosu Hospital of Showa University, 4-1-18
Toyosu, Koto-ku, Tokyo 135. Tel: +81 3 (534) 1151.
**Tsukigase Rehabilitation Center of Keio
University**, 380-2 Tsukigase, Yugashima-machi,
Amagi, Tagata-gun, Shizuoka 410-32.
Tel: +81 588 5 1701.
Tsukushi Hospital of Fukuoka University,
377-1 Ooaza-Zokumyou-in, Chikushino-shi,
Fukuoka 818. Tel: +81 92 921 1011.

Special national hospitals that are functionally equivalent/superior to university hospitals:

Konodai Hospital, National Center of Neurology and Psychiatry, 1-7-1 Kono-dai, Ichikawa-shi, Chiba 272. Tel: +81 473 72 0141.

Musashi Hospital, National Center of Neurology and Psychiatry, 4-1-1 Ogawahigashi-machi, Kodaira-shi, Tokyo 187. Tel: +81 423 41 2711.

National Cancer Center, 5-1-1 Tsukiji, Chuo-ku, Tokyo 104. Tel: +81 3 542 2511.

National Cardiovascular Center, 5-7-1 Fujishiro-dai, Suita-shi, Osaka 565. Tel: +81 6 833 5012.

National Children's Hospital, 3-35-31 Taishido, Setagaya-ku, Tokyo 154. Tel: +81 3 414 8121.

Hospitals designated for clinical training for medical practitioners in Japan:

Akita Red Cross Hospital, 1-4-36 Nakadori, Akita-shi, Akita 010. Tel: +81 188 34 3361.

Asahikawa Municipal Hospital, 1-1-65 Kanehoshi-cho, Asahikawa-shi, Hokkaido 070. Tel: +81 166 24 3181.

Chiba Rosai Hospital, 2-16 Tatsumidai-higashi, Ichihara-shi, Chiba 290. Tel: +81 436 74 1111.

Chugoku Rosai Hospital, 1-5-1 Hiro-Tagaya, Kure-shi, Hirochima 737-01. Tel: +81 823 72 7171.

Ehime Pefectural Central Hospital, 83 Kasuga-cho, Matsuyama-shi, Ehime 790. Tel: +81 899 47 1111.

First Nagoya Red Cross Hospital, 3-35 Michishita-cho, Nakamura-ku, Nagoya-shi, Aichi 453.

Fukuoka-Chuo National Hospital, 2-2 Jiyo-nai, Chuo-ku, Fukuoka-shi, Fukuoka 810. Tel: +81 92 714 01.

Gifu Prefectural Hospital, 4-6-1 Noitsushiki, Gifu-shi, Gifu 500. Tel: +81 582 46 1111.

Hiraga General Hospital, 64-2 Inukawara, Yathuhashi, Akita-shi, Akita 013. Tel: +81 182 32 5121.

Hirosaki National Hospital, 1 Ooaza-Tomino-cho, Hirosaki-shi, Aomori 036. Tel: +81 172 32 4311.

Hiroshima Prefectural Hiroshima Hospital, 1-5-54 Ujina-Kanda, Minami-ku, Hiroshima-shi, Hiroshima 734. Tel: +81 822 54 1818.

Hiroshima Railroad Hospital, 3-1-36 Futabanosato, Higashi-ku, Hiroshima-shi, Hiroshima 732. Tel: +81 82 262 1170.

Hyogo Prefectural Amagasaki Hospital, 1-1-1 Higashi-Oumono-cho, Amagasaki-shi, Hyogo 660. Tel: +81 6 482 1521.

Ishikawa Prefectural Central Hospital, Nu-153 Minami-Shinbo-cho, Kanazawa-shi, Ishikawa 920-02. Tel: +81 762 37 82.

Iwakuni National Hospital, 2-5-1 Kuroiso-machi, Iwakuni-shi, Yamaguchi 740. Tel: +81 827 31 7121.

Iwate Prefectural Central Hospital, 1-4-1 Ueda, Morioka-shi, Iwate 020. Tel: +81 196 53 1151.

Kagoshima Municipal Hospital, 20-17 Kajiyacho, Kagoshima-shi, Kagoshima 892. Tel: +81 992 24 2101.

Kameda General Hospital, 929 Higashi-machi, Kamogawa-shi, Chiba 296. Tel: +81 4709 2 2211.

Kanazawa National Hospital, 3-1-1 Ishibiki, Kanazawa-shi, Ishikawa 920. Tel: +81 762 62 4161.

Kansai Denryoku Hospital, 2-1-7 Fukushima, Fukushima-ku, Osaka-shi, Osaka 553. Tel: +81 6 458 5821.

Kawasaki Municipal Hospital, 12-1 Shinkawadori, Kawasaki-ku, Kawasaki-shi, Kanagawa 210. Tel: +81 44 233 5521.

Kobe Municipal Central Hospital, 4-6 Minatoshima-nakamachi, Chuo-ku, Kobe-shi, Hyogo 650. Tel: +81 78 302 4321.

Kochi Municipal Hospital, 1-7-45 Marunouchi, Kochi-shi, Kochi 780. Tel: +81 888 22 6111.

Kochi Prefectural Central Hospital, 2-7-33 Sakurai-cho, Kochi-shi, Kochi 780. Tel: +81 888 82 1211.

Kokuho Asahi Chuo Hospital, 1-1326 Asahi-shi, Chiba 289-25. Tel: +81 4796 3 8111.

Koritsu Showa Hospital, 2-450 Tenjin-cho, Kodaira-shi, Tokyo 187. Tel: +81 424 61 0052.

Kumamoto Municipal Hospital, 1-1-60 Koto, Kumamoto-shi, Kumamoto 862. Tel: +81 96 365 1711.

Kumamoto National Hospital, 1-5, Ninomaru, Kumamoto-shi, Kumamoto 860. Tel: +81 96 353 6501.

Kurashiki Central Hospital, 1-1-1 Miwa Kurashiki-shi, Okayama 710. Tel: +81 864 22 0210.

Kure Kyosai Hospital, 2-3-28 Nishi-Chuo, Naka-ku, Kure-shi, Hiroshima 737. Tel: +81 823 22 2111.

Kure National Hospital, 3-1 Aoyama-cho, Kure-shi, Hiroshima 737. Tel: +81 823 22 3111.

Kyushu Rosai Hospital, 1-3-1 Kuzuharatakamatsu, Kokuraminami-ku, Kita-Kyushu-shi, Fukuoka 800-02. Tel: +81 93 471 1121.

Maebashi Red Cross Hospital, 3-21-36 Asahi-cho, Maebashi-shi, Gunma 371. Tel: +81 272 24 4585.

Matsudo Municipal Hospital, 4005 Kamihongo, Matsudo-shi, Chiba 271. Tel: +81 473 63 2171.

Mitsui Kinen Hospital, 1 Izumi-cho, Kanda, Chiyoda-ku, Tokyo 101. Tel: +81 3 862 9111.

Miyazaki Prefectural Hospital, 5-30 Kita-Takamatsu-cho, Miyazaki 880. Tel: +81 985 24 4181.

Musashino Red Cross Hospital, 1-26-1 Kyonan-cho, Musashino-shi, Tokyo 180. Tel: +81 422 32 3111.

Nagasaki Chuo National Hospital, 2-1001-1 Hisahara, Omura-shi, Nagasaki 856. Tel: +81 957 52 3121.

Nagasaki Municipal Hospital, 6-39 Shinchi-macji, Nagasaki-shi, Nagasaki 850. Tel: +81 958 22 3251.

Nagoya Ekisaikai Hospital, 4-66 Shonen-cho, Nakagawa-ku, Nagoya-shi, Aichi 454. Tel: +81 52 652 7711.

Nagoya National Hospital, 4-1-1 Sannomaru, Naka-ku, Nagoya-shi, Aichi 460. Tel: +81 52 951 1111.

Nara Prefectural Nara Hospital, Hiramatsu-cho, Nara-shi, Nara 631. Tel: +81 742 46 6001.

National Medical Center Hospital, 1-21-1 Toyama-cho, Shinjuku-ku, Tokyo 162.

Niigata Municipal Hospital, 2-6-1 Shichikuyama, Niigata-shi, Niigata 950. Tel: +81 25 241 5151.

NTT Kanto Teishin Hospital, 5-9-22 Higashi-Gotanda, Shinagawa-ku, Tokyo 141. Tel: +81 3 448 6651.

Oita Prefectural Hospital, 2-37 Takasago-cho, Oita-shi, Oita 870. Tel: +81 975 32 5141.

Okayama Red Cross Hospital, 65-1 Aoe, Okayama-shi, Okayama 700. Tel: +81 862 22 8811.

Okayama Saiseikai General Hospital, 1-17-18 Ifuku-cho, Okayama-shi, Okayama 700. Tel: +81 862 52 2211.

Okinawa Prefectural Central Hospital, 208-3 Miyazato, Gushikawa-shi, Okinawa 904-22. Tel: +81 997 3 4111.

Oomuta Municipal Hospital, 3-3, Shiranui-cho, Oomuta-shi, Fukuoka 836. Tel: +81 944 53 1061.

Osaka-Minami National Hospital, 677-2 Kido-machi, Kawachinagano-shi, Osaka 586. Tel: +81 721 53 5761.

Osaka Prefectural Hospital, 3-1-56 Mandai-higashi Sumiyoshi-ku, Osaka-shi, Osaka 558. Tel: +81 6 692 1201.

Osaka Prefectural Nakamiya Hospital, 3-16-21 Miyanosaka, Hirakata-shi, Osaka 573. Tel: +81 720 47 3261.

Osaka Red Cross Hospital, 5-53 Fudegasaki-machi, Tennouji-ku, Osaka-shi, Osaka 543. Tel: +81 6 771 5131.

Osaka Teishin Hospital, 2-6-40 Karasugatsuji, Tenouji-ku, Osaka-shi, Osaka 543. Tel: +81 6 771 0545.

Rissho Koseikai Fuzoku Kosei Hospital, 5-25-15 Yayoi-cho, Chuo-ku, Tokyo 194. Tel: +81 3 383 1281.

St Luke International Hospital, 10-1 Akashi-cho, Nakano-ku, Tokyo 104. Tel: +81 3 541 5151.

Sakai Municipal Hospital, 2-1-1 Nishi, Shukuin-machi, Sakai-shi, Osaka 590. Tel: +81 722 38 5521.

Saku General Hospital, Ooaza-Usuda, Usuda-cho, Minami-Saku-gun, Nagano 384-03. Tel: +81 278 82 3131.

Sanraku Hospital, 2-5 Kanda-Surugadai, Chiyoda-ku, Tokyo 101. Tel: +81 3 292 3981.

Sapporo National Hospital, 2 Kikusui, Shijo, Shiraishi-ku, Sapporo-shi, Hokkaido 003. Tel: +81 11 811 9111.

Sasebo Municipal General Hospital, 10-3 Shimaji-cho, Sasebo-shi, Nagasaki 857. Tel: +81 956 24 1515.

Second Nagoya Red Cross Hospital, 2-9 Myoken-cho, Showa-ku, Nagoya-shi, Aichi 466. Tel: +81 52 832 1121.

Second Tokyo National Hospital, 2-5-1 Higashigaoka, Meguro-ku, Tokyo 152. Tel: +81 3 411 0111.

Sendai Municipal Hospital, 3-1 Shimizu-koji, Sendai-shi, Miyagi 980. Tel: +81 22 266 7111.

Shakai Hoken Hiroshima Municipal Hospital,

7-33, Moto-machi, Naka-ku, Hiroshima-shi, Hiroshima 730. Tel: +81 82 221 2291.

Shakai Hoken Kokura Hospital, 1-1 Kibune-cho, Kokurakita-ku, Kitakyushu-shi, Fukuoka 802. Tel: +81 93 921 2231.

Shizuoka Municipal Hospital, 10-93 Oute-machi, Shizuoka-shi, Shizuoka 420. Tel: +81 542 53 3125.

Shizuoka Prefectural General Hospital, 4-27-1, Kitayasu-Higashi, Shizuoka-shi, Shizuoka 420. Tel: +81 542 47 6111.

Shizuoka Red Cross Hospital, 8-2 Oute-machi, Shizuoka-shi, Shizuoka 420. Tel: +81 542 54 4311.

Shizuoka Saiseikai General Hospital, 1-1-1 Kojika, Shizuoka-shi, Shizuoka 422. Tel: +81 542 85 6171.

Sumitomo Hospital, 5-2-2 Nakanoshima, Kita-ku, Osaka-shi, Osaka 530. Tel: +81 6 443 1261.

Tachikawa Hospital, 4-2-22 Nishiki-cho, Tachikaw-shi, Tokyo 190. Tel: +81 425 23 3131.

Takayama Red Cross Hospital, 3-11 Tenma-cho, Takayama-shi, Gifu 506. Tel: +81 577 32 1111.

Takeda General Hospital, 3-27 Yamashika-machi, Aizuwakamatsu-shi, Fukushima 965. Tel: +81 242 27 5511.

Tenri Yorozu Soudansho Hospital, 20 Mishima-cho, Tenri-shi, Nara 632. Tel: +81 7436 3 5611.

Tochigi National Hospital, 1-10-37 Nakatomatsuri, Utsunomiya-shi, Tochigi 320. Tel: +81 286 22 5242.

Tokyo Metropolitan Hiroo Hospital, 2-34-10 Ebisu, Shibuya-ku, Tokyo 150. Tel: +81 3 444 1181.

Tokyo Metropolitan Komagome Hospital, 3-18-22 Honkomagome, Bunkyo-ku, Tokyo 113. Tel: +81 3 823 2101.

Tokyo Teishin Hospital, 2-14-23 Fujimi, Chiyoda-ku, Tokyo 102. Tel: +81 3 238 7144.

Tokyo-to Saiseikai Central Hospital, 1-4-17 Mita, Minato-ku, Tokyo 108. Tel: +81 3 451 8211.

Tottori Prefectural Hospital, 730 Gotsu, Tottori-shi, Tottori 680. Tel: +81 857 26 2271.

Toyama Prefectural Central Hospital, 2-2-78 Nishi-Nagae, Toyama-shi, Toyama 930. Tel: +81 764 24 1531.

Tranomon Hospital, 2-2-2 Toranomon, Minato-ku, Tokyo 105. Tel: +81 3 588 1111.

Tsu National Hospital, 1022 Shin-machi, Hisai-shi, Mie 514-11. Tel: +81 5925 5 3120.

Wakayama Red Cross Hospital, 4-1 Komatsubaradori, Wakayama-shi, Wakayama 640. Tel: +81 734 22 4171.

Yamaguchi Prefectural Central Hospital, 77 Ooaza-Ozaki, Hofu-shi, Yamaguchi 747. Tel: +81 835 22 4411.

Malaysia

Population: 20 million
Language: Malay
Capital: Kuala Lumpur
Currency: Ringgit
Int Code: +60

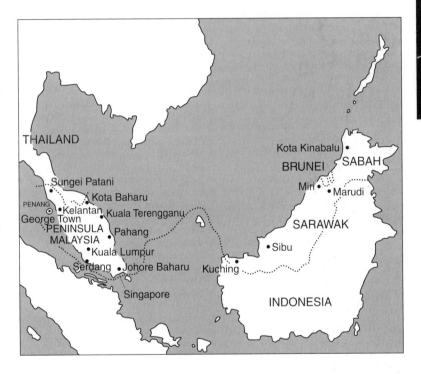

Malaysia consists of three territories: Malaya, Sarawak and Sabah. In recent years its economy has boomed and people in cities have become a lot richer, whereas those in rural areas have remained the same. It has some beautiful beaches and national parks to visit. There are three main races in Malaysia (Malay, Chinese and Indian), each with their own language and dialects. About 30% speak English, although this obviously varies between rural and city areas. This can prove some barrier in history-taking, but don't let this put you off. Most doctors and nurses speak English.

✪ Medicine:

In the cities, Western medicine is the norm, and a state-funded system exists. In rural areas, traditional medicine is still commonly practised. TB, HIV, malaria and dengue fever are relatively common.

⊃ Visas and work permits:

Commonwealth citizens do not require a visa for stays of up to 60 days. Some students however, have found that their host institution has required them to get a student visa, available either on arrival or before they went. You need four passport-sized photos and an introduction letter from the hospital (the cost is £30). Others have been told to get professional study passes. The majority, however, have been told they don't need anything. Check with your host institution and the embassy as it obviously varies.

USEFUL ADDRESSES:

Ministry of Health, Jalan Cenderasari, Kuala Lumpur 50590. Tel: +60 3 298 5077. Fax: +60 03 291 1436.

Malaysian Medical Council – address as Ministry of Health.

Malaysian Medical Association, 4th Floor, Bangunan MMA, No 124 Jalan Pahang, 53000. www.mma.org.my.

Malaysian Dental Association, 69-2, Medan Setia, 1, Plaza Damansara, Bukit Damansara, 50490 Kuala Lumpur. Tel: +60 3 255 1532/1495. Fax: +60 3 254 4670. www.mda.org.my.

Malaysian Nurses Association, PO Box 11737, GPO 50756, Kuala Lumpur. Tel: +60 3 254 3846.

West Malaysia
Kuala Lumpur

Kuala Lumpur is the capital of Malaysia and has recently undergone an economic boom. This is very evident from the abundance of huge new buildings. It is also a good base to explore the rest of peninsular Malaysia, offering easy access to Taman Nagara (the National Park) and Singapore.

University Kebangsaan Malaysia (UKM)

Faculty of Medicine, Jalan Yaacob Latiff, Bandar Tun Razak, 56000, Kuala Lumpur. Tel: +60 3 9173 3333. Fax: +60 3 9172 4568. www.medic.ukm.my.

This is the central medical school and uses:

Hospital Kuala Lumpur

Jalan Pahang, 50586 Kuala Lumpur. Tel: +60 3 292 1044. Fax: +60 3 298 9845.

The hospital: A government-run tertiary referral centre and teaching hospital for the UKM right in the city centre. It is thought to be one of the biggest hospitals in Asia with 2585 beds on over 80 wards. The doctors (200 consultants) work for either the Ministry of Health or the university. The wards are divided into first, second and third class. A general medical ward has around 60 beds with three house officers. Ward rounds start at 7 am and last about four hours.

O Elective notes: The teaching is mainly bedside during the round. Interesting cases include TB, tropical fevers (dengue and typhoid) and filariasis. AIDS and subsequent diseases are also common. There's lots of blood-taking, venflons and arterial blood gases to do but not many other practical procedures. The third-class obstetrics department sees around 80 deliveries a day, offering excellent experience. There is good teaching, although there is a question over whether it will remain a teaching hospital. Students have free rein of the second- and third-class wards. Not that many patients speak English.

Accommodation: Not provided but easily arranged and cheap. A hostel is typically 30 MYR (£4–5) a night. If you apply through the university (*see* the address above), they may be able to obtain accommodation with the residents.

Universiti Malaya

Faculti Perubatan, Lembah Pantai 59100, Kuala Lumpur. Tel: +60 3 750 2429. Fax: +60 3 755 7740. www.cc.um.edu.my.

This is the older medical school situated just outside the city. It uses:

University Hospital

Lembah Pantai 59100, Kuala Lumpur.

The hospital: This is 10 km from the city centre of Kuala Lumpur and is the teaching hospital for medical students at the University of Malaysia. It is a major tertiary referral centre. It has a friendly feel, and more patients speak English than at Hospital Kuala Lumpur. The emergency department has a five-bed resuscitation room and is one of the largest emergency departments in the country.

O **Elective notes:** There is plenty to do, with many procedures in the emergency department. The local medical students have tutorials that you are welcome to attend. The school has a very good teaching programme. Teaching is in English.

Accommodation: May be arranged on the university campus if you are persistent. Alternatively, there is a YMCA.

National Heart Institute

145 Jalan Tun Razak, 50400 Kuala Lumpur.
Tel: +60 3 298 1333. Fax: +60 3 298 2824.
The hospital: Founded in 1992 and sees increasing cardiac disease. It is in the centre of Kuala Lumpur, with 300 beds and all the facilities of a modern hospital. It is a training centre for cardiothoracic surgeons and a tertiary referral centre for all of Malaysia. The cardiology department is the largest in the country, with 10 consultants. There is a great deal of rheumatic as well as ischaemic heart disease.

Accommodation: Not provided, but cheap places are available nearby.

OUTSIDE KUALA LUMPUR

Hospital Sultanah Aminah

Jalam Skudai, 80100 Johore Bahru, Johor, West Malaysia.
The hospital: Hospital Sultanah Aminah is a 1000-bed district general hospital in Johore Baharu, a busy, thriving town in the southern-most tip of the Malaysian peninsula. Facilities and investigations are limited. Owing to the high incidence of rheumatic heart disease in Malaysia, cardiology is busy and a good place to go to practise hearing murmurs. Diseases to be seen include dengue fever, viral hepatitis, typhoid fever and TB. These often present late and at an advanced stage.

O **Elective notes:** Since it is not a teaching hospital, there are no local medical students so you have free rein through the departments.

Johore Specialist Hospital

39b Jln Abdul Samad, 80100 Johore Baharu, Johor, Western Malaysia.
The hospital: A specialist private hospital, it's very friendly. There are usually no other students.

Hospital Sungei Patani

08000 Sungei Patani, Kedah Darulaman.
The hospital: Sungei Patani is about 3 km from the town centre and easily reached by regular buses. It is the largest district hospital in the south of Kedah and acts as a secondary referral centre for the surrounding smaller towns. It has three medical wards each receiving about 200 admissions a month. There is also a six-bed ITU. There are four specialists (medical, surgical, O&G, and radiology). There are also visiting physicians from Penang.

O **Elective notes:** There are no house officers so the presence of medical students is very much appreciated. The specialists and medical officers are very keen to teach. Diseases are like those in the rest of Malaysia … TB, hepatitis B, HIV, snake bites and odd fevers. Sungei Patani is the second largest town in the state of Kedah (the 'rice-pot' of Malaysia). It is a fast-developing town (in the golden triangle of the north), with a population of 30 000. There is very little to do in Sungei Patani, but there is plenty to see in the surrounding areas.

Hospital Kuala Terengganu

Jalan Sultan Mohammed, Kuala Terengganu.
The hospital: A relatively modern busy district general hospital in the capital of Terengganu state on the east coast of peninsular Malaysia. It is a very Muslim area. The doctors and nurses speak English but the patients do not. There is lots of TB, HIV, CVAs, MIs and dengue fever.

O **Elective notes:** Very friendly. Thursday afternoons and Fridays are the weekend, but there is plenty of time off. There's not much 'hands on' practice.

There's not actually that much to do in the vicinity, but a nearby beach offers scuba diving. Four weeks may be enough.

Penang and Kelantan

Kelantan is a state on the north-east coast of peninsular Malaysia bordering Thailand. Islam is the main religion and it is the poorest state in Malaysia. Kota Baharu is the capital of Kelantan but is actually quite small. Penang is a tropical island, mainly wooded, off the west coast of Malaysia. The population totals 500 000, most of whom live in George Town where the state general hospital is situated. For an elective in Penang, write to the State Health Department for permission (The Director, Health Department, Pulau Pinang, Tingkat 37, Komtar 10590, Pulau Pinang). You will need to get an immigration visa from the office in Penang during your first week. You need a letter from the hospital, and a letter from the Department of Health.

Hospital Universiti Sains Malaysia (HUSM)

16150 Kubang Kerian, Kelantan Draul Naim. Tel: +60 9 765 1700. Fax: +60 9 765 3370. www.kck4.usm.my.

The hospital: Founded in 1979, the school of medical sciences runs its pre-clinical years on the Penang campus and the clinical years in the Kelantan campus that houses the USM teaching hospital. HUSM is the referral centre for the east coast states of peninsular Malaysia. It has 50 beds over 22 wards providing most major specialities. There is also an emergency department. Write to the chairman of the electives committee for an application form.

Penang General Hospital (Hospital Pulau Pinang)

Jalan Residensi 10990, Pulau Pinang.
The hospital: The second-largest hospital in Malaysia with all specialities; it is, for example, one of only two centres performing invasive cardiology. It is just becoming a university hospital. Equipment is sparse, but there is enough to get by. Dengue and other fevers are common, as are malaria, TB and HIV.
O **Elective notes:** It is well set up for electives; write to the deputy director at the above address. There is not much formal teaching but plenty of bedside education.
Accommodation: A wide variety is available in Penang from 12 MYR (£2) a night for a dormitory to 72 MYR (£12) a night for an air-conditioned room with shower. The YMCA is five minutes from the hospital and costs 48 MYR (£8) a night.

Hospital Lam Wah Ge

Jalan Tan Sri The Exe Him, 11600 Penang.
The hospital: Lies about an hour out of the main tourist area of Penang. It is a charity hospital where patients are means tested for the amount they can pay. Accordingly, they are classed into first-, second- and third-class patients.
O **Elective notes:** It is a very friendly hospital and, as it is not government run, there are no local students. Everyone speaks immaculate English.
Accommodation: In the college of nursing in the hospital grounds and very cheap.

Hospital Tengky Ampuan Afzan

Jalan Tanah Puteh, 25100 Kuantan, Pahang.
The hospital: A DGH with departments including emergency, paeds and O&G.
O **Elective notes:** Lots of 'hands on' experience can be gained here.
Accommodation: Can be arranged.

East Malaysia

Sarawak

Sarawak and Sabah are the Malaysian parts of Borneo. There is some beautiful countryside and it's excellent for mountaineers (as Sabah has the highest mountains in south-east Asia). In Sarawak you can visit Bako National Park, Damai Beach and Wind Cave.

USEFUL ADDRESS:

State Health Department, Tun Abang Haji Openg Rd, 93590 Kuching, Sarawak, East Malaysia.

There is a medical school on Sarawak:

Universiti Malaysia Sarawak, Faculty of Medicine

94300 Kota Samarahan, Sarawak. Tel: +60 82 671 000 ext. 208. Fax: +60 82 427 090. www.unimas.my/fmhs.

Sarawak General Hospital (Hospital Umum Sarawak)

Jalan Tun Ahmad Zaidi Adruce, 93586 Kuching, Sarawak, East Malaysia.
Tel: +60 82 257 555. Fax: +60 82 242 751.
The hospital: A relatively large, modern, busy teaching hospital in Kuching, the beautiful capital of Sarawak, well known for its rich history of culture and tradition. The emergency department admits an average of 160 patients per day and is one of the most advanced units in Malaysia.
O Elective notes: Elective students are allowed out on the ambulances where there is plenty of opportunity to practise resuscitation. In the emergency department there are histories to be taken (if you can understand them), patients to examine and minor procedures (e.g. stitching) to be done. The general medical wards (four in total) are, like the rest of Malaysia, divided into first, second and third class. Again, there are many opportunities for practical procedures. Cardiology outpatients is excellent for murmurs (as there is a high prevalence of rheumatic fever).

There is a village healthcare team that goes out to visit different villages (e.g. Batu Nah 400 km north of Kuching, 100 km south of Marudi, five hours up river through dense rainforest) providing primary healthcare. You can travel with them by either boat or jeep, a must if you really want to sample Malay life, food and hospitality. It is often the elective highlight. It is becoming more difficult to organize these trips with the healthcare teams since some Aussie students overdid it with the rice wine in one of the villages a few years back. Officially, the elective coordinator has stopped students going with them … just ask the healthcare team directly once you are there. More people tend to speak English here than in other parts of Malaysia.
Accommodation: Easy to organize as Kuching is popular with elective students and tourists. Many stay at St Thomas' Anglican Rest house (Jalan McDougall, Kuching. Tel: +60 82 414 027). There are many other elective students from Australia and Germany.

Sibu General Hospital

Batu 5 1/2, Jalan OYA, Sibu, Sarawak, East Malaysia. Tel: +60 88 434 333.
The hospital: Has two consultants covering 40 beds and offers the opportunity to see many diseases rare to the West. Diseases seen include rheumatic and dengue fever, malaria, TB and amoebic abscesses.
O Elective notes: There's 'hands on' experience in a number of procedures, including ECHO. The teaching is good, and there are usually other elective students there so you can get yourself into groups. The food is great and the locals friendly (although few speak English). Sibu itself is 2½ hours by bus from the Niah caves and a five-hour ride from Miri.

Marudi Hospital

Miri Division, East Sarawak, East Malaysia.
The hospital: A small rural hospital in a frontier town about five hours' express boat journey from Miri. It is deep in jungle. It serves not only Marudi but the local Kelabit, Kayan and Penan tribes that live along the river and in the deep interior. The hospital has four wards: male, female, paeds and maternity, each with eight to ten beds. There is a basic operating theatre, a basic X-ray department and lab facilities. The three doctors tend to be very junior (a few months to a couple of years out of school). The hospital also runs public health programmes. Lots of tropical diseases (malaria, Japanese B encephalitis) here.

Malaysia

Sabah

Queen Elizabeth Hospital

Locked Bag No 2029, 886500 Kota Kinabalu, Sabah, East Malaysia.
Tel: +60 88 218 166. Fax: +60 88 211 999.
The hospital: The Queen Elizabeth is the main teaching hospital for Sabah, with approximately 500 beds, but some have found it a bit grotty and overcrowded, although it is fairly well equipped. It has most specialities (popular ones with elective students are dermatology, paeds, O&G, ophthalmology, medicine, TB, emergency medicine, surgery, orthopaedics and radiology).
O Elective notes: You can decide what to do when you get there or rotate around. It is very busy and a good place for seeing big livers, spleens, TB, malaria etc. Kota Kinabulu is a large city (population 200 000) so there is a great deal to do. There is good teaching but not much responsibility. The local ophthalmologist takes a special interest in medical students and organizes trips to the interior and smaller district general hospitals. You'll also go out with the Lion Club (a bit like Rotary) to take free medical services to the villages in the jungle ... this has excellent reports. You get as much out as you put in. Ward rounds are in English. Half the doctors are Indian and don't speak Malay so it's not essential for you to learn it. However, like most places in Malaysia, the locals don't speak English.

There are many islands a short boat trip from Kota Kinabulu. Sipadan Island is a tiny coral island nearby, advertised as the top scuba-diving spot in the world ... it is well worth a visit but can be pricey so be prepared to haggle. Also go to Sepilok Orangutan Sanctuary, Poring Volcanic Springs and Turtle Island and climb Mount Kinabulu (4267 m). This elective is repeatedly highly recommended.

Note: To work here you have to pay MYR 100 (£25) to the hospital library.
Accommodation: Try Jack's B&B (Jalan Karamunsing Karamungsing Warehouse Lot 17, KK, Sabah. Tel: +60 88 232 367; see the Lonely Planet guide; 25 MYR (£4.50) a night. It's just 15 minutes from the hospital, clean and serves fresh pancakes for breakfast.

OTHER MALAYSIAN MEDICAL SCHOOLS:

Melaka-Manipal Medical College, Jalan Batu Hampar, Bukit Baru 75159, Melaka. Tel: +60 6 292 5851. Fax: +60 6 292 5852. www.manipal.edu.my.
International Medical University, Universiti Perubatan Antarabangsa, Sesama Centre, Plaza, Komanwel Bukit Jalil, 57000, Bukit Jalil, 57000, Kuala Lumpur. Tel: +60 38 656 7228. Fax: +60 38 656 7229. www.imu.edu.my.
Universiti Putra Malaysia, Faculty of Medicine and Health Sciences, 47400 UPM, Serdang, Selangor Darul Ehsan. Tel: +60 38 948 6101. Fax: +60 38 942 6957. www.medic.upm.edu.my.

The Maldives

Population: 300 000
Language: Dhivehi
Capital: Male
Currency: Rufiyaa
Int Code: +960

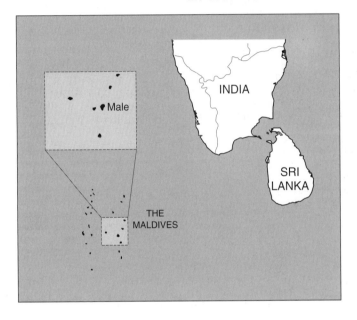

The Maldives is one of the world's poorest countries although it has become a well-known tourist destination because of its beaches. This is an Islamic country so alcohol is allowed only in expensive tourist resorts (and not even in your own home). It is not a popular elective or voluntary work destination.

✛ Medicine:

Medical care has been very poor, but things have improved dramatically over the past ten years. In 1986, the infant death rate was 63 per 1000 births; now it is less than 30. There are no medical schools. Hypertension, diabetes and infectious diseases such as typhoid, are fairly common. There is a central hospital in Male, four regional hospital and 27 Atoll health centres. Some students have found universal precautions rather lacking so it may be worth taking your own gloves and goggles.

USEFUL ADDRESSES:

Ministry of Health, Ghaazee Building, Ameer Ahmed Magu, Male 20-05. Tel: +960 323 820. Fax: +960 328 889.

Maldives Medical Council: address as Ministry of Health. www.maldivesmedicalcouncil.gov.mv.

MAIN HOSPITAL:

Indira Gandhi Memorial Hospital
Kanbaa Aisa Rani Hingun, Male. Tel: +960 316 647. Fax: +960 330 049.
The hospital: The tertiary referral hospital for the islands. It has 200 beds and most specialities.

REGIONAL HOSPITALS:

Seenu Regional Hospital
S. Hithadhoo, Addu Attoll. Tel: +960 575 045.
The hospital: Founded in 1984 with 15 beds, it now has 50 and acts as a referral centre for the whole Attoll. It has one operating theatre, laboratory facilities and an X-ray machine. It is staffed by six doctors. The patients speak Divehi, although the doctors speak English.

O **Elective notes:** As the hospital is so small, you get to know everyone very quickly. The day usually finishes about 2 pm, giving plenty of time for exploring, diving or sunbathing. There are some excellent dive spots, although the novelty of a tropical island does eventually wear off.

Accommodation: Usually provided free in a shared house a few minutes from the hospital.

Other regional hospitals are in Haa Dhaalu Kulhuduffushi, Raa Atoll Ungoofaaru and Meemu Atoli Muli (totalling 125 beds). A fifth is being built on Gaafu Dhaalu Atoll.

Nepal

Population: 21.4 million
Language: Nepali
Capital: Kathmandu
Currency: Nepalese rupee
Int Code: +977

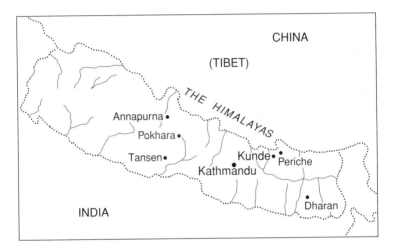

Nepal is one of the poorest countries in the world (the average income being US$150 a year), but the economy is rapidly improving. Eighty per cent of people rely on subsistence farming (hence there is no shortage of food). Seventy-four per cent are illiterate. Working here provides not only the opportunity to practise basic medicine where it is very much needed, but also some spectacular scenery in the Himalayas.

✛ Medicine:

Until recently, medicine was very primitive. There is only one doctor per 16 110 people but 100 *dharmi-jhankri* (faith healers) for every doctor. Maternal and infant mortality are very high owing to dangerous traditional birth practices. This is being tackled by a re-education programme for midwives. Patients have to pay for their healthcare. They seem small sums to us, but it often means they have to sell animals to raise the money. Infectious diseases such as TB, malaria and Japanese encephalitis are common. HIV has become a problem, mainly in the intravenous drug-using population. The incidence of leprosy is 6 per 1000 and average life expectancy is 54 years.

Most elective students go to the main hospitals in Kathmandu, but there are plenty of opportunities in rural Nepal, the Himalayas and other towns. There are a great number of charities that also do work here (*see* Section 4). Five years ago, there was only one medical school. Now there are five.

◎ Climate:

Monsoon season is July to October,

causing many floods in the Terai plain. The rest of the year is fairly warm and sunny. It can get cold between December and February.

➲ Visas and work permits:

Visitors' visas are easily obtained form the Royal Nepalese Embassy. A 60-day visa costs £30. These can be extended in Kathmandu/Pokhara. Allow two to three weeks for the visa to be processed if posted (they can do it in 24 hours if by hand). They say that no special permit is required for elective students. If you hold a medical degree from a recognized institution, you can register with the Nepal Medical Council.

USEFUL ADDRESSES:

Nepal Medical Association: www.nma.org.np.
Nepal Medical Council, Ministry of Health, Ram Shah Path, Kathmandu.
Nepal Dental Association, Kantipath, Kathmandu. Tel: +977 1 245572. Fax: +977 1 266859.

Kathmandu

Kathmandu is a big, bustling city, rapidly becoming a popular tourist destination. The people are extremely friendly. A trip in to the mountains from here is a must. The mountain villagers are very welcoming. There is jungle in the south where you can go elephant riding.

MEDICAL SCHOOLS:

Nepal Medical College, Jorpati PO Box 13344, Kathmandu. Tel: +977 1 471875. Fax: +977 1 473118. www.nmcth.edu.
Tribhuvan University, Institute of Medicine, Maharajgung, PO Box 1524, Kathmandu. Tel: +977 1 412798. Fax: +977 1 418186. (This was the country's original medical school.)

HOSPITALS:

Bir Hospital

Tundikhel, Kathmandu. Tel: +977 1 221800 (A&E 223807).
The hospital: Bir Hospital is a large, busy general hospital receiving patients from all over Nepal. It is overcrowded and dirty. All the doctors are very friend-

ly and speak good English, although few of the patients do.
O Elective notes: You are encouraged to do minor procedures and there are plenty of unusual conditions. The medical ward rounds last for ever and are mostly conducted in Nepali ... however, interesting patients are translated for you. Working here for four weeks costs $100, with $50 for each week after that. It sounds like a lot, but the hospital really does need the funds (registrars are paid £40 a month) and you get great teaching and experience in the emergency department. You can visit other hospitals, and there is time off to go trekking, etc.
Accommodation: Not provided, but there are plenty of cheap hostels and hotels in Thamel, which is close to the hospital and where most restaurants and bars are located. Food and drink are very cheap.

Kanti Children's Hospital

Maharajgunj, Kathmandu, PO Box 2664. Tel: +977 1 411550/414798.
The hospital: A large (170-bed), modern, busy government-run paediatric hospital located on the north side of Kathmandu. It is the only paediatric hospital in Nepal and provides all specialities bar orthopaedics and ENT. It has two medical wards, two surgical wards, four theatres, a neonatal ITU, a paediatric ITU, a burns unit and an emergency department. Reasonable facilities are available, including ultrasound and ECHO. There are no doctors' fees, but patients have to pay for medication (except at the doctor's discretion). Common conditions include malnutrition, congenital hip dysplasia, malaria, typhoid, Jap B encephalitis, meningitis, TB, childhood cancers and rheumatic fever. The outpatient department is chaotic, with doctors duty bound to see all patients who have paid their 6R (5p) and registered by 11 am.
O Elective notes: The teaching is excellent (the doctors speak English) and the cases interesting. A charge of $25 a week is made. When you see how desperate the patients are, you realize how much it is needed. The staff are incredibly friendly.

Electives can be in medicine, surgery or emergency medicine, or you can rotate. There are not many other students, and the day finishes around 2 pm (the doctors have to do private work as they are only paid £50 a month by the government). It has been repeatedly highly recommended. Try to get out with the Social Action Volunteers, who run clinics in the villages.

Accommodation: Not provided but easy to find.

Prasuti Griha Government Maternity Hospital

Thapathali, PO Box 5307, Kathmandu. Tel: +977 1 211243/214205.

The hospital: Nepal's main maternity hospital, with over 12 000 deliveries a year (i.e. 40 a day). There is also a small SCBU. It is well run and clean, although very lacking in resources.

O Elective notes: Lots of experience and the opportunity to do a research project.

Patan Hospital

United Mission to Nepal, PO Box 126, Patan, Kathmandu. Tel: +977 1 522266. (Work and electives here can be arranged through Interserve.)

The hospital: A district general hospital run by the government and the United Mission to Nepal (UMN). It is in a rural area of south Kathmandu. It was built in 1982 and has 150 beds, with medical, surgical, paeds and O&G wards. There is a busy outpatients seeing 200 000 patients a year. COPD (± chest infections), caused by pollution in Kathmandu valley, smoking and smokey fires is very common. TB, meningitis, rheumatic heart disease and gastroenteritis are also common. Outreach clinics take place.

Accommodation: Previously provided in a UMN guesthouse.

Pokhara

Pokhara is Nepal's second city and lies 200 km west of Kathmandu. It is an excellent base for trekking the Annapurna circuit.

MEDICAL SCHOOL:

Manipal College of Medical Science

PO Box 155, Upallo Deep, Pokhara 16. Tel: +977 6 121387. Fax: +977 2 122160. www.manipalgroup.com/mcoms.

The college is relatively new, having taken its first students in 1994. It is currently building its own 700-bed hospital, which will be made into the local teaching hospital. They also run 'eye camps', going out into the hills for a couple of weeks. All notes and medical discussions are in English.

HOSPITALS:

Western Regional Hospital

Pokhara. Tel: +977 6 120066/120461.

The hospital: Is run by the Nepali government and the International Nepal Fellowship (INF; *see* below). It has a good reputation. Surgical procedures often arise from leprosy and road traffic accidents.

Green Pastures Hospital

Pokhara.

The hospital: A tertiary leprosy referral hospital for the western region of Nepal. It is financed and staffed by the INF. It has 100 acute and 20 long-stay beds, as well as theatre facilities for reconstructive surgery. Owing to the stigma, patients with leprosy are often thrown out by their families. The hospital can arrange marriages between patients.

O Elective notes: After some teaching about leprosy, students are given jobs to do and patients to look after. There is quite a bit of responsibility. This elective is well recommended. Apply through the INF VERY EARLY (*see* page 163).

Drug Education Programme

PO Box 5, Pokhara.

The project: An 'outreach' project, going out and befriending drug addicts and alcoholics, giving out needles and condoms and trying to prevent drug use.

The language barrier can be a mild problem, but don't let that put you off. People who have worked here have found in very rewarding.

RURAL HOSPITALS:

BP Koirala Institute of Health Sciences
Dharan.
The hospital: Is on the site of a former British military hospital but is now under government control and incorporates a medical school and school of nursing. It has 150 beds. Rare diseases that are common here include TB, malaria, kala-azar, rabies and tetanus.

Amda Hospital
Damak, Jhapa.
The hospital: A welfare centre on the flatland of Nepal in Damak. Amda was set up by a Japanese-based charity for several thousand Bhutanese refugees. The UN now controls these camps.

United Mission to Nepal Hospital
Tansen.
The hospital: A mission hospital on a hill overlooking a flood plain in southwest Nepal.

UMN Okhaldunga Hospital
c/o UMN Post Box 126, Kathmandu.
The hospital: A 40-bed mission hospital built on a hillside in beautiful eastern Nepal. It is three hours' walk from the airstrip and three days' walk from the nearest road. The hospital community comprises a few Western doctors (GPs) and a few Nepali hospital workers. There are four wards and a rudimentary outpatients clinic. Common conditions include TB, pneumonia, typhoid, diarrhoea, abscesses, trauma, burns and obstetric emergencies. The language is pretty much Nepalese, although the doctors speak English.
O **Elective notes:** This elective is very highly recommended, although you may

feel isolated. There is a local bazaar 45 minutes' walk away. In theatre there is plenty to be seen and assist in. The hospital does have e-mail.
Accommodation: A guesthouse is on site.

Kunde Hospital
Kunde, near Makhe Bazaar. Postal address: c/o Himalayan Trust, PO Box 224, Kathmandu.
The hospital: Kunde Hospital is run by a charitable organization (the Himalayan Trust), set up by Sir Edmund Hilary for the Sherpa people in the Everest region. It is more of a clinic with seven long-stay and two short-stay beds but is run very well. There is an operating table/examination couch and limited X-ray machine. Sherpa people are reluctant to stay in hospital as they believe that ghosts transmit illnesses and therefore hospitals are teeming with them. An impressive immunization scheme has been successful. They will not normally take elective students.

OTHER MEDICAL SCHOOLS:

B.P. Koirala Institute of Health Sciences, Faculty of Medical and Health Science, PO Box 7053 (Kathmandu), Ghopa Camp Dharan, Sunsari District. Tel: +977 25 21017. Fax: +977 25 20251. www.bpkihs.edu.
Kathmandu University, College of Medical Sciences, PO Box 23, Bharatpur, Chitwan. Tel: +977 56 21861. Fax: +977 56 21527.

OTHER HOSPITALS:

ARGHAKHANCHI: Arghakhanchi Hospital, Arghakhanchi. Tel: +977 77 20188.
BANEPA: Scheer Memorial Mission Hospital, Banepa, PO Box 88. Tel: +977 11 61111/61112.
BHADRAPUR: Mechi Zonal Hospital, Bhadrapur. Tel: +977 23 20024/20172/20011.
BHAIRAHAWA: Lumbini Eye Hospital, Siddhartha Nagar, Bhairahawa. Tel: +977 71 20265/20668.
BIRATNAGAR: Koshi Zonal Hospital, Biratnagar. Tel: +977 21 22900/21234/25619.
Rab Lal Golcha Eye Hospital, Biratnagar. Tel: +977 21 23706/22022.
BIRGUNJ: Kedia Eye Hospital, Lipani, Birgunj. Tel: +977 51 21382.

Narayani Zonal Hospital, Birgunj.
Tel: +977 51 21993/22153.
BUTWAL: Lumbini Zonal Hospital, Butwal.
Tel: +977 73 20201/20200.
CHITWAN: Bharatpur Hospital, Bharatpur,
Chitwan. Tel: +977 56 20022.
King Mahendra Memorial Eye Hospital,
Bharatpur, Chitwan. Tel: +977 56 20333.
DAMAULI: Public Health Centre, Damauli,
Tanahun. Tel: +977 65 60119.
DANG: Mahendra Hospital, Dang.
Tel: +977 82 60119.
Rapti Eye Hospital, Tulsipur, Dang.
Tel: +977 82 20165.
**DHANGADHI: Far Western Regional Eye
Hospital**, Dhangadhi. Tel: +977 91 21112.
Seti Zonal Hospital, Dhangadhi.
Tel: +977 91 21171/21111/21271.
DHARAN: Dharan Hospital, Dharan-4.
Tel: +977 25 20134/20119.
Eastern Regional Hospital, Dharan.
Tel: +977 25 20839/20845.
GORKHA: Amppipal Mission Hospital,
Amppipal, Gorkha, PO Box 126, KTM.
Gorkha Hospital, Gorkha. Tel: +977 64 20288.
GULMI: Tamghas Hospital, Gulmi, Lumbini.
Tel: +977 79 20188.
ILAM: Ilam Hospital, Ilam. Tel: +977 27 20044.
INARUWA: Inaruwa Hospital, Inaruwa.
Tel: +977 25 20044.
JALESHWOR: Jaleshwor Hospital, Jaleshwor.
Tel: +977 44 20170/20070.
JANAKPUR: Janakpur Zonal Hospital,
Janakpurdham. Tel: +977 41 20133.
Shree Janaki Eye Care Centre, Janakpurdham.
Tel: +977 41 20133/20397.
KAPILVASTU: Taulihawa Hospital, Kapilvastu.
Tel: +977 76 60200.
**LAHAN: Sagarmatha Chaudhari Eye
Hospital**, Lahan, Siraha. Tel: +977 33 20102.
**MAHENDRANAGAR: Mahakali Zonal
Hospital**, Mahendranagar, Nepal
Tel: +977 99 21111.
MALANGAWA: Sarlahi Hospital, Malangawa,
Sarlahi. Tel: +977 46 20133/20183.
NAWALPARASI: Prithivi Chandra Hospital,
Nawalparasi. Tel: +977 78 20188.
NEPALGUNJ: Bheri Zonal Hospital,
Nepalgunj. Tel: +977 81 20158/20183/20193.
Fathe Bal Eye Hospital, Fultekra, Nepalgunj.
Tel: +977 81 20598.
PALPA: Palpa Mission Hospital, Palpa.
Tel: +977 75 20154.
POKHARA: Himalaya Eye Hospital, Dhari
Patan, Pokhara PO Box 78. Tel: +977 61 20352
Fax: 977 061 20352.
RAJBIRAJ: Sagarmatha Zonal Hospital,
Rajbiraj. Tel: +977 31 20196/20034.
SURKHET: Surkhet District Hospital,
Surkhet. Tel: +977 83 20200.
TRISHULI: Trishuli Hospital, Nuwakot, Trishuli.
Tel: +977 10 60188.

Kathmandu valley:

Anand Ban Leprosy Hospital, Tika Bhairab, Lele,
Lalitpur, GPO Box 151. Tel: +977 1 290545/290538.
Fax: +977 1 290538.

Ayurved Hospital, Naradevi, Kathmandu.
Tel: +977 1 220764/228182.
Bankali Hospital, Gaushala, Kathmandu.
Tel: +977 1 470302.
Bhaktapur Hospital, Dudhpati, Bhaktapur.
Tel: +977 1 610676/610798.
Birendra Military Hospital, Chhauni,
Kathmandu. Tel: +977 1 271940/271941/271965.
Birendra Police Hospital, Maharajgunj,
Kathmandu. Tel: +977 1 412430/412530/412630.
Central Jail Hospital, Bagh Durbar,
Tripureshwor, Kathmandu. Tel: +977 1
212442/212443.
Chest Hospital, Kalimati, Kathmandu.
Tel: +977 1 270329.
Hospital for Disabled Children, Dhobighat,
Jawalakhel, Lalitpur, GPO Box 2430.
Tel: +977 1 525578.
Infectious Diseases Hospital, Teku, Kathmandu.
Tel: +977 1 211344/211112/21294.
Maternity Hospital, Thapathali, Kathmandu,
PO Box 5307. Tel: +977 1 211243/214205.
Mental Hospital, Lagankhel, Lalitpur.
Tel: +977 1 521333.
Nepal Anti TB Hospital, Sanothimi, Bhaktapur.
Tel: +977 1 610033/610706.
Nepal Eye Hospital, Tripureshwor, Kathmandu.
Tel: +977 1 215466/213317/212102.
Patan Hospital, Lagankhel, Lalitpur, PO Box 252.
Tel: +977 1 521048/521034/522266.
Shree Pashupati Homeopathic Hospital,
Harihar Bhawan, Pulchowk, Lalitpur.
Tel: +977 1 522092.
TU Teaching Hospital, Maharajgunj, Kathmandu
PO Box 3578. Tel: +977 1
412303/412404/412505/412707.
Tokha Hospital, Tokha, Kathmandu.
Tel: +977 1 213228.

International Nepal Fellowship

69 Wentworth Road, Harborne,
Birmingham B17 9SS, UK. Tel: +44 121 427
8833. Fax: +44 0121 428 3110.
www.inf.org.np. In Nepal, their address is:
PO Box 1230, Kathmandu. E-mail:
lp@nf.wlink.com.np.

The fellowship: They are involved in
agricultural development and medical
care throughout Nepal. It is not supposed
to convert the Nepalis to Christianity,
and volunteers don't need to be Christian
but just to respect their beliefs. They run
leprosy hospitals and rural clinics in
Pokhara.

O Elective notes: There are some elective places, but these are often booked up
over a year in advance. Doing a rural
clinic elective with them comes highly
recommended. It can involve trekking
through to many villages with a couple
of nurses to do a specific project.

Accommodation: Can be arranged for a minimal cost. The INF looks after elective students well. APPLY EARLY.

United Mission to Nepal
PO Box 126, Kathmandu.
The UMN runs four hospitals in Nepal; for electives contact their UK Headquarters (*see* Section 4).

SOMETHING DIFFERENT:

For the **Himalayan Rescue Association**, *see* Section 3, 'Adventure Medicine'.

Pakistan

Population: 140.5 million
Language: Urdu
Capital: Islamabad
Currency: Pakistani rupee
Int code: + 92

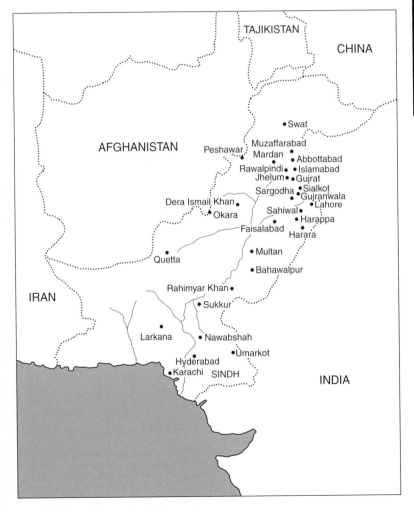

Pakistan has many political and domestic problems that unfortunately overshadow this beautiful country. It was originally created in 1947 as an independent Muslim Indian state. However, the disputes with India over Kashmir still exist and, as Islamic militancy increases, so does discrimination against other religious minorities. There is a very large social gap between the rich and the poor. The average annual income is $370, 1.7% of the average US income. Women's role in society is also very second-rate. There is a high male:female ratio, implying that female neglect and infanticide still occur. The religious make-up is 97% Muslim, 1.7% Christian and 1.5% Hindu.

Warning: Think very seriously if you intend to go to Pakistan as a single white female. The cultural differences can cause many problems. Try to go in a pair or with a male colleague. At the time of writing, there has recently been a military coup. You should probably enquire with the Foreign Office before going.

✪ Medicine:

Pakistan is the ninth most populous country. Despite population growth falling, 50% of the population is under 15 years old. The official literacy rate is 40%, but there is a wide variation. Healthcare is very poor, with a shortage of staff, equipment and medicine. Infectious diseases (malaria, TB, diarrhoea and meningitis) are common causes of death. Infant mortality is among the highest in the world. The doctor:patient ratio is 1:1918. Because of high illiteracy and it being difficult to reach isolated women who do not leave their homes, family planning and education have been difficult. Government hospitals provide free treatment to the poor. However, no medicine is supplied; it has to be purchased by the family.

Pakistan vastly overproduces doctors, many of whom leave for greener pastures. In contrast, there are very few nurses trained (approximately one for every 20 doctors). Doctors do not want to work in rural areas and there are very few female doctors.

◎ Climate and crime:

The climate can vary considerably from the north (cold) to the south (hot – over 30°C). Rainfall peaks between July and August. Crime is frighteningly high compared with other Islamic countries. There is a high incidence of murder, rape, robbery and drugs crime. Abuse of women is also a major problem.

➲ Visas and work permits:

Visas are needed for electives. You need an application form, a letter from your clinical school and two passport photos. You also need to register with police at your destination. Visas for study purposes are given after proof of acceptance at an organization in Pakistan has been demonstrated. Short-term work offers are considered on the basis of qualifications, experience, eligibility and the specific needs of the country. Doctors trained abroad usually have no problems, but check that your degree is recognized by the Pakistan Medical and Dental Council.

USEFUL ADDRESSES:

Ministry of Health, Block C, Pakistan Secretariat, Islamabad. Tel: +92 51 213 933.
Pakistan Medical Association, PMA House, Garden Road, Karachi 3. www.pma.org.pk.
Pakistan Medical and Dental Council, 30 Attaturk Avenue, Islamabad.
Pakistan Dental Association, Flat # 3, 2nd Floor, 31-C, Zamzama Commercial Lane-2, phase V, D.H.A., Karachi. Tel: +92 21 582 3196. Fax: +92 21 587 3075. www.pda.org.pk.
College of Physicians and Surgeons Pakistan, 7th Central Street, Defence Housing Authority, Karachi. Tel: +92 58 928 0110. Fax: +92 8 875 137 5500. www.cpsp.edu.pk.

Lahore

Lahore has been described as the 'Paris of Asia', like no other city. It is an excellent place for sightseeing, the Lahore Fort, Badshahi Mosque and Iqbal Park as well as the city centre. There is a great deal of Mughal history.

MEDICAL SCHOOLS AND THEIR HOSPITALS:

King Edward Medical College
University of the Punjab, Nila Gumband, Anarkali, Lahore 54000. Tel: +92 42 735 4005. Fax: +92 42 723 3796. www.kemc.edu.

Founded in 1860, this is the oldest medical school in Pakistan. It uses a number of hospitals, including the **Mayo Hospital**, **Lady Willingdon** and **Lahore General Hospitals**. The **Mayo Hospital**, one of the largest in the country, was founded in 1870 and named after the then-Viceroy of India. All specialities are available. There is an excellent range of pathologies in all subjects and a busy emergency department. Friendly staff and students.

O **Elective notes:** There are enthusiastic teachers but not much in the way of practical procedures as everyone is too busy.

Allama Iqbal Medical College
University of the Punjab, 6 Birwood Road, Lahore 54550. Tel: +92 42 516 0107. Fax: +92 42 516 0771. www.iqbalians.com.

The medical school uses the **Jinnah Hospital** as its main teaching hospital. It is relatively new, clean and not over-crowded.

O **Elective notes:** There is a great deal of pathology and opportunity to investigate and manage people under supervision in the emergency department. There is also daily teaching with the local medical students.

Accommodation: Free, but very basic.

Fatima Junnah Medical College for Women
University of the Punjab, Shahrah-e-Fatima Jinnah, Lahore 54000. Tel: +92 42 636 9469. Fax: +92 42 636 6058. www.welcome.to/fjmc.

The hopsital: Founded in 1948 as more Muslim women doctors were desperately needed. Its teaching hospital is the near 1000-bed Fatima Jinnah Hospital. It is still women only.

OTHER HOSPITALS IN LAHORE:

Shaukhat Khanum Cancer Hospital
Lahore. www.shaukatkhanum.org.pk.

The hospital: Built in 1989 by Imran Khan in memory of his mother who died of cancer. It is a first-class institution that diagnoses and treats those with cancer, irrespective of their ability to pay. It has a massive catchment area of 640 km. Most of the consultants are from the US and it has MRI and CT facilities.

O **Elective notes:** Their website has an elective application form that can be downloaded. It is incredibly well organized.

Accommodation: Very plush, with a nominal charge of 6000R (£80). Go with a friend if you can. There is a hospital car that previous students have used to go to the centre of town.

Services Hospital
Lahore.

The hospital: A government hospital. Some reports describe it as being understaffed and not that clean.

Sheikh Zayed Hospital
Lahore.

The hospital: A postgraduate hospital with many specialities. Patients have to pay a small fee to be seen here.

O **Elective notes:** Recommended for the wide range of pathology, but there is very little practical exposure.

Islamabad

Islamabad, the capital of Pakistan, is a beautiful, clean and pleasant city. It is surrounded by the Margalla Hills and Rawal Lake, making it a very enjoyable place to work. Travel to Muree, a scenic hill station, or Lahore. Hop across into India if you have a visa.

Margalla Institute of Health Sciences
Pitrus Bokhari Road, H-8/1. Tel: +92 51
443 0260. Fax: +92 51 443 0264.
www.margalla.com.
The medical school has both clinical and academic activities on the same campus. Its teaching hospitals are:

Dar-ul-Shifa Hospital, H–8/1, Islamabad. This has 150 beds expanding to 500, and all major specialities. It is for the 'poor and needy'.
Margalla Welfare Hospital, Pirwadhai, Rawalpindi. Pirwadhai is a densly populated area with some very poor pockets.
Glora Welfare Hospital (Ghosia-Mahria Trust), Gloria, Islamabad. The main campus is 15 minutes from the airport.

Quaid-I-Azam Postgraduate Medical College
Pakistan Institute of Medical Sciences, Islamabad.
The hospital: A government-run tertiary referral hospital and part of the postgraduate medical college. It is busy and overcrowded. Doctors here get paid £100 a month.

Children's Hospital
Pakistan Institute of Medical Sciences, Sector G-8, Islamabad.
The hospital: A tertiary referral hospital taking children from most of north Pakistan and Azad Kashmir. There is a wide range of illness in this multiracial society. There are many Afghanistani and Sudanese refugees. Encephalomyelitis and malnutrition are common causes of admission.
O **Elective notes:** If pushy, you can get to do procedures such as lumbar punctures and liver biopsies. Clinics also throw up a whole range of petty to life-threatening conditions. The hospital is a postgraduate teaching centre so there is plenty of teaching if you want it.
Accommodation: Provided and excellent by Pakistani standards, but the food is a bit monotonous.

OTHER MEDICAL SCHOOLS IN ISLAMABAD:

Shifa College of Medicine
Sector H-8/4, Islamabad Tel: +92 51 446 801 ext. 3367. Fax: +92 51 446 879.
www.shifacollege.edu.

Karachi

Karachi is the largest city in Pakistan.

Aga Khan University Medical College
PO Box 3500, Stadium Road, Karachi 74800. Tel: +92 21 493 0051 Fax: 21 494 6623. www.akuweb.com/medicalcollege.
The medical school was founded in 1983 and has a strong commitment to community medicine. Forty per cent of Karachi's population live in *Katchi abadis* (slums) so this, and medicine in rural Pakistan, are important areas of learning.
O **Elective notes:** There are many other students and lots of 'group seminars and tutorials' if you are into that kind of thing. The work can be quite intense. Once a week, there is community medicine. The emergency department is busy, with quite a few gunshots and punishment beatings.

Dow Medical College
University of Karachi, Baba-e-Urdu Road, Karachi. www.dmc.edu.
This is a large medical school (founded in 1945) with a 1400-bed hospital.

Sindh Medical College and Jinnah Postgraduate Medical Centre
University of Karachi, Rafiqui HI Shaheed Road, Karachi 75510. Tel: +92 21 519 00609.
This is one of the biggest teaching hospitals in Pakistan and comes under the University of Karachi. Hospitals used include the **Jinnah Postgraduate Medical Centre**, the **National Institute of Cardiovascular Diseases** and the **National Institute of Child Health**.

Liaquat National Hospital
Stadium Road, Karachi 5. Tel: +92 41 961 21314.
The hospital: Started as an outdoor hospital in 1958. It is a non-profit making, privately managed public hospital. It has 475 beds, and the outpatient department sees 550 patients a

day. There are nine operating theatres and a CT scanner. All surgical specialities, including chest and neurosurgery, are carried out.

Imam Clinic and General Hospital
ST-5 Block-I North Nazimabad, Karachi SD 74700. Tel: +92 21 662 5111.

OTHER MEDICAL SCHOOLS IN KARACHI:

Baqai Medical University, Faculty of Medicine, 51 Deh Tor Road, Baqai Chowk, PO Box 2407, Karachi 18. Tel: +92 21 635 0433. Fax: +92 21 661 7968.
Hamdard University, Hamdard College of Medicine and Dentistry, Madinat al Hikmah, Muhammad Bin Qasim Avenue, Karachi 74600. Tel: +92 21 690 0000. Fax: +92 21 699 6002. www.hamdard.edu.pk.
Karachi Medical and Dental College, F.B. Area Block 16, Karachi 75950. Tel: +92 21 632 0020.
Sir Syed College of Medical Sciences for Girls, ST-32, Block-5, Boating Basin, Clifton, Karachi. Tel: +92 21 583 5682. Fax: +92 21 583 8682. www.sscms.edu.pk.

Rawalpindi

Rawalpindi Medical College
University of the Punjab, Tipu Road, Rawalpindi 46000. Tel: +92 51 552 819. Fax: +92 51 502 148. www.rmc.edu.pk. The medical school and its hospitals serve Islamabad and Rawalpindi and act as a referral centre for Northern Punjab and Azad Kashmir. The teaching hospitals are:

Rawalpindi General Hospital (Murree Road, Rawalpindi). This is a major teaching hospital offering the basic specialities as well as psychiatry, orthopaedics, urology and cardiology. It has Rawalpindi's only CT scanner.
Holy Family Hospital. This has 400 beds (soon to increase to 800) and is all air-conditioned. It is advanced with an MRI scanner.
District Headquarters Hospital. This is in the inner city and has a trauma centre, neurosurgery and chest department.

Al Shifa Eye Hospital
Jhelum Road, Rawalpindi. www.alshifa-eye.org.pk.

The hospital: Next to the Pakistani Institute of Ophthalmology and near the city centre. Islamabad is about 30 minutes by car. The hospital receives from all of north Pakistan.
Accommodation: Cheap.

Hamdard University
Islamic International Medical College, Hummak-Islamabad, Old Supreme Court Building, 274 Peshawar Road, Rawalpindi. Tel: +92 51 556 5981. Fax: +92 51 556 5980. www.iimc.edu.pk.

Quaid-e-Azam University
Army Medical College, Abid Majid Road, Rawalpindi 46000. www.amcollege.cjb.net.

OTHER MEDICAL SCHOOLS IN PAKISTAN:

Ayub Medical College, University of Peshawar, Abbottabad. www.amc.8k.com.
Bolan Medical College, University of Baluchistan, Quetta. www.uob.cjb.net.
Chandka Medical College, University of Sind, Jamshoro, Larkana.
Gandhara Institute of Medical Sciences, Peshawar, Kabir Medical College, 57 Gul Mohar Lane, University Town, Peshawar. Tel: +92 91 844 429. Fax: +92 91 277 010. www.gandhara.edu.pk.
Khyber Medical College, University of Peshawar, Peshawar. Tel: +92 52 184 1425. Fax: +92 52 184 1598.
Liaquat Medical College, University of Sind, Jamshoro, Larkana. Tel: +92 22 177 1239. Fax: +92 22 177 1303. www.lmc.edu.pk/.
Nawabshah Medical College for Girls, University of Sind, Nawabshah.
Nishtar Medical College, Bahuddin Zakaria University, Nishtar Road, Multan. Tel: +92 61 72979. Fax: +92 61 571 648. www.nmc.paklinks.com. (Founded in 1951, it uses the Nishtar Hospital.)
Punjab Medical College, Sargodha Road, Faisalabad. Tel: +92 41 72970. Fax: +92 41 762 846. (Founded in 1970, the school uses the Allied Hospital (1150 beds) and the DHQ Hospital (500 beds) to serve Faisalabad, Pakistan's third-largest city.)
Quaid-e-Azam Medical College, Islamia University, Circular Road, Bahawalpur. Tel: +92 621 884 289. Fax: +92 621 7189. (Founded in 1970, the school uses the Bahawalpur Victoria Hospital with 1300 beds, a CT scanner and cardiac, hand and limb transplant surgery.)

Pakistan

RURAL HOSPITALS:

Kunri Christian Hospital
Kunri, Umarkot, Sindh 69160.
The hospital: Kunri is a small 'desert town' in south-east Pakistan. It is very hot (up to 40°C). It has 60 inpatient beds as well as wards for ophthalmology and TB. The hospital tends to concentrate on women and children (75% of admissions being female). Malaria, malnutrition, TB, tetanus and rickets are common. There is a busy theatre and outpatient department and a large O&G workload. It's a friendly place. All the doctors operate and it's a good place to see a wide variety of surgery, all of which is done under ketamine. There is a huge TB programme at present. It is a Christian hospital (Church of Pakistan) in a very Muslim area. This is very restrictive, especially if you are female (do not go into town alone, and make sure you wear Pakistani dress). Men can't eat with female staff. Most of the staff are Pakistani, with a couple of Westerners.
O Elective notes: A hard elective but a good experience.
Accommodation: Provided, with bed, bathroom and kitchen for 50R (80p) a night. Food is chapattis and curry for 15R.

Bach Christian Hospital
PO Qulandarabad, Abbotabad District, Harara. (Contact Interserve.)
The hospital: A mission hospital in the foothills of the Himalayas with plenty of unusual pathology.
O Elective notes: Staff very friendly and welcoming. Lots to explore, and you can visit local clinics.
Accommodation: Excellent apartment available.

Tank Christian Hospital
Tank, near Dera Ismail Khan, NWFP, Pakistan. (Contact Interserve.)
The hospital: A well-staffed and very friendly mission hospital. Tetanus, TB, malaria and gunshot wounds are relatively common. It is in a very remote area, next to the tribal homeland of the Pathans.
O Elective notes: It's a mission hospital so you should at least be sympathetic to the Christian faith. It's well staffed so there are not many procedures to do, but students have had good teaching in the past. There's not much responsibility. Excellent exploring to be done nearby.
Accommodation: Excellent flat available.

Memorial Christian Hospital
Paris Road, Sialkot 51310. Tel: +92 432 265 868. Fax: +92 432 265 869.
The hospital: Sialkot is a busy industrial town in north-east Pakistan, 10 km from the volatile Kashmir/India border. It can get VERY hot (45°C) in June and cool in winter (5–10°C). The hospital was established by the Presbyterian Church of the USA in 1886 and moved to its current site in 1932. It is run by 20 Pakistani doctors and a couple of Westerners. It has 300 beds (but 400 patients, including those in the corridors). It has basic laboratory and radiology facilities. The hospital provides care to 120 villages in a rural outreach programme. There is also a school of nursing and midwifery. Although it is charity-run, a small charge of 20p for a consultation and £2 for an admission is requested. Relatives cook meals on stoves provided by the hospital. The 'intensive care unit' has one pulse oximeter. There's plenty to see and do in outpatients.
O Elective notes: Students are supposed to be 'committed Protestant Christians in sympathy with the hospital's aims'.

Shilokh Mission Hospital
Jalapur Jattan, Gujrat District. Tel: +92 4 331 592 113.
The hospital: A 150-bed rural mission hospital run by the Sialkot Diocese Church of Pakistan. It has medical, surgical, O&G and ophthalmology services.

HOSPITALS IN PAKISTAN APPROVED BY THE PAKISTAN MEDICAL AND DENTAL COUNCIL FOR HOUSE JOB/INTERNSHIP IN ADDITION TO TEACHING HOSPITALS:

ABBOTTABAD: Civil Hospital Combined Military Hospital.
DERA ISMAIL KHAN: District Headquarters Hospital.
GUJRANWALA: Combined Military Hospital Faisal Shaheed Memorial Hospital Trust.
ISLAMABAD: Federal Government Services Hospital.
Pakistan Institute of Medical Sciences.
JHELUM: Combined Military Hospital.
District Headquarters Hospital.
KARACHI: Abbasi Shaheed Hospital.
Akhter's Eye Hospital.
Baqai Hospital.
KV Site Hospital.
Lady Dufferin Hospital.
Liaquat National Hospital.
LRBT Hospital.
Mary Adelaide Leprosy Centre.
Masoomeen Hospital.
National Institute of Child Health.
Naval Surgery.
PAF Hospital, Mauripur.
PNS Shifa.
Sind Government Hospital, Liaquatabad.
Skin and Hygiene Centre.
Social Security Hospital, Landhi.

Sobraj Maternity Home.
Spencer Eye Hospital.
SRS Hospital.
KHARIAN: Combined Military Hospital.
LAHORE: Cairns Hospital, PWR.
Combined Military Hospital.
Data Darbar Hospital.
Fatima Memorial Hospital.
Gulab Devi Hospital for Chest Diseases.
Ittefaque Hospital.
OPD Society of Rehabilitation of Disabled.
Shaikh Zayed Hospital.
Shalamar Hospital Trust.
United Christian Hospital.
LARKANA: District Headquarters Hospital
MARDAN: District Headquarters Hospital.
MULTAN: Combined Military Hospital.
MUZAFFARABAD: Combined Military Hospital.
OKARA: Combined Military Hospital.
PESHAWAR: Combined Military Hospital.
Health Care Medical Centre.
Marhaba Hospital.
QUETTA: Combined Military Hospital.
Sardar Bahadur Khan TB Sanatorium, PWR.
RAHIMYAR KHAN: District Headquarters Hospital.
RAWALPINDI: Cantonment General Hospital.
SAHIWAL: District Headquarters Hospital.
SARGODHA: District Headquarters Hospital.
PAF Base Hospital.
SIALKOT: Combined Military Hospital.
District Headquarters Hospital.
SUKKUR: District Headquarters Hospital.
SWAT: Saidu Group Hospitals.
WAH CANTT: POF Hospital.

Papua New Guinea

Population: 4.5 million
Languages: English and Motu
Capital: Port Moresby
Currency: Kina
Int Code +675

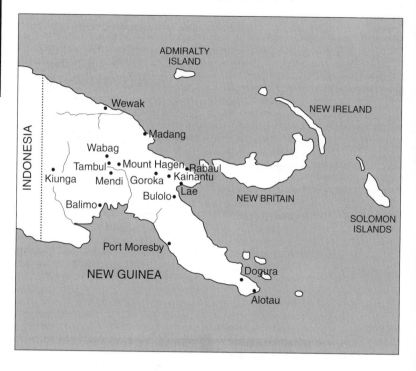

Papua New Guinea is a fascinating place. It consists of 600 islands 160 km north of Australia. It has great diversity, from volcanic highlands to tropical beaches and swamps. It has more languages (over 700) than any other country in the world. Most people, however, can speak Pidgin. Since it gained independence from Australia in 1975, not a lot has changed. Many areas are still

extremely remote and do not have easy access to medical care.

✛ Medicine:

In each province there is a government-run hospital, but this doesn't amount to much. A number of missionary hospitals provide care in deep jungle. Very few Westerners go to the government-run ones so the latter will be concentrated on here. The health system makes best use of the few doctors, and nurses often treat patients alone, only asking the doctor if they are unsure. Infectious diseases, for example TB (of every part of the body), malaria, leprosy and elephantiasis, are extremely common, especially in the Western Province. In paeds, it's malnutrition and pneumonia. In some areas, hypertension and type II diabetes are increasing as the diet is becoming westernized. Orthopaedics is busy because of the country's outdoor work, houses on stilts and passion for rugby. There are, however, very few orthopaedic operations for risk of infection. Cases are all treated with traction. Trauma and violence are very common for a number of reasons:

- Alcohol (since it was legalized with independence) has created a major problem. There is a culture of going out and getting completely trashed. Marijuana use is also increasing. Violence stems directly from the alcohol as well as from the need for money to fund it.
- Women get a rough time, as shown by the fact the government has had to produce a leaflet entitled 'Wife Beating is Illegal'. In many parts of the country, women are not allowed to initiate a conversation with a man; they don't eat at the same table or even sleep in the same house as men (including their husband). A wife has to be bought by her husband, but with high unemployment and low pay, many cannot afford 20 pigs, etc., so rape has become a major problem. It isn't reported, not that the authorities would do anything anyway.
- 'Payback' is an inherent part of the culture. If your clan has a grievance with a member of another clan, you all get together and knife him (or anyone in his clan), sparking a vicious cycle. Sixty per cent of the population is under 24, and many of these young men are unemployed, with no social role and nothing else to do.

○ Visas and work permits:

A visa (£7) is required for an elective, and a work permit to work here. Contact the High Commission.

Note: Girls, beware ... most of the smaller communities are fine (although it is advisable to wear a long skirt), but the capital (Port Moresby) is not that safe for single white females. Try to observe local customs. Use common sense: Friday (pay-day) is not a good day to go to town as all the locals will be getting pissed and rowdy.

USEFUL ADDRESSES:

Department of Health, PO Box 3991, Boroko, Port Moresby. Tel: +675 324 8600. Fax: +675 325 0826.
Papua New Guinea Dental Association, Department of Health, PO Box 807, Waigani. Tel: +675 301 3781. Fax: +675 323 1640.

Port Moresby

The capital has Papua New Guinea's only medical school.

University of Papua New Guinea

Faculty of Medicine, PO Box 5623, Boroko. www.upng.ac.pg.
This has a busy teaching hospital (**Port Moresby General Hospital**, Free Mail Bag, Boroko 111. Tel: +675 324 8200. Fax: +675325 0342) with 600–700 deliveries a month. It's the only tertiary referral centre in the country.

RURAL HOSPITALS:

Sopas Adventist Hospital

PO Box 112, Wabag, Enga Province. Fax: +675 54 71231.
The hospital: A busy hospital with around 100 beds and floor space. Outpatients is also very busy. There are usually only one or two doctors so students are very much appreciated and will find they are running clinics fairly quickly. There are many bush-knife and gunshot wounds as the locals here still

believe in payback and tribal fighting despite their conversion the Christianity. Two full days a week are devoted to surgery.

O **Elective notes:** The hospital is pretty isolated and it is only really safe to go out with hospital staff. Try to go with someone else. It is all friendly, but everyone is very busy. Overall, people have thoroughly enjoyed it. You do not need to be an Adventist or a Christian to go here. There are also nursing students. Enga Province is remote and in the beautiful cool tropical rainforest highlands. It was one of the last areas to be 'discovered'. Most of the locals are subsistence farmers. It is a 'dry' province so leave the duty free at home (cars are occasionally searched).

Wewak General Hospital

PO Box 395, Wewak, East Sepik Province.
The hospital: Wewak is one of the main hospitals (365 beds) on the north coast of Papua New Guinea and receives referrals from smaller hospitals in the region. Specialities include medicine, surgery, O&G, and paeds. There is a severe lack of facilities. Mobile clinics are also run from here. The only way to get to the villages along the Sepik River is by canoe. Conditions seen include: malaria (+++), TB, broken limbs (wife- and daughter-beating), asthma, meningitis and pneumonia. The staff are incredibly welcoming and friendly.

O **Elective notes:** There are plenty of practical procedures in the emergency department and loads of deliveries and operations in O&G. It's excellent for surgery too. The hospital is on a beautiful coastline with golden sand and blue sea.
Accommodation: A backpackers' lodge is in town, but something usually becomes available in the hospital.

St Barnabus Health Centre

PO Box 21, Dogura, Milne Bay Province.
The hospital: Dogura is a very small rural village with one basic store, a school and the health centre. The health centre consists of an outpatients, a theatre and four wards. The facilities are very poor. There are beds but few mattresses. There's a very old X-ray and ultrasound machine. The centre is currently run by one VSO doctor (who also does surgery), one VSO midwife and six local nurses. The 'patrol' goes out into the mountains (for days) to do rural clinics and immunization. The hospital has electricity for three hours a day. The phone is (intermittently) run from a car battery. Malaria is the major problem here with 30% of cases being chloroquine resistant.

O **Elective notes:** This elective comes extremely highly recommended if you want a bit of responsibility with the chance to practise clinical skills in a friendly developing world setting. There are excellent beaches and it's a good spot for snorkelling and walking. This is a beautiful part of the country. Dogura is a ten-minute flight from Alotau, i.e. very isolated. Alotau itself is a small town with one hotel (expensive £40 a night). Get anything you may need here before going to Dogura.
Accommodation: Has previously been provided.

Nazarene Hospital

PO Box 456, Mount Hagen, WHP.
The hospital: A 100-bed general mission hospital, consisting of medical, surgical, paeds and O&G wards. There is one operating theatre, an outpatients, emergency department and pharmacy. It's run by three or four doctors (mainly American missionaries).

O **Elective notes:** There are excellent opportunities for students in both outpatients and theatre with plenty of responsibility when on call without the feeling of being left alone or dumped on. Learn Pidgin before you go as it means you can converse directly with patients. Note: this is a Christian mission run by an American missionary. You should probably be Christian if applying. No smoking or drinking is allowed on site. Girls need to wear a skirt. Also, the surrounding areas are not safe so you shouldn't go out alone. Highly recommended though.
Accommodation: Provided.

OTHER HOSPITALS:

Angau Memorial Hospital, PO Box 457, Lae.
Tel: +675 432100. Fax: +675 423015.
Goroka Base Hospital, PO Box 393, Goroka. Tel:
+675 712100. Fax: +675 721081. (Goroka is anoth-
er hospital that's well recommended.)
Kainantu Hospital. (Kainantu is in the highlands.
It has 125 beds.)
Madang General Hospital, PO Box 2115,
Madang. Tel: +675 822022. Fax: +675 823038.
Mendi Hospital. (Mendi in the highlands has a
good student programme and comes recommend-
ed.)
Nonga Base Hospital, Free Mail Bag, Rabaul. Tel:
+675 927333. Fax: +675 927331.
Veiferi'a Hospital, Veiferi'a. (This is a Catholic
mission hospital.)

UFM-RUN HOSPITALS:

Contact UFM Worldwide, 47a Fleet
Street, Swindon, Wiltshire SN1 1RE, UK.
Tel: +44 1793 432255. www.ufm.org.uk
A Christian faith is a prerequisite to work
here. They will usually want to meet
you. They can provide accommodation
at their hospitals.

Rumginae Health Centre

PO Box 41, Kiunga, Western Province.
Fax: +675 583416.
The hospital: Rumginae is in a tropical
jungle near the source of the Fly River.
The hopsital has 60 beds with three doctors serving 20 000 people. Resources
are limited, but it provides a good service. It has medical, TB, antenatal and

postnatal wards. There is a minor operation theatre but major stuff goes to
Tabubil (100 km away). There is a busy
outpatients run entirely by nurses and
community healthcare workers. X-rays
and ultrasound can be done.

Balimo Health Centre

PO Box 4, Balimo, Western Province. Fax:
+675 661492.
The hospital: Set in the flood plain of
the Aramia River (with crocodiles).
Balimo is a health centre rather than a
government-run hospital. However, it
has a surgeon (unlike the government-
run hospital) and a school of nursing
(nurses being trained to diagnose and
refer). Balimo has 100 beds, with wards
for surgery, general medicine, acute
admissions, nutrition, leprosy and TB. It
has a well-equipped operating theatre. It
serves 30 000 but receives referrals from
all over the Western Province. There is a
busy outpatients. Medical patrols extend
the work to villages upstream. Some of
these are up to nine hours away in a
dugout canoe. TB, malaria and leprosy
are common.
O Elective notes: In addition to ward
rounds and clinics, radio 'sked' is a
lunchtime affair in which doctors in
Balimo give advice to surrounding
health workers in other villages via
short-wave radio. Students can also carry
out a few minor procedures.

Philippines

Population: 70 million
Languages: Pilipino and English
Capital: Manila
Currency: Philippine peso
Int Code: +632

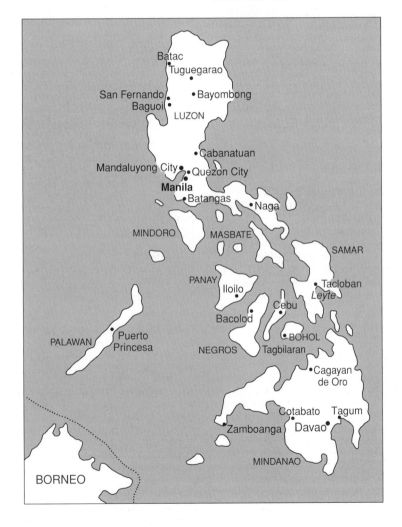

The Philippines are in the west of the Pacific Ocean and comprise over 7000 separate islands in three main groups (the Luzon, Visayan and Mindanao/Sulu islands). It's a land where earthquakes and volcanoes tend to keep the people poor. Most in the country are Catholic, although Islamic in the south. Very few of the local population can speak English. This and the lack of translators does not make the Philippines a popular elective destination.

✪ Medicine:

Most people have to pay for healthcare, which even then is pretty poor. Most hospitals are private although there are few government ones. Infectious diseases, including TB and typhoid, are common. Malaria however, has been successfully reduced.

➲ Visas and work permits:

A temporary non-immigrant visitor's visa should be applied for in person at the embassy. You will need a passport, one photo, proof you can fund yourself and, ideally, a letter from the hospital where you're going. Visas can usually be picked up the next day. They will deal with postal applications if a registered SAE is enclosed. A student visa is required if enrolling on a course. Tell the embassy that you are only shadowing for a few weeks and ensure that they are happy that you don't need a student visa (which is a lot more hassle and cost). Work permits require a petition from the institution employing you.

USEFUL ADDRESSES:

Department of Health, San Lazaro Compound, Rizal Avenue, Sta. Cruz, Manila. Tel: +632 711 9502/9503. Fax: +632 743 1829. www.doh.gov.ph. (This website provides details on all hospitals in the Phillipines and also has links to every medical organization – from the Phillipine College of Surgeons to the Phillipine Society of Climacteric Medicine! It even has a National Health Atlas.)
Philippine Medical Association, Secretariat PMA Building, North Avenue, Quezon City. PO Box 4039 Manila. Tel: +632 929 3514. Fax: +632 929 4974. www.pmasite.org.ph.
Philippine Nurses Association, 1663, FT Benitez Street, Malate, Manila 1004. Tel: +632 258 3092.

Philippine Dental Association, Ayala Avenue, Cor Komagong Street, Makati, Metro Manila 1200. www.pda.org.ph.

Organizations for doctors:
Philippine College of Surgeons Corporate Address, 3rd Floor PCS Building, 992 Edsa, Quezon City 1005. Tel: +632 929 2359. Fax: +632 929 2297. www.pcs.org.ph.
Philippine College of Physicians, Unit 2201–2203, 22nd Floor, 1 San Miguel Avenue, cor Shaw Boulevard, Ortigas, Pasig City 1600. Tel: +632 910 2250. Fax: +632 910 2251. www.pcponline.home.ph.
Check the Philippines Department of Health's website for more links.

Manila

Manila is a huge city with a major traffic problem. There are plenty of cinemas, restaurants and shops. There are some nice beaches nearby while inland are rainforests and volcanoes. The people are friendly, with a great sense of humour. There are 27 medical schools in the Philippines, five of which are in Manila. It is usually best to arrange an elective directly with the hospital and therefore all of the major regional hospitals are listed below. The oldest medical school in Manila is:

University Santo Tomás
Catholic University of the Philippines, Faculty of Medicine and Surgery, España Street, Manila 2801.
It uses:

Philippines General Hospital
Taft Avenue, Manila. Tel: +632 521 8450. Fax: +632 524 2221. www.pgh.gov.ph.
The hospital: A tertiary referral centre receiving patients from all over the country. It also acts as a teaching hospital for a number of universities. It has nearly 2000 beds crammed into wards of 50 patients and sees 700 000 patients a year. It is a government hospital but patients have to pay for medications; otherwise, doctors or charities pay. It is very poorly equipped. TB, rheumatic fever and heart diseases are fairly common.
✪ **Elective notes:** Write to the Clinical Director. Patients don't speak English,

but the doctors do (albeit with an American accent).

SPECIALITY AND MAJOR HOSIPTALS:

Dr Jose Fabella Memorial Hospital, Lope de Vega, Santa Cruz, 1003 Manila. Tel: +632 734 5561. www.doh.ph/quert/jfmh.
Lung Center of the Philippines, Quezon Avenue, Quezon, Metro Manila. Tel: +632 924 6101. Fax: +632 924 0696. www.doh.gov.ph/quert/lcp.
National Center for Mental Health, Nueve de Febrero Street, Mandaluyong City, Metro Manila. Tel: +632 531 8682.
National Kidney Institute, East Avenue, Quezon City, Metro Manila. Tel: +632 924 3601. Fax: +632 924 0701. www.kidney.gov.ph.
Philippine Children's Medical Center, Quezon Avenue, Quezon City, Metro Manila. Tel: +632 924 6601. Fax: +632 924 0840. www.doh.gov.ph/quert/pcmc.
Philippine Heart Center, East Avenue, Quezon City, Metro Manila 1100. Tel: +632 923 1301. Fax: +632 922 0551. www.phc.gov.ph.
Philippine Orthopaedic Center, Banawe Avenue, Quezon City, Metro Manila. Tel: +632 712 4569. Fax: +632 712 4746.
San Lazaro Hospital, Quiricada Street, Santa Cruz 1003, Manila. Tel: +632 732 3776. Fax: +632 711 6966.

RESEARCH HOSPITALS:

Institute for Tropical Medicine, Alabang, Muntinlupa. Tel: +632 842 2828. Fax: +632 842 2245.
Schistosomiasis Control and Research Hospital, Palo, North Leyte. Tel: +632 53 323 3083.

OTHER HOSPITALS IN MANILA:

Capitol Medical Center, Scout Magbanua St, Quezon City. Tel: +632 99 15 71. Fax: +632 928 1571.
Cardinal Santos Medical Center, Wilson St, San Juan. Tel: +632 721 3361. Fax: +632 78 5 60.
Children's Medical Center, Phils, Inc, 11 Banawe St, Quezon City. Tel: +632 712 0845. Fax: +632 712 0801.
Chinese General Hospital, 286 Blumentritt, Manila. Tel: +632 711 4141. Fax: +632 711 3967.
De Los Santos Medical Center, 201E Rodriguez Sr. Boulevard, Quezon City. Tel: +632 78 70 11.
Dr Jesus C. Delgado Memorial Hospital, 7 Kamuning Road, Quezon City. Tel: +632 96 53 63 Fax: +632 926 53 63.
Makati Medical Center, 2 Amorsolo St, Makati. Tel: +632 815 99 11.
Medical Center Manila, 1122 Gen Luna St, Ermita, Manila. Tel: +632 59 16 61. Fax: +632 59 00 21.

Medical City General Hospital, Lourdes Drive, Ortigas Business Complex, Mandaluyong. Tel: +632 631 8626.
Olivarez General Hospital, Sucat Road, Paranaque. Tel: +632 828 7966. Fax: +632 827 8747.
St Luke's Medical Center, 279 E Rodriguez Sr Boulevard, Quezon City. Tel: +632 722 6161.

MEDICAL CENTRES:

Baguio General Hospital and Medical Center, Baguio City 2600. Tel: +632 74 442 3738.
Davao Medical Center, Davao City, Davao del Sur. Tel: +632 082 73974.
Dr P. Garcia Memorial Research and Medical Center, Cabanatuan City, 3100 Nueva Ecija. Tel: +632 44 463 1607.
East Avenue Medical Center, East Avenue, Diliman, Quezon City, Metro Manila. Tel: +632 98 0611.
Jose R. Reyes Memorial Medical Center, Rizal Avenue, Sta Cruz, 1003 Manila. Tel: +632 711 9491. Fax: +632 732 1077.
Mariano Marcos Memorial Hospital and Medical Center, Batac, Ilocos Norte. Tel: +632 77 792 3144.
Rizal Medical Center, Pasig, Rozal, Metro Manila. Tel: +632 671 4216. Fax: +632 671 4216.
Vicente Sotto Sr Memorial Medical Center, Cebu City. Tel: +632 72801.
Western Visayas Medical Center, Mandurriao, Iloilo City. Tel: +632 33 77742.
Zamboanga Medical Center, Zamboanga City. Tel: +632 62 991 0573.

Palawan

Palawan is a small island on the west of the Philippines. It has been largely unspoilt by Western influence. Travel around the island can be slow with many roads closed. The alternative method of transport is by sea.

Palawan Provincial Hospital

Puerto Princesa, Palawan.

The hospital: The people in the hospital (100 beds) are very friendly and keen to practise their English. There is a fair bit of malaria, TB and gastroenteritis. In the emergency department you'll need an interpreter as the locals do not speak enough English. Most of the illnesses are fairly basic (e.g. dehydration) but in the extreme.

O Elective notes: The clinical director is a top chap from Ipswich.

OTHER REGIONAL HOSPITALS:

Batangas Regional Hospital, Batangas City.
Tel: +632 43 725 2011.
Bicol Regional Hospital, Naga City, Camarines
Sur. Tel: +632 5421 332 775.
Cagayan Valley Regional Hospital, Tuguegarao,
Cagayan. Tel: +632 78 446 1410.
Cotabato Regional Hospital, Cotabato City
9600. Tel: +632 64 212 373.
Davao Regional Hospital, Tagum, Davao Del
Norte. Tel: +632 82 701 0747.
Eastern Visayas Regional Medical Center,
Tacloban City, Leyte. Tel: +632 38 321 3129.
Governor G. Galleres Memorial Hospital,
Tagbiliran City, Bohol. Tel: +632 38 3165.

Ilocos Regional Hospital, San Fernando, Ilocos.
Tel: +632 72 412 691.
Jose B. Lingad Memorial General Hospital,
San Fernando, La Union. Tel: +632 44 961 3921.
**Mariano Marcos Veterans Memorial
Hospital**, Bayombong, 3700 Nueva Vizcya.
Tel: +632 321 2090.
**Northern Mindanao Regional Training
Hospital**, Cagayan de Oro City.
Tel: +632 8822 3646.
Quirino Memorial Medical Center, Quirino
Compound, Project 4, Quezon City.
Tel/fax: +632 721 3089.
Tondo Medical Center, Balut, Tondo.
Tel: +632 251 8420.
Western Visayas Regional Hospital, Bacolod
City. Tel: +632 34 74131.

Singapore

Population: 2.8 million
Official Languages: Malay, Chinese,
Tamil and English
Capital: Singapore City
Currency: Singapore dollar
Int Code: +65

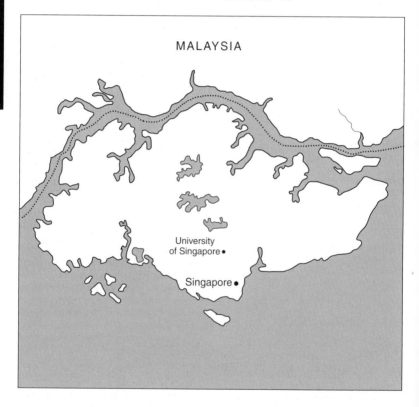

MALAYSIA

University
of Singapore •

Singapore •

Singapore is a lovely island country in south-east Asia with nearly three million inhabitants in a space less than the distance from Edinburgh to Glasgow. Despite this, there are many green areas, and the environment is very clean.

✛ Medicine:

Singapore has an advanced, efficient health system. This is due partly to its wealth but also to the fact that the people are encouraged to preserve the extended family and therefore care for elderly relatives at home. There's one medical school and three major government-subsidized general hospitals: **Singapore General**, **Tan Tock Seng** and the **National University Hospital**. The **Eastern General Hospital** is just being completed. Primary care consists of private GPs and government polyclinics. Private practice is very much on the rise in Singapore.

The government has introduced a scheme of mandatory saving so that a proportion of salary goes into a fund that can be used for a pension or healthcare. The proportion of the bill to be paid by patients is set at a different level depending on their 'class': class A patients also get better rooms; class C gets the same treatments without the frilly bits (typically 30 beds to a ward). Older patents speak only their Chinese dialect or Malay or Tamil. Communication between staff is usually in English. The leading causes of mortality are heart/cerebrovascular diseases and cancers.

◒ Visas and work permits:
Any foreigner wishing to study in Singapore needs a student pass. To obtain one of these you need to:
- Fill in a student pass application form (Form 16, available from the Singapore High Commission (*see* below))
- Send two passport-sized photographs
- Send two copies of your passport
- Send two copies of the acceptance letter from the college/university in Singapore.

Note: It can take up to six weeks to process your application. They may then ask you to pay a security deposit. The cost of a student pass is S$15 a year.

The dispensing of employment passes has recently changed from the Ministry of Home Affairs to the Ministry of Manpower (contact the Work Permit Department at +65 5383033 or Singapore Immigration and Registration at +65 3916100). As a doctor, you will probably need a P pass; as a paramedical professional, you may need a Q pass. Full details are available from the High Commission or MOM's Employment Pass Department (Fifth Floor, SIR Building, 10 Kallang Road, Singapore 208718).

USEFUL ADDRESSES:

For employment opportunities, contact the centre director in London at **Contact Singapore** (Charles House, Lower Ground Floor, 5–11 Regent Street, London SW1Y 4LR, UK. Tel: +44 20 7976 2090. Fax: +44 20 7976 2091. E-mail: cslondon@sings.demon.co.uk).

A licence to practise medicine is available after completing 1 year as a houseman at an approved hospital; it can be obtained from the **Singapore Medical Council** (address below).

Ministry of Health, College of Medicine, 16 College Road, Singapore 169854. Tel: +65 325 9220. Fax: +65 224 1677. www.gov.sg/moh.
Singapore Medical Association, 2 College Road, Level 2, Alumni Medical Centre, Singapore 169850. Tel: +65 223 1264. Fax: +65 224 7827. www.sma.org.sg.
Singapore Medical Council, College of Medicine Building, 16 College Road, Singapore 169854. Tel: +65 223 7777. Fax: +65 224 1677.
Singapore Nurses Association, 77 Maude Road, Singapore 208353. Tel: +65 392 0770. Fax: +65 392 7877. www.sna.org.sg.
Singapore Dental Association, 2 College Road, Singapore 169850. Tel: +65 220 2588. Fax:+65 6224 7967. www.sda.org.sg.
Singapore Physiotherapy Association, Tanglin, PO Box 442, Singapore. Tel: +65 329 0331. Fax: +65 227 3738.
Singapore Association of Occupational Therapists, Orchard, PO Box 0475, Singapore.

MEDICAL SCHOOL:

National University of Singapore
Faculty of Medicine, 10 Medical Drive, Singapore 117597. Tel: +65 874 3297. Fax: +65 778 5743. www.med.nus.edu.sg.
This was founded in 1905 and has access to over 5000 beds. The language of instruction is English. They have a very well-organized elective programme and will send you a list of hospitals (including the three big ones) and departments you can choose from. They can arrange accommodation at minimal cost (the

National being nearest to the halls). Some students have previously arranged electives directly with the hospital.

Note: Singapore students have a summer holiday between March and June and some departments won't take students between these months. For those that do, there will be little structured teaching. Between November and February is a good time to go as the students have finals and there are therefore many revision sessions. By March (when they have finals) everyone is too stressed to care!

Another useful address is:

Graduate School of Medical Studies

National University of Singapore, Blk MD5, Level 3, 12 Medical Drive, Singapore 117598. Tel: +65 874 3353. Fax: +65 773 1462.

HOSPITALS:

National University Hospital

5 Lower Kent Ridge Road, Singapore 119074. Tel: +65 6779 5555. Fax: +65 6779 5678. www.nuh.com.sg.

The hospital: A large 957-bed tertiary hospital (opened in 1985) that also has the National University Children's Medical Centre on its grounds. Both have every speciality imaginable, right down to hand and reconstructive microsurgery.

Singapore General Hospital

Outram Road, Singapore 169608. www.sgh.com.sg.

The hospital: The country's largest (1600-bed) teaching hospital catering for a huge proportion of the Singapore population. It is divided into seven blocks of eight floors each. It is very busy and there is a wide range of pathology. All specialities, including emergency medicine and a department of forensic medicine, are here. The doctors have heavy workloads.

O Elective notes: Try to go in term time. Highly recommended.

Accommodation: Previously available in a houseman's quarters for S$818 (£300) for seven weeks.

Tan Tock Seng Hospital

11 Jalan Tan Tock Seng, Singapore 308433. Tel: +65 256 6011. Fax: +65 252 7282. www.ttsh.com.sg.

The hospital: One of the hospitals affiliated to the National University of Singapore. It was established in 1844 as the first and only local hospital for the sick and poor. It is in fairly old buildings but a new, modern, 14-storey block (providing 1211 beds) has just been built. It is well known for its stroke centre (neurology, neurosurgery and rehab) and respiratory medicine. It is the second-largest general hospital in Singapore. It is not far from the city centre and next to an SMRT train station. Most conditions are similar to those of other developed countries, although type II diabetes is more prevalent. There is usually excellent teaching with the local students. The surgery department is reputed to be the best in Singapore. The head of the department is extremely amiable and approachable, and an excellent teacher. This elective is great revision for surgical finals, although most time is spent in outpatients, not theatre.

Alexandra Hospital

Alexandra Road, Singapore 159964. Tel: +65 473 5222 Fax: +65 479 3183. www.alexhosp.com.sg.

The hospital: You can take a vitual tour of this 400 bed hospital from the website!

Changi General Hospital

2 Simei Street 3, Singapore 529889. Tel: +65 6788 8833. Fax: +65 6788 0933. www.cgh.com.sg.

The hospital: This nine-storey, 801-bedded hospital provides all specialities from sports medicine to neurosurgery.

Woodbridge Hospital

Institute of Mental Health, 10 Buangkok Green, Singapore 539747.

SOME SPECIALIST AREAS:

KK Womens and Childrens Hospital, 100 Bukit Timah Road, Singapore 229899. Tel: +65 293 4044. Fax: ++65 293 7933. www.kkh.com.sg. (This is Singapore's principal paediatric and O&G hospital.)
National Cancer Centre, 11 Hospital Drive, Singapore 169610. Tel: +65 436 8000. Fax: +65 225 6283. www.nccs.com.sg.
National Heart Centre, Mistri Wing, 17 Third Hospital Avenue, Singapore 168752. Tel: +65 436 7800. Fax: +65 221 0944. www.nhc.com.sg.
National Neuroscience Institute, 11 Jalan Tock Seng, Singapore 308433. Tel: +65 357 7153. Fax: +65 256 4755. www.nni.com.sg.
Singapore National Eye Centre, 11 Third Hospital Avenue, Singapore 168751. Tel: +65 227 7255. Fax: +65 227 7290. www.snec.com.sg. (This is the principal specialist eye facility in Singapore and in the compound of Singapore General Hospital.)

HOSPICE CARE:

Hospice Care Association, 6 Dunearn Road, Singapore 1130.

SOMETHING DIFFERENT:

Institute of Science and Forensic Medicine

11 Outram Road, Singapore 169078. Fax: +65 229 0749. www.gov.sg/moh/isfm.
The institute has seven forensic pathologists and deals with the gruesome and not-so-gruesome aspects of forensic pathology.

Sri Lanka

Population: 19 million
Language: Sinhalese
Capital: Colombo
Currency: Sri Lanka rupee
Int Code: +94

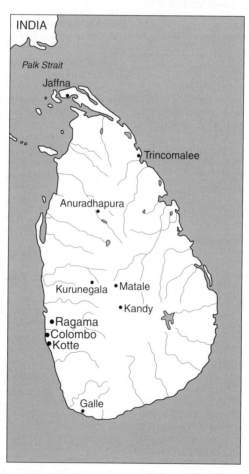

INDIA

Palk Strait

Jaffna

Trincomalee

Anuradhapura

Kurunegala •Matale

•Kandy

•Ragama
•Colombo
•Kotte

Galle

Sri Lanka is definitely worth a visit. It's small enough to explore thoroughly in a relatively short time but there is plenty to do. The capital, Colombo, is dirty and typically developing world, but further south the beaches are astonishingly beautiful. To the north there are many tourist attractions. Kandy is a very pretty city set up high in the hills and therefore relatively cool. It's an ideal base for seeing the rest of the island. The bus and train services are very good and cheap. With 1000 miles of beaches, Sri Lanka offers superb snorkelling and diving. There is also a very rich history. Visit Anuradhapura, the ancient capital from 380BC, and Polonnaruwa from AD 1100. The rugged central uplands offer a number of mountains with shrines and fortresses on the summit. Go on safari in Yalla and Wilpattu. In Nuwala Eliya, if you're smart enough (jacket and tie) you can visit the Hill Club. The cost of living is generally much higher than you might have expected … beware of touts and con merchants. The civil war in which the Tamils are fighting for an independent state is in the north-east area of the island. DO NOT GO THERE.

✪ Medicine:

Medical training follows the British system since it is a former colony. Therefore notes are written in English and all the doctors speak it. Many people in large towns can also speak it; if they can't, there is usually someone around to translate. There are two systems of medicine:

- Western medicine, practised by fully qualified doctors who have done five years of training at one of the five medical schools. They are aided by assistant medical practitioners (AMPs or apothecaries) who have done two years of Western training and practise mainly in rural areas
- Auyrvedic (indigenous) medicine practised by many rural people.

The primary care service is provided by Western-style GPs and small surgeries run by AMPs in rural areas. These provide good maternity and paediatric care. Secondary healthcare consists of remote 'one-man stations' with a doctor or AMP and 'base' hospitals in towns. These provide general medical, surgical, obs and paeds facilities. Tertiary care is provided by one of the big town hospitals. They are often poorly equipped and overcrowded. A few people pay for private care. Infectious diseases including malaria and TB are pretty common.

➲ Visas and work permits:

A visitors' visa is required for an elective. Contact the embassy for details on this and work permits.

USEFUL ADDRESSES:

Ministry of Health, 385 'Suwasiripaya', Dean Road, Colombo 10. Tel: +94 698475. Fax: 692913. www.gov.lk/Ministry/health. (This website lists many hospitals throughout Sri Lanka.)
Sri Lankan Medical Association, Wijerama House, No 7 Wijerama Avenue, Columbo 7. (The Medical Association's journal website is www.infolanka.com/CMJhome.)
Sri Lankan Dental Association, Professional Centre, 275/75 Bauddhalloka, Mawatha, Colomba 7. Tel: +94 1 59 51 47.

MEDICAL SCHOOLS AND THEIR TEACHING HOSPITALS:

Colombo

University of Colombo
Faculty of Medicine, PO Box 271, Kynsey Road, Colombo 8. Tel: +94 1 695 300. Fax: +94 1 691581. www.infolanka.com/people/shyam/ClinMed6.htm.
This is the oldest (1870) and largest medical school in Sri Lanka.

National Hospital Columbo General Hospital
Ward Place, Colombo.
www.infolanka.com/people/shyam/ClinMed7.htm.
The hospital: Is the largest teaching hospital (3000 beds) in Sri Lanka, and the quality of care and teaching is high. The hospital is government run, very busy and has limited resources. Common problems are diabetes, malaria, dengue fever, TB, valve disease and leprosy.
O Elective notes: In the mornings, there are ward rounds, tutorials and case presentations. The teaching is excellent, however, the 'hands on' experience is somewhat limited unless you speak Sinhalese. The students are very happy to translate. Surgery has also come highly recommended. It is possible to go on a

variety of outpatient clinics, for example leprosy clinics, paeds visits and to TB hospitals. Electives here are well organized, and you can do what you want when you arrive. Medical student hours are about 8 am to 2 pm. The website above has a downloadable application form.

Accommodation: Mrs Peiris (62/2 Park Street) comes recommended.

Lady Ridgeway Hospital for Children

Borella Colombo 10.

The hospital: The paediatric hospital for the medical school. Much of the pathology is tropical disease. Congenital problems are also common. Community clinics to shanty towns are run from here.

O Elective notes: A number of other students are often around though not normally elective students. Everyone is friendly and welcoming. The hospital has limited facilities but it is a good learning experience.

De Soysa Maternity Hospital

Colombo 8.

The hospital: This is the specialist maternity hospital for Sri Lanka.

Peradeniya

University of Peradeniya

Faculty of Medicine, Peradeniya 20400, Kandy. Tel: +94 8 388 315. Fax: +94 8 232 572. www.pdn.ac.lk/med.

Peradeniya General Hospital, University of Peradeniya

Peradeniya, Kandy.

The hospital: Perandeniya Teaching Hospital is the largest hospital outside the capital. It consists of a medical unit comprising two wards and a complement of 150–200 patients. There are usually upwards of 60 admissions per day. Mornings consist of consultant ward rounds (huge) and teaching (all in English).

O Elective notes: Very few locals speak English so liaise closely with the 'home'

students, of whom there are around 40. There are plenty of heart murmurs to hear and spleens to feel. Owing to the pressures of numbers, practical procedures are not plentiful.

Kandy General Hospital

Kandy. Tel: +94 8 233337. Fax: +94 8 233343.

Galle

University of Ruhuna

Faculty of Medicine, PO Box 70, Galle. Tel: +94 9 34801. Fax: +94 9 22314. www.ruh.ac.lk/Uni/medicine/Medicine. (The school uses Karapitiya Hospital at the same address.)

The hospital: A major, 1200-bed teaching hospital (the third-biggest in Sri Lanka). It lies 6.5 km (4 miles) from old town Galle. It is a tertiary referral centre for southern Sri Lanka. An excellent range of pathologies from many congenital/rheumatic heart disorders through to tropical diseases (malaria, filariasis, leprosy and tropical splenomegaly).

O Elective notes: Few patients speak English, but they are more than happy for you to examine them. There is no formal teaching, but the bedside teaching is all in English. There are plenty of students about (30 in a clinic!) so there is not much 'hands on' experience, although the teaching is good. Go to Unawatuna beach in the afternoons. The university charges US$40 a week to do an elective here. Forms are downloadable on able link.

Accommodation: Cheap family houses can be arranged through the university, but a tourist place (such as Seaview Guesthouse) on the beach may be better.

Galle General Hospital

Karapitiya, Galle. Tel +94 9 32176.

OTHER MEDICAL SCHOOLS:

University of Jaffna, Faculty of Medicine, Adiyapatham Road, Kokuvil, Thirunelvely, Jaffna. Tel: +94 21 238 38. www.jaffna.tripod.com/jaffnafront.

University of Kelaniya (North Colombo Private Medical College), Faculty of Medicine, PO Box 6, Thalagolla Road, Ragama. Tel: +94 1 958 219. Fax: +94 1 958 337. www.schin.ncl.ac.uk/medkel/.
University of Sri Jayewardenepura, Faculty of Medicine, Gangodawila, Nugegoda. Tel: +94 1 852 695. Fax: +94 1 852 604. www.sjp.ac.lk/med. (This uses Sri Jayawardanapura Hospital, Thalapathpitya Road, Kotte.)

SOME RURAL HOSPITALS:

Kurunegala Hospital
Kurunegala.
The hospital: This is in the hill country and has a great deal of tropical medicine (malaria, typhoid and dengue fever).
O **Elective notes:** Although interesting, students have complained of endless ward rounds.

Matale Base Hospital
Matale.
The hospital: Excellent for surgery, although facilities are extremely poor. There are two operating tables in one theatre.

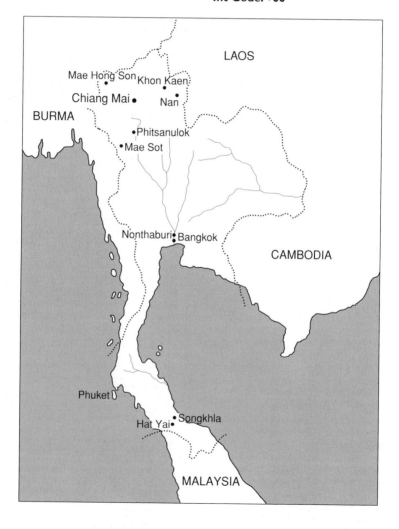

Thailand

Population: 60 million
Language: Thai
Capital: Bangkok
Currency: Baht
Int Code: +66

Thailand lies between the Indian and Pacific Oceans and has Burma, Laos, Cambodia and Malaysia as its neighbours. In recent years, business in Bangkok has been booming however, the north still remains very poor. Although Thailand is not a very popular destination, most medics and students head for these northern parts. Because of the problems in Burma, a number of refugee camps are set up just over the border in Thailand. This area has provided some very interesting electives.

✪ Medicine:

Specialist medical care can really only be found in Bangkok. Improvements have, however, occurred in rural areas. This has been achieved by training more primary healthcare workers rather than more doctors. A system runs by which the poor can obtain a certificate so that they do not have to pay for healthcare. HIV is a major problem in Bangkok, especially among the many prostitutes (over 80% prevalence in this group).

➲ Visas and work permits:

A visa is required to enter Thailand for more than 15 days. Enquire with the embassy for more details. Most students do not require special permits, but check with the embassy. Work permits are required for anything more than voluntary work. A very helpful source of information for electives is the **Foreign Medical Student Exchange Committee** (6th Floor, Aduly Adejvikrom Building, Faculty of Medicine, Siriraj Hospital, Mahidol University, 2 Prannok Road, Bankoknoi, Bangkok 10700. Tel: +66 2 411 3087 ext 6421. Fax: +66 2 411 0100. An elective application form can be downloaded from www.si.mahidol.ac.th/eng/student-for.htm)

USEFUL ADDRESSES:

Ministry of Health, Tiwanon Road, Amphoe Muang, Nonthaburi, Bangkok. Tel: +66 2 591 8141. Fax: +66 2 591 8492.
Medical Association of Thailand, 67/9 Soi Soonvichai, New Petchburi Road, Bangkok. Tel: +66 2 314 4333. Fax: +66 2 314 6305. www.masean.org/thailand.

Thailand Medical Council, Office of Permanent Secretary Building, Ministry of Health, Nonthaburi 11000.
Nurses Association of Thailand, 12/21 Rang Nam Road, Bagkok 10400. Tel: +66 2 247 4463. Fax: +66 2 247 4470.
Dental Association of Thailand, PO Box 355, Samsennai Post Office, Bankok 10400. www.welcome.to/thaidental.

SOME MEDICAL SCHOOLS AND TEACHING HOSPITALS:

Bangkok

Chulalongkorn University
Faculty of Medicine, 1873 Rama IV Road, Bangkok 10330. Tel: +66 2 256 4244. Fax: +66 2 252 4963. www.md2.md.chula.ac.th. Founded in 1947, the school uses Chulalongkorn and Siriraj hospitals (over 1000 beds).

Mahidol University
Faculty of Medicine, Siriraj Hospital, 2, Phan Nok Road, Bangkok 10700.
Tel: +66 2 411 1429. Fax: +66 2 412 1371. www.mahidol.ac.th.
This is the oldest medical school in Thailand and has two faculties – one based at Ramathibodi Hospital, the other at Siriraj Hospital.

Bangkok Metropolitan Medical College, 681 Samsen Road, Dusit, Bangkok 10300. Tel: +66 2 241 5129. Fax: +66 2 241 5129. www.vajira.ac.th.
Pramongkutklao Hospital and College of Medicine, 315 Rajavithee Road, Rajadevi, Bangkok 10400. Tel: +66 2 248 3391. Fax: +66 2 247 9559. www.pmk.ac.th.
Rangsit University, Faculty of Medicine, Phya Thai 2 Hospital, 943 Pahalyothin Road, Phya Thai, Bangkok 10440. Tel: +66 2 270 1847. Fax: +66 2 271 2306. www.rsu.ac.th.
Srinakharinwirot University, Faculty of Medicine, Prasarnmit Campus, Sukhumvit 23, Klong Toei, Bangkok 10110. Tel: +66 2 260 2124. Fax: +66 2 260 0125. www.swu.ac.th.

Chiang Mai

Chiang Mai University
110 Intawaroros Road, Muang District, Chiang Mai 50200. Tel: +66 53 221122. Fax: +66 53 217144.
www.medicine.cmu.ac.th.

Founded in 1959, this is the only medical university in the north and uses the largest hospital, the Maharaj Nakorn Chiang Mai Hospital. This has 1800 beds and all major specialities in three buildings. The school was originally designed to produce more doctors for rural Thailand and there is a close cooperation with rural health centres. The campus (including hospital) is in west Chiang Mai at the base of Doi Suthep (1000 m). It is 5 km from the airport.

MEDICAL SCHOOLS OUTSIDE BANGKOK:

Khon Kaen University, Faculty of Medicine, 123 Mitraparp Highway, Maung, Khon Kaen 40002. Tel: +66 43 237909. Fax: +66 43 348375. www.kku.ac.th.
Naresuan University, Faculty of Medicine, Amphur Wang, Phitsanulok 65000. Tel: +66 55 261071. Fax: +66 55 261057. www.med.nu.ac.th.
Prince of Songkhla University, College of Medicine, PO Box 5, Khohong, Hat Yai, Songkhla 90112. Tel: +66 74 212070. Fax: +66 74 212900. www.medinfo.psu.ac.th.
Thammasat University, Faculty of Medicine, Rangsit Campus, 99 Mhu 18, Paholyothin Rd., Klong Luang, Pathum Thani 12121. Tel: +66 2 564 4440. Fax: +66 2 516 9403. www.med.tu.ac.th.

SOME RURAL HOSPITALS:

Fang Hospital
Amphur Fang, Chiang Mai 50110.
The hospital: Is a 150-bed hospital in a relatively rural area close to Chiang Mai. The doctors are all extremely friendly. Frequent problems include HIV, TB, typhoid, malaria and gunshot wounds. Road traffic accidents are also common. Visits to local hill tribes are carried out. The hospital only has very basic equipment (X-ray being the only imaging).

Srisungwan Hospital
Mae Hong Son.
The hospital: Has 140 beds and seven doctors. Wards include O&G, male and female medical and surgical, paeds, an ITU and a monk's ward. There are two operating theatres, ultrasound and X-ray

facilities. It is a highly respected hospital in Thailand despite its small size. It has public and private wards. The public have malaria, TB, meningitis, heroin addictions and gunshot wounds. The private wards have the diseases of the West: type II diabetes, MIs and cancer. Malaria is a huge problem in the region accounting for 50% of hospital admissions.

O **Elective notes:** You will need to attempt to learn some Thai. This is not a holiday elective but very educational. You can get out to trek and also to visit Burmese refugee camps.

Nan Hospital
Nan.
The hospital: Nan is a provincial, secondary referral hospital for surrounding rural hospitals. Nan itself is remote in the north of Thailand close to the Thai–Laos border. All the doctors are incredibly friendly and good at teaching. Trauma (from motorbike accidents), dengue fever, malaria, snakebites, TB, hepatocellular cancer and HIV are all common.

O **Elective notes:** Beautiful surroundings and excellent opportunities for practical procedures and theatre work. Just be aware of the high HIV prevalence.

Phya Thai Phuket International Hospital
28/36–37 Sri Sena Road, Tambol Taladyai, Amphur Muang, Phuket 83000. Tel: +66 76 252603/252604/252605/252606. Fax: +66 76 252646/252647. www.phyathai.com.
The hospital: Has first-class facilities and equipment as a significant percentage of patients are overseas tourists. It has all major specialities. The hospital is a 15-minute walk from the town. However, sometimes there are not so many patients. Local patients often don't speak English. All the doctors do and they are very friendly.

O **Elective notes:** Phuket is a lovely island but if you don't have transport, the actual area around the hospital can get a bit dull. There's plenty of time to explore.

Accommodation: Furnished rooms adjacent to the hospital are provided for 2000 baht (£33) a month. They have fridge, freezer and air-conditioning but NO HOT WATER.

NORTHERN THAI HEALTH STATIONS:

The Thai German Highland Development Project is a German organization that donates money towards the development of hill tribes. The Thai government contributes 20%. There are a number of Health Stations, usually run by around three paramedics, providing basic health needs, treatment of malaria, TB, etc. Contact the **Foreign Medical Student Exchange Committee** for more details.

A SPECIAL NOTE ON THE SITUATION WITH BURMA:

Due to the poverty (despite it being the top heroin exporter in the world) and civil war, Burma's healthcare is almost non-existent, and hospitals tend to only cater for military personnel. There are no hospitals in rural areas. There is high infant mortality and many people have TB, malaria and/or HIV. The intense fighting has resulted in many people fleeing to the jungle (not without its dangers). Others have crossed the border as refugees into Thailand. In total, there are over 100 000 such refugees in many camps along the border. They are not recognized as refugees by the Thai Government or the UN and so are dependent on NGOs such as Médecins sans Frontières (MSF), the Red Cross and the Burmese Border Consortium. The camps are often attacked by Burmese soldiers who cross the border. If you are thinking of working here, up-to-date information is vital. Contact one of these groups. The Foreign Medical Student Exchange Committee can also give advice. An example of one of the camp health centres is the tremendously successful Dr Cynthia's clinic in Mae Sot.

Mae Sot

An area in north-west Thailand 7 km from the Burmese border. It has 50 000 people in it, including Thai and Burmese refugees. Mae Sot has a huge gem trade and is a lively border town with day and night markets, restaurants and bars. MSF and Shoklo Malaria Research Unit (SMRU) crowds hang out here in the evenings.

Dr Cynthia's Clinic
PO Box 67, Mae Sot, Tak 63110.
Tel: +66 55 533644 Fax: +66 55 544655.
E-mail: win7@loxinfo.co.th.
The clinic: This was set up by Dr Cynthia Maung, originally from Karen, who had to flee during the student uprising in 1988. Many of her colleagues with her in the jungle died from malaria. She has now set up a clinic for the refugees in Mae Sot. It relies on money from NGOs to function. Many volunteer doctors, medical students and teachers come to help. Dr Cynthia, her brother (also a doctor) and 50 medical assistants (refugees), who are trained at the clinic, run it.

The clinic works as an outpatients but also has 15 beds (with no nurses – the relatives have to do that), a basic lab, maternity and child health clinics and a computer (with Internet access). All services are free. It trains 50 medics a year, who go to other camps and across into the Burmese jungle to give treatment to those with no access to healthcare. There is a great deal of malaria and drug resistance is a major problem. TB, peptic ulcers and worm infestations are also common. There is basic education into personal hygiene. To organize an elective or work here write or e-mail to the above address.

Note: Dr Cynthia is (obviously) incredibly busy so don't expect a quick reply. It is also expensive for them to e-mail back so you may only get one reply. Ring before you go to ensure all is OK.
O Elective notes: Medical students run clinics with medics trained in the clinic. They act as translators. When there are no students, the medics run the clinics themselves so are very experienced.

Thailand

Students are also involved in teaching the local medics. There is a great deal of responsibility in going here and it is exhausting work. Mae Sot itself is a pleasant, safe town, and the people are very warm-hearted, but venturing into the jungle is dangerous. Gunfire can be heard at night and tourists have been kidnapped. There are many languages. Make attempts to learn a bit of each.

Accommodation: Has previously been in the clinic. As there is the possibility it may be attacked, and as it is now crowded with refugees, you are best staying in a guesthouse in town (see the Lonely Planet guide). No. 4 Guest House comes recommended.

Shoklo Malaria Research Unit

PO Box 46, Mae Sot, Tak Province, 63110.
Tel: +66 55 531531. Fax: +66 55 544442.

(It has close links with the Centre for Tropical Medicine, University of Oxford, John Radcliffe Hospital, Headington, Oxford OX3 9DU, UK.) Alternatively get in touch with the faculty of Tropical Medicine, Wellcome–Mahidol University, 420/6 Rajvithi Road, Bangkok 10400.
Tel: +66 2 246 0832. Fax: +66 2 246 7795.
SMRU is made up of an international group of scientists and physicians, and researches into resistant strains of malaria. Most of its work is done in the Maela refugee camp on the Thai–Burmese border (the MSF has a hospital in the camp).

Accommodation: Provided by the SMRU in their base camp. It is now too dangerous to stay in the border camps for fear of raids. The cost is about 2000 baht (£33).

AUSTRALIA and NEW ZEALAND

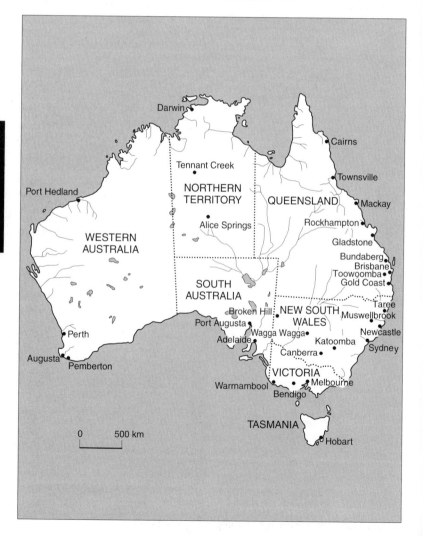

Australia

Population: 19.4 million
Language: English
Capital: Canberra
Currency: Australian dollar
Int Code: +61

Darwin

Cairns

Tennant Creek

Port Hedland

Townsville

NORTHERN
TERRITORY

QUEENSLAND

Mackay

Alice Springs

Rockhampton

WESTERN
AUSTRALIA

Gladstone

Bundaberg
Brisbane
Toowoomba
Gold Coast

SOUTH
AUSTRALIA

Taree
Muswellbrook

Broken Hill

NEW SOUTH
WALES

Port Augusta

Newcastle

Wagga Wagga

Katoomba

Perth

Adelaide

Canberra

Sydney

Augusta
Pemberton

VICTORIA

Warrnambool

Melbourne

Bendigo

TASMANIA

0   500 km

Hobart

The world's sixth-largest country comprises six states and the Northern Territory. Its variety of landscapes range from snowy mountains to magnificent beaches, arid deserts to tropical rainforests. Most Australians live on the coast; indeed, all cities bar Canberra are on the coast. Working in Australia can therefore almost guarantee some sun, sand and surf as well as spectacular diving and a multitude of water sports.

✪ Medicine:

Australia has an impressive public health system with high standards and short waiting lists. There are many world-renowned city hospitals as well as the well-known Royal Flying Doctor Service serving the outback communities.

Despite massive efforts to increase community health provision, there is still a great deal of disparity. The Aboriginal community is under-represented in society with higher rates of alcoholism, trauma and medical conditions compared with their white counterparts. The average life expectancy of an Aboriginal male is only 47 years. Australia's main health priorities at present include Aboriginal health, cancer prevention (especially skin, lung, cervical and breast), heart disease and injury prevention.

There is less distinction between private and public healthcare with many people having some form of health insurance. The national insurance scheme is called Medicare. A normal consultation with a GP costs about AU$30 (£15), for which Medicare gives a rebate of AU$24 (£12). The patient therefore has to pay about AU$6 (£3) to see a GP. Emergency care is free so some people go to the emergency department with what should really be conditions for the GP. There's one doctor per 434 people and the leading causes of death are cardio/cerebrovascular diseases and cancer.

While on the subject of health, it is worth mentioning something about the demography of HIV in the Asia–Pacific region. The rapid increase in HIV in countries such as Thailand is of great concern to its neighbours. In Australia by the mid-1990s there were approaching 3000 reported cases of AIDS, 96% of which were males. There are two main populations. Most is known about the city group, especially prevalent in inner Sydney. The Aboriginal community is the other group. They are experiencing a massive increase, especially in areas such as Palm Island. Hepatitis C is also a major problem among intravenous drug users in Sydney, in some areas reaching 60% prevalence in this group. For general information on Australian healthcare, visit www.health.gov.au.

Working in Australia as a doctor, nurse, physiotherapist or medical student provides the opportunity to practise a wide range of medicine – from advanced First World medicine in the cities to almost Third World medicine in the Aboriginal communities.

◎ Climate and crime:

The north of Australia is warm all year round and particularly humid during the summer monsoon. The east and southeast are fairly temperate. The warmest months are December to February (25–30°C), the coolest June to August. Although Australia is not a violent country, crime is increasing in some inner city and Aboriginal areas.

○ Elective notes:

Australia is a very popular destination. Early planning is vital as most hospitals work on a 'first come, first served' basis. It is also worth noting that Australian students have a massive summer holiday between November and February. This can mean that the hospitals get a bit quiet – brilliant if you want individual attention and the chance to do procedures, not so good if you want formal teaching and to make friends. If you have to go at this time of year, think about going with a friend.

If you want to do Aboriginal work, aim for the Northern Territories and Darwin. If you are planning to travel around Oz, book flights before you go as this can work out half the price of booking them once you are there. Aussies are proud of their country and will want you to go and see it.

Australia

➲ Visas and work permits:

Electives: To do an elective in Oz you require a visitor's visa ('tourist' class (class 676)), available free of charge from the High Commission (*see* Section 4). Some schools, however, recommend an occupational training visa (sub-class 442). If you're staying for more than an elective and are enrolling on a full time course, you will need a student visa (currently £130). You need to fill in forms, get letters, send money, etc. Full details (including details on immigration) are now available on the websites www.australia.org.uk and www.immi.gov.au.

Working holiday visas: If aged between 18 and 30, you may well be elegible for a working holiday visa (class 417), which means you can work for three months (for a single employer) and stay in Australia for a total of a year. You can apply on line at www.immi.gov.au – make sure your destination is happy to employ you on a working holiday visa.

Longer-term work:

● *Doctors*: For work of up to a year, you will need a medical practioners' visa (class 422)

● *Nurses and other health professionals*: A temporary residence visa can usually be obtained, but it depends on how much your services are needed. Sometimes a specialist visa (class 414) is more appropriate.

Immigration: WARNING – you are entering a minefield! Unless you want to work in remote 'area of need', this will be difficult – especially if you are a doctor (*see* below). Full details can be found on www.australia.org.uk.

Getting registered: Whatever your profession, you have to get registered with the appropriate Professional Council (coordinated by the **National Office of Overseas Skills Recognition** (NOOSR), GPO Box 1407, Canberra, ACT 2601. Tel: +61 6 240 8111. Fax: +61 6 240 7636. www.dest.gov.au/noosr) and then get registered with the appropriate state board.

The Australian government has established a number of very comprehensive websites with details on hospitals, schools and job vacancies for each region (*see* the first column in Table 1).

	State/territory health department and website	Medical board (for doctors to register with)	Nursing board (for nurses to register with)	Remote medical agency (especially for remote GP work)
ACT	GPO Box 825, Canberra, ACT 2601. Tel: +61 2 6205 5111. Fax: +61 2 6205 0830. www.health.act.gov.au	Po Box 976, Civic Square, Canberra, ACT 2608. Tel: +61 2 6205 1600. Fax: +61 2 6205 1602. www.healthregboards. act.gov.au. E-mail: bob.bradford@act.gov. au	PO Box 976, Civic Square, Canberra, ACT 2608. Tel: +61 2 6205 1599. Fax: +61 2 6205 1602. www.healthregboards. act.gov.au	
New South Wales	Locked Mail Bag 961, North Sydney, NSW 2059. Tel: +61 2 9391 9000. Fax: +61 2 9391 9101. www.health.nsw.gov.au	PO Box 104, Gladesville, NSW 2111. Tel: +61 2 9879 6799. Fax: +61 2 9816 5307. www.nswmb.org.au	Level 2, 28–36 Foveaux Street, Surry Hills, Sydney, NSW 2010. Tel: +61 2 9219 0222. Fax: +61 2 9281 2030. www.nursesreg.nsw.gov .au. E-mail: nursesreg@doh.health. nsw.gov.au	New South Wales Rural Doctors Network, Suite 19, Level 3, 133 Kings Street, Newcastle, NSW 2300. Tel: +61 2 4929 1811. Fax: +61 2 4929 1911. E-mail: icameron@nswrdn.aust. com

Northern Territory	GPO Box 40596, Casuarina, NT 0811. Tel: +61 8 8999 2400. Fax: +61 8 8922 8233. www.health.nt.gov.au	PO Box 4221, Darwin, NT 0801. Tel: +61 8 8999 4157. Fax: +61 8 899 4196. E-mail: healthprofessions.ths @nt.gov.au	PO Box 4221, Darwin, NT 0801. Tel: +61 8 8946 9545. Fax: +61 8 8946 9550. E-mail: nurses.board@nt. gov.au	Northern Territory Remote Health Workforce Agency, P.O. Box 1195, Alice Springs, NT 0871. Tel: +61 8 8952 3881. Fax: +61 8 8952 3536. E-mail: ntrwa@octa4.net.au
Queensland	GPO Box 48, Brisbane, QLD 4001. Tel: +61 7 3234 0111. Fax: +61 7 3234 0062. www.health.qld.gov.au	19th Floor, Forestry House, 160 Mary Street, Brisbane, QLD 4000. Tel: +61 7 3227 2515. Fax: +61 7 3225 2527. www.medicalboard.qld. gov.au	GPO Box 2928, Brisbane, QLD 4001. Tel: +61 7 3223 5111. Fax: +61 7 3223 5115. www.qnc.qld.gov.au	Queensland Rural Medical Support Agency, PO Box 167, Kelvin Grove DC, QLD 4059. Tel: +61 7 3356 1860. Fax: +61 7 3352 7557. E-mail: nlawrence@gpnetwork. net.au
South Australia	PO Box 39, Rundle Mall, SA 5000 Tel: +61 8 8226 7000. Fax: +61 8 8226 6649. www.health.sa.gov.au	91 Payneham Road, St Peters, SA 5069. Tel: +618 8362 7811. Fax: +61 8 8362 7906. www.medicalboardsa. asn.au	GPO Box 7176, Adelaide SA 5000. Tel: +61 8 8223 9700. Fax: +61 8 8223 9717. www.nursesboard.sa.g ov.au E-mail: registrations@nursesb oard.sa.gov.au	South Australian Rural and Remote Medical Support Agency, Calvary Hospital, 89 Strangeways Terrace, North Adelaide, SA 5006. Tel: +61 8 8239 1222. Fax: +61 8 8239 1777. E-mail: sarrmsa@sarrmsa.com.au
Tasmania	GPO Boz 125B, Hobart, TAS 7001. Tel: +61 3 6233 8011. Fax: +61 3 6233 6392. www.dhhs.tas.gov.au	2 Gore Street, South Hobart, TAS 7004. Tel: +61 3 6223 5400. Fax:+61 03 6223 7986. E-mail: mct@our.net.au	15 Princes Street, Sandy Bay, PO Box 847, TAS 7006. Tel: +61 03 6224 3991. Fax: +61 3 6224 3995. www.nursingboardtas. org.au	Tasmanian General Practice Divisions Limited, PO Box 104, Newstead, TAS 7250. Tel: +61 3 6334 3255. Fax: +61 3 6334 3651. E-mail: pbarns@tgpd.com.au
Victoria	GPO Box 4057, Melbourne, VIC 3001. Tel: +61 3 9616 7777. Fax: +61 3 9616 7350. www.health.vic.gov.au	Level 16, 150 Lonsdale Street, Melbourne, VIC 3000. Tel: +61 3 9655 0500. Fax: +61 3 9655 0580. www.medicalboardvic. org.au	GPO Box 4932, Melbourne, VIC 3001. Tel: +61 3 8635 1200. Fax: +61 3 8635 1248. www.nbv.org.au	Rural Workforce Agency of Victoria, Suite 8, Level 4, 458 Swanson Street, Carlton, VIC 3053. Tel: +61 3 9349 7800. Fax: +61 3 9349 4211. www.rwav.com.au E-mail: rwav@rwav.com.au
Western Australia	PO Box 8172, Stirling Street, Perth, WA 6849. Tel: +61 8 9222 4222. Fax: +61 8 9222 4009. www.health.wa.gov.au	London House, 216 St Georges Terrace, Perth, WA 6805. Tel: +61 8 9481 1011. Fax: +61 8 9321 1744. www.medicalboard.com. au	165 Adelaide Terrace, East Perth, WA 6892. Tel: +61 8 9421 1100. Fax: +61 8 9421 1022. www.nbwa.org.au	Western Australia Centre for Rural and Remote Medicine, 328 Stirling Highway, Claremont, WA 6010. Tel: +61 8 9384 2811. Fax: +61 8 9385 2938. E-mail: gregdown@cyllene.uwa. edu.au

Australia

Australia

✪ Working in Australia as a doctor:

This can require a great deal of planning. There are two options: temporary work (up to a year) and permanent work. A good place to start is www.health.gov.au/workforce/overseas/overseas.htm.

Temporary work: Six months or a year in a speciality in Australia as either an SHO or a registrar is very attractive and commonly done. It is also relatively easy to get jobs, especially in 'areas of need' in the rural outback. It is far more difficult to get a pre-registration job, however. You are better to wait and register at home. Look at individual hospital websites as they often advertise jobs that are or will be available. To obtain a visa for temporary work as a medical practitioner you need to have a medical and a chest X-ray. You do not have to have sat the Australian Medical Council (AMC) exams. Most contracts however, will require you to return to home at the end of your contract and not apply to sit the AMC exams. They really don't want you to stay! Breaking these rules will make it extremely difficult for you to apply for more/permanent work out there at a later date.

Permanent work: This has become extremely difficult to obtain over the past few years. Australia has been flooded with overseas doctors, hence they are making it as difficult as possible. Again, pre-registration house jobs are virtually impossible to get. Once registered, you can either migrate immediately and join a postgraduate training scheme or, alternatively, complete your SHO training and membership and then leave. Either way, there are a number of obstacles – immigration and exams being the main ones.

Immigration: If wanting to stay you will need to obtain residency status from the Department of Immigration and Multicultural Affairs before you can apply to sit the AMC exams. Allow up to a year (or even longer) for a migration application to be accepted. You need proof of identity (birth certificate), education (school and degree certificates), health (medical and chest X-ray) and character (no convictions – you may get away with the odd one; after all, they used to be compulsory!). It's all done on a points system, and as a doctor you score minus 25 for skills (they *really* don't want you!). It can be made a bit easier if you marry an Australian. Check out www.immi.gov.au.

Exams: You may well need to sit the Australian Medical Council (AMC) exams. These are the Australian 'finals' and hence test undergraduate as well as graduate knowledge. They consist of an MCQ and a clinical component. They also cover the specialities so you are best to sit these as soon as possible after qualifying while it is all still fresh (you can't sit it before qualifying, as you can the American exams). If you have already completed your specialist training you often don't have to get 'general registration' via the AMC exam route. The AMC forwards your application to the relevant college for assessment. If they are happy, they can then give you 'specialist registration'. Full details on the examination and on how they assess overseas doctors can be obtained from the AMC (address below), which has an excellent website: www.amc.org.au.

Registration: You will need to register with the appropriate state board (listed in Table 1). This is usually fairly simple, requiring a letter of good standing from your home medical council, a small fee and about a week. Registration can be with or without conditions. Graduates of Australian or New Zealand medical schools or those who have completed AMC exams and have obtained migrant status can obtain registration without conditions. For eveyone else (e.g. those wanting temporary work), registration will have conditions.

Provider numbers: If working in the private sector (for example as a GP) you will also need to apply for a provider number – this enables you to receive payment from the government for treating patients under the Medicare scheme. It is obtained through the Health Insurance Commission. Doctors working in governmental hospitals do not need a number.

Indemnity insurance: You may find that your home idemnity provider has a reciprocal arrangement with governmental hospitals in Australia and New Zealand. If so, ask for written confirmation and take it with you. If you intend to do private work (and that includes GP work) you will need to organize your own cover when there. There are plenty of providers – ask a colleague to recommend one.

Finding a job: Look at the *Medical Journal of Australia*, hospital websites, www.bmj.com and www.medicstravel.org.

Working in Australia as a nurse:

Australia is much more receptive to nurses than doctors, possibly because of the shortage in both cities and remote areas. You will need to obtain a visa as outlined above and get registration/ enrolment with the appropriate state nursing board (*see* Table 1). If you go through a recruitment agency, this should all be done for you. In short, registered nurses can practise unsupervised; enrolled nurses, however, have to be supervised. The process by which you are assessed varies from state to state. Some will assess you simply from what you have done before. Others will want you to undergo a period of 'bridging', in which you are supervised before registration. You need to apply through the **Australian Nursing Council Inc**. (address below). It may be worth going out initially on a working holiday visa to get assessed and then changing the visa type if your registration is succsesful.

Working as a dentist:

You will need to register with the board of the state in which you want to work (check the NOOSR website). For most Western dentists this is relatively easy, however, if your qualification is not recognized you will need to sit the Australian Dental Coucncil exams.

PROFESSIONAL ORGANIZATIONS:

Doctors: Australian Medical Council, PO Box 4810, Kingston, ACT 2604. Tel: +61 2 6270 5400. Fax: +61 2 6270 9799. E-mail: amc@amc.org.au. www.amc.org.

Nurses: Royal College of Nursing, 1 Napier Close, Deakin, ACT 2600. Tel: +61 2 6282 5633. Fax: +61 2 6282 3565. www.rcna.org.au.
Australian Nursing Federation, Level 2, 21 Victoria Street, Melbourne, VIC 3000. Tel: +61 3 9639 5211. Fax: +61 3 9652 0567.
Australian Nursing Council Inc, 1st Floor, 20 Challis Street, Dickson, ACT 2602. Tel: +61 2 6257 7960. Fax: +61 2 6257 7955. www.anci.org.au.
Dentists: Australian Dental Association, PO Box 520, St Leonards, NSW 1590. Tel: +61 2 9906 4412. Fax: +61 2 9906 4917. E-mail: adainc@ada.org.au. www.ada.org.au.
Australian Dental Council, Suite 1, Level 2, 112 Wellington Parade, Melbourne, VIC 3002. Tel: +61 3 9415 1638. Fax: +61 3 9415 1669.
Physiotherapists: Australian Physiotherapy Association, PO Box 6465, Melbourne, VIC 3004. Tel: +61 3 9534 9400. Fax: +61 3 9534 9199.
Occupational therapists: Australian Association of Occupational Therapists, 6 Spring Street, Fitzroy, VIC 3065. Tel: +61 3 9416 1021. Fax: +61 2 9416 1421. E-mail: otausnat@ozemail.com.au.
Radiographers: Australian Institute of Radiography, PO Box 1169, Collingwood, VIC 3066. Tel: +61 3 9419 3336. Fax: +61 3 9416 0783.
Speech therapists: Speech Pathology Association of Australia, 2nd Floor, 11–19 Bank Place, Melbourne, VIC 3000. Tel: +61 3 9642 4899. Fax: +61 3 9642 4922.
Dietitians: Dietician's Association of Australia, 1/8 Phipps Close, Deakin, ACT 2600. Tel: +61 2 6282 9555. Fax: +61 2 6282 9888. www.daa.asn.au.

ADDITIONAL PROFESSIONAL ORGANIZATIONS FOR MEDICAL/SURGICAL SPECIALISTS:

Anaesthetics: Australian and New Zealand College of Anaesthetists, 630 St Kilda Road, Melbourne, VIC 3000. Tel: +61 3 9510 6299. Fax: +61 3 9510 6786. E-mail: ceoanzca@anzca.edu.au. www.anzca.edu.au.
Dermatology: Australasian College of Dermatologists, PO Box 2065, Boronia Park, NSW 2111. Tel: +61 2 9879 6177. Fax: +61 2 9816 1174. E-mail: admin@dermcoll.asn.au. www.dermcoll.asn.au.
Emergency medicine: Australasian College for Emergency Medicine, 17 Grattan Street, Carlton, VIC 3053. Tel: +61 3 9663 3800. Fax: +61 3 9663 8013. E-mail: acemadmin@acem.org.au. www.acem.org.au.
General practice: Royal Australian College of General Practitioners, 1 Palmerston Crescent, South Melbourne, VIC 3205. Tel: +61 3 9214 1414. Fax: +61 3 9214 1400. E-mail: racgp@racgp.org.au. www.racgp.org.au.
Obstetrics and gynaecology: Royal Australian and New Zealand College of Obstetricians and Gynaecologists, 254 Albert Street, East Melbourne, VIC 3002. Tel: +61 3 9417 1699. E-mail: ranzcog@ranzcog.edu.au. www.ranzcog.edu.au.

Australia

Occupational health: Australasian Faculty of Occupational Medicine, 145 Macquarie Street, Sydney, NSW 2000. Tel: +61 2 9256 5400. E-mail: afom@racp.edu.au. www.racp.edu.au/afom.

Opthalmology: Royal Australian and New Zealand College of Ophthalmologists, 94–98 Chalmers Street, Surry Hills, NSW 2010. Tel: +61 2 9690 1001. Fax: +61 2 9690 1321. E-mail: ranzco@ranzco.edu. www.ranzco.edu.

Paediatrics: Paediatrics and Child Health Division, Royal Australasian College of Physicians, 145 Macquarie Street, Sydney, NSW 2000. Tel: +61 2 9256 5409. E-mail: paed@racp.edu.au. www.racp.edu.au.

Pathology: Royal College of Pathologists of Australasia, 207 Albion Street, Surry Hills, NSW 2010. Tel: +61 2 8356 5858. Fax: +61 2 8356 5828. E-mail: rcpa@rcpa.edu.au. www.rcpa.edu.au.

Physicians: Royal Australasian College of Physicians, 145 Macquarie Street, Sydney, NSW 2000. Tel: +61 2 9256 5444. Fax: +61 2 9252 3310. E-mail: racp@racp.edu.au. www.racp.edu.au.

Psychiatry: Royal Australian and New Zealand College of Psychiatrists, 309 La Trobe Street, Melbourne, VIC 3000. Tel: +61 3 9640 0646. Fax: +61 3 9642 5652. E-mail: ranzcp@ranzcp.org. www.ranzcp.org.

Public health: Australian Faculty of Public Health Medicine, 145 Macquarie Street, Sydney, NSW 2000. Tel: +61 2 9256 5404. E-mail: afphm@racp.edu.au. www.racp.edu.au/afphm.

Radiology: Royal Australian and New Zealand College of Radiologists, Level 9, 51 Druitt Street, Sydney, NSW 2000. Tel: +61 2 9268 9777. Fax: +61 2 9264 7799. E-mail: warden@ranzcr.edu.au. www.ranzcr.edu.au.

Rehabilitation: Australasian Faculty of Rehabilitation Medicine, 145 Macquarie Street, Sydney, NSW 2000. Tel: +61 2 9256 5402. E-mail: afrm@racp.edu.au. www.racp.edu.au/afrm.

Remote and Rural medicine: Australian College of Remote and Rural Medicine, Level 1, 467 Enoggera Road, Alderley, QLD 4051. Tel: +61 7 3352 8600. Fax: +61 7 3356 2167. E-mail: acrrm@acrrm.org.au. www.acrrm.org.au.

Surgery: Royal Australasian College of Surgeons, Spring Street, Melbourne, VIC 3000. Tel: +61 3 9249 1200. Fax: +61 3 9249 1219. E-mail: College.sec@surgeons.org. www.surgeons.org or www.racs.edu.au.

AUSTRALIAN UNIVERSITIES AFFILIATED TO MEDICAL SCHOOLS:

South Australia:
Flinders University, School of Medicine, Flinders University of South Australia, Bedford Park, SA 5042 (or GPO 2100, SA 5001). Tel: +61 8 8 204 4160. Fax: +61 8 8 204 5845. www.flinders.edu.au. University of Adelaide Medical School, Frome Road, Adelaide, SA 5000. Tel: +61 8 8 303 5193. Fax: +61 8 8 303 3788. www.health.adelaide.edu.au.

Victoria:
Monash University, Faculty of Medicine, Monash University, Wellington Road (PO Box 64), Clayton, Melbourne, VIC 3168. Tel: +61 3 9 905 4318. Fax: +61 3 9 905 4302. www.med.monash.edu.au.
University of Melbourne, Faculty of Medicine, University of Melbourne, Gratton Street, Parkville, Melbourne, VIC 3052. Tel: +61 3 9 344 5894. Fax: +61 3 9 347 7854. www.unimelb.edu.au.

Queensland:
James Cook University, School of Medicine, Townsville, QLD 4811. Tel: +61 7 4 781 6232. Fax: +61 7 4 781 6986. www.jcu.edu.au.
University of Queensland Medical School, Herston Road, Herston, Brisbane, QLD 4006. Tel: +61 7 3 365 5316. Fax: +61 7 3 365 5433. www.uq.edu.au.

Tasmania:
University of Tasmania, Faculty of Medicine, University of Tasmania, 43 Collins Street, Hobart, TAS 7000 (or GPO Box 252-71). Tel: +61 3 6 226 4860. Fax: +61 3 6 226 4816. www.healthsci.utas.edu.au/medschool/index.html.

New South Wales:
University of Newcastle, Faculty of Medicine, University of Newcastle, Newcastle, NSW 2308. Tel: +61 2 4 921 5678. Fax: +61 2 4 921 5669. www.newcastle.edu.au/department/fmhs.
University of New South Wales, Faculty of Medicine, University of New South Wales, PO Box 1, Kensington, Sydney, NSW 2033. Tel: +61 2 9 385 2454. Fax: +61 2 9 385 1874. www.unsw.edu.au.
University of Sydney, Faculty of Medicine, University of Sydney, Sydney, NSW 2006. Tel: +61 2 9 351 4579. Fax: +61 2 9 351 3196. www.usyd.edu.au.

Western Australia
University of Western Australia, School of Medicine, University of Western Australia, 1st Floor, N Block, Queen Elixabeth Medical Centre, Monash Avenue, Nedlands, Perth, WA 6009. Tel: +61 8 9 346 3876. Fax: +61 8 9 346 2369. www.meddent.uwa.edu.au.

NEW SOUTH WALES

Sydney

Sydney is Australia's largest city with the largest suburban area of any city in the world (twice the size of Beijing, six times the size of

Rome). It has the famous Opera House, harbour and plenty of beaches. Nightlife is superb with many shows on Oxford Street (student tickets being available 30 minutes before the performance). There is a fantastic beach culture in the summer (which shuts down between May and September), and the temperature can reach 40°C with high humidity. Outside Sydney there are some excellent national parks, blue marines and, in the winter, skiing. A trip to the Blue Mountains is a must. Coaches to Brisbane (12 hours) and Melbourne (10 hours) overnight are much cheaper than flights (about £25 one way).

There is a fantastic website, www.health.nsw.gov.au, which gives a tremendous amount of detail on hospitals, GP surgeries and medical schools througout New South Wales. It provides comprehensive details on jobs for GPs, specialists, nurses and other health professionals, especially in areas of need. Another useful website for the area north of Sydney is the Hunter health site: www.hunter.health.nsw.gov.au.

UNIVERSITIES IN SYDNEY:

There are two universities based in Sydney: the University of New South Wales and the University of Sydney. Each has specific hospitals (and clinical schools) affiliated to it. There is also the University of Newcastle futher north.

University of New South Wales (UNSW)
Faculty of Medicine, Anzac Parade, Sydney 2052. www.unsw.edu.au. Tel: +61 2 9385 2454. Fax: +61 2 9385 1874.
It uses the following hospitals:

St Vincent's
St George's
Prince of Wales Hospital
Sydney Children's Hospital
Women's Hospital
Liverpool Hospital

University of Sydney
The Secretary, Faculty of Medicine, Edward Ford Building (A27), University of Sydney, NSW 2006. Tel: +61 2 9351 3132. Fax: +61 2 9351 6645. www.usyd.edu.au. This uses the:

Royal Prince Alfred Hospital (home to the Central Clinical School)
Royal North Shore Hospital (part of Northern Clinical School, www.ncs.usyd.edu.au)
Concord Hospital
Westmead Hospital
Nepean Hospital
Children's Hospital at Westmead
Canberra Hospital (see Australian Capital Territory)

To do a medical elective at any of the above hospitals you have to write to the affiliated clinical school (not the university, as used to be the case). APPLY EARLY. Most schools have downloadable forms and links can be found from www.medfac.usyd.edu.au/s-info/ electives.html for the University of Sydney. Visit the UNSW main site for links to their schools (or look below).

The University of Sydney will want:
- To know the areas of work which are of special interest to you
- The precise dates during which you require an attachment
- A letter from your dean
- A recent passport photo
- A curriculum vitae
- A bank cheque drawn on an Australian bank for AU$100 (about £40).

The earlier you apply, the more likely you are to get what you want. The clinical schools have an administrative fee (e.g. Concord and Northern charges AU$500 for four weeks and AU$650 for four to eight weeks). It's all very expensive but well organized. Some electives can be time-limited to a maximum of eight weeks. Also note that elective places are often not available between December and January. www.usyd.edu.au/su/accom/welcome is a useful place to look for short-term accommodation. Most of the schools affiliated with the UNSW do not charge.

HOSPITALS AND CLINICAL SCHOOLS AFFILIATED TO THE UNSW:

St Vincent's Hospital

Hospital: Victoria Street, Darlinghurst, Sydney, NSW 2010. Tel: +61 2 9339 1111.
Fax: +61 2 9332 4142.
www.stvincents.com.au.
Clinical School: Level 9, Cator Building, Victoria St, St Vincent's Hospital, Darlinghurst, Sydney, NSW 2010.
Tel: +61 2 8382 2024. Fax: +61 2 8382 3229.
E-mail: m.jordan@unsw.edu.au.
www.stvcs.med.unsw.edu.au.

The hospital: A medium-sized teaching hospital of UNSW (approximately 400 beds) right in the city centre (20 minutes' walk from the Opera House and Harbour Bridge). It's between Sydney's red light district (King's Cross) and the gay district (Oxford Street). Not surprisingly, the area is therefore always buzzing, day and night. Also not surprisingly, there is a high incidence of HIV among patients (1 in 20) and Darlinghurst has the highest concentration of homeless people in Sydney. The hospital covers internal medicine, surgery, trauma and psychiatry. WARNING: This is a dangerous area at night (mainly muggings); it is, however, perfectly safe during the day.

O Elective notes: The consultants are pretty relaxed and it's not too difficult to get the afternoons off to get down the beach (they'll encourage you to see Australia). The casualty teams are happy for you to see patients first and do minor procedures such as suturing. Most major trauma goes to other hospitals, however, no Australian students go here so you have free rein. GI surgery also has good reports. It doesn't charge tuition fees.

Accommodation: No private accommodation in the hospital and they recommend you stay in a local hostel (AU$100–150 a week). However, most elective students stay in a place called Lavinus Nolan House (433 Bourke Street, Darlinghurst, NSW 2030); this is approximately ten minutes' walk from the hospital, just off Taylor square. It's a residence in the grounds of St Margaret's Womens' Hospital (a private hospital) and costs about AU$120 (£60) a week for your own room and good facilities. It is well situated for buses to Circular Quay and the beaches (Bondi beach being a 30 minute bus ride away). The nun who runs the residence is pretty strict (especially on the no visitors rule!) but it is thoroughly recommended as you'll be hard pushed to find a place so central so cheaply. Some elective students stay at a youth hostel in Coogee Beach (about 30 minutes away by bus). They also report this as a good option. The youth hostel by the coach station is good for short-term accommodation.

St George's Hospital

Hospital: Belgrave Street, Kogarah, Sydney, NSW 2217. Tel: +61 2 9350 1111.
Fax: +61 2 9350 3960.
Clinical school: Clinical Sciences Building, Short Street, St George Hospital, Kogarah, Sydney, NSW 2217. Tel: +61 2 9350 2992.
Fax: +61 2 9350 3998.
E-mail: d.reid@unsw.edu.au.
www.stgcs.med.unsw.edu.au.

The hospital: A large, high-tech hospital in the south-eastern suburbs of Sydney (five minutes to the station and then 15 minutes on the train).

O Elective notes: The emergency department is busy, and in other specialities it's all advanced stuff. You are welcome to attend the Sydney students' tutorials, but in some specialities (e.g. orthopaedics) reports suggest that consultants have been very keen that students explore Oz.

Accommodation: Has been provided in a flat a couple of minutes from the hospital at a rather expensive rate. The hospital can supply a list of local guesthouses. The more central hospitals in Sydney (Royal Prince Alfred or St Vincent's) may be more sociable. Bondi beach is a short train and bus ride away.

Prince of Wales Hospital

Hospital: High Street, Randwick, Sydney, NSW 2031. Tel: +61 2 9282 2222.
Fax: +61 2 9382 2033.

Clinical School: 1st Floor, Edmund Blacket Building, Prince of Wales Hospital, Randwick, Sydney, NSW 2031.
Tel: +61 2 9382 2645. Fax: +61 2 9382 2650.
E-mail: j.ryall@unsw.edu.au.
www.powcs.med.unsw.edu.au.

The hospital: A tertiary referral centre next to Sydney's Children's Hospital and the Royal Hospital for Women. Originally a destitute children's asylum, it was converted into a military hospital during the World Wars. It was converted back to civilian use in 1953. There are 313 000 people in its catchment population, although nearly half of its patients come from outside this area. The Randwick campus is currently under redevelopment to include facilities such as a new acute service, a helipad, the new Royal Hospital for Women and a hyperbaric unit. It is fairly central (a 20-minute bus ride from the centre).

O **Elective notes:** The emergency department is typical of any Western hospital, and you can do as much as you want. Note: If you're doing orthopaedics and want to see sporting injuries, most go to private clinics; however, the professor is very keen that you explore Oz. This is highly recommended if you're wanting more of a laid-back elective.

Accommodation: At the Prince Henry Hospital (*see* below). They may be able to arrange accommodation on site but not until you arrive.

Sydney Children's Hospital
High Street, Randwick, Sydney, NSW 2031. www.sch.edu.au.
Clinical school: Same address. Tel: +61 2 9382 1799. Fax: +61 2 9382 1401.
E-mail: carolyn.green@unsw.edu.au.
www.swch.med.unsw.edu.au.

The hospital: A modern hospital (next to the adult Prince of Wales (*see* above)) in the suburbs of Sydney, but not too far from the city centre (6 km).

O **Elective notes:** Very easy going, and you can choose to do as much or as little as you wish.

Accommodation: Again this is at the Prince Henry Hospital (some have not been impressed by it; *see* below).

Royal Hospital for Women
Clinical school: Locked Bag 2000, Randwick, Sydney, NSW 2031.
Tel: +61 2 9382 6777. Fax: +61 2 9382 6444.
E-mail: v.hammond@unsw.edu.au.
www.swch.med.unsw.edu.au.

Prince Henry Hospital
Anzac Parade, Little Bay, Sydney, NSW 2036. Tel: +61 2 9382 5555.
Fax: +61 2 9382 5029.

The hospital: Was founded in 1881 during an outbreak of smallpox in Sydney. The Coastal Hospital was erected at 'sufficient distance from Sydney to ensure safety and confidence'. It was renamed Prince Henry in 1934 and since 1959 has been affiliated with the Prince of Wales as part of the UNSW teaching hospitals. The acute services of this hospital are currently being relocated to the Randwick campus (*see* Prince of Wales above) while the Prince Henry is becoming a centre of excellence for rehabilitation and aged care.

Accommodation: The Prince of Wales and Sydney Children's Hospitals both have their accommodation on the Prince Henry site. The plus points are that it is cheap and next to a lovely golf course and beach. The major problem is that it is 6 km from these other hospitals and in the opposite direction to the city (making it about an hour's bus ride from the centre). You may be better organizing your own accommodation.

Liverpool Hospital
Elizabeth Street, Liverpool, Sydney, NSW 2173. Tel: +61 2 9828 3000.
Fax: +61 2 9828 3307.
www.swsahs.nsw.gov.au/livtrauma/ (trauma department).

The hospital: Has a good trauma unit as well as the regional perinatal centre (the Caroline Chishom Centre).

The UNSW also has a:

School of Rural Health
Wagga Wagga Base Hospital (HQ), PO Box 5695, Wagga Wagga, NSW 2650. Tel: +61 2 6938 6586. Fax: +61 2 6938 6587.
www.sorh.med.unsw.edu.au.

Australia

Australia

HOSPITALS AND CLINICAL SCHOOLS AFFILIATED TO THE UNIVERSITY OF SYDNEY:

Royal Prince Alfred Hospital

Hospital: Missenden Road, Camperdown, Sydney, NSW 2050. Tel: +61 2 9515 6111. Fax: +61 2 9515 6133.

www.cs.nsw.gov.au/rpa.

Clinical school: Central Clinical School, RPA. Same address.

E-mail: duriyev@gmp.usyd.edu.au.

The hospital: Being linked to Sydney University, this is one of the Bohemian student areas of Sydney, 10–20 minutes' bus ride from the city centre. It's a friendly hospital with specialities in breast cancer and liver transplantation. There is a very busy emergency department.

O **Elective notes:** With the busy emergency department, there's plenty of opportunity for practical procedures and doing early investigations. Reports show that the cardiology firm is intense work (cardiology ward rounds starting at 7 am). There is a specialist breast cancer unit (the **Sydney Breast Cancer Institute**) based within the hospital. If this is your specialist interest, it is well worth writing to them. There is a specialist liver transplant unit. They will give you a radio pager and expect you to be ready within two hours' notice to go on an organ retrieval. Great if it involves helicopters or fast jets to New Zealand … not so good if you wanted to go for a night out in Sydney.

Accommodation: For elective students, accommodation is in the nurses' home (Queen Mary's) with other students so there is the opportunity to meet many new people. There are, however, only two rooms available for medical students (AU$35 (£18) a week). If you don't get a room, ask one of the local students … many go away and are happy to rent out their room for a month or so. Failing that, Billerbong Gardens Hostel (AU$100 (£50) a week) is the next nearest. There's also a superb gym with aerobics classes and outdoor pool. There are lots of cafés and bars close by.

Royal North Shore Hospital (RNSH)

Hospital: Pacific Highway St Leonard's, North Sydney, NSW 2065. Tel: +61 2 9226 7111. Fax: +61 2 9926 7779.

www.nsh.nsw.gov.au/rnsh.

Clinical school: Northern Clinical School (which also uses Hornsbey, Maly, Mona Vale and Ryde Hospitals) is at the RNSH. Same address. www.ncs.usyd.edu.au.

The hospital: The RNSH is a large (950-bed), modern teaching hospital in north Sydney (St Leonard's), 15 minutes by train (four stops across Harbour Bridge) from the city centre and 40 minutes from Manly Beach. There are many students present. This area is very safe.

O **Elective notes:** The busy emergency (with helicopter service) and oncology departments come particularly recommended. The intensive care department can provide a well-organized elective. Like the rest of Australia, it seems that the staff are very keen for you to go out and see Oz while you are there (although vascular surgery may be the exception to this)! Oncology (it would appear) is very relaxed. There's no formal teaching for elective students, but you can attend the Sydney medical students' tutorials, which are very good, and also the weekly medical grand round (free lunch provided). The staff and other medical students are very friendly and you can do something different every night.

Note: Apply early here as it fills up quickly. Repeatedly highly recommended.

Accommodation: The nurses' home, costing AU$70 (£35) a week (the price has actually come down over the years), varies between grotty and reasonable (many have noted cockroaches in the kitchen). You meet many other students. There is a canteen close by and a couple of cheap restaurants. Another place you can stay is Billy Blue Palace (expensive, but the accommodation is good and food is provided) or the rather extravagantly named St Leonard's Mansions (AU$100 (£50) a week; 7 Park Road, St Leonard's. Tel: +61 2 9439 6999. Fax: +61 2 9437 5890), which may well have the largest population of funnel web spiders in

Sydney (always wear shoes!) There is a good gym and heated outdoor swimming pool on the hospital site and the hospital is conveniently on a bus route to the beach.

Advice for electives: Some have found it beneficial to write directly to the department they want to work in (emergency being the most popular) and *then* to the clinical school elective coordinator. If you write directly to the clinical school, they will give you four choices and allocate you where available. Either way, you won't be exempt from the AU$100 (£50) registration fee to the University of Sydney, or the AU$250 (£125) administration fee of the Northern Clinical School.

Concord Hospital

Hospital: Hospital Road Concord, Sydney, NSW 2005. www.cs.nsw.gov.au/concord. Clinical school: Concord Repatriation Hospital, Hospital Road, Concord, NSW 2139. www.concord.med.usyd.edu.au.

The hospital: A large teaching hospital in one of Sydney's western suburbs. It was founded to repatriate soldiers after World War II but was later handed over to the local authority. Although not far away, it can take a little while to get into Sydney. There are very friendly staff in a lovely hospital.

O Elective notes: It can get very quiet and dull, especially when the students are not there. The upper GI team is good, keen to give informal teaching and get you assisting in theatre. The formal teaching for the Aussie students is on a Friday afternoon and well worth attending.

Accommodation: In the hospital and cheap (about AU$60 (£30) a week), but remember that it can be difficult to get in and out of Sydney, especially at night. Some have stayed in the Queen Mary Building at the Royal Prince Alfred Hospital (20 minutes from Sydney, 45 from Concord).

Westmead Hospital

Hawksbury Road, Westmead, Sydney, NSW 2145. Tel: +61 2 9845 5555. www.westmead.nsw.gov.au. Clinical school: E-mail: sondrae@westgate.wh.usyd.edu.au.

The hospital: A large (900-bed) teaching hospital in a suburb of Sydney (a 45-minute train ride from the city). It claims to be the largest teaching hospital in the southern hemisphere (covering 95 acres). It has both state and private divisions. The hospital covers many specialities but is especially known for its neonatal and paediatric medicine (there is a 30-bed unit for emotionally disturbed children). There is a busy emergency department.

O Elective notes: There is excellent teaching and many clinics to attend. The cardiologists are keen to teach but expect you to turn up to the catheter lab, which can get a bit repetitive. Some units (such as oncology) may expect a small project. The emergency department is well organized. With the neonatal and paediatric group they run something called ISAM (intravenous substance-abusing mothers) clinics. There is an affiliated dental school.

Accommodation: Pretty basic (AU$20 (£10) a week) so plan to spend your weekends in Sydney. Having said that, it's cheap, and there's nowhere else to stay in Westmead. The cooking facilities are good and it is convenient for the train station. There is a pool and some tennis courts. Bondi Beach is an hour away.

Nepean Hospital

PO Box 63, Penrith, Sydney, NSW 2751.

The hospital: About an hour's train ride from Sydney at the foot of the Blue Mountains. It provides most general specialities to the local area.

O Elective notes: The consultants are fairly relaxed ... put in what you want. It's good, but if it's Sydney you want, remember the distance. The train can get dodgy late at night.

Accommodation: Provided in the nurses' home at about AU$20 (£10) a week. It's fine but a bit quiet.

Children's Hospital at Weastmead

Hawkesbury Road, Westmead, Sydney, NSW 2145. Tel: +61 2 9845 0000. Fax: +61 2 9845 3489. www.chw.edu.au.

The hospital: This is the major paediatric hospital (350 beds) for New South Wales and the South Pacific. It is the home of the University of Sydney's department of paediatrics and was purpose-built in 1996. It has superb facilities for staff, patients and relatives. There is a special paeds emergency department. This hospital is also superb for other medical professionals, for example speech therapists (Tel: +61 2 9845 2076), physiotherapists (Tel: +61 2 9845 3369), nurses (Tel: +61 2 9845 3023) and teachers (Tel: +61 2 9845 2813). Briefly, some of the departments include the gene therapy research unit, the **Children's Hospital Insitute of Sports Medicine** (8% of children in the emergency department have sports injuries), cardiology/cardiac surgery, clinical genetics, the cochlear implant centre, emergency, endocrinology, immunology and infectious diseases, intensive care, psychological medicine, respiratory medicine, rheumatology, spina bifida, surgery and trauma. It is also associated with the **Neonatal and Paediatric Emergency Transport Service** (NETS), a Flying Doctor service especially for kids transporting 1500 children a year by helicopter.

The hospital is 28 km west of Sydney, accessible by the Sydney metro (get off at Parramatta). A direct shuttle bus goes from the airport. Full details are available on their incredible website. This also displays current job opportunities.

O **Elective notes:** The opportunities in an elective here are vast and can be decided upon arrival. NETS is worth a special mention. They are happy for elective students to go on retrieval, but it takes a couple of days to train up before you can go on the helicopter. The views of Sydney, however, make it well worthwhile. Elective places here are hard to come by … you really should apply 12 months in advance. Write to the elective coordinator at the above address.

Note: It is a long way out of Sydney (45 minutes on the tube). The hospital has close links with the King George V Hospital in central Sydney, a tertiary referral maternity hospital delivering 4700 babies a year.

Accommodation: Available at about $35 (£17) a week and has air-conditioning and a swimming pool. However, there are no cooking facilities. Tel: +61 2 9845 2958. E-mail: hostel@nch.edu.au.

Sydney Hospital and Sydney Eye Hospital

Macquaire Street, Sydney, NSW 2000. Tel: +61 2 9382 7111. Fax: +61 2 9382 7320.

The hospitals: The oldest in Australia, dating back to 1788. There are currently 113 inpatient beds, and three academic departments are affiliated with Sydney University and/or UNSW. Services include general medicine, surgery, orthopaedics, ENT, hand surgery, ophthalmology and drug, alcohol and sexual health. It has an emergency department and specialist eye emergency department.

O **Elective notes:** A nice central hospital (a 10 minute walk to the Opera House). The general part of the hospital is pretty small. It's excellent if you're interested in eyes.

OTHER HOSPITALS IN NEW SOUTH WALES:

The only university outside Sydney in New South Wales is the:

University of Newcastle

Faculty of Medicine, University of Newcastle, Medical Sciences Building Room 613, Callaghan, Newcastle, NSW 2308. Tel: +61 2 4921 567. Fax: +61 2 4921 5071.
E-mail: Health-Enquiries@newcastle.edu.au. www.newcastle.edu.au..
Newcastle is on the coast about 170 km north of Sydney.

John Hunter Hospital

Lookout Road, New Lambton, Newcastle, NSW. Tel: +61 2 4921 3000. Fax: +61 2 4921 3999. www.hunter.health.nsw.gov.au.
The hospital: John Hunter Hospital (with 550 beds) is the principle referral centre and teaching hospital and a com-

munity hospital for Newcastle, Lake Macquarie and beyond. It is the only trauma centre in New South Wales outside Sydney and has the busiest emergency department in the state. Its specialities include O&G, respiratory medicine, emergency medicine, trauma, cardiology and cardiac surgery, gastroenterology, nephrology, kidney transplants, anaesthesia and intensive care, neonatal intensive care, neurology and neurosurgery, and endocrinology.

Royal Newcastle Hospital
Pacific Street (PO Box 664J), Newcastle, NSW 2300. Tel: +61 2 4923 6000.
Fax: +61 2 4923 6204.
The hospital: The Royal Newcastle used to be the major teaching hospital for the university it is now a scaled-down (95-bed) public hospital with specialist departments (urology, diabetes, rheumatology, ophthalmology and orthopaedics). Note: It is situated right on the coast!

Belmont District Hospital
Croudace Bay Road, Belmont, Newcastle, NSW 2280. Tel: +61 2 4923 2000.
Fax: +61 2 4923 2106.
The hospital: A 75-bed acute facility. The services include general medicine, general surgery, day surgery, a coronary care unit, gynaecology, neonatal, obstetrics and a 24-hour emergency department. Allied services include physiotherapy, occupational therapy and speech therapy.

Cessnock District Hospital
View Street (PO Box 154), Cessnock, Newcastle, NSW 2325. Tel: +61 2 4991 0555. Fax: +61 2 4991 0563.
The hospital: Is a 68-bed acute facility. Services include general medicine, general surgery, orthopaedics, urology, gynaecology, obstetrics and a 24-hour emergency department.

Kurri Kurri District Hospital
Lang Street, Kurri Kurri, Newcastle, NSW 2327. Tel: +61 2 4936 3200.
Fax: +61 2 4936 3239.
The hospital: A 41-bed acute and transi-

tional care facility. Services include general medicine, general surgery, ear/nose and throat, ophthalmology and a 24-hour emergency department. Allied services include physiotherapy, dietetics, speech pathology and occupational therapy.

Maitland Hospital
550–560 High Street, Maitland, Newcastle, NSW 2320. Tel: +61 2 4939 2000.
Fax: +61 2 4939 2270.
The hospital: Is a referral facility for the Upper and Lower Hunter Regions. Services include medical and rehabilitation, surgical and day surgery, and maternity and child services. There is a busy emergency department and a coronary care/high-dependency unit.

Muswellbrook District Hospital
Brentwood Street (PO Box 120), Muswellbrook, Newcastle, NSW 2333.
Tel: +61 2 6542 2000.
Fax: +61 2 6542 2002.
The hospital: Provides the communities of Muswellbrook and the surrounding district with quality health services that include surgical, medical, emergency, obstetrics, paediatrics, aged care and oncology.

Newcastle Mater Misericordiae Hospital
Edith Street, Waratah, Newcastle, NSW 2298. Tel: +61 2 4291 1211.
Fax: +61 2 4960 2673.
The hospital: The Newcastle Mater is a 192-bed public teaching hospital owned by the Sisters of Mercy Singleton and managed by Catholic Health Care. It provides services such as emergency care, general medical and surgical, plastic and oncology specialities. There is easy access to beaches, lakes and vineyards. The surrounding economy is based on industry, mining and tourism.

Manly Hospital
Darley Road, Manley, Sydney, NSW 2095.
Tel: +61 2 9977 9611.
Fax: +61 2 9977 8907.
The hospital: A small district general hospital serving the northern beach

towns and coastal commuter belt of north-east Sydney, it's three-quarters of a mile north of the area of Ventremup. It's on a steep slope and has a magnificent view of Sydney Harbour. It was founded in the late 19th century and has been built up since. Serious cases are, however, referred to the **Royal North Shore Hospital** 8 km away.

O **Elective notes:** By applying here, you can do a number of specialities. They can also arrange general practice for you.

Broken Hill Base Hospital

PO Box 457, 174 Thomas Street, Broken Hill, NSW 2880. Tel: +61 8 8088 0333. Fax: +61 8 8088 1715.

The hospital: Is in the outback of New South Wales, over 1000 km from Sydney, with a half-hour time difference from the rest of the state. The nearest large town is Adelaide (five hours' drive away). Broken Hill ('Silver City') allegedly has a population of 27 000, but you may feel that most of them have gone away. The hospital has 100 beds. The town's claim to fame is that it appears in the film *Priscilla, Queen of the Desert* (the hotel with the gaudy paintings). The hospital serves the Far West Health Region, covering a vast area of desert and countryside (one and a half times the size of the UK). It has one consultant surgeon and one consultant physician, all other specialities being covered by visiting specialists from all over the state.

O **Elective notes:** You can do whatever you want, rotating from one week to the next. If you are persistent, there is the opportunity to fly with the Flying Doctors (this is where the Royal Flying Doctors are based). It's also worth going out into one of the outlying Aboriginal communities for a day or two.

Accommodation: Costs approximately AU\$70 (£35) a week and is in the nurses' home, where most people who work in the hospital live. Food is also provided cheaply from the canteen. It's very friendly, and there's always something going on. Someone will have a car or if you talk to the right people you might be able to borrow a hospital car. There is lots of beer to drink. Sydney is 16–18 hours away by coach, two-and-a-half hours by plane. Things to do in the vicinity include camel riding, go down a disused mine, visit Silverton (and go down active silver mines), visit Menindee caves, bush camping or the locals' favourite . . . sunset watching. You can go on the postal round with the postman for AU\$230 (£115) – he flies to the different houses, making 50–70 landings en route.

Wagga Base Hospital

20 Docker Street, Wagga Wagga, NSW 2650.

The hospital: Wagga is actually the largest inland town in New South Wales so is fairly busy. It's friendly but freezing cold in the winter. The hospital is a fairly typical district general.

O **Elective notes:** The medical students extradited there from Sydney consider it some sort of Siberia. The staff are friendly and the consultants keen to teach. It's great if you like skiing. Overall advice: it's good, but if you're only visiting one place in Australia, try somewhere else.

Accommodation: Free, and the town is nice, if unexciting.

Blue Mountains District Anzac Memorial Hospital

Locked Bag No 2, Katoomba, NSW 2780.

The hospital: Katoomba is a quiet town in the Blue Mountains, surrounded by stunning scenery and only two hours (109 km) by train (AU\$10 (£5)) from Sydney. The hospital has 95 beds covering general surgery and medicine, paeds, O&G, care of the elderly and emergency medicine. The emergency department receives from several towns and a very large area of National Park. You will mainly see outdoor activity injuries (fractures, etc.). This is, however, a great place to go if you are the outdoor type with rock climbing, caving, pot-holing and horse riding easily accessible.

Note: While the rest of Oz is in sunshine, this place is usually in mist. It is also home to many funnel web and red back spiders.

Accommodation: Free for students in the nurses' home but a little run-down. It may be a bit lonely if you're on your own.

Manning Base Hospital

PO Box 35, Taree, NSW 2430.
The hospital: Manning Base Hospital is located in Taree, a three-and-a-half hour drive north of Sydney just off the highway to Brisbane. The area is popular with tourists and the retired. Taree itself has a high unemployment rate and considerable social problems among the local Aboriginal cluster. The hospital has approximately 180 beds providing emergency medicine, surgical, medical, paeds, O&G as well as psychiatric services.
O Elective notes: It does have a few medical students from Newcastle (Australia) on their rural attachment. The staff are friendly, but there may be some lack of supervision for elective students, and you may well find yourself out on a limb. There may be little opportunity to practise practical procedures. Transport here is limited, but the staff are friendly and will offer lifts.
Accommodation: Available in the nurses' quarters for AU$60 (£30) a week.

OTHER HOSPITALS:

Auburn Hospital, Norval Street, Auburn, NSW 2144. Tel: +61 2 9563 9500. Fax: +61 2 9563 9510.
Balmain Hospital, Booth Street, Balmain, NSW 2041. Tel: +61 2 9395 2111. Fax: +61 2 9395 2119.
Bankstown Hospital, Eldridge Road, Bankstown, NSW 2200. Tel: +61 2 9722 8000.
Fax: +61 2 9722 8316.
Blacktown Hospital, Blacktown Road, Blacktown, NSW 2148. Tel: +61 2 9830 8000.
Fax: +61 2 9830 8020.
Canterbury Hospital, Canterbury Road, Campsie, NSW 2194. Tel: +61 2 9789 9111.
Fax: +61 2 9789 3450.
Gladesville Hospital, Victoria Road, Gladesville, NSW 2111. Tel: +61 2 9477 9123.
Fax: +61 2 9477 2005.
Hornsby Ku-Ring-Gai Hospital, Palmerston Road, Hornsby, NSW 2077. Tel: +61 2 9477 9123.
Fax: +61 2 9477 2005.
Lismore Base Hospital, 60 Uralba Street, Lismore, NSW 2480. Tel: +61 2 6621 8000.
+61 2 6621 708S8.

Orange Base Hospital, Sale Street, Orange, NSW 2800. Tel: +61 2 6362 1411.
Fax: +61 2 6362 0306.
Royal Womens Hospital, 188 Oxford Street, Paddington, NSW 2021. Tel: +61 2 9382 6111.
Fax: +61 2 9382 6513.
Rozelle Hospital, Cnr Church and Glover Streets, Leichardt, NSW 2040. Tel: +61 2 9556 9100.
Fax: +61 2 9818 5712.
Sutherland Hospital, 430 Kingsway Street, Caringbah, NSW 2299. Tel: +61 2 9540 7111.
Fax: +61 2 9540 7197.
Tamworth Base Hospital, Dean Street, Tamworth, NSW 2340. Tel: +61 2 6766 1722.
Fax: +61 2 6766 6638.

PRIVATE HOSPITALS:

Cape Hawke Community Private Hospital, Breckenridge Street, Forster, NSW 2428.
Tel: +61 65 546077. Fax: +61 65 558750.
www.midcoast.com.au/prof/medical/hosp/chcph.html.
Hills Private Hospital, 499 Windsor Road, Baulkham Hills, NSW 2153. Tel: +61 639 3333.
Fax: +61 639 5950. www.midcoast.com.au/prof/.
medical/hosp/hills.html.
Mayo Private Hospital, Potoroo Drive, Taree, NSW 2430. Tel: +61 65 521466.
Fax: +61 65 626759. www.midcoast.com.au/prof/.
medical/hosp/mayo.html.
Sydney Adventist Hospital, 185 Fox Yalley Road, Wahroonga, NSW 2076. Tel: +61 2 9487 91. Fax: +61 2 9487 92. www.sah.org.au/sahwelc.htm. (The South Pacific flagship of the Seventh-day Adventist health care system. It operates a 324 bed unit.)

SOMETHING DIFFERENT:

NSW Institute of Forensic Medicine

42–50 Parramatta Road, PO Box 90, Glebe, NSW 2037. www.forensic.org.au.
The institute: For some gruesome murders, appalling suicides (and the odd natural death), this can at least be described as an interesting elective. Not great for communication skills with patients! The chappy to contact is the Associate Professor, Director of the NSW Institute of Forensic Medicine, at the above address. Alternatively, write to the Elective Coordinator, Department of Clinical Education, Royal Prince Alfred Hospital, Missenden Road, Camperdown, NSW 2050.

Australia

VICTORIA

Melbourne

Melbourne is the 'culture capital' of Oz, with great shops, restaurants and theatres. It's also the sports capital, being home to Aussie Rules football, Grand Prix and the tennis open. Travel around the city is easy and cheap. Beaches are a 45-minute tram ride from the centre (there is an excellent transport system). The weather is hottest in January and February, but it can be unpredictable. Out of the city, things to do consist of: the Coreal Ocean Road, Grampians National Park, Philip Island (see the penguins) and Yarra and Clare Valleys. There is also excellent skiing.

There are two universities in Victoria, one in Melbourne, the other in Clayton (20 km outside Melbourne).

University of Melbourne

Faculty of Medicine, University of Melbourne, Gratton Street, Parkville, VIC 3052. Tel: +61 3 9 344 5894. Fax: +61 3 9 347 7854. www.unimelb.edu.au. (This has three teaching hospitals.)

Monash University

Faculty of Medicine, Monash University, Wellington Road, Clayton, Melbourne, VIC 3168. Tel: +61 3 9 905 4318. Fax: +61 3 9 905 4302. www.med.monash.edu.au. (With 4145 beds.)

HOSPITALS IN MELBOURNE:

Royal Melbourne Hospital

132 Grattan Street, Parkville, Melbourne, VIC 3050. Tel: +61 3 9342 7031. Fax: +61 3 9342 7802. www.mh.org.au. **The hospital:** A large, busy inner city hospital with several hundred beds and all specialities affiliated to the University of Melbourne.
O Elective notes: It's a very friendly place, at least for nephrology and vascular surgery, gastroenterology, endocrinology (mainly outpatients), neurology and cardiology and you can do as much or as little as you want. You won't be able to do general medicine, surgery, paeds or O&G as these are full with Aussie students. The staff are very keen for you to explore Australia. Not so good for practical skills as there are loads of other students around, but on the other hand this makes the social life good. There are many lectures and tutorials for you to attend if you want. It's a 15-minute walk into the centre of Melbourne. Psychiatry has had some very good reports. You must apply to the dean of the clinical school, Royal Melbourne Hospital.
Accommodation: There is excellent accommodation for elective students at only AU$ 11.50 a week (contact the clinical school Charles Cornibere Residence). A swimming pool and sauna are in the residence; the university gym is just a short walk away ($29 (£15) a month membership).

St Vincent's Hospital

41 Victoria Parade, Fitzroy, VIC 3065. Tel: +61 3 8288 2211. Fax: +61 3 9288 3399. www.svhm.org.au.
The hospital: Founded in 1883, this is one of the three teaching hospitals in Melbourne. It is modern and right in the city centre.
O Elective notes: The clinical school takes in 80 students per year who tend to be hard-working but good fun. There is a high doctor:patient ratio so the staff have plenty of time for teaching. In dermatology, like the rest of Oz, malignant melanomas are the hot topic. This hospital has often been thoroughly recommended.
Accommodation: The clinical school has its own building, with 14 bedrooms and excellent facilities. It's AU$25 (£10) a week, with free washing machine, drier, tea, coffee, cleaning lady, free local calls, etc.

Royal Children's Hospital

Flemington Road, Parkville, Melbourne, VIC 3052. Tel: +61 3 9345 5522 (switchboard). Fax: +61 3 9345 5789. www.rch.unimelb.edu.au.
The hospital: A very busy tertiary refer-

ral centre (330 beds) and great if you're into paediatrics. The hospital is affiliated to the Royal Women's Hospital, University of Melbourne and has all the rarities of a tertiary referral centre as well as the usual illnesses as it's the local children's hospital. Melbourne city centre (2 km away) is 30 minutes on foot or ten minutes by tram.

O **Elective notes:** There are loads of students so it's good on social life but poor on practical skills. The teaching programme is excellent. You get into small tutorial groups ('tutes') and get regular lectures, quiz sessions and case presentations.

Accommodation: A flat for elective students is situated just a short walk from the hospital. There are two bedrooms, each sleeping two, plus a bathroom, kitchen and living room. The rent is AU$10 (£4) a night. It's clean but the appliances have a habit of breaking. The hospital is famous for its McDonalds in the foyer, but don't worry, there are plenty of good pubs and restaurants close by. As the accommodation only takes four, it's important to apply early (a year in advance is advisable); however, if it is full, you can try Brookes Gillespie House (part of the University: Brookes Gillespie House, 740 Swanson Street, Carlton, Melbourne, VIC).

To apply to the hospital, you can either contact the elective coordinator (and risk being charged an administration fee of AU$250 (£125)) or apply directly to one of the consultants.

Royal Women's Hospital

132 Grattan Street, Carlton, VIC 3053. Tel: +61 3 9344 2000. Fax: +61 3 9348 1840. www.rch.unimelb.edu.au.

The hospital: A 400-bed obstetric, gynaecological and neonatal paediatric hospital. It is the largest Australian hospital specializing in women's and infant's health and is a major teaching hospital.

Monash University

Faculty of Medicine, Monash University, Wellington Road, Clayton, VIC 3168. www.med.monash.edu.au.

Monash University is situated approximately 20 km outside Melbourne. It incorporates the Alfred and Box Hill Hospitals as well as the Monash Medical Centre in Clayton.

Alfred Hospital

PO Box 315, Commercial Road, Prahran, VIC 3181. Tel: +61 3 9510 2000/2513. Fax: +61 3 9276 2222.

The hospital: This is one of the big teaching hospitals in Melbourne a ten minute bus ride from the city centre. The Alfred has big research interests in trauma, intensive care, diving medicine and chest medicine. This wide range of interests means that there are many interesting patients to see. The main beach (St Kilda) is a 15-minute walk away.

O **Elective notes:** The consultants and registrars are friendly and keen to teach. They are also as keen for you to see Australia as you are.

Accommodation: Not always provided however, some units will try their best to find you some cheaply.

Monash Medical Centre

246 Clayton Road, Clayton, Melbourne, VIC 3168.

www.southernhealth.org.au/mmc.

The hospital: Is about 20 km outside Melbourne and accepts patients from the southern suburbs.

O **Elective notes:** For paediatrics at least, it is very friendly, but it can be quiet in the summer.

HOSPITALS IN COUNTRY VICTORIA:

Austin Hospital

Studley Road, Heidelberg, Melbourne, VIC 3081. Tel: +61 3 9496 5000. Fax: +61 3 9458 4779.

The hospital: Is a well-advanced centre of excellence, having a PET scanner, a liver transplant unit, cardiac surgery, neurosurgery, cardiology, neurology, endocrinology, oncology, gastroenterology and a spinal injuries unit. There is a very good physiotherapy department. The psychiatry department sees a number of patients with post-traumatic stress disorder from Vietnam. The hospital is 10 km north-east of Melbourne.

O **Elective notes:** The hospital is very busy, but the staff are keen to teach.

Accommodation: Provided on-site for around AU$20 (£10) a week and has a gym and pool.

Bendigo Hospital

Lucan Street, PO Box 126, Bendigo, VIC 3550.

The hospital: Bendigo is an old gold-mining town two hours north of Melbourne and a tourist destination in its own right. The hospital is medium-sized serving a large surrounding area. Bendigo itself is a lovely place. From here you can travel to Melbourne, the Great Ocean Road, Philip Island, Healesville, the Yarra Valley, the Dandenong Mountain range and Sydney for a long weekend.

O **Elective notes:** You can do emergency and general medicine, surgery, orthopaedics, O&G or oncology. There are Aussie students there in term time; they and the other staff are all friendly. The interns and registrars rotate from Melbourne so there's always a bit of a party atmosphere as people come and go and it's easy to get lifts to Melbourne. You can do as much or as little as you wish. There is no fee to the hospital.

Accommodation: Cheap – AU$25 (£12) a week in the nurses' home in the hospital.

Warrnambool and District Base Hospital

Ryot Street, Warrnambool, VIC 3280. Tel: +61 3 5564 1666. Fax: +61 3 5564 9660.

The hospital: Warrnambool is a small city on the south coast of Victoria towards the end of the Great Ocean Road (population 28 000). It's a relatively quiet, medium-sized hospital.

O **Elective notes:** There are few Aussie medical students so you can quickly become a member of the team and get doing practical skills. You can choose any speciality and the consultants are willing to teach, although there is no formal teaching. As you might expect, the nightlife is fairly quiet, but there are plenty of good, cheap places to eat and drink. The local bay is good for swimming and surfing but can get cold and windy in the winter.

Accommodation: In the nurses' home opposite the hospital and costs AU$50 (£25) a week. There's a decent canteen. Warrnambool is pretty remote, especially if you don't have a car. It's three hours from Melbourne, but it's easy to get to Great Ocean Road and the Grampians.

Mornington Peninsula Hospital/ Frankston Community Hospital

8–10 Hastings Road, Frankston, Melbourne, VIC 3199. Tel: +61 3 9783 6077.

The hospital: This is a modestly sized, acute general hospital with 344 beds, of which 140 are surgical. There are four general surgeons in the professorial unit.

Geelong Hospital

Geelong, Melbourne, VIC.

The hospital: A fairly small DGH one hour from Melbourne.

O **Elective notes:** There are no students here so you have free rein. It is very close to some famous surf beaches.

OTHER HOSPITALS IN VICTORIA:

Ballarat Base Hospital, Drummond Street, Ballarat, VIC 3350. Tel: +61 3 5320 4000. Fax: +61 3 5333 1562.

Box Hill and District Hospital, Nelson Road, Box Hill, VIC 3128. Tel: +61 3 9895 3333. Fax: +61 3 9895 3176.

Caufield Hospital, 260 Kooyong Road, Caufield, VIC 3162. Tel: +61 3 9276 6000.

Dandenong and District Hospital, David Street, Dandenong, VIC 3175. Tel: +61 3 9791 6000. Fax: +61 3 979 5709.

Fairfield Hospital, Yarra Bend Road, Fairfield, VIC 3078. Tel: +61 3 9345 5522. Fax: +61 3 9482 6572.

Frankston Community Hospital, 8–10 Hastings Road, Frankston, Melbourne, VIC 3199. Tel: +61 3 9783 6077.

Goulburn Valley Base Hospital, Shepparton, VIC 3630.

Melbourne Clinic, 130 Church Street, Richmond, VIC 3121. Tel: +61 3 9429 4688.

Mildura Base Hospital, Thirteenth Street, Mildura, VIC 3500. Tel: +61 3 5022 3333. Fax: +61 3 5023 3470.
Peter MacCallum Cancer Clinic, 481 Little Lonsdale Street, Melbourne, VIC 3000. Tel: +61 3 9641 5555.
Preston and Northcote Community Hospital, 205 Bell Street, Preston, VIC 3072. Tel: +61 3 9285 2222. Fax: +61 3 9487 2524.
Repatriation General Hospital, Heidelberg, Banksia St West, Heidelberg, VIC 3081. Tel: +61 3 9496 2111. Fax: +61 3 9862 3658.
St George's Hospital, 283 Cotham Road, Kew, VIC 3101. Tel: +61 3 9272 0444.
Tallangatta Hospital, Tallangatta, VIC 3700.
Wangaratta District Base Hospital, Green Street, Wangaratta, VIC 3677. Tel: +61 3 5722 0111. Fax: +61 3 5722 0105.
Western Hospital, Gordon Street, Footscray, VIC 3011. Tel: +61 3 9319 6666. Fax: +61 3 9317 7815.
Wimmera Base Hospital, Baillie Street, Horsham, VIC 3400. Tel: +61 3 5381 9111. Fax: +61 3 5382 0829.

SOMETHING DIFFERENT:

Victorian Institute of Forensic Medicine
Kavanagh Street, Southbank, Melbourne, VIC. Tel: 61 3 9684 4444.
For those wishing to study forensic/coronial services, contact the professor at the above address. They expect a small project to be done while you're there.
Accommodation: Sometimes provided; if not, there are plenty of youth hostels in central Melbourne.

SOUTH AUSTRALIA

Adelaide

Although considered by many to be more of a 'country town' than a city, Adelaide has wonderful beaches, wines and a good music scene. It's not usually on the tourist route and hence is not so often visited on electives. This is a good place to go, however, if you've 'done' Australia before and want to work in a very friendly major teaching hospital.

There are two universities in South Australia, both in Adelaide.

University of Adelaide
Medical School, Frome Road, Adelaide, SA 5000. Tel: +61 8 8303 5193. Fax: +61 8 8 303 3788. www.health.adelaide.edu.au. (With 2179 beds.)

Flinders University
School of Medicine, Flinders University of South Australia, Bedford Park, SA 5042 (or GPO 2100, SA 5001). Tel: +61 8 8204 4160. Fax: +61 8 8204 5845. www.flinders.edu.au. (With 775 beds.)

Royal Adelaide Hospital
North Terrace, Adelaide, SA 5000. Tel: +61 8 8222 4000. Fax: +61 8 8223 4761. www.rah.sa.gov.au.
The hospital: Is a very friendly major hospital. You can walk to the city centre in two minutes and it's surrounded by botanical gardens and parks. It is a centre for diving medicine and a world centre for training in baromedicine. The hospital itself came from a humble background, starting as the Colonial Infirmary in 1837. Three of its four patients died, but it is now one of Australia's largest teaching hospitals.
O Elective notes: There is high-quality teaching in both medicine and surgery. It's great if you are a bit of a diver. As an elective student you are given a great deal of responsibility.
Accommodation: Costs AU$22 (£11) a week in the nurses' home.

Adelaide Women and Children's Hospital
72 King William Road, North Adelaide, SA 5006. Tel: +61 8 8204 7000. Fax: +61 8 8239 0417. www.wch.sa.gov.au.
The hospital: A major hospital providing extensive services both within the hospital and on rural outreach clinics. Departments include cardiology, child development, endocrine and diabetes, gastroenterology, neurology, oncology, orthopaedic, paediatric intensive care and renal. They are currently developing Telehealth services to facilitate videoconferencing to the rural and remote areas.

Flinders Medical Centre
Bedford Park, Adelaide, SA 5042.
Tel: +61 8 204 5511. Fax: +61 8 204 5450.
www.flinders.sa.gov.au.
The hospital: Being a teaching hospital for Flinders University, nearly all specialities are catered for. This 430-bed hospital is superb for emergency medicine – it has a very modern emergency department with a CT scanner next door. The hospital itself is outside the city centre, but buses are cheap. It allegedly has a better working atmosphere than the Royal Adelaide.
O **Elective notes:** Lots of teaching and responsibility and many opportunities to do practical procedures such as suturing. Aussie medical students actually go here to do their electives. There are many things to do: Kangaroo Island, many wineries (Coonawwarra, Clare, McLaren, Barossa Valleys ... a one-hour drive).
Accommodation: Can be arranged within the hospital.

HOSPITALS OUTSIDE ADELAIDE:

Pika Wiya Health Service
PO Box 2021 Port Augusta, Perth, SA 5700.
The hospital: In the outback of South Australia 200–300 km north of Adelaide. The town's population is about 17 000, with a large Aboriginal community. Pika Wiya is a health service specifically for Aboriginal people and is run in general practice style. There is an 80-bed hospital, however, but no resident doctors so the Pika Wiya doctors have to cover that too. Clinics are in Port Augusta and Davenport, both giving lots of 'hands on' medicine.
O **Elective notes:** Spend time with the child health service and paediatrician as both go out into the local communities, providing real experience of Aboriginal life. The Flying Doctors in Port Augusta are willing to take students up so there's even more opportunity to get to meet real Australians.
Accommodation: Is in Port Augusta.

The social life is not as bad as you may think. People are often happy to lend you a car or give you a lift and there is often the odd student from Adelaide. You must visit the nearby Flinders Mountain Range. Warning: You may get lonely.

HOSPITALS IN SOUTH AUSTRALIA:

Mount Gambier Hospital Inc, Lake Terrace West, Mount Gambier, SA 5290. Tel: +61 8 8724 2211. Fax: +61 8 8723 0008.
Queen Elizabeth Hospital, Woodville Road, Woodville, SA 5011. Tel: +61 8 8222 6000. Fax: +61 8 8222 6010.
Queen Victoria Hospital, 160 Fullerton Road, Rose Park, SA 5067. Tel: +61 8 8332 4888. Fax: +61 8 8333 9171.
Whyalla Hospital, Wood Terrace, Whyalla, SA 5600. Tel: +61 8 8645 8300. Fax: +61 8 8645 3007.

QUEENSLAND

Brisbane

With a population of 1.4 million, Brisbane is Australia's third-largest city. It's a relaxed city, 25 km upstream from the mouth of the Brisbane River, with many places to eat, drink and watch sport. It has good weather, and there are loads of things to do on the 2000 km of Queensland coast: Fraser Island, Byron Bay, Surfer's Paradise, Whitsunday Islands, the Sunshine Coast and the Great Barrier Reef. Magnetic Island is a good place to try jetskiing at a reasonable price, and for white water rafting, try the Tully River at Mission Beach. If you are in Cairns for a day and have a sense of humour, try 'Uncle Brian's Fun, Falls and Forest' day trip. Around Brisbane itself are the beautiful Hinterlands, superb for those interested in bush walking or mountaineering (but remember that Australia has eight of the world's ten most poisonous snakes!). September to October is a good time to visit as the weather is starting to get hot but box jellyfish are not yet out so it's safe to swim in the sea. Despite Australia's 'Slip, Slap, Slop' policy, malignant melanomas and other skin conditions are still highly prevalent. Brisbane has become the skin capital of the world. Therefore dermatology and skin surgery are good specialities here. Expect loads of hassle if you turn up in the melanoma clinic with a tan.

MEDICAL SCHOOL:

University of Queensland Medical School

Herston Road, Herston, Brisbane, QLD 4006. Tel: +61 7 3365 5316.
Fax: +61 7 3365 5433. www.uq.edu.au.

To do your elective in Queensland you MUST apply to the **Postgraduate Medical Education Foundation of Queensland Ltd**, at the above address. Apply AT LEAST SIX MONTHS IN ADVANCE and pay the AU$150 (£75) administration fee. They can then place you somewhere in Queensland (the earlier you apply the more chance you will get your first choice). Also request accommodation at this time. The University of Queensland can then levy further charges (which can be pretty steep – up to AU$700 (£350) for four weeks).

Again, as in the case for Sydney, you can put yourself at an advantage by writing to your desired destination before writing to the Postgraduate Medical Education Foundation. It's much better to say that 'Dr X from Y hospital has said he would be delighted to have me do an elective in his department'.

Royal Brisbane Hospital

Herston Road, Herston, Brisbane, QLD 4006. Tel: +61 7 3253 8111.
Fax: +61 7 3857 4462.
www.health.qld.gov.au/royal.

The hospital: A large (800-bed, 500 000 admissions a year) hospital, it is a 15-minute bus ride (3 km) from the city centre. It is right next to the Queensland Medical School on the northern side of Brisbane and shares its campus with the **Royal Children's Hospital**, **Royal Women's Hospital** and **Queensland Institute of Medical Research**. All specialities are covered bar cardiology and transplant surgery, which are catered for at the Prince Charles hospital.

O **Elective notes:** There is a laid-back, welcoming attitude but also excellent teaching, with a library and computer lab on site that you are free to use. Units such as gastroenterology may be a bit too specialized, and you learn nothing. It's a 25-minute walk to the city centre and a 20-minute bus ride to the airport. If you want to travel Oz, this is a good start as the Greyhound bus stops at the front gates and the staff are keen that you explore.
Note: This is a popular place, so make enquires early.

Accommodation: The Lady Lamington Home Nurses' Quarter is quaint (AU$70 (£35) a week or AU$11.50 (£5.75) a night, although prices may be going up), and there's a swimming pool and gym for residents. The canteen's not great, but it's only five minutes' walk to the food store in Fortitude Valley.

Royal Children's Hospital Brisbane

Herston Road, Herston, Brisbane, QLD 4006. Tel: +61 7 3253 8111.
Fax: +61 7 3857 4462. www.rchf.org.au.

The hospital: Part of a site of three hospitals situated in the Herston area of Brisbane (the other two being the **Royal Brisbane** and the **Royal Women's Hospital**). Each year, it admits 16 000 children to its wards, sees 18 000 children in the emergency department, and 99 800 outpatients and has 3600 admissions for cancer. The 168 beds comprise 12 for transplants, 24 for neurosurgery and 20 neonatal beds.

Accommodation: In the nurses' home. It's comfortable and cheap (AU$10 (£5) a night). It's friendly as all the elective students stay here.

Note: Think about the Mater Misericordiae Hospital if you are staying some time as that is free.

Mater Misericordiae Hospital

Raymond Terrace, South Brisbane, QLD 4101. Tel: +61 7 3840 8111/8518.
Fax: +68 7 3840 3846/1548.
www.mater.org.au.

The hospital: The Mater is one of

Brisbane's teaching hospitals. Located on the South Bank of Brisbane, it's within walking distance (20 minutes) of the city centre.

O **Elective notes:** As an elective student, you are attached to a group of finalists therefore you get some excellent teaching and opportunities to do minor procedures. There are also X-ray and pathology meetings but not much ward-based activity.

Accommodation: Provided free to students by the hospital, although kitchen facilities are poor. You can buy meal tickets for the canteen.

Mater Children's Hospital

Department of Paediatrics and Child Health, South Brisbane, QLD 4101.

The hospital: This is part of the Mater Misericordiae Hospital. It's fairly large and good for developing skills in examining and assessing children. Neonatology, emergency medicine, general paediatrics and child psychiatry (mainly emotional and behavioural disorders) departments have all been praised. The paediatrics is very similar to that in any Western hospital. It's close to the city centre so there's plenty to do in your time off.

Accommodation: Free to students and has a pool. There's a man-made beach nearby.

Princess Alexandra Hospital

Ipswich Road, Woolloongabba, Brisbane, QLD 4102. Tel: +61 7 3240 2111/5346. Fax: +61 7 3240 2420/5399.

The hospital: A large (900-bed), modern general (tertiary referral) hospital on the south side of the Brisbane river. It covers all major adult specialities with the exception of cardiac surgery. It is nationally recognized for spinal injuries and solid organ transplants. It's affiliated to the University of Queensland and sees 60 000 inpatients a year. The hospital is a couple of miles from the city centre, a 10–20-minute train ride from the nearby station (500 yards). There are many job opportunities for doctors, radiographers and nurses. Check their website for the latest details.

O **Elective notes:** The doctors are friendly and enthusiastic, with a realistic attitude to the amount of work that you should do! Ward rounds on the general surgery side start at 7.30 am, but the accommodation is only two minutes from the ward. There's a large hepatobiliary department and the opportunity to assist in liver and kidney transplants. In orthopaedics there are ten consultants, each with their own special interest. There are many motorcyclists in Queensland, so this tends to be a busy department. This elective comes well recommended.

Accommodation: AU$11 (£5.50) a night in the nurses' home (Diamantina House), with good facilities, including a 25 m outdoor swimming pool. Other sports facilities are available at the St Lucia campus of Queensland University, a ten-minute walk and five-minute ferry ride across the Brisbane River. There are regular 'kegs' (free beer nights) for doctors and medical students.

MEDICAL SCHOOLS AND HOSPITALS OUTSIDE BRISBANE:

James Cook University

School of Medicine, Townsville, QLD 4811. Tel: +61 7 4781 6232. Fax: +61 7 4781 6986. www.jcu.edu.au.

This is a new medical school and home to the **Mount Isa Centre for Rural and Remote Health**.

Townsville General Hospital

Eyre Street Townsville, QLD 4810. Tel: +61 7 4781 9211 Fax: +61 7 4772 1373

The hospital: A large modern(ish) hospital with many specialist departments. It's even more relaxed than many other Aussie hospitals, allowing you to do what you want at a slightly slower pace. Not that much to do in Townsville, but Magnetic Island is only 15 minutes away by ferry. This is a lovely island and offers some of the best diving in Australia ... the courses are pretty cheap here as well.

Accommodation: Basic, but is in the hospital grounds and not expensive.

Gladstone Hospital

PO Box 299, Gladstone, QLD 4680.

The hospital: A small hospital in a rather bleak looking industrial town. There are only nine doctors but many visiting consultants. It is busy, and the doctors are keen for you to do practical procedures, minor operations and suturing. The staff are friendly.

Accommodation: Free in the (condemned!) but quaint nurses' home. The canteen varies in standard.

Mackay Base Hospital

Bridge Road, Mackay, QLD 4740.

The hospital: Mackay is a small town in north Queensland. The hospital is a 220-bed, very busy, sociable hospital. There are usually about 12 students (mostly Australian) present. This is a popular hospital for British doctors on a 'working holiday' so the social life is very good.

O Elective notes: The emergency department has a quite a reasonable turnover and they are keen for you to do minor surgery and suturing. General medicine, ITU and coronary care have also been very popular with previous visitors. They are a bit more serious about attendance than other Australian hospitals but are keen to teach. The town has a number of pubs and clubs and is very pretty. Note, however, that public transport is very limited so you have to rely on (expensive) taxis to get about. If you can borrow a car you are only two hours from Airlie Beach, opening the gateway to the Whitsunday Islands and Barrier Reef. The Eungella National Park is fairly close to town.

Accommodation: Free and is in the newly renovated nurses' home. There is a swimming pool outside the quarters, with palm trees and a barbecue. The food in the canteen is expensive and not great so most people cook in the quarters. The Aussie students live there too so the social life is good.

Gold Coast Hospital

108 Nerang Street, Southport, QLD 4215.

The hospital: Gold Coast Hospital is a teaching hospital about 70 km south of Brisbane in a very popular holiday strip of Queensland. It has recently undergone some major improvement. It provides all major specialities except cardiothoracic surgery, radiotherapy and burns. There are a number of UK doctors working throughout the hospital. The emergency department is busy and an excellent experience if you get stuck in. There are many surfing injuries as the Gold Coast is otherwise known as 'surfer's paradise'.

O Elective notes: If there when the Queensland students are on holiday (e.g. September/October) you'll get more experience (but fewer lectures); however, make sure that you spend some time in the emergency department or it can get a bit boring. If the students are around you are welcome to go to their teaching. The respiratory department has been popular with time off to explore the local areas. The Gold Coast is well suited for exploring the eastern coastline. There's loads to do and plenty of nightlife. The beach is a 20-minute walk away.

Accommodation: Accommodation in the nurses' quarters costs AU$19.50 (£8) a week, and there's a swimming pool.

Bundaberg Base Hospital

Bourbong Street, Bundaberg, QLD 4670. Tel: +61 7 4152 0222. Fax: +61 7 4173 1779.

The hospital: Bundaberg is a coastal town of 32 000. Its main industry is sugar cane farming, mainly for the production of Bundaberg rum. The hospital is friendly and laid back, many of the doctors being British. If doing emergency medicine, quite a few of the injuries are work related.

Accommodation: In the hospital with the other doctors. Bundaberg is the cheapest place in Queensland to do a scuba diving course, and there is easy access to the coral Whitsunday Islands and Fraser Island.

Rockhampton Base Hospital

Canning Street, Rockhampton, QLD 4700. Tel: +61 7 4931 6211.

The hospital: Rockhampton is a mining community and the beef capital of Australia, just inland of the south Queensland coast. The hospital is friendly and the medics are keen to teach. There are many lunchtime tutorials (and free lunch). Many of the doctors are Brits. There's little to do in Rockhampton itself so you have to rely on the interns for your social life.

Accommodation: Basic but costs only AU$60 (£30) a week. There's an on-site swimming pool and tennis court.

Cairns Base Hospital

The Esplanade, Cairns, North Queensland.

The hospital: Is currently undergoing renovation. The emergency department has four major trauma beds, eight minor cubicles and a four-bed observation ward. The usual trauma, overdoses, etc. are common, but there are also box jellyfish stings, snake bites and barotrauma in local divers. It's not wildly busy though. There is the occasional bit of tropical medicine to see and quite a bit of diabetes. Outreach clincs are run (by plane) into the bush.

O Elective notes: This is a good place for the Barrier Reef, but the weather is unpredictable and there's no beach nearby (ten minutes by car). The elective is organized through the University of Queensland, and there is a AU$150 (£75) fee.

Accommodation: None at present, but this may change.

Toowoomba Base Hospital

Private Mailbag No 2, Toowoomba, QLD 4350. Tel: +61 7 6316 310. Fax: +61 7 6391 098.

The hospital: Toowoomba (population 80 000) is 100 km west of Brisbane, lying on a plateau that defines the Darling Downs. It has 485 beds serving the 500 000 people between Queensland's border and the eastern Darling Downs. There is general medicine and surgery, orthopaedics, O&G,

paeds, anaesthetics, psychiatry and emergency medicine.

O Elective notes: They are very keen to have students.

OTHER HOSPITALS IN QUEENSLAND:

Ipswich Hospital, East Street, Ipswich, QLD 4305. Tel: +61 7 3810 1111. Fax: +61 7 3812 1419.
Maryborough General Hospital, 185 Walker Street, Maryborough, QLD 4650. Tel: +61 7 4123 8222. Fax: +61 7 4123 1606.
Repatriation General Hospital, Newdegate Street, Greenslopes, QLD 4120. Tel: +61 7 3394 7111. Fax: +61 7 3394 7745.
Royal Women's Hospital, Bowen Bridge Road, Herston, QLD 4006. Tel: +61 7 3253 8111. Fax: +61 7 3857 4462.

PRIVATE HOSPITALS:

Greenslopes Private Hospital, Newdegate Street, Greenslopes, QLD. Tel: +61 7 3394 7284. Fax: +61 7 3394 7789.
Park Haven Private Hospital, 9–13 Bayswater Road, Hyde Park, QLD 4812. Locked Bag 913, TMC Townsville, QLD 4810. Tel: +61 7 422 8822. Fax: +61 7 4721 3365.

WESTERN AUSTRALIA

Larger than western Europe, Western Australia exports 60% of Australia's gold and 11% of the world's iron ore and has Perth as its capital.

Perth

With a population just over one million, Perth is Australia's fourth-largest and most isolated city. It is clean with plenty to do: try sandsurfing, take a day trip to Rottnest Island, taste wine in Swan Valley and camel ride through the Bush. There are heaps of good pubs and clubs in Perth, and the weather is extremely pleasant even in the winter. South of Perth you have the Margaret River area, home to some of Oz's finest wines, limestone caves and surf. The town of Augusta has whale-watching cruises during the season and at Pemberton you can climb one of the tallest trees in the world (the Gloucester Tree, at 61 m high).

USEFUL ADDRESSES:

Government of Western Australia, European Office, 5th Floor, Australia Centre, Corner of Strand and Melbourne Place, London WC2B 4LG, UK. Tel: +44 20 7240 2881. Fax: +44 20 7240 6637.
Health Department of Western Australia, 189 Royal Street, East Perth, WA 6004.
Avon Health Service, combining Northam Regional Hospital (a 40 bed unit; Robinson Street, Northam, WA 6401. Tel: +61 8 9690 1300. Fax: +61 8 9690 1319), York District Hospital (a 12 bed unit; Trews Road, York, WA 6302. Tel: +61 8 9641 1200. Fax: +61 8 9641 1706) and Avon Community Heath (222 Fitzgerald Street, Northam, WA 6401. Tel: +61 8 9622 5080. Fax: +61 8 9622 2734). www.avon.net.au/~health\.

There is one university in Western Australia:

University of Western Australia
School of Medicine, University of Western Australia, 1st Floor, N Block, Queen Elizabeth Medical Centre, Monash Avenue, Nedlands, Perth, WA 6009.
Tel: +61 8 9346 3876. Fax: +61 8 9346 2369. www.meddent.uwa.edu.au. (The elective fee is currently around AU$250 (£125).)

Royal Perth Hospital
Wellington Street/Box 2213, Perth, WA 6000. Tel: +61 8 9224 2244.
Fax: +61 8 9224 3511. www.rph.wa.gov.au.
The hospital: Claims to be Western Australia's premier teaching hospital and is located in the city centre. Its history traces back to the first colonial hospital in a tent on Garden Island in June 1829. Today, the 855-bed hospital, seeing 67 000 admissions a year, is on two separate sites: Wellington Street in the city of Perth and Shenton Park 8 km away (Royal Perth Hospital, Selby Street, Shenton Park, WA 6008. Tel: +61 8 9224 2244. Fax: +61 8 9224 3511). It is also associated with the Royal Perth Rehabilitation Hospital (address below).

Services include emergency services, coronary angioplasty, cardiothoracic surgery, stroke treatment, bone marrow transplantation, immunodeficiency diseases, interventional neuroradiology, burns treatment, plastic and max-fax, rehab and a spinal unit.
O Elective notes: General medicine is a friendly department and you are encouraged to attend ward rounds and outpatient clinics. All in all … fairly laid back. There's good teaching and the grand round has a free lunch. An elective here is arranged through the University of Western Australia. Beaches and nightlife are nearby. There are some wonderful nursing opportunities here.
Accommodation: Costs around AU$50 (£25) a week for an air-conditioned room, lounge and kitchen in the hospital.

Sir Charles Gardiner Hospital (Queen Elizabeth II Medical Centre)
Verdun Street, Nedlands, Perth, WA 6009. Tel: +61 8 9346 3333. Fax: +61 8 9389 2534. www.scgh.health.wa.gov.au.
The hospital: A large, modern teaching hospital in the suburbs of Perth. Both general medicine and surgery are reported to be very friendly and well organized and there is a newly refurbished emergency department. The hospital is a short bus ride (about an hour's walk) from the city centre.
O Elective notes: The department of respiratory medicine offers good opportunities to specialize and do projects if you wish. In the emergency department, you'll see one red back spider/scorpion bite a day. It's a good place to get procedures under your belt. The staff are keen for you to go off and explore Oz.
Accommodation: Pretty basic (in Anstey House) and only AU$60 (£30) a week with the overseas doctors, nurses and other students. The hospital is very close to King's Park, which has walks through natural bushland and great barbecuing facilities. The University of Western Australia (very picturesque) is about ten minutes' walk away and has an excellent gym. At night during the

summer months an open-air cinema also runs here. The beaches are accessible by bus. Some students have found they can't use the computers and there aren't many pubs nearby.

Princess Margaret Children's Hospital

Roberts Road, Subiaco, Perth, WA 6009.
Tel: +61 8 9340 8222. Fax: +61 8 940 8111.
www.pmh.wa.gov.au.

The hospital: The Princess Margaret is a pleasant, friendly place, reasonably busy and the only specialized paediatric hospital in Western Australia. The paediatrics is fairly similar to that in the UK, with the exception of Aboriginal children, who are often flown in from the communities. The hospital is in one of the nicest areas of Perth and is not far from the city centre.

O Elective notes: There are fifth- and sixth-year students on attachment here and elective students are free to join any of their teaching.

Accommodation: No accommodation here, but it is provided at the Charles Gardiner Hospital, a short bus journey away. The Princess Margaret has a good doctor's room with a pool table and free muffins every day.

Fremantle General Hospital

Alma Street, Fremantle, Perth, WA 6160.
Tel: +61 8 9431 3333.

The hospital: A modern hospital, relaxed and friendly in a suburb of Perth. The professorial unit is great if you're after intensive medicine followed by intensive relaxation.

OTHER HOSPITALS IN WESTERN AUSTRALIA:

Armadale–Kelmscott Memorial Hospital, Albany Highway, Armadale 6112, WA.
Tel: +61 8 9391 2000.
Bentley Health Service, Bentley Hospital, Mills Street, Bentley, WA 6102. Tel: +61 8 9334 3666.
Graylands Hospital, Brockway Road, Mt Claremount, WA 6010. Tel: +61 8 9347 6600.
Hawthorn Hospital, 100 Flinders Street, Mount Hawthorn, WA 6016. Tel: +61 8 9444 8166.
Joondalup Health Campus, Shenton Avenue, Joondalup, WA 6027. Tel: +61 8 9405 2211.

Kalamunda District Community Hospital, Elizabeth Street, Kalamunda, WA 6076.
Tel: +61 8 9293 2122.
King Edward Memorial Hospital for Women, Bagot Road, Subiaco, WA 6008.
Tel: +61 8 9340 2222.
La Salle Hospital, Eveline Road, Middle Swan, WA 6056. Tel: +61 8 9347 5500.
Lemnos Hospital, Selby Street, Shenton Park, WA 6008. Tel: +61 8 9382 0760.
Mount Henry Hospital, Cloister Avenue, Como, WA 6152. Tel: +61 8 9313 1555.
Fax: +61 8 9450 1036.
Osbourne Park Hospital, Osbourne Place, Stirling, WA 6021. Tel: +61 8 9346 8000.
Perth Dental Hospital, 196 Goderich, Perth, WA 6000. Tel: +61 8 9220 5777.
Repatriation General Hospital, Hollywood, Monash Avenue, Nedlands, Perth, WA 6009.
Tel: +61 8 9346 6000. Fax: +61 8 9386 3153.
Rockingham–Kwinana District Hospital, Elanora Drive, Rockingham, WA 6168.
Tel: +61 8 9527 2777.
Royal Perth Rehabilitation Hospital, Selby Street, Shenton Park, WA 6008.
Tel: +61 8 9382 7171.
Swan District Hospital, Eveline Road, Middle Swan, WA 6056. Tel: +61 8 9347 5244.
Woodside Maternity Hospital, 18 Dalgety, Fremantle, WA 6160. Tel: +61 8 9339 1788.
Wooroloo Hospital, Linley Valley Road, Wooroloo, WA 6558. Tel: +61 8 9573 1228.

PRIVATE HOSPITALS IN WESTERN AUSTRALIA:

Attadale Hospital, 21 Hislop Road, Attadale, WA 6156. Tel: +61 8 9330 1000.
Bethesda Hospital Inc, 25 Queenslea Drive, Claremont, WA 6010. Tel: +61 8 9340 6300.
Bicton Hospital, 220 Preston Point Road, Bicton, WA 6157. Tel: +61 8 9339 1133.
Colin Street Day Surgery, 51 Colin Street, West Perth, WA 6005. Tel: +61 8 9321 4256.
Fremantle Kaleeya Hospital, Staton Road, East Fremantle, WA 6158. Tel: +61 8 9339 1655.
Glengarry Hospital, 53 Arnisdale Road, Duncraig, WA 6023. Tel: +61 8 9447 0111.
Gosnells Family Hospital, 2 Hamilton Court, Gosnells, WA 6110. Tel: +61 8 9490 1333.
Hollywood Private Hospital, Monash Avenue, WA, Perth, WA 6009. Tel: +61 8 9346 6000.
Mercy Hospital, Thirlmere Road, Mount Lawley, WA 6050.
Mount Hospital, 150 Mounts Bay Road, Perth, WA 6000. Tel: +61 8 9480 1822.
Mount Lawley Private Hospital, 14 Alvan, Mount Lawley, WA 6050. Tel: +61 8 9370 2500.
Niola Private Hospital, 61–69 Cambridge, Leederville, WA 6007. Tel: +61 8 9380 1833.
Perth Surgicentre, 38 Ranelagh Cresent, South Perth, WA 6151. Tel: +61 8 9367 4322.
St John of God Hospital Murdoch, 100 Murdoch Drive, Murdoch, WA 6150.

St John of God Hospital Subiaco, 175
Cambridge, Subiaco, WA 6008. Tel: +61 8 9382
6111. Fax: +61 8 9381 7180.
South Perth Community Hospital Inc, South
Terrace, Como, WA 6152. Tel: +61 8 9367 7966.
Stirling Community Hospital, 32 Spencer
Avenue, Yokine, WA 6060. Tel: +61 8 9276 5244.
Undercliffe Hospital Complex, 20 Coogan
Avenue, Greenmount, WA 6056. Tel: +61 8 9294 1211.

NORTHERN TERRITORY

Royal Darwin Hospital

Rocklands Drive, Casuarina, NT 0810. Tel:
+61 8 8922 8888. Fax: +61 8 8920 8286.
www.royaldarwinhospital.nt.gov.au.
The hospital: The hospital has 300 beds
and is a teaching hospital for Flinders
University. Twenty-five per cent of the
population is Aboriginal. It is close
(300 km) to the Kakadu National Park
World Heritage Area. There are many
Aboriginal settlements.
O **Elective notes:** It's a very relaxed and
friendly lifestyle. Darwin's population is
about 60 000 so there's plenty to do.

Alice Springs Hospital

Gap Road/ PO Box 2234, Alice Springs,
NT 0870. Tel: +61 8 8951 7777.
Fax: +61 8 8952 2712.
The hospital: Has just under 200 beds,
and departments including paeds, O&G,
surgery, medicine, emergency medicine,
psychiatry and anaesthetics. Half the
patients are Aboriginal. On the paeds
wards, you'll see lots of gastroenteritis,
pneumonia and failure to thrive. There is
also a flying doctor base. The emergency
department is very busy especially on a
Friday night.
O **Elective notes:** The doctors are
friendly and encourage you to do practical procedures (especially in the emergency department) and take long weekends to explore Ayers Rock, Kings
Canyon and Western MacDonnells. They
are good teachers. The town has shops,
banks restaurants, etc. but is by no means
big. Note: Apply well in advance if you
want to go.

Accommodation: This was previously a
problem, but now it's free and very good.

Tennant Creek Hospital

PO Box 346, Tennant Creek, NT 0861. Tel:
+61 8 8962 3132. Fax: +61 8 8962 4399.
Tenant Creek is 12-hour bus ride from
Darwin, and many would ask why the
hell go there. Tennant Creek has the
dubious claim to fame of being one of
the few towns in the world with a population of 3500 to appear on most world
maps. This is because it's the only real
settlement between Darwin and Alice
Springs. It's halfway between the two
and (according to unreliable Australian
legend) was founded when a beer wagon
bound for one of the local telegraph stations broke down. This attracted others,
but as the golden liquid began to dry up,
they had to explore the area around. One
lucky chap discovered a different type
of golden stuff and even more people
came in. It became a gold-mining town
and to this day there are still two gold
mines, which provide most of the
employment. The town also provides the
administration centre for the Barkley
region (about the size of England) and a
supply centre for many of the cattle stations and Aboriginal settlements in this
region.
The hospital: Serves an area about the
size of England and has just over 20 beds
(12 general medical, four paediatric and
four O&G), and they are always full.
There are usually four doctors: the medical superintendent, two district medical
officers (running bush clinics and most
of the patient management in the hospital) and a resident medical officer on
eight weeks' rotation from Alice Springs
(running the emergency department and
some bush clinics). There's a one-man
path lab, a radiographer and a community care team (doing immunizations,
screening and health awareness programmes (HIV, diabetes and skin cancer)
in the Bush. There is a six-seater air
ambulance that can transport patients
from the settlements in the Barkley
region to either Tennant Creek or Alice
Springs. The town has one GP.

O **Elective notes:** There are many great experiences to be had, emergency medicine, ward work and frequent clinics, either reached by many days' four-wheel-drive cross-country driving or flying. These clinics provide an excellent insight into Aboriginal life and health as well as being amazingly sociable and relaxing. Contact the superintendent to organize this. Don't give up (fax) – it's a great elective.

ANOTHER HOSPITAL IN NORTHERN TERRITORY:

Katherine Hospital, Gorge Road, Katherine, NT 0850. Tel: +61 8 8973 9211. Fax: +61 8 8973 9375.

AUSTRALIAN CAPITAL TERRITORY (ACT)

Canberra

Canberra Clinical School

Canberra, ACT. Tel: +61 2 6244 3649.
Fax: +61 2 6281 5616.
www.canberrahospital.act.gov.au/
education/clinical_school/clinsch.htm.
The Canberra Clinical School is affiliated to the University of Sydney and is a popular destination for elective students from Europe, Japan, Canada, New Zealand and Australia itself. Elective students can attend for a maximum of eight weeks (contact the University of Sydney). There is a university enrolment fee of AU$100 (£50; covering insurance and other costs) and an administration fee of AU$300 (£150) for elective periods of up to four weeks, and AU$500 (£250) for those of four to eight weeks. These fees are payable to the Canberra Clinical School before arrival. To apply, write, stating which discipline you prefer, to the elective officer at the clinical school.

Canberra Hospital

Yamba Drive, Garran, Canberra, ACT 2605. Tel: +61 2 6244 2930. Fax: +61 2 6281 3935.
www.canberrahospital.act.gov.au.
The hospital: A large teaching hospital with 500 beds in the centre of Canberra (population 300 000). It's three hours from snowfields, beaches and outback Australia. This is a friendly, cosmopolitan, political city (as well as being the national capital). The hospital itself is a little isolated, being 20 minutes' walk from the shopping centre.
O **Elective notes:** An elective with the cardiothoracic or neurosurgery unit comes thoroughly recommended. There's plenty of time for sightseeing. The staff and other students are friendly and welcoming. The elective officer is very efficient.
Accommodation: On-site in the Canberra Hospital, this costs AU$4.70 (£2.50) a night (student rate), with a redeemable bond of AU$50 (£25) to be paid on arrival, together with two weeks' rent payable in advance. There's a pool for residents.

OTHER HOSPITALS IN ACT:

Calvary Public Hospital, Haydon Drive, Bruce, ACT 2617. Tel: +61 2 6201 6111.
Fax +61 2 6252 9201.
Jindalee Nursing Home, Goyder Street, Narrabundah, ACT 2604. Tel: +61 2 6295 5511.
Fax: +61 2 6239 6686.

TASMANIA

Tasmania is a large island off the south coast of Australia. It offers some spectacular scenery and diving.

University of Tasmania

Faculty of Medicine, University of Tasmania, 43 Collins Street, Hobart, TAS 7000 (or GPO Box 252-71). Tel: +61 3 6226 4860. Fax: +61 3 6226 4816.
www.healthsci.utas.edu.au/medschool/
index.html.

HOSPITALS IN TASMANIA:

Douglas Parker Rehabilitation Centre, 31
Tower Road, Newtown, Hobart, TAS 7008.
Tel: +61 3 6228 1801. Fax: +61 3 6278 1373.
Launceston General Hospital, Charles Street,
Launceston, TAS 7250. Tel: +61 3 6332 7111.
Fax: +61 3 6332 7018.
Queen Victoria Hospital (Maternity), Charles
Street, Launceston, TAS 7250. Tel : +61 3 6337
2777. Fax +61 3 6337 2729.
Royal Hobart Hospital (General), 48 Liverpool
Street, Hobart, TAS 7000. Tel: +61 3 6222 8308.
Fax: +61 3 6231 2043.

TORRES STRAITS

*The Torres Straits (population 8500) are a
group of over 70 islands just north of Cape
Horn, Queensland, Australia. It's not a
common elective destination, principally
because of difficulty in finding information
and because of its remote location. This
section aims to give some details of formal
organizations on the islands.*

HOSPITALS AND HEALTHCARE SERVICE:

Torres Straits has two hospitals and a
number of primary healthcare facilities.

The Torres Strait and Northern
Peninsula Health Service District is run
from **Thursday Island Hospital**
(Douglas Street, PO Box 391, Thursday
Island, QLD 4875. Tel: +61 7 4069 0200
(for the health service), +61 7 4069 1109
(for the hospital). Fax: +61 7 4069
1603). This is the main hospital for the
region and has 36 beds (a 30-bed general ward, which contains two high-dependency and four paediatric beds). There is
also an eight-bed maternity unit and an
emergency department, all of which
cater for the needs of the residents of
Thursday Island and the Outer Islands of
the Torres Straits. There's an operating
suite and emergency, general medical

and maternity services. Specialist services include diabetes, paeds, adult mental health and surgery. There are a number of visiting specialities such as ophthalmology, vascular surgery and gynaecology.

Thursday Island also has the area's
main primary healthcare centre:
**Thursday Island Primary Health Care
Centre** (Douglas Street, PO Box 624,
Thursday Island, QLD 4875. Tel: +61 7
4069 0400. Fax: +61 7 4069 2045). A
number of other much smaller primary
healthcare centres can be found on the
other islands. Contact Thursday Island
Primary Health Care Centre for details of
visiting the smaller units.

The second hospital for the region is
Bamaga Hospital (Sagaukaz Street,
QLD 4876. Tel: +61 7 4069 3166. Fax:
+61 7 4069 3314). This is a new 14-bed
hospital providing general medical,
emergency, maternity and paediatric care.

The main referral hospitals for these
regions are **Cairns** (850 km), **Townsville**
(1200 km) and the **Royal Brisbane**
(2900 km). If you're thinking of visiting
these islands for an elective, but don't
want to spend your entire time there, it
may well be worth arranging an elective
at one of these referral hospitals and
organizing a trip with a team that does
visiting clinics.

ROYAL FLYING DOCTOR SERVICE

See Section 3 for full details.

FURTHER READING:

Working in Australia by Steve Kisely
and Judy Jones, *BMJ* Classified, 2
January 1999, pp 2–3.

New Zealand

Population: 4 million
Language: English
Capital: Wellington
Currency: New Zealand dollar
Int Code: +64

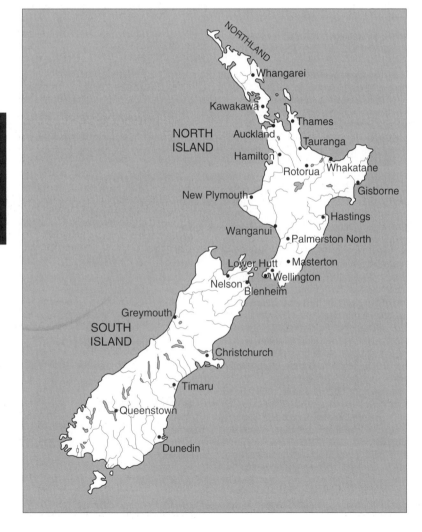

New Zealand, 1600 km (1000 miles) off the coast of Australia, comprises the North and South Islands as well as a number of smaller islands. North Island has a larger population, hot springs and geysers, whereas the (adrenaline) South is more mountainous and is the place to be based if you're an outdoors type. Nearly half the population lives in one of the three big cities (Auckland, Wellington and Christchurch).

✪ Medicine:

New Zealand is a world leader in public health services, having been the first to introduce a welfare state. They did try to charge for hospital beds, but the move was so unpopular that it was scrapped. The vast majority of conditions are as for any developed country (cardiovascular diseases and cancers); the big exception, however, is in the Maori population. A number of hospitals, mainly in Northland on North Island, serve areas rich in Maori people. They tend to suffer more with infectious diseases, such as rheumatic fever, and diseases resulting from their Westernization, such as diabetes and hypertension. Trauma, both deliberate and accidental, is also more common. Primary healthcare is funded by a combination of public subsidy and private contribution. Secondary (hospital) healthcare is provided free, although as the system is gradually becoming stretched, waiting lists have developed. Because of this, around 50% of New Zealanders have private insurance.

New Zealand medical practice, at least in the peripheral hospitals, can be very relaxed ... t-shirts and definitely no white coats. New Zealand medical students spend their final (sixth) year as trainee interns. They have done all their finals and spend a year rotating through medicine, surgery, O&G, paeds and psychiatry. It's similar to being a house officer without the on call or prescribing. They are paid half a house surgeon's salary, but since they are still paying school fees, the gain is negligible. Most elective students are given a similar role (without pay!).

◎ Climate and crime:

The climate varies greatly from an almost subtropical north to a cold, windy south. The best weather is after Christmas. The crime rate is incredibly low, making *Crimewatch* more of a 'lost and found' service.

➲ Visas and work permits:

British students are not required to obtain visas and British citizens can stay up to six months if not taking paid work. A few students have previously paid £45 for a visa. A temporary work permit allows work for up to three years. For up-to-date information on visas and work permits, either ring the embassy on their rip-off line (*see* Section 4) or look on www.immigration.govt.nz. Australian citizens are free to travel between Oz and NZ.

Jobs for all health professionals can be found on www.everybody.co.nz, www.nzhealth.co.nz and www.southern doctor.co.nz. For a list of health and hospital services (but not hospital addresses), visit www.hospitals.co.nz/public.html.

○ Elective notes:

There are two universities in New Zealand: the University of Auckland and the University of Otago (based in Dunedin). There are, however, four clinical schools: Auckland (www.auckland.ac.nz), Wellington (www.wnmeds.ac.nz), Christchurch (www.chmeds.ac.nz) and Dunedin. The last three are the clinical schools of the University of Otago (www.otago.ac.nz). There are big summer holidays in the run-up to Christmas so there are not many students around: you lose on the social life but get a bit more attention.

Working as a doctor:

New Zealand (like Australia) is oversupplied with 'foreign doctors. Four thousand have entered since 1992, and the country as a whole requires only 6000. They got in because a loose immigration policy did not check whether a person's overseas qualification was recognized locally. Many of these doctors are now sitting exams to register or are unemployed.

New Zealand

Legislation is tightening quickly. You should therefore have a job offer before leaving for New Zealand and should have your contract checked by the **Association of Salaried Medical Specialists** (PO Box 5251, Wellington. Tel: +64 4 499 1271. Fax: +64 4 499 4500).

You will need to register (or gain temporary registration) with the **Medical Council of New Zealand**. Visiting doctors can stay for up to three years for educational reasons or to supply an area of need – however, it is only on the understanding that they will return home. If attempting to gain full registration, you may well need to sit the New Zealand Registration Exams (NZREX) or enter vocational training. The NZREX exam consists of steps I and II of the USMLE exams (*see* the section on the USA), an English language test and clinical examination. This provides provisional registration which leads to a 12-month probationary period. Visit www.moh.govt.nz/bridging.html for more information. Australian graduates are free to enter without examination.

Working as a nurse:
To work in New Zealand, you have to register with the **Nursing Council of New Zealand** (address below) – they will require evidence of your training and experience.

Working as a dentist:
British- and Australian-trained dentists can register without the need for further examination, but the situation varies for other countries. Check with the **Dental Council of New Zealand**.

USEFUL ADDRESSES:

New Zealand Ministry of Health: www.moh.gov.nz.

PROFESSIONAL ORGANIZATIONS AND BOARDS:

Note: many organizations are joined with those in Australia.

Doctors: New Zealand Medical Association, PO Box 156, Wellington. Tel: +64 4 472 4741. Fax: +64 4 471 0838. www.nzma.org.nz.
Medical Council of New Zealand, 139–143 Willis Street, PO Box 11-649, Wellington. Tel: +64 4 384 7635. Fax: +64 4 385 8902. www.mcnz.org.nz.
Nurses: Nursing Council of New Zealand, PO Box 105 483, Auckland. www.nursingcouncil.org.nz.
New Zealand Nurses Organisation, PO Box 2128, Wellington. Tel: +64 4 386 0847. Fax: +64 4 382 9993. www.nzno.org.nz.
Nurses Association Inc, PO Box 2128, Wellington. www.nram.org.nz.
Dentists: New Zealand Dental Association, PO Box 28 084, Auckland 5, Tel: +64 9 524 2778. Fax: +64 9 520 5256. E-mail: nzda@nzda.org.nz. www.nzda.org.nz.
New Zealand Dental Therapists Association, 9 Miriam Corban Heights, Henderson, Auckland. www.nzdta.co.nz.
Dental Council of New Zealand, Level 8, 108 The Terrace, PO Box 10-448, Wellington. Tel: +64 4 499 1668. www.dentalcouncil.org.nz.
Physiotherapists: New Zealand Society of Physiotherapists, PO Box 27 386, Level 5, Wang House, 195–201 Willis Street, Wellington. Tel: +64 4 801 6500. Fax: +64 4 801 5571. E-mail: nzsp@physiotherapy.org.nz. www.physiotherapy.org.nz.
Physiotherapy Board, PO Box 10 734, Wellington Tel: +64 4 471 2610. Fax: +64 4 471 2613. E-mail: physio@physioboard.org.nz. www.physioboard.org.nz.
Occupational therapists: New Zealand Association of Occupational Therapists, PO Box 12-506, Royal Society of New Zealand Offices, 4 Halswell Street, Thorndon, Wellington 6001. Tel: +64 4 473 6510. Fax: +64 4 473 1841. www.nzaot.com.
Occupational Therapy Board, PO Box 10-140, Wellington. Tel: +64 4 499 7979. Fax: +64 4 472 2350. www.occupationaltherapyboard.org.nz.
Pharmacists: Pharmacy Guild of New Zealand, PO Box 27139, 124 Dixon Street, Wellington. Tel: +64 4 802 8200. Fax: +64 4 384 8055. E-mail: p.guild@pharmacy-house.org.nz. www.pgnz.org.nz.
Speech therapists: New Zealand Speech-Language Therapists Association, Suite 369, 63 Remuera Road, Newmarket, Auckland. Tel: +64 3 235 8257. Fax: +64 3 235 8850. E-mail: nzsta@clear.net.nz. www.nzsta-speech.org.nz.
Dieticians: New Zealand Dietetic Association, PO Box 5065, Wellington. Tel: +64 4 473 3061. Fax: +64 4 473 3062. E-mail: nzda@dietitians.org.nz. www.dietitians.org.nz.
Dieticians Board, PO Box 10-140, Wellington. Tel: +64 4 499 7979. Fax: +64 4 472 2350.

MEDICAL SPECIALIST ORGANIZATIONS:

A full list can be found at www.mcnz.org.nz/registration/overseastrained/branchmedicine.asp.

Australian and New Zealand College of Anaesthetists, Ulimaroa, 630 St Kilda Road, Melbourne VIC 3004, Australia. Tel: +61 3 9510 6299. Fax: +61 3 9510 6786. www.anzca.edu.au.
New Zealand General Practitioners' Association, PO Box 10 789, 28 The Terrace, Wellington. Tel: +64 4 472 8992. Fax: +64 4 499 360704.
Royal Australasian College of Physicians, 5th Floor, St John House, 99 The Terrace, Wellington. Tel: +64 4 472 6713. Fax: +64 4 472 6718. E-mail: jo.jones@racp.org.nz. www.racp.edu.au.
Royal Australian and New Zealand College of Radiologists (New Zealand), St John House, Terrace Level, 99 The Terrace (PO Box 10-424), Wellington. Tel: +64 4 472 6470. Fax: +64 4 472 6474. www.ranzcr.edu.au.
Royal New Zealand College of General Practitioners, PO Box 10 440, The Terrace, Wellington. Tel: +64 4 496 5999. Fax: +64 4 496 5997. E-mail: rnzcgp@rnzcgp.org.nz. www.rnzcgp.org.nz.

NORTH ISLAND

Auckland

Auckland (New Zealand's largest city) is about the size of Los Angeles but has only 800 000 people. Transport can therefore be tricky without a car. There is plenty to do in the city which also has a pretty good nightlife. It does have some outdoor activities (white and black water rafting, swimming with dolphins, volcano walking, skydiving) … but if that is specifically what you're after, Christchurch or somewhere else in the South Island is probably better. Check out www.adhb.govt.nz/akhealth/ for details on hospitals and all their departments throughout Auckland.

University of Auckland

School of Medicine, Private Bag 92019, Auckland. Tel: +64 9 373 7521. Fax: +64 9 373 7482. www.health.auckland.ac.nz.

The medical school's principal hospital is Auckland Hospital and electives here should be arranged through the elective coordinator at the above address. There is an administration fee of around NZ$350. They are very helpful, but NZ is a popular place … apply very early. Some people have avoided going

through the university and gone direct to hospitals to save the fee, however, the university says you must go through them to make it official. The main hospitals in Auckland are: Auckland, Green Lane, National Women's, North Shore and Middlemore.

Auckland Hospital

Private Bag 92 024, Park Road, Grafton, Auckland. Tel: +61 9 379 7440.
Starship Children's Department: Private Bag 92 189, Park Road, Grafton, Auckland. Tel: +61 9 307 8900. www.starship.org.nz

The hospital: Auckland Hospital is the main tertiary referral centre for the North Island (and some Pacific islands) and is therefore very busy. It's right in the middle of the city. The emergency department receives a great deal of trauma. On-site there is also the **Starship Hospital** (almost a theme park), an impressive, busy specialist paediatric hospital that serves the whole of New Zealand and the South Pacific Islands. There is also a specific Maori health service. Other specialist services include liver and bone marrow tranplantation.

O Elective notes: In the emergency department, you'll get to do many minor procedures. There are eight-hour shifts and students can come in for any shift. Formal teaching occurs twice a week in the form of X-ray meetings and journal clubs. Elective students are very much encouraged to take the weekends off for exploring. In January and February there are no local students and you're probably made to feel more part of the team because of this. Neurology rarely has students and is highly recommended.

Accommodation: Provided in the on-site residency with other students and staff. Good (NZ$110 a week).

Green Lane Hospital

Green Lane, Auckland 1005.
The hospital: Green Lane is a small hospital to the south of the city centre (15–20 minutes by bus). This is New Zealand's premier centre for cardiac surgery, respiratory medicine and otolaryngology.

New Zealand

O **Elective notes:** It's well-equipped, with friendly doctors and helpful staff, but it can get a bit quiet. There are Auckland students, so there is consistent teaching and exploring is encouraged. As this is the day surgery unit for Auckland, it's great for assisting with or performing many relatively minor operations.

Accommodation: On-site in a hostel that is also open to the general public (NZ$80 a week). This means you meet a wide variety of people, although many are not young and the night-life can be pretty poor.

National Women's Hospital
Claude Road, Epsom, Auckland.
Tel: +64 9 630 9943. Fax: +64 9 630 9761.
The hospital: This is the largest women's hospital in Australasia, providing comprehensive obs and gynae care. There are around 8000 deliveries a year.

North Shore Hospital
Shakespeare Road, Milford, Takapuna, Auckland.
The hospital: North Shore lies north across the Waitemata Harbour from the main city (approximately 35 minutes by bus). It has acute medical, surgical, obstetric and psychiatric services. There's a fantastic urology department, although there are no paeds or acute orthopaedic departments. An ITU has just been built. The emergency department offers a wide variety of experience, although most major trauma goes to the main Auckland Hospital.

O **Elective notes:** There's plenty of opportunity to suture wounds, set fractures and attend resuscitations. It has its own local facilities and a beach.

Accommodation: In the nurses' home with occupational and physiotherapists. All facilities are available, and it's very relaxed and friendly. Book early as some have left it too late to get accommodation (in which case stay in Central City Backpackers, 26 Lorne St, for £30 a week).

Middlemore Hospital
Private Bag 93311, Auckland.
The hospital: This is a trauma centre, situated in the rough end of town and home to the **South Auckland Clinical School**.
O **Elective notes:** This is a very friendly hospital with very good teaching. With many people arriving here from the Pacific Islands, there's quite a bit of unusual pathology to be seen.

Wellington

For the capital city, Wellington is fairly small, but it's friendly and there's a lot going on. It has a beautiful harbour and many tourist attractions, including the 'Bee-hive' parliament complex, museums, gardens and cable car.

Wellington School of Medicine
23A Mein St, Newtown, Wellington, PO Box 7343, Wellington South.
Tel: +64 4 385 5541. Fax: +64 4 385 5725.
www.wnmeds.ac.nz.
To do an elective in Wellington, contact the Overseas Elective Coordinator at the above address (or e-mail wsmelectives@wnmeds.ac.nz). You have to fill in a form stating what you have already done, stick a photo on it, get malpractice insurance, tick subjects you would like to do (from paediatric surgery to neurology; research, general practice, public health and psychiatry are also available) and send it back.

Wellington Hospital
Mein Street, Newtown, Wellington, PO Box 7343. www.ccdhb.org.nz.
The hospital: Wellington Hospital is in Newtown, about a 30-minute walk (five-minute bus ride) from the city centre. It's a tertiary referral centre and teaching hospital so has most specialities.
O **Elective notes:** You tend to follow one of the interns and gradually take on their work! Lots of tutorials and lectures if you wish. This is good experience and Wellington is a good base in the centre of New Zealand. The students are very

friendly and invite you out to parties, etc. You partially act as a trainee intern but get to sit in on clinics (which the real ones don't). Paeds is highly recommended. It is in **Wellington Children's Hospital**, which is two wards off the main hospital.

Accommodation: Sometimes arranged in the residency. Other times, it is in the Riddleford Hostel next to the hospital (NZ$90 a week). Free tea and coffee for medical students!

Hutt Hospital
High Street, Lower Hutt.
Tel: +64 4 566 6999. Fax: +64 04 570 4401.
www.huttvalleydhb.org.nz.
The hospital: This is a small friendly hospital, 30 minutes' drive from Wellington. Specialities include medicine, paeds and general surgery. It's more laid back than Wellington and there are usually only a couple of students around so teaching is much more personal.

Porirua Hospital
Kenepuru Drive, PO Box 50-233, Porirua.
The hospital: This is a psychiatric centre about 30 minutes from Wellington. It has both acute and long-term patients and is set in very large grounds. They are often looking for people to work here.

Kenepuru Hospital
Kenepuru Drive, Porirua.
Tel: +64 4 237 0179.
The hospital: Situated next to Porirua and provides elective orthopaedic and general surgical specialities. It is very isolated.

Palmerston North Hospital
Ruahine Street, Palmerston North.
Tel: +64 6 356 9169. Fax: +64 6 355 0616.
The hospital: A large hospital covering most specialities, with enthusiastic staff who are happy to teach. Palmerston North is a university (of agriculture) town so it's usually pretty lively (although it quietens off between November and January).

Masterton Hospital
Te Ore Ore Road, Masterton.
Tel: +64 6 946 9800. Fax: +64 6 946 9801.
The hospital: Small but friendly and (possibly more importantly) close to some of the best wine regions in New Zealand (Martinborough). The hospital is about 90 minutes from Wellington and has most specialities. There are rugged beaches and this is a good place for outdoor activities. They often recruit overseas doctors.

Taranaki Base Hospital
David Street, New Plymouth.
Tel: +64 6 753 6139.
The hospital: Is situated on the west coast of the north island with excellent surf, windsurfing and tramping.
O Elective notes: Not many students go here so they tend to get good 'hands on' experience.

Wanganui Hospital
Heads Road, Wanganui.
www.wdhb.org.nz/Mcontect.htm.
The hospital: Is a small friendly unit, popular with those who enjoy the outdoors. It's an excellent base if you like tramping, kayaking or skiing in the winter.

NORTHLAND REGION

Northland has some beautiful beaches and is excellent for diving (with dolphins), fishing and sailing. It has some amazing countryside and is great if you're an outdoors type. The Bay of Islands is particularly impressive. There are many Maori people here, making interesting folklore and medicine.

Check out the Northland's extensive health website (which includes job vacancies): www.northlanddhb.org.nz.

Note: Two other small hospitals in this area are **Kaitaia** and **Daraville**.

New Zealand

Whangarei Area Hospital

Northland Health Limited, PO Box 742, Whangarei. Tel: +64 9 430 4100.
Fax: +64 9 430 4110.
www.northlanddhb.org.nz/NHL/whangarei hospital.htm.

The hospital: Whangarei Area Hospital is a modern hospital with a busy emergency department. Whangarei (a two-hour drive from Auckland) is Northland's largest city. It is the major referral centre for Northland, with surgical, medical, intensive care, coronary care, paeds, psychiatric, oncology, renal, O&G, and emergency services. Opened in 1901, it now has 255 beds. There is a helicopter service to bring in referrals. It is also a training centre for Auckland Medical School so trainee interns (but not students) get sent here. There's quite a lot of trauma from road traffic accidents. There is a large Maori population who often practise 'home kills' of animals and sustain lacerations in the process … lots of nerve blocks and suturing practice. There's a busy paeds ward (18 beds) and a paeds emergency department. There's also a great deal of orthopaedics.

O Elective notes: They have previously tried to arrange a helicopter ride in the air ambulance for visiting students. Only elective students are here so it's not over-crowded. There are quite a few British doctors and nurses. Write to the Medical Staff Coordinator at the above address. A fee of NZ$75 is charged. Whangarei is not very picturesque, although the harbour is quite nice. It is, however, a great base from which to explore the Northland and the Bay of Islands. There is a good bus service. This is recommended as a good elective.

Accommodation: Provided at NZ$70 a week (£30) and good, although the cooking facilities leave a lot to be desired. There's a good canteen and a swimming pool for residents.

Bay of Islands Hospital

PO Box 290, Kawakawa. Tel: +64 9 404 0280.
www.northlanddhb.org.nz/NHL/BayofIslands Hospital.htm.

The hospital: Bay of Islands is a small (22-bed) rural hospital with a day surgical ward and a general medical ward with some paediatric beds. It's run by four doctors. There is also a small maternity unit and an emergency department. Kawakawa itself is a pretty small, mainly Maori village, 15 km from the coast. The population is around half Maori/ Polynesian and half white, with many from poor social circumstances. Specialists (from Whangarei) visit and run clinics.

O Elective notes: Write to the medical secretary to organize a trip here. You can get to do some minor procedures. The staff are friendly and offer lifts to local areas to see the sites. This is recommended for four to five weeks. GP work can be arranged on arrival. Transport is tricky, although easy enough if you want to get to Auckland (four hours south). Kawakawa has a few shops, a pub and a vintage railway. Borrow a bike to get to the lovely beach at Paitia (famous for dolphin and whale watching, watersports and boogy boarding down giant sand dunes).

Accommodation: Free. It can either be in the nurses' home or in a cottage with other medical staff. The canteen food isn't great but again is free (make sure you book it with the kitchen). There's a good sports centre 15 minutes from the hospital.

Whakatane Hospital

Stewart Street, Whakatane, Bay of Plenty, North Island.

The hospital: This is a 200-bed general hospital with a 40% Maori population. All the major specialities are here and the staff are helpful both in and out of the hospital.

O Elective notes: You'll probably be the only student and you can do as much or as little as you want. There are tutorials and the opportunity to visit community clinics. The area has quite a lot of thermal activity (volcanoes and hot springs). Organize this elective early.

Accommodation: Provided free of charge in the old nurses' home.

Rotorua

Rotorua is a brilliant place for an elective or work. It lies centrally in North Island so is a good base to explore from and has a lot of geothermal activity. Things to do include hot spa pools, naturally warm rivers to swim in, bush walks and mountain biking. This also makes for some pretty novel therapies (see Queen Elizabeth Hospital below). Nearby there is white and black water rafting, caving and skydiving. The ski fields are two hours away (but can be closed if the local volcanoes are covering them in ash). There are lots of fast food places, cafés and a five-screen cinema. Night-life is quiet, but if you like rugby this is paradise.

Rotorua Hospital

Lakeland Health, Private Bag 3023, Rotorua Tel: +64 7 348 1199.

The hospital: A small friendly district hospital with 120 beds. It has two medical, a surgical, orthopaedics, paeds, O&G, psychiatry and geriatrics wards. Most of the patients are Maori so you see lots of diabetes and its complications. Other common conditions in Maori paeds are malnutrition and rheumatic fever. Amoebic meningitis is also a problem because of the thermal baths (two cases a year). Don't put your head under water! The luge and mountain bike trail provide a decent bit of trauma.

O Elective notes: There are no New Zealand medical students, only trainee interns who are willing to teach. It's all pretty laid back … the hospital day starts at 8 am but yours starts whenever you get out of bed! Ward rounds are conducted in polo shirts. Apply very early (up to 18 months in advance).

Accommodation: And food (not great) are provided at the hospital for NZ$100 a week (about £40). You share accommodation with trainee interns from Auckland Medical School.

Queen Elizabeth Hospital for Rheumatology and Rehabilitation

PO Box 1342, Whakaue Street, Rotorua. Tel: +64 7 348 0189. Fax: +64 7 348 4266. www.qehospital.co.nz.

The hospital: Situated on the edge of Lake Rotorua, it has 50 patients and is run by three consultants. It has two rheumatology and one orthopaedic ward. Common conditions include rheumatoid arthritis, osteoarthritis, gout, scleroderma, psoriasis, fibromyalgia and SLE. There is also an outpatient department. Treatments (given for three weeks) include exercise, physiotherapy, occupational therapy, balneotherapy (the use of hot mud, mud baths, hot springs, massage, steam treatment or wax therapy), counselling, relaxation and drugs. This is a highly specialized and different type of hospital. It is highly recommended for physio- and occupational therapists (jobs are available via their website).

Gisborne

Gisborne Hospital

Tairawhiti Healthcare Ltd, Private Bag 7001, Gisborne.

The hospital: Located on the outskirts of the town (population 30 000) on the east coast of North Island. There are two medical and two surgical wards, an ITU, a paeds and an emergency department. There is a large Maori population in the East Cape, which is reflected in the medicine, with a high percentage of rheumatic fever, diabetes and renal dysfunction. The general medical wards are covered by three consultant physicians and students tend to be allocated to one. There are no middle-grade staff but numerous house officers.

O Elective notes: There's plenty of teaching on the rounds, in lunchtime sessions and in practical procedures. The consultants also go on outreach clinics offering a great opportunity to see the countryside and GP-run hospitals north of Gisborne. This is a good elective, but you may feel a bit out of the way and it has a slower pace of life than others. There's a lot to explore around Gisborne (which has a cinema). Note: The hospital is about an hour's walk from anywhere – get a bike!

Accommodation: Free. The house officers all live in and the social life is actually quite good.

Thames

Thames Hospital
Waikato Area Health Board, Thames,
PO Box 707.
The hospital: Thames is a small district general hospital with both medical and surgical wards.
O **Elective notes:** You can choose to spend your time in one area or rotate. The busiest time is their summer (i.e. over Christmas). Most action is in the emergency department, where all admissions are seen first. This is a relaxed, friendly elective with good teaching, but the staff are also keen for you to go and explore the surrounding countryside. There are some lovely walks and beaches nearby. Thames itself (one-and-a-half hours by bus from Auckland) is a small, quiet town, but the people are genuine and there's plenty to do. Try to go with someone or visit somewhere else as well.
Accommodation: The nurses' hostel costs around NZ$50 (£20) week and is usually pretty full so there is plenty of life.

Tauranga Hospital
Cameron Road, Tauranga. (Run by Pacific Health, Private Bag 12024, Tauranga. Tel: +64 7 577 8000. Fax: +64 7 577 8487.)
The hospital: A large modern hospital with enthusiastic and friendly staff. Specialities include general medicine and surgery, orthopaedics, ENT and urology. The hospital is often frequented by overseas doctors and nurses.
O **Elective notes:** Tauranga is a reasonably sized town with quite a few things to do. There's an airport for flights to South Island. The beaches are excellent for swimming, surfing, diving, windsurfing and fishing. Described as an excellent elective.
Accommodation: Can usually be arranged on-site, although you may wish to find digs near the beach!

Hastings Memorial Hospital
c/o Health Care, Hawkes Bay, Hastings.
The hospital: A small hospital with a good range of services (surgery, orthopaedics, O&G, paeds and medicine).
O **Elective notes:** An immensely friendly hospital well worth visiting. There's responsibility if you want it, time off if you don't.
Accommodation: Provided.

Waikato Hospital
Private Bag 3200, Hamilton.
Tel: +64 7 839 8880. Fax: +64 7 839 8897.
www.waikatodhb.govt.nz.

SOUTH ISLAND
Christchurch

Christchurch (population 300 000) is a top base from which to start exploring New Zealand. If you go in winter, the skiing is supposed to be excellent in the Southern Alps. Since it's in South Island, it's also very convenient if you are after the silly sports (bungee jumping, skydiving, etc.). Christchurch itself is very 'British' and although, there is a great deal outside, it's not so great for wild nights out.

Christchurch School of Medicine
Christchurch School of Medicine, Christchurch Hospital, PO Box 4345, Christchurch. Tel: +64 3 364 0824.
Fax: +64 3 364 0935. www.chmeds.ac.nz.
The school is in and uses Christchurch Hospital for its clinical training. It is the major teaching hospital of the University of Otago (based further down the coast). They can arrange electives in all specialities (for a charge of NZ$500), although some students have found that they can't do general medicine or surgery as these are full with their own students. This is an extremely popular destination. Write incredibly early to the above address. Full details can be found at http://healthsci.otago.ac.nz/division/medicine/elective.htm.

The two health service providers in this area are:

Canterbury Health, Private Bag 4710, Christchurch. Tel: +64 3 364 0137. Fax: +64 3 364 0438.
Healthlink South, 3rd Floor, 10 Oxford Terrace, Christchurch. Tel: +64 3 364 0150. Fax: +64 3 364 0318.

Christchurch Hospital

Riccarton Avenue, Private Bag 4710, Christchurch, South Island.
Tel: +64 3 364 0640. Fax: +64 3 364 0453. www.cdhb.govt.nz/christchurch.htm.
The hospital: Christchurch Public Hospital is the major acute hospital (650 beds) for the city and surrounding area. It has many large and well-organized departments. Quite a few British doctors work here. There are many local as well as elective medical students.
○ **Elective notes:** Elective students tend to be treated as trainee interns. Departments include:
● *Cardiology:* comprising a 30-bed long-stay ward, a day ward, coronary care unit, intensive care, catheter lab and outpatient department, all of which you can rotate through.
● *Emergency:* a busy friendly unit seeing 65000 patients a year with a 40% admission rate. This is arguably one of the best attachments. Not much planned teaching but plenty by the bedside.
● *Bone marrow transplant:* the team look after those with an underlying haematological problem. Students have previously been able to do lumbar punctures and bone marrow biopsies and give intrathecal medication. **Warning:** Young people die, be prepared for this.
● *Oncology:* highly recommended, but there is less practical experience.
● *Neurosurgery, endocrinology and dermatology.*
● *Orthopaedics* (only acute and trauma here): offers some excellent teaching and the opportunity to visit the **Burwood Spinal Injuries Unit**, world renowned for treating tetraplegics and for reconstruction surgery (*see* below); the department is

also pretty relaxed allowing plenty of time to go exploring.
Accommodation: Not provided. There is a local YMCA right opposite the hospital, costing NZ$90 (£40) a week for a shared room and another NZ$70 (£30) a week for cafeteria food as there are no self-catering facilities. If you are there for more than a couple of weeks, you might be able to haggle and get it cheaper. Sports facilities in the YMCA are good. Book well in advance.

Spinal Injuries Unit

Burwood Hospital, Private Bag 4708, Christchurch.
The hospital: This is one of two in New Zealand dealing with a whole spectrum of spinal injuries. Acute spinal patients are rapidly transported here for their acute management and then extensive rehabilitation lasting two to four months.
○ **Elective notes:** The consultants are very knowledgeable and keen to teach however, for obvious reasons, clinical experience can be slow. The patients are the ones who teach you the most. The unit itself is 11km outside the city centre, with an excellent bus service.
Accommodation: Provided in a nurses' hostel on-site or can be arranged in the city. Sports facilities are available in hospital.

Princess Margaret Hospital

Private Bag, Christchurch.
The hospital: A smaller hospital in Christchurch that mainly provides healthcare for the elderly. A number of British doctors work here.

Dunedin

Dunedin is a relatively isolated town, not a city, in South Island. The total population is 115 000, of whom 15 000–20 000 are students. The people often have Scottish relatives, and there are many Scottish street names. All the student night-life is pub based and a good laugh. Queenstown and Janaka (skiing) are close (snowboarding is booming), and there are many glaciers to explore.

Otago Medical School

PO Box 913, Gt King Street, Dunedin. Tel:
+64 3 479 7454. Fax: +64 3 479 5459.
www.otago.ac.nz/facmed.
Otago has three clinical schools:
Christchurch, Wellington (*see* above) and
Dunedin. The Dunedin school can
arrange electives in its main teaching
hospital, **Dunedin**, or a number of others,
including the **Wakari**, **Balclutha**,
Oamaru, **Dunstan**, **Southland** and
Lakes District Hospitals. Write to the
Overseas Elective Coordinator at the
administration office at the above address
(or look on http://healthsci.otago.ac.nz/
dsm/electives.htm). Note: There is a
charge of NZ$500.

Dunedin Hospital

Dunedin. (Run by Healthcare Otago,
Private Bag 1921, Dunedin.
Tel: +64 3 474 0999. Fax: +64 3 474 7623).
The hospital: A teaching hospital with
all specialities (neurosurgery, cardiotho-
racics, a good anaesthetics department –
with pain team – orthopaedics, ENT,
etc.).
O **Elective notes:** Elective students are
often given positions as trainee interns.
In anaesthetics, students have previously
done quite a few procedures.
Accommodation: No hospital accommodation is available, but they help you
arrange some.

Southland Hospital

Invercargill, Dunedin, South Island.
The hospital: Is also part of the medical
school on the south side of town and
acts as a district general hospital with
200 beds. It has a good neurology
department. This is a very friendly hospital.
O **Elective notes:** You can either act as
a trainee intern or go to clinics. The
emergency department is very 'hands
on' with respect to minor injuries. The
elective is highly recommended however, the hospital is about an hour's walk
from the town centre. Apply through
Otago Medical School.
Accommodation: In the doctors' residence.

Nelson

*Nelson is a small coastal town (population
45 000) located in the extreme north of
South Island. There's plenty to do ... walks,
kayaking, skydiving, skiing, river surfing,
bungee jumping, jet boating and horse riding.
The Marlborough Sounds and Abel Tasman
National Parks are not too far away. This is
New Zealand's sunniest city, and the weather
is hottest around January and February ...
take a raincoat in November/December. The
night-life is not great but the locals are
friendly. Surrounding Nelson there are
fantastic golden beaches.*

Nelson Hospital

Private Bag, Nelson, South Island.
Tel: +64 3 546 1800. Fax: +64 3 546 1680.
The hospital: Nelson Hospital is medium-sized (100 beds) with friendly (but
no middle-grade) staff. It is the largest
hospital for over 500 km.
O **Elective notes:** Students are treated as
trainee interns, and there are plenty of
practical procedures to do. There's lots of
teaching as there are no local students
(although there can be quite a few elective students). You can do as much or as
little as you want. The emergency department doesn't get much major trauma but
does see lots of minor injuries. This is a
more relaxed elective than in the cities.
You also get to do more. This (repeatedly) comes very highly recommended.
Accommodation: Has been provided at
NZ$140 (£60) a week sharing with other
elective medical students. However, it
has occasionally been closed. There are
youth hostels in town (Dave's Palace
does special medical student discounts,
costing around NZ$60 (£25) a week).
There are a small gym and swimming
pool in the hospital grounds.

Timaru

Timaru Public Hospital

Health South Canterbury, High Street,
Private Bag 911, Timaru. Tel: +64 3 688
1079. Fax: +64 3 688 0238.

The hospital: As the only medical centre between Dunedin and Christchurch, Timaru has a wide catchment area extending up into the Southern Alps and including Mount Cook and Mount Aspiring National Park. It covers all basic specialities and has 250 beds and three theatres. There is a maternity hospital with a further 50 beds.

O **Elective notes:** It is a very friendly hospital and students can usually do a few procedures and assist in theatre.

Accommodation: Up to three students can stay in the inexpensive hospital flats.

OTHER HOSPITALS:

Wairau Hospital
Hospital Road, Blenheim. Tel: +64: 3 520 9914. Fax: +64 3 578 9517.

The hospital: Covers the general specialities and is situated at the top of South Island in the middle of a wine region. Malborough Sounds are about 30 minutes away.

Grey Base Hospital
High Street, Greymouth. Tel: +64 3 768 0499.
The hospital: Often recruits overseas staff and is great if you like the great outdoors.

Lakes District Hospital
Douglas Street, Frankton, Queenstown.
Tel: +64 3 442 3053. Fax: +64 3 442 3305.
The hospital: Relatively small and run mainly by GPs. It is however situated in Queenstown, which, as any backpacker will tell you, is the heart of the adrenalin South Island. Jet boating, paragliding, mountain climbing – it's all here.

THE
CARIBBEAN

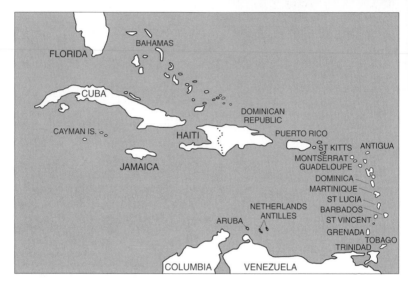

The Caribbean is an idyllic place to work if you like the sun and beautiful beaches. Beware, however, as the islands are very different. Some have wonderful health facilities, whereas others can be classed as Third World. Even within an island itself (e.g. Jamaica), the wide disparity can mean superb private care for a minority and very poor conditions for others. This chapter goes through the islands from west to east. Some are independent. Some still have ties to America or Europe. Look at the map above to find out their relations. You may well be able to offer your services to various boats travelling between islands in return for free transport (look out for notices at the dockyards). It should be noted that HIV is an increasing problem, especially in some of the Islands of the West Indies, a few of the islands having the world's highest rates for heterosexual transmission.

◎ Climate:

The Caribbean as a whole has a subtropical climate with very mild winters. It's hottest between June and September (30°C), but this is also when rainfall tends to peak. Hurricanes seem to be an increasing threat between July and December.

To do an elective at one of the hospitals that are affiliated with the University of the West Indies (Antigua, Dominica, St Vincent, St Lucia, Grenada, Martinique, Jamaica, Guadalope, St Joseph, St Martin and Barbados), you can write directly to the university. However, to give yourself a head start, write to where you want to go first and then (if they require it) write to the university stating that you have been offered an elective placement. The University of the West Indies itself is based on three campuses: Cave Hill (Barbados – www.cavehill.uwi.edu), Mona (Jamaica – www.uwimona.edu.jm) and St Augustine (Trinidad – www.uwi.tt).

The eastern Caribbean states (St Lucia, St Vincent and the Grenadines, and St Christopher and Nevis) are part of the Commonwealth. Most information is given below but if you need more details contact the **High Commission for Eastern Caribbean States** (10 Kensington Court, London W8 5DL, UK. Tel: +44 20 7937 9522. Fax: +44 20 7937 5514) or the **Ministry of Health** (Chausee Road, Castries, St Lucia).

Note: A number of the Islands have other medical schools – many of these are offshore American Medical Schools that have preclinical components on the island and clinical components in affiliated hospitals in the US and UK. The only hospitals in the Carribean commonly used by these students are in Kingston and Grenada.

The Bahamas

Population: 300 000
Official Language: English
Capital: Nassau
Currency: Bahamian dollar
Dialing Code: +1 242

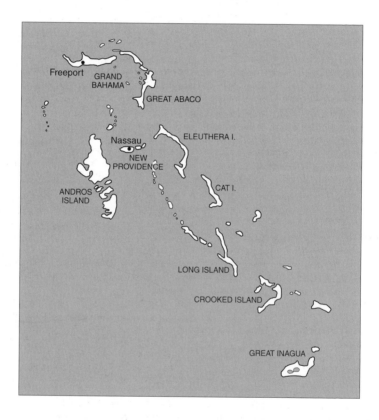

Freeport
GRAND BAHAMA
GREAT ABACO
ELEUTHERA I.
Nassau
NEW PROVIDENCE
ANDROS ISLAND
CAT I.
LONG ISLAND
CROOKED ISLAND
GREAT INAGUA

The Bahamas are a group of 700 islands and 2400 cays of the south Florida coast. However, only 30 islands are inhabited. As well as a large tourist industry, the Bahamas has more recently become a major offshore financial centre.

✪ Medicine:

The Ministry of Health and the Environment is responsible for the provision of general healthcare in the Bahamas. There are both private and government-maintained hospitals, providing a modern and comprehensive healthcare system. The system is not free, but curative treatment is generally available to all residents in the government-maintained hospitals notwithstanding their ability to pay. The government healthcare system is funded by a national insurance scheme paid by employers and employees on the Bahamas. It covers those employed and those previously employed on the islands.

Hospitals are maintained only on the two most populated islands – Nassau and Grand Bahama (over 83% of the population resides on these two islands, with over 67% living in Nassau alone) – but general clinics with resident physicians are available on all the major islands. A rapid response emergency Air Sea Rescue programme is available throughout the islands, provided with the assistance of the American Coast Guard. Private boats can also transport patients. The doctor:population ratio is 1:692, but for every inhabitant, there are six tourists per year. Leading causes of mortality are heart disease, cancers, crime, accidents and obstetric problems. The prevalence of HIV is around 4%.

➲ Visas and work permits:
Contact the **High Commission of the Commonwealth of the Bahamas** (Bahamas House, 10 Chesterfield Street, London W1X 8AH, UK. Tel: +44 20 7408 4488. Fax: +44 20 7499 9937).

No clear information is available regarding the need for students to obtain a study visa. UK and American citizens can land as visitors with just a passport and stay for up to eight months, although anyone staying longer than an 'average holiday' has to apply for an extension.

In most lines of work, the government of the Bahamas has to offer the job to a suitably qualified Bahamian before an outsider; if it is then given to an expatriate, a costly work visa is obtained. For nurses, doctors and kindred services, however, no work permit is required. Write to the Ministry of Health. The Bahamas government website (www.bahamas.gov.bs) has many useful links.

◎ Crime:
Illegal weapons are easily obtainable, hence gunshot injuries and murders occasionally occur.

USEFUL ADDRESSES:

Ministry of Health, Victoria Gardens, PO Box N-3729, Nassau. Tel: + 1 242 322 7425. Fax: +1 242 322 7788.
Bahamas Medical Council, PO Box N-9802, Nassau. Tel: +1 242 328 2260. Fax: +1 242 328 1211.
Medical Association of the Bahamas, PO Box N3125, Nassau. Tel: +1 242 356 3536. Fax: +1 242 324 3141.
Bahamas Dental Association, PO Box CB-13420, Nassau. Tel: +1 242 322 8589. Fax: +1 242 326 3577.
Health Professionals Council, PO Box N7528, Nassau. Tel: +1 242 326 7740/0566. Fax: +1 242 326 0537. (For everything from acupuncture and dietetics to radiology.)

HOSPITALS IN NASSAU:

Princess Margaret Hospital
Shirley Street, PO Box N-3730, Naussau. Tel: +1 242 322 2861. Fax: +1 242 325 0048. www.doctors-hospital.com.
The hospital: A government-maintained hospital providing 484 beds. Its departments include emergency medicine, medical, surgical, maternity, paeds, intensive care, eye and chest medicine, speciality clinics and dialysis. It is the trauma centre for the country and also provides a GP service.
O Elective notes: There are plenty of patients and things to see. Although everything is conducted in English, it can be difficult to understand. There are quite a few friendly local students.
Accommodation: Not provided, but the Sunshine Guesthouse is recommended.

The Doctors Hospital
PO Box N-3018, Collins Ave and Shirley Street, Nassau. Tel: +1 242 322 8411. Fax: +1 242 322 3284.
The hospital: An acute care, privately operated hospital with 72 beds. Medical specialities include emergency medicine, ENT, general surgery, orthopaedics, O&G, ophthalmology, internal medicine, gastroenteology, urology, cardiology and

paeds. The hospital has recently been renovated.

Sandilands Rehabilitation Centre
Nassau.

The hospital: A government-maintained geriatric and psychiatric hospital with 477 beds. The facility includes a security unit, a family guidance centre and a combined substance abuse centre for drug and alcohol abuse. The occupational therapy department runs a 'Very Special Arts' programme.

Lyford Cay Hospital/Bahamas Heart Institute
PO Vox N-7776, Naussau. Tel: +1 242 362 4025. Fax: +1 242 362 4493.

The hospital: A private hospital specializing in plastic and reconstructive surgery. There's a cardiac diagnostic centre providing Doppler echocardiography, 24-hour ECGs, exercise ECGs and pacemaker implants.

HOSPITALS IN FREEPORT, GRAND BAHAMA:

There's one general hospital and two specialist medical centres.

Rand Memorial Hospital
PO Box F-40071, East Atlantic Drive, Freeport, Grand Bahama. Tel: +1 242 352 6735. Fax: +1 242 352 6791.

The hospital: A government-owned, community-type hospital providing general medical care broadly similar to that offered by the Princess Margaret Hospital. It has 103 beds and a full medical staff.

Sunrise Medical Centre
PO Box 42575, Freeport, Grand Bahama. Tel: +1 242 373 3333. Fax: +1 242 373 3342.

The hospital: A private medical facility providing specialist services in general medicine, dental, O&G, oral and max-fax surgery, orthodontics and optometry.

Lucayan Medical Centre
Freeport, Grand Bahama. Tel: +1 242 373 7400.

The hospital: A private medical facility offering specialist services in family medicine, internal medicine, obstetrics, gastroenterology, kidney diseases, ophthalmology, paeds, psychiatry, surgery, urology and anaesthetics.

Cuba

Population: 11.1 million
Language: Spanish
Capital: Havana
Currency: Cuban peso
Int Code: +53

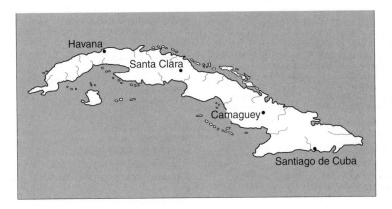

The Caribbean's largest island is also its only Communist one. It is a former Spanish colony, and the culture, language and traditions have persisted. The USA put sanctions on Cuba in 1962 in response to the presence of Soviet nuclear weapons on the island. Despite the collapse of Communism in the Soviet Union, the restrictions remain, making life pretty tough financially. The social life is, however, excellent, with street and beach parties, beer and rum. There is a lot to see around the island.

✪ Medicine:

Although it has limited resources, Cuba has a very impressive healthcare system. Life expectancy (76 years) is the highest in Latin America. Basic drugs and materials (such as X-ray films) are in very short supply owing to the US blockade. Havana's large pharmaceutical industry manages to supply what is needed. Cuba's ophthalmalogical services are world-renowned as being very advanced.

The doctor:patient ratio is 1:333. Despite the stretched resources, the doctors tend to be very friendly and keen to teach. Leading causes of death include heart disease, cancers and malnutrition. The prevalence of HIV is around 0.03%.

Note: Medical students here train for a particular speciality, for example to become a paediatrician and hence they don't need to study other subjects.

✪ Elective notes:

Ask the hospital if there is anything they want you to bring. Also take a bike (and a lock!) with you as there isn't much in the way of public transport. Most elective students have had to stay in hotels which has proved expensive.

➲ Visa requirements:

For £15 you can get a six-month visa for Cuba that allows you to stay as a tourist for 30 days, although this can be extended to six months when there. This visa is available 'instantly' from the embassy. The embassy's official line on electives is that you require a student visa (£47), which requires two passport photos and an invitation from the school and takes a couple of days to process. Visit the embassy in the UK between 9:30 and 12:30 Monday to Friday (167, High Holborn, London, UK. Tel: +44 20 7240 2488). To work, you must register with the Cuban Ministry of Health.

USEFUL ADDRESSES:

Ministerio de Salud Pública, Calle 23 y N, Vedado, Habana.
Cuban Medical Association – Doctors for Free Cuba, Colegio Médico Cubano Libre, PO Box 141016, Coral Gables, FL 33114-1016, USA. Tel: +1 305 446 9902. Fax: +1 305 445 9310.
Cuban Dental Association, 23YN Vedado, Habana. Tel: +53 7 33 32 99.

MEDICAL SCHOOLS AND HOSPITALS:

An extremely useful website is www.infomed.sld.cu. This lists a number of specialist as well as general hospitals. It provides web links for many of these as well as for some medical schools. The website is, however, only in Spanish so if you aren't yet fluent (and it's a good idea to have a good working knowledge if you are planning an elective in Cuba), translate the page using the translate function on medicstravel.com or altavista.com.

There are 13 areas with medical schools, although each listing may have a number of medical institutions within it (for example, 11 in Havana).

Instituto Superior de Ciencias Medicas de La Habana, Calle 146 y Avenida 31, Playa, Habana 11600. Tel: +53 7 218 545. Fax: +53 7 336 257. www.sld.cu/instituciones/iscmh/index.htm. (This is the oldest and largest Cuban medical school, using many hospitals in the area.)
Facultad de Ciencias Medicas Ciego de Avila, Circunvalacion y Carretera de Moron, Ciego de Avila 65100.
Facultad de Ciencias Medicas Cienfuegos, Calle 51 Entre 36 y 38, Cienfuegos 55100.
Facultad de Ciencias Medicas Granma Celia Sanchez Mandulay, Avenida Camilo Cienfuegas, Esquina Carretera Campechuela, Manzanillo 87510.

Facultad de Ciencias Medicas Guantanamo, Calle 5 Oeste Entre 8 y 9 Norte, Guantanamo 95100.
Facultad de Ciencias Medicas Holguin, Avenida Lenin No. 4 Esquina A Aguilera, Holguin 80100.
Facultad de Ciencias Medicas Las Tunas, Avenida de La Juventud s/n, Las Tunas 75100.
Facultad de Ciencias Medicas Matanzas, Carretera de Quintanilla Km 101, Matanzas 40100.
Facultad de Ciencias Medicas Pinar Del Rio, Carretera Central Km 89, Pinar Del Rio 20100.
Facultad de Ciencias Medicas Sancti Spiritus, Carretera Circunvalacion Norte, Banda, Sancti Spiritus 60100.
Instituto Superior de Ciencias Medicas Carlos J. Finlay, Carretera Central Oeste y Madame Curie, Camaguey 70100. Tel: +53 7 989 10. Fax: +53 7 615 87.
Instituto Superior de Ciencias Medicas de Santiago de Cuba, Avenida de Las Americas y Calle E, Santiago de Cuba 90100.
Instituto Superior de Ciencias Medicas de Villa Clara, Carretera de Acueducto y Circunvalacion, Santa Clara 50200.

A SELECTION OF HOSPITALS AND PRIMARY CARE UNITS:

Hospital Nacional Ameijeiras
Havana.
The hospital: Is one of the main hospitals. It has most major specialities, however, as with most of Cuba, the facilities and drugs are limited.

Hospital Clinico Quirlurgico
Dr Gustavo Aldereguia Lima', Avenida 5 de Septiembre y Calle 51 A, Cienfuegos.
The hospital: A DGH, friendly and offering a full range of services. Resources are poor but the healthcare still manages to be very good.
O Elective notes: Medical students, especially from South American countries, come here and there is plenty of teaching.

Civa Garcia International Clinic
Havana. Tel: +53 7 332 605.
Fax: +53 7 331 633.

Hospital Fajardo
Zapata YD, Vedado, Havana CR 10400.

Polyclinico Plaza de la Revolucion
Havana. (This is like a GP surgery, i.e. primary healthcare.)

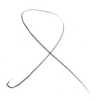

The Cayman Islands

Population: 35 000
Language: English
Capital: George Town
Currency: Dollar
Int Code: +1 345

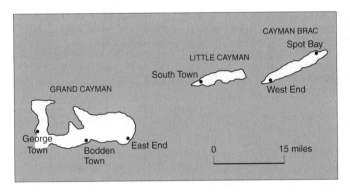

The three islands that make up the Caymans are situated 300 km north-west of Jamaica. Tourism is the major economy here; however, the Caymans are also a major financial centre because of the absence of tax and foreign exchange controls.

The two largest islands have hospitals. Grand Cayman has a modern, well-equipped 120-bed hospital. Cayman Brac (the second largest island) has a small cottage hospital.

⊃ Visas and work permits:
Very few medical students have done electives in the Cayman Islands. Approach the hospital directly to find out more about visa requirements and accommodation.

Those holding British, Commonwealth or US qualifications are able to practise in the Cayman Islands once they have been locally licensed through the Health Practitioners Board (the Chief Medical Officer is the chairman of the board). Persons employed at the George Town Hospital are on a government contract – equivalent to a work permit. It's worth mentioning that the government has a policy of having to try to give the job to a Caymanian before an outsider. With such a small population, however, it shouldn't be a problem for medics.

USEFUL ADDRESSES:

Public Health Services: The equivalent of the Ministry of Health is based at George Town Hospital.
Cayman Islands Medical and Dental Society, PO Box 1785 GT, George Town, Grand Cayman. Tel: +1 345 949 6066. Fax: +1 345 949 4447.

George Town Hospital

PO Box 915, Grand Cayman.
Tel: +1 345 949 8600.
Fax: +1 345 945 1754.
The hospital: A modern, well-equipped 120-bed hospital. It has a wide range of services and a number of specialists on the staff. In cases where specialist treatment is not available locally, patients are airlifted to Miami, where the government has an arrangement with certain hospitals. The hospital also houses the local decompression chamber.

Faith Hospital

PO Box 85, State Bay, Cayman Brac.
Tel: +1 345 948 2248.
Fax: +1 345 948 2460.
The hospital: Has 16 beds and emergency facilities.

OTHER MEDICAL ORGANIZATIONS ON THE ISLANDS:

Other organizations are the Cayman Islands Red Cross, Cayman Island Medical and Dental Association, Cayman Against Substance Abuse (CASA), Alcoholics Anonymous and Cayman Island Cancer Society.

There are also many private practitioners. The three major private centres are listed below:

Cayman Medical Centre, PO Box 30618SMB, Rankin's Plaza, Eastern Avenue, Grand Cayman. Tel: +1 345 949 8150. Fax: +1 345 949 7855.
Chrissie Tomlinson Memorial Hospital, George Town, Grand Cayman. Tel: +345 949 6066. Fax: +345 945 1695. www.chrissietomlinsonhospital.com. (This is a state-of-the-art, privately owned and run, brand new 18 bed hospital providing emergency, obstetric, surgical and intensive care facilities.)
Professional Medical Centre, Walkers Road, George Town, Grand Cayman. Tel: +1 345 949 6066. Fax: +1 345 945 1695.

Jamaica

Population: 2.7 million
Language: English
Capital: Kingston
Currency: Jamaican dollar
Int Code: +1 876

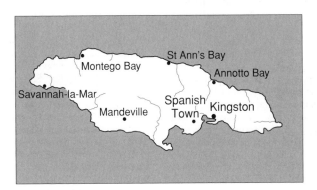

Jamaica is one of the larger islands in the Caribbean, separated from the southern coast of Florida by Cuba. It is the peak of one of the great volcanic mountains that form the seabed and therefore consists of central mountainous jungle surrounded by a strip of flat land around the coast. The idyllic beaches and exclusive holiday resorts that are associated with Jamaica are mainly on the north coast. The capital, Kingston, is a city of about 1 million people and is on the much poorer south coast. The University of the West Indies and the associated teaching hospital, University Hospital West Indies, sit on two adjacent sites in the northern outskirts of the city. After gaining independence in 1962, Jamaica underwent great political changes resulting in massive inflation and a large disparity between rich and poor.

In the early 1990s, 50% of households did not have a WC and 29% did not have electricity. These disparities are reflected in Jamaica's health problems.

Kingston has a well-earned reputation for violence, with a murder rate of 15 per 100 000 a year (two murders a day), one of the highest in the world. The violence tends to be in certain areas. Most of this is confined to gangland feuds, but foreigners are occasionally targeted, usually for money. Jamaicans equate white with rich, so if you're white, expect to be plagued by beggars and drug pushers. Women get even more hassle, with proposals of marriage as well. Despite all this, the university, hospital and surrounding areas are relatively safe, especially during daylight hours.

There is much to see and do outside Kingston. The best way to travel around the island is by car. However, this can be expensive so you may have to cram into the minibuses that make the five-hour trip across the mountains to the north coast. You may think that Jamaica is an English-speaking country: it is, but you may well have difficulty understanding the history in Patois and local dialect.

✪ Medicine:

Both tropical and Western diseases are common. Trauma, from both violence and road traffic accidents (50% each), is regularly seen. Cancers, heart and cerebrovascular disease are the most common causes of death. The prevalence of diabetes mellitus has increased by 300% since the 1960s, presumably through Western influence. The complications of this are putting a major strain on the health service. Child malnourishment is common and 90 clinics around the island try to deal with it. Approximately 15 000 children live on the streets of Kingston. Gastroenteritis is the most common cause of hospital admission. Other infectious diseases are also common. The prevalence of HIV is around 1%.

A few diseases are interesting to see. Malaria and yellow fever have now both been wiped out by mosquito eradication. Vomiting sickness is a common disease in the winter months that is unique to Jamaica. Vomiting occurs approximately three hours after a meal and can be fatal in a few days. It has been found to be due to eating undercooked ackee (a fruit introduced by Captain Bligh in 1793). Ingestion of Barracuda fish sometimes also causes poisoning. Jamaican neuropathy (tropical spastic paraparesis) is now known to be due to HTLV-1, present in 5% of the population and 28% of Jamaican prostitutes. Veno-occlusive disease of the liver as a result of drinking *Crotalaria retusa* bush tea is also seen. One in ten Jamaicans carries the sickle cell gene, reflecting their African descent and the previous prevalence of malaria in Jamaica.

The Jamaican psychiatrist also has a different job from most. There are a number of reasons for this: the social backdrop, cultural differences and the financial constraints under which they work. Although Christianity is very strong in Jamaica, many children are born without any commitment between their parents. It is common for a young woman to have children and leave them with the grandmother while she goes out to work. The father has no responsibilities. Single parenting is therefore part of the norm, one woman having several children by two or three 'babyfathers'. Another cultural difference is the widespread use of cannabis and, to a lesser extent, cocaine. Drug-induced psychoses are therefore more common. Also, because of the poor funding in the healthcare system, physical treatments are used very early on to expedite discharge. This means higher doses of antipsychotics and early ECT.

The **University Hospital**, **Kingston Public Hospital** and the **Cornwall Regional Hospital** in Montego Bay are class A secondary and tertiary referral centres. Class B hospitals (providing in- and outpatient services in general surgery, internal medicine, O&G, and paeds) are located in St Ann's Bay, Savannah-la-Mar, Mandeville and Spanish Town. There are also about a dozen smaller class C hospitals that are parish based, two or three doctors providing general medicine, child and community care.

Specialist hospitals include the **Victoria Jubilee** (maternity), the **Bustamante Children's Hospital**, the **Mona Rehabilitation Centre** (physiotherapy and occupational therapy for sufferers of polio, spasticity, amputation and paraplegia), the **Bellevue** (psychiatry), the **National Chest Hospital** and the **Hope Institute** (palliative care). About 450 doctors work in the public hospital and health centres. Elsewhere there are 750 doctors working within the private healthcare system.

USEFUL ADDRESSES:

Jamaican Ministry of Health, 2–4 King Street, Kingston. Tel: +1 876 967 1101. Fax: +1 876 967 7293. www.moh.gov.jm.
Medical Association of Jamaica, 3a Pisley Avenue, Kingston 5. Tel: +1 876 929 9227. Fax: +1 876 929 5829. www.maj.org.jm.
Jamaican Dental Association, PO Box 19, Kingston 5. Tel: +1 876 978 0440. Fax: +1 876 978 4728. www.jamaicadentalassn.com.

University of the West Indies – Jamaica

Faculty of Medical Sciences, The Registry, Kingston. Tel: +1 876 927 1297. Fax: +1 876 927 2556. www.uwimona.edu.jm.

The University of the West Indies was initially a university college associated with the University of London. Due to the lack of medics on the island, the faculty of medicine was the first faculty to be established. It proved impossible to adapt Kingston Public Hospital into a teaching hospital so a new university hospital was specially designed.

The university has a well-organized elective programme both in Jamaica and on other islands. It can send an application form on which you request a speciality. It can also help with accommodation by suggesting private residences. One address that comes recommended is that of Mrs Soares (16 Beverly Drive, Beverly Hills, Kingston 6. Tel: +1 809 978 3806). She is an elderly Jamaican lady living in an affluent part of Kingston. A number of local students live there. The usual cost is around £10 a day. Another is Mrs S. Grant (43 University Crescent, Kingston 6).

University Hospital of the West Indies

Mona, St Andrew, Kingston 7. Tel: +1 876 927 1620. Fax: +1 876 927 2101.
The hospital: Is the major teaching hospital and is situated on the Mona campus. It has just over 400 beds, making it larger than Kingston Public Hospital. It has pretty good facilities and caters for most specialities, although there are specialist hospitals. The department of psychiatry has a 20-bed ward, which, due to different approaches to psychiatric management in Jamaica, is rarely much more than half full. There is also a day ward. There are connections with the large long-stay psychiatric hospital, **Bellevue Hospital** (*see* below). There is an MRC sickle cell laboratory on the Mona Campus (mrcjamaica.nimr.mrc.ac.uk).
O Elective notes: It's a busy hospital, with plenty to see and do in the emergency department. There's a high standard of well-organized teaching.
Accommodation: Can be difficult. The Dean's office can put you in touch with people who run boarding houses for students (*see* above).

Cornwall Regional Hospital

Mount Salem, Montego Bay, St James. Tel: +1 876 952 5100. Fax: +1 876 952 4149.
The hospital: The main public hospital in Montego Bay. It is busy, especially for O&G, emergency medicine and surgery. The emergency department sees quite a lot of penetrating injuries. There are fewer shootings than in Kingston, and it is a nicer area.
O Elective notes: It provides good experience but not loads of responsibility.
Accommodation: They try to provide it, but no guarantees.

St Ann's Bay Hospital

St Ann's Bay PO Centre, St Ann's Bay. Tel: +1 876 972 0150. Fax: +1 876 972 1736.
The hospital: It is a type B, secondary-level hospital with 155 beds.

Annotto Bay Public Hospital

Annotto Bay, St Mary. Tel: +1 876 996 2222.
The hospital: A very busy (type C) rural hospital. It is pretty isolated but has all main specialities (surgery, medicine, O&G, paeds). It is poorly funded.
O Elective notes: There's good teaching on the wards and plenty of chance to practise clinical skills. You can visit St Ann's Bay Public Hospital or Port Antonio Public Hospital (Tel: +1 876 993 2646), which are nearby. The hospital is fairly isolated.

Bellevue Hospital

Kingston. Tel: +1 876 928 1380.
The hospital: The largest psychiatric hospital in the Caribbean. It is a state-funded hospital in deepest downtown. It is part of Jamican folklore and is like something out of a horror film. It has 23 wards spread out over extensive grounds and houses 1500 patients – yardies from the neighbouring ganglands, drugs-runners, pimps and prostitutes. All bar seven of the wards are long-stay wards and Bellevue also acts as a dumping ground for old Jamaicans whose relatives have emigrated. This is a place of institutionalization – schizophrenics lying in bed all day, mentally

retarded patients not even getting sanitary care. Some patients can be very violent. The hospital, however, has guards who carry assault rifles. There are only four or five doctors and one nurse per ward. The doctor sees about 60 outpatients in the morning and 90 in the afternoon. Most patients are probably incorrectly diagnosed. WARNING: This is a dangerous place ... if you are white, think seriously before going here.

Haiti

Population: 7.1 million
Language: French and French Creole
Capital: Port-au-Prince
Currency: Gourde
Int Code: +509

Due to the political unrest in Haiti (the western third of Hispaniola) it is difficult to find out information. It is an incredibly poor country, and most people cannot afford healthcare, instead getting help from voodoo priests. This is reflected in a life expectancy of only 57 years. Malnutrition, infectious diseases, such as malaria and TB, and political killings are the big killers. There is only one doctor for every 7040 people. The prevelance of HIV is around 5%. Of note, Haiti is the most mountainous region of the Caribbean, with three mountain ranges.

USEFUL ADDRESSES:

Ministry of Health: Ministère de la Santé publique et de la Population, Palais des Ministères, Port-au-Prince. Tel: +509 22 1248. Fax: +509 22 4066.
Haiti Medical Association: Association Médicale Haitienne, 1ère Avenue du Travail, Bois Verna, Port-au-Prince. Tel: +509 245 2060. Fax: +509 511 0253. www.amhhaiti.org.
For information on hospitals, doctors and NGOs in Haiti, check out: www.haitimedical.com.

MEDICAL SCHOOLS:

Ecole de Médecine et de Pharmacie, Université d'Etat d'Haiti, Rue Oswals Durand 89, Port-au-Prince. Tel: +509 220 488. Fax: +509 573 974.
Université Catholique Notre Dame d'Haiti, Faculté de Médecine, 6 Rue Sapotille, Port-au-Prince.

HOSPITALS:

Port-au-Prince:
Centre Obstetrico Gynecologique Isaie Jeanty-Leon Audain, Chancerelles, Port-au-Prince. Tel: +509 222 2757.

Clinique de la Santé, 102, Ave Poupelard (Après Ruelle Chrétien), Port-au-Prince. Tel : +509 245 9906/244 093.
Hôpital du Canape-Vert, Route du Canape-Vert, Port-au-Prince. Tel: +509 245 1053.
Hôpital Francais (Asile Francais), Rue du Centre, Port-au-Prince. Tel: +509 222 4242.
Hôpital-Maternité Sapiens, Avenue Christophe # 120, Port-au-Prince. Tel: +509 245 8349.
Hôpital Ofatma, Cité Militaire, Port-au-Prince. Tel: +509 222 3846.
Hôpital Saint François de Sales, Rue Chareron, Port-au-Prince. Tel: +509 222 5033.
Hôpital de l'Université d'Etat d'Haiti, Rue Monseigneur Guilloux, Port-au-Prince. Tel: +509 222 1221.

Petion-Ville:
Citymed – Petion-Ville, 27 Rue Darguin, Petion-Ville. Tel: +509 257 1084.
Hôpital de la Communauté Haitienne, Rue Audant, Route de Freres, Freres. Tel: +509 257 7505.
Maternité de Pétion-Ville, 1 Rue Goulard, Pétion-Ville (Derriere la Place Boyer). Tel: +509 257 0857.

Delmas:
Grace Children's Hospital, Delmas 31.

Carrefour:
Hôpital Adventiste de Diquini, Carrefour. Tel: +509 234 0521.
Hôpital Saint Charles (Mariani), Carrefour. Tel: +509 34 0130.

Nord:
Hôpital de Bienfaisance de Pignon. www.pignon.org.
Hôpital Justinien – Cap Haitien, Rue 17 Q, Cap Haitien. Tel: +509 262 1877.

Sud:
Hôpital Immaculée Conception (Les Cayes). Tel: +509 286 0041. Fax: +509 286 0116.
Hôpital Sainte Anne, Camperrin. Tel: +509 286 0249.

Artibonite:

Hôpital La Providence (Gonaives), Rue C. Imbert, Gonaives. Tel: +509 274 0322.
Hôpital Albert Schweitzer (Deschapelles), BP 1744, Port-au-Prince. www.hashaiti.org.

Ouest (except metro Port-au-Prince):

Hôpital Sainte Croix de Leogane, Leogane. www.hopital-stecroix.org.
Hôpital Wesleyen de La Gônave (La Gonave Wesleyan Hospital).

Sud-Est:

Hôpital Saint Michel de Jacmel.
Tel: +509 288 2151.

Nord-Ouest:

Hôpital de Port-de-Paix.

Centre:

Clinique Bon Sauvéur de Cange.
Hôpital de la Nativite de Belladere.
Hôpital Sainte Thérèse de Hinche.

Grand'Anse:

Hopital Saint Antoine (JEREMIE), Bordes, Jeremie. Tel: +509 284 5260.

Dominican Republic

Population: 8.6 million
Language: Spanish
Capital: Santo Domingo
Currency: Dominican Republic peso
Int Code: +1 809

The Dominican Republic occupies the other two-thirds of Hispaniola and is mountainous and forested. It is a popular tourist destination with Italians and Germans. Since 1996 they have had free elections.

○ Medicine:

Tropical diseases are relatively common. The prevalence of HIV is in the region of 4%. There are a number of medical schools.

USEFUL ADDRESSES:

Ministry of Health: San Cristoval Avenue, Santo Domingo. Tel: +1 809 541 3121.
Dominican Republic Medical Association: Asociación Médica Dominicana, Calle **Paseo de los Médicos Esquina Modesto Diaz Zona Universiteria**, Santo Domingo.
Tel: +1 809 533 4602. Fax: +1 809 535 7337.

MEDICAL SCHOOLS

Pontificia Universidad Católica Madre y Maestra, Facultad de Ciencias de la Salud, Autopisto Duarte Km 1 1/2, Apartado 822, Santiago de Los Caballeros. Tel: +1 809 580 1962 ext. 226. Fax: +1 809 241 5128.
www.pucmmsti.edu.do/academica/fcs.htm.
Universidad Autónoma de Santo Domingo, Facultad de Ciencias de la Salud, Calle Correa y Cidron, Ciudad Universitaria, Cidron, Santo Domingo. Tel: +1 809 685 7597.
Fax: +1 809 687 1449.
Universidad Central del Este, Facultad de Ciencias Medicas, Avenida Francisco Alberto Camaño #1, San Pedro de Macorís. Tel: +1 809 529 3562. Fax: +1 809 529 5146. www.uce.edu.do.
Universidad Iberoamericana, Escuela de Medicina, Avenida Francia 129, Santo Domingo. Tel: +1 809 689 4111. Fax: +1 809 686 5821. www.unibe.edu.do. (This is a new medical school (founded in 1982) also in the nation's capital. It trains a number of foreign students.)
Universidad Instituto Tecnológico de Santo Domingo, Facultad de Ciencias de la Salud, Avenida de los Próceres, Los Jardines del Norte, Santo Domingo. Tel: +1 809 567 9271. Fax: +1 809 566 3200. www.intec.edu.do.
Universidad Nacional Pedro Henríquez Ureña, Facultad de Ciencias de la Salud – Escuela de Medicina, Avenida John F. Kennedy Km 5½, Apartado Postal 1423, Santo Domingo. Tel: +1 809 562 6601. Fax: +1 809 563 2254. www.unphu.edu.do.
Universidad Nordestana, Faculty of Medical Sciences, 27 de Febrero No. 19, Apartado Postal 239, San Francisco de Macoris. Tel: +1 809 588 3239. Fax: +1 809 244 1647. www.unne.edu. (This is a much smaller teaching hospital to the north of the island.)
Universidad Tecnologica de Santiago, Facultad de Ciencias de la Salud, Campus Central de Herrera, Isabel Aguiar No. 61 Apartado Postal No. 21243, Santo Domingo. Tel: +1 809 530 1080. Fax: +1 809 682 0200. www.utesa.edu.
Universidad Tecnologica del Cibao, Escuela de Medicina, Avenida Universitaria, Apartado Postal No 401, La Vega. Tel: +1 809 573 1020. Fax: +1 809 573 6194. www.uteci.edu.do.

The two main hospitals in Santo Domingo are:

Hospital Dr Dario Contreras, Santo Domingo. Tel: +1 809 596 3686.
Hospital Dr Francisco Moscoso Puello, Santo Domingo. Tel: +1 809 681 6922.

Puerto Rico

Population: 3.7 million
Language: Spanish, English
Capital: San Juan
Currency US Dollar
Int code: +1 787

The Commonwealth of Puerto Rico comprises Puerto Rico itself and the smaller islands of Vieques and Culebra. There is a hot tropical climate, but cool trade winds keep the temperature bearable all year round.

✚ Medicine:

Tropical diseases including schistosomiasis do occur, as does the flu-like illness 'la manga', but Western diseases are the common cause of death.

USEFUL ADDRESS:

Department of Health, PO Box 70184, San Juan Tel: +1 787 274 7621. Fax: +1 787 250 6547.

MEDICAL SCHOOLS:

Puerto Rico has four medical schools:

Ponce School of Medicine

PO Box 7004, Ponce, PR 00732. Tel: +1 787 840 2511. Fax: +1 787 840 9756.
Initially the Catholic University of Puerto Rico School of Medicine, the name changed in 1980. **Damas Hospital** (356 beds) is the main teaching hospital. **La Playa Diagnostic Center**, **Ponce District Hospital** (550 beds), **Dr Pila Hospital** (160 beds) and **St Luke's Hospital** (160 beds) are also used. In San Germán, the **Concepcíon Hospital** (188 beds) and **Yauco Regional Hospital** (140 beds) are also linked.

San Juan Bautista School of Medicine

Interamerican Hospital for Advanced Medicine, Ground Floor, Avenida Luis Munoz Marin, Caguas 68465. Tel: +1 787 743 3038. Fax: +1 787 746 3093. www.sanjuanbautista.edu.

Universidad Central del Caribe School of Medicine

PO Box 60-327, Bayamón, PR 00960–6032. Tel: +1 787 740 1611. Fax: +1 787 269 7550. www.uccaribe.edu.
Founded in 1976, the school uses the **Dr Ramón Ruíz Arnau University Hospital** as its principal teaching hospital in the city of Bayamón.

University of Puerto Rico School of Medicine

PO Box 365067, San Juan, PR 00936–5067. Tel: +1 787 758 2525. Fax: +1 787 282 7117.
Founded in 1949, the University School of Medicine is affiliated with the **Puerto Rico Medical Center** and the **Hospital Consortium**. It is based next to the **University District Hospital**.

HOSPITALS IN PUERTO RICO:

University District Hospital, Puerto Rico Medical Center, San Juan. Tel: +1 787 754 3654.
University Paediatric Hospital, Puerto Rico Medical Center, San Juan. Tel: +1 787 754 3700.
Carolina Area Hospital, PO Box 38691, Carolina. Tel: +1 787 757 1800.

St Kitts and Nevis

Population: 41 000
Language: English
Capital: Basseterre
Currency East Caribbean dollar
Int Code: +1 869 (St Kitts) and
+ 1 978 (Nevis)

St Kitts is a small beautiful island and a popular tourist destination. It is a former British colony and lies at the top of the Leeward Islands chain. The government provides a basic health service. Some developments were put on hold after Hurricane George, but improvements are being made.

Two American-run preclinical medical schools are on St Kitts, and one school is on Nevis (addresses below) – to organize electives, write directly to the hospitals.

USEFUL ADDRESS:

Ministry of Health, Government Headquarters, Church Street, Basseterre. Tel: +1 869 465 2521. Fax: +1 869 465 1316.

HOSPITALS:

Joseph N. France General Hospital
Buckley's Site, Basseterre, St Kitts.
Tel: +1 869 465 2551.
Fax: +1 869 466 6681.
The hospital: A small hospital. It's very friendly and has recently opened an ITU and neonatal ITU. Tuberculosis, HIV, diabetes, thyroid disorders and hypertension are very common.

Hospital Molineux
St Kitts. Tel: +1 869 465 7398.

Pogson Hospital
Mount Idle, Sandy Point, St Kitts.
Tel: +1 869 465 6231.
The hospital: An old hospital scheduled for demolition.

Alexandra Hospital
Government Road, Charlestown, Nevis.
Tel: +1 978 469 5473.
Fax: +1 978 469 5956.
The hospital: Is a 52-bed hospital on Nevis.

MEDICAL SCHOOLS:

They do not have clinical components on the islands, hence full details are not given here.

On St Kitts:
International University of the Health Sciences, School of Medicine. www.iuhs.edu/. Windsor University, School of Medicine. www.windsor.edu.

On Nevis:
Medical University of the Americas. www.medicaluniversity.org.

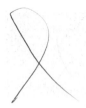

Guadeloupe

Population: 387 000
Official Language: French
Capital: Pointe-à-Pitre
Currency: French Franc/Euro
Int Code: +590

Guadeloupe is a group of islands comprising Guadeloupe, Grande Terre and five smaller islands. All have beautiful palm-fringed beaches and lush mountain areas.

✛ Medicine:
Tropical diseases such as dengue fever, leishmaniasis and schistosomiasis are all present, but Western diseases are also common.

HOSPITALS:

Centre Hospitalier Régional Universitaire
Route de Chauvel, Pointe-à-Pitre Cedex 97159. Tel: +590 89 10 10. Fax: +590 89 10 29.
The hospital: This is the main hospital and possesses a recompression chamber for diving accidents and a CT scanner.

Centre Hospitalier general de Basse-Terre/Saint Claude
Rue Danial Beauperthuy, Basse Terre 97100. Tel: +590 80 54 54. Fax: +590 80 54 28.

Centre Hospitalier Maurice Selbonne
Pigeon, Bouillante 91125. Tel: +590 80 49 00. Fax: +590 80 49 15.

Centre Hospitalier Louis Daniel Beauperthuy
Mahault, Pointe Noire 97116. Tel: +590 80 59 59. Fax: +590 80 59 27.

HOSPITALS ON TWO SMALLER ISLANDS:

Hôpital de Bruyn, Gustavia 97133, Saint Barthelemy. Tel: +590 27 60 35. Fax: +590 27 85 78.
Hôpital de Saint Martin, Marigot 97150, Saint Martin. Tel: +590 29 57 57. Fax: +590 87 50 72.

Antigua and Barbuda

Population: 65 000
Official Language: English
Capital: St John's
Currency: East Caribbean dollar
Int Code: +1 283/268

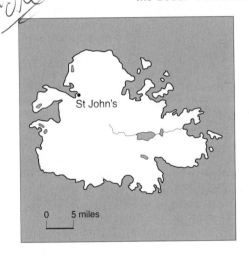

St John's

0   5 miles

Antigua and Barbuda

Antigua and Barbuda comprise three islands (the third uninhabited island being Rehona). They have been a colony of the Spanish, French and British. Tourism is the islands' main industry and accounts for about half the workforce. Approximately 65 000 people live on Antigua, of whom 90% are of African descent but the British influence is clear in their passion for cricket. There are beautiful beaches that are all open to the public. Prime beaches to visit are located on the east coast, Dickenson and Runaway beaches, Deep Bay and Hawksbill Beach to the west of St John's, and Darkwood beach to the south. Antigua has some excellent diving, with coral canyons, the most popular diving site being at Cades Reef. The going rate is about £20 for a single tank and £175 for a

certification course. Snorkelling from the shore is readily available, wrecks and many shoals of fish being easily visualized. Windsurfing schools are located at Dickenson Bay. The main places to visit on the island are Nelson's Dockyard, Jolly Harbour and Shirley Heights. Nelson's Dockyard is the island's main port of entry for yachts; it has many restaurants, a small market, a museum and various other historical buildings with a colonial atmosphere. Jolly Harbour is a new marina with various shops and boutiques located on the quay. At night, there are many bars and discos. Shirley Heights is an 18th century fort ruins with a wonderful hilltop view. Within the ruins is a bar that offers a public barbecue on Sundays with a live steel band. Other places of interest include Devil's

Bridge, a coastal sea arch and Fig Tree Drive, a road that passes by pineapple patches and tall plants.

To get around you can hire a bike or car or use the bus service. The roads, however, are very poor with many potholes. In order to drive on Antigua, you will need a temporary 90-day driving licence which costs about £8. Car rental is about £20 a day. Taxis are government run, but always confirm the price with the driver before the journey. When you've done all that, head to Barbuda, Antigua's dependency 50 km north-east with even more beautiful beaches.

✪ Medicine:

The standard is pretty good for the Caribbean. Western conditions of malignancy and cardio/cerebrovascular disease are the common causes of death. There are state-run hospitals providing treatment free. GPs are not free so everything comes to hospital.

USEFUL ADDRESSES:

Ministry of Health, St John's Street, St John's. Tel: +1 283 462 1600. Fax: +1 283 462 5003.
Antigua and Barbuda Medical Association, 2nd Avenue, Gambels Terrace, PO Box 18, St John's. Tel: +1 283 462 1838., Fax: +1 283 462 3105.

Holberton Hospital

PO Box 2797, St Johns. Tel: +1 283 462 0251. Fax: +1 283 462 6073.
The hospital: Located in St John's, which is the island's capital. From the outside it looks like a small, rundown warehouse. It has 220 beds, comprising four wards and an 'intensive care unit'. Although poorly sanitized, it does have a good X-ray department, including a CT scanner. The beds are huddled close to each other on crumbling wards often without curtains around them. There are ants and insects everywhere, including the theatres.

✪ **Elective notes:** There is a ward round in the morning, after which there are few doctors on-site. The hospital is run by three casualty officers and the on-call teams who work from home. By 7 am the emergency department waiting room is full. There is quite a bit of trauma because of the state of the roads and the lack of road law. Local anaesthetic is reserved for children. Consultants conduct one clinic a week from a shed at the bottom of the main hospital drive. To arrange this elective, contact the hospital administrator MONTHS before you intend to go. It works out cheapest and quickest to fax.

Accommodation: Hospital accommodation is basic. There are many insects and the shower consists of a high-up tap. No mosquito nets are provided. Try Mrs E. Murphy (Murphy's Apartments, All Saint's Road, St Johns), although this can be expensive.

OTHER HOSPITALS:

Adelin Medical Centre, Fort Road, Box 1123, St John's. Tel: +1 268 462 0866. (This is the private hospital on Antigua.)
Fiennes Institute, Queen Elizabeth Highway, St John's. Tel: +1 268 462 0419. (This is a 100 bed care of the elderly hospital.)
St John's Hospital Project Team, Camacho's Avenue, St John's. +1 268 562 1115.

There is an American-style preclinical medical school also on the island:

University of Health Sciences Antigua

School of Medicine, Downhill Campus, Piccadilly, PO Box 510, St John's.
Tel: +1 268 1 460 1391.
Fax: +1 268 1 460 1477. www.uhsa.ag.

Montserrat

Population: 10 700
Official Language: English
Capital: Plymouth
Currency: East Caribbean dollar
Int Code: +664

Montserrat is one of the Leeward Islands and is about 90 km north of Guadeloupe. Most recently it has been known for its volcanic activity, which has forced some of the country's popultion to resettle in the north. Note: An HIV test is necessary for working here.

USEFUL ADDRESS:

Ministry of Health, Parliament Street, Plymouth. Tel +664 481 2880.

HOSPITAL:

Glendon Hospital
PO Box 24, St John's. Tel: +664 491 2552.
The hospital: This is a general hospital with 70 beds and around eight doctors.

OFFSHORE MEDICAL SCHOOL:

American University of the Caribbean
School of Medicine, PO Box 400, Plymouth. Tel: +1 305 446 0600. www.aucmed.edu.
Note: This medical school has been relocated to the Netherlands Antilles because of volcanic activity on Montserrat.

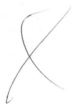

Dominica

Population: 71 000
Language: English
Capital: Roseau
Currency: East Caribbean dollar
Int Code: +1 767

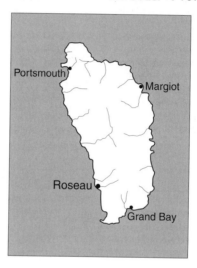

Dominica is a small island in the eastern Caribbean measuring only 46 km by 25 km. The volcanic mountains rise spectacularly out of the sea and are richly forested. The highest peak is Morne Diablotin, 1447 m high and is within the Northern Forest reserve. There is an abundance of rivers, lakes and impressive waterfalls which make excellent swimming. The east coast is very dramatic, being washed by the fierce Atlantic waves, in great contrast to the west which faces onto the Caribbean sea and is more typically sandy beaches and palm trees. A third of the population live in Roseau. Most of the islanders are of African descent, with about 3000 native Caribs, who reside in a large reserve on the eastern side of the island. The Caribs settled in the 14th century and called the island 'Waitikubuli'. It was rediscovered by Christopher Columbus and pronounced a British colony until its independence in 1978. There is still a strong Carib and Creole tradition found in the art and basketwork, music and clothes. This is combined with the Rastafarians and Catholic religions that have superseded. The local language is Patois, but English is mostly spoken. There is high unemployment and most women are involved in the upbringing of at least five children. Agriculture is the main income, and there is an effort to export bananas, chillies and bay leaves although the annual hurricanes destroy many of the crops. Subsistence farming and local produce provide enough food for most people and, despite a low standard of living compared with other Caribbean islands, none seems to suffer from malnutrition. Tourism is increasing rapidly and this island is sure to change.

○ Medicine:

Medical care is provided from 44 health centres, the main hospital being in the capital. There is private healthcare, but most have to make do with the government's cover.

USEFUL ADDRESSES:

Ministry of Health and Social Security,
Government Headquarters, Kennedy Avenue, Roseau. Tel: +1 767 448 2401. Fax: +1 767 448 6086.
Dominica Medical Association, PO Box 1956, Princess Margaret Hospital, Roseau. Tel: +1 767 448 2231.

Princess Margaret Hospital

Roseau.
The hospital: The main hospital on the island, with 800 beds. It is mostly an old building, but the French have constructed a new wing (foyer, radiology and emergency department). The staff, most of whom trained in the University of the West Indies in Jamaica or Cuba, are very friendly. There are also VSO workers. Despite the lack of facilities, lab tests, imaging and drugs, the standard of care is very impressive. Common disorders include diabetes, hypertension, TB, intestinal parasites and yaws.
Accommodation: Available in a local bed and breakfast for $12 a night.

OTHER HOSPITALS:

Portsmouth Hospital, Portsmouth.
Tel: +1 767 445 5237.
Marigot Hospital, Marigot. Tel: +1 767 445 7091.

FOR PRIMARY CARE:

Grand Bay Health Centre, Grand Bay.
Tel: +1 767 446 3706.

AMERICAN-STYLE PRECLINICAL SCHOOL:

Ross University, School of Medicine,
PO Box 266, Roseau. Tel: +1 767 445 5355.
Fax: +1 767 445 5583. www.rossmed.edu.

Martinique

Population: 371 000
Language: French and Creole
Capital: Fort-de-France
Currency: French franc
Int Code: +596

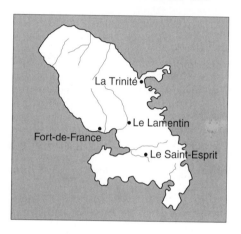

La Trinité

Le Lamentin

Fort-de-France

Le Saint-Esprit

Martinique is a beautiful small French island next to St Lucia. There are plenty of white, sandy beaches and clear blue sea … perfect if you want to learn to dive or windsurf. The people are mostly black Caribbeans, although there are many French settlers. So if you want to hit the beach, enjoy Creole food, get a tan and practise your French, this is the place to go. You will need good French to converse with patients. There are 14 hospitals.

La Meynard Hospital
BP 632, Chu De Fort-De-France, 97261 Fort-De-France. Tel: + 596 55 20 00. Fax: +596 75 50 60.
The hospital: Relatively large. The emergency department has a helicopter service, and the hospital covers all the main specialities.

O Elective notes: The medical wards are extremely laid back. Turn up in the mornings, do a ward round and a few procedures (e.g. bone marrow aspirates, pleural drains, ECGs, blood gases, etc.) and then go explore. One of the consultants has an interest in haematology so you can see advanced cases of leukaemia, Hodgkin's lymphoma and AIDS.

OTHER HOSPITALS:

Lamentin Hospital, Boulevard Fernand Guilon, Le Lamentin 97232. Tel: +596 57 11 11. Fax: +596 51 63 66.
Saint-Esprit Hospital, Borg, Saint Esprit 97270. Tel: +596 56 61 03. Fax: +596 56 55 59.
Saint Joseph Hospital, Rue Pelceee, Saint-Pierre 97250. Tel: +596 78 14 93. Fax: +596 78 18 24.
Trinité Hospital, Route du Stade, Trinité 97222. Tel: +596 66 46 00. Fax: +596 66 46 06.

Population: 145 000
Language: English
Capital: Castries
Currency: East Caribbean dollar
Int Code: +1 758

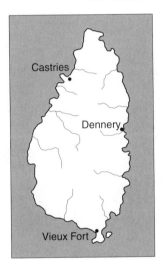

Castries

Dennery

Vieux Fort

St Lucia is a beautiful island (possibly the most beautiful in the Caribbean) with good beaches and amazing rainforests. It has been both a French and a British colony and retains the character of both. Today it relies on tourism, mainly from cruise ships, and banana-growing.

St Jude Hospital
PO Box 331, St Jude Highway, Vieux Fort.
Tel: +1 758 454 6041. Fax: +1 758 454 6684.
The hospital: St Jude's is St Lucia's largest hospital and is situated by the town Vieux Fort. It was previously a charity hospital run by the Sisters of Mercy but has recently been sold, patients now being charged for eveything (from ambulance call-outs to nebulizers). There is plenty of interesting pathology, but reports suggest that the hospital is not well run.

O Elective notes: A few years ago, this was an excellent elective destination. They now charge students to go there, and, from recent reports, it appears that the hospital has become preoccupied with making money. Volunteers are treated well, but until things improve, think twice about going here.

OTHER HOSPITALS:

Dennery Hospital, Hospital Road, Dennery.
Tel: +1 758 453 3310.
Golden Hope Hospital, La-Toc Road, Castries.
Tel: +1 758 452 7393.
Victoria Hospital, Hospital Road, Castries.
Tel: +1 758 452 2421. Fax: +1 758 453 0960.

St Vincent and the Grenadines

Population: 111 000
Language: English
Capital: Kingstown
Currency: East Caribbean dollar
Int Code: +1 784

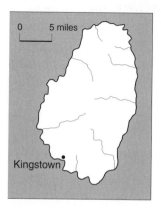

0   5 miles

Kingstown

St Vincent is a beautiful volcanic island that relies mainly on banana production and elite tourism. Associated with it are a group of mainly coral islands, the Grenadines. Kingstown itself is a little run down, and the people can be a bit rude if you are a single white female, but this is not true of the other Grenadine islands. There is a lot to do around St Vincent – botanical gardens, volcanoes, rainforests, waterfalls, etc. However, the best places to go for deserted paradise are the smaller Grenadine islands, with their white sands, palm trees and clear blue water, ideal for diving and snorkelling.

USEFUL ADDRESSES:

Ministry of Health, Governement Building, Kingstown. Tel: +1 784 456 1111.

Medical Association of St Vincent and the Grenadines, PO Box 815, Granby Street. Tel: +1 784 457 2023. Fax: +1 784 456 1186.

Kingstown General Hospital

Kingstown. Tel: +1 784 456 1185.
The hospital: Kingstown General Hospital has 210 beds and serves the whole of St Vincent and the Grenadines. Specialities include emergency and general medicine and surgery, paeds, O&G, ophthalmology, ENT and radiology. The hospital has most of the necessary equipment, although much is old and in short supply. They also lack simple things such as tourniquets and make do with gloves and catheters. X-ray and ultrasound are the only imaging techniques.
O Elective notes: Most of the doctors

are friendly and helpful. They come from many nationalities, mainly Indian. They don't give much formal teaching but are keen to answer questions. The hospital is always busy, especially in the after-noons, when medical students from the nearby American offshore medical school descend in huge numbers. This is your cue to escape as nothing much happens once they arrive. This elective is thoroughly recommended if you want a stress-free, relaxing time.

Accommodation: Provided in the nurses' hostel, a five-minute walk from the hospital. It is cheap and convenient, and meals can be provided very cheaply if you like rice.

HOSPITALS ON THE GRENADINES:

Bequia District Hospital, Port Elizabeth, Bequia. Tel: +1 784 458 3294.
Union Island District Hospital, Clifton, Union Island. Tel: +1 784 458 8339.
Mesopotamia District Hospital, Mesopotamia. Tel: +1 784 458 5245.

AMERICAN PRECLINICAL SCHOOL:

Kingstown Medical College, PO Box 585, Ratho Mill, Saint Vincent. Tel: +1 809 458 4832. www.sgu.edu.

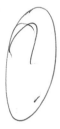

Barbados

Population: 260 000
Language: English
Capital: Bridgetown
Currency: Barbados dollar
Int Code: +1 246

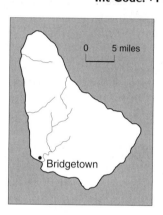

Barbados is one of the larger islands that comprise the West Indies. It is made of coral, unlike the other Caribbean islands, which are volcanic. Measuring 35 km by 22 km, it has a resident population of about 260 000 which, during peak season, reaches roughly 400 000. As part of the Commonwealth (independence granted in 1966), the Queen is still the monarch, but a separate parliament operates here. The island is divided into 'parishes', like counties in the UK. The majority of Barbadians (colloquially Bajans) are black of African descent, the other 5% being white, of Scottish/English descent. The island's economy consists of tourism, sugar and rum. Bridgetown is the capital and is not the typical capital you would expect from a developing world country. Crime is not really a problem here although in recent years people have had to start locking doors and there is the occasional mugging. Occasionally you will be bothered by a VERY friendly Bajan offering to 'walk you home safely'. He will ask for money

at some point. It's best just to say that you're a doctor at the hospital and fed up with being asked. Tourist attractions include Welchman Hall gully, Harrison's cave, the picturesque coastline at Bathsheba, Farley Hill National Park and the Barbados wildlife reserve. An abundance of water sports is available. Barbados is the place to learn to scuba-dive (five-day PADI courses). Tell them you work in the hospital as this can give you up to 50% off courses. There's also water-skiing, jetskiing, windsurfing, sailing and fishing on many beaches. The cricket is a must-see. Other events include the races at Garrison Savannah, Oistins Easter fish festival, Congaline Carnival, open-air opera, the Jolly Roger cruise and the Mount Gay rum tour. As you might expect, the night-life is pretty active with a number of clubs along the coastline (drink as much as you can for about £6). Transport is provided cheaply by government taxis or private ZR vans (50p a ride). WARNING … there is no law against drink-driving.

Barbados

✪ Medicine:

Medical care is provided by both government-subsidized hospitals/clinics and private hospitals. Western diseases are the killers, although type II diabetes with a prevalence of 20% in the general population) and HIV are on the increase.

USEFUL ADDRESSES

Ministry of Health, Jemmott's Lane, St Michael. Tel: +1 246 426 4669. Fax: +1 246 426 5570.
Barbados Association of Medical Practitioners, BAMP Complex, Spring Garden, St Michael. Tel: +1 246 429 7569. Fax: +1 246 435 2328.
Barbados Dental Association, 17 Pine Road, Belleville, St Michael. Tel: +1 246 228 6488.

The University of the West Indies has the Cave Hill Campus on Barbados:

Cave Hill Campus

School of Clinical Medicine and Research, Queen Elizabeth Hospital, Martindale's Road, Bridgetown. Tel: +1 246 429 5112. Fax: +1 246 429 6738.
www.cavehill.uwi.edu.

Queen Elizabeth Hospital

Martindales Road, St Michael, Bridgetown. Tel: +1 246 429 5112 or +1 246 436 6450. Fax: +1 246 429 6738.
The hospital: The QEH is the main hospital on the island and is situated 10 minutes' walk from the centre of Bridgetown. There are other smaller hospitals on the island, although there are no other surgical theatres except at the private hospital, 'Bayview'. The wards are all male or female. The decor can also leave a bit to be desired. The lattice brickwork on one of the wards allows a pleasant draught but doesn't keep the birds out! There is also a lack of comforts for the visiting doctor, although the place is very relaxed (7.30 am clinics may not start until 10.30). Medications are flown in from Florida. The hospital has a (temperamental) CT scanner, but this contrasts with the fact that they regularly run out of steroids, saline, blood and aspirin. Orthopaedics is very busy with trauma because of the lack of seat-

belts. There is also a lack of hip prostheses for the ageing population, and amputation is becoming more common. If you can't afford to go privately, you can order your new hip by mail from Miami and bring it with you on the day of your operation.

✪ **Elective notes:** It is difficult for visiting students to do much in theatre (chances are, you won't get to scrub up), but the teaching makes up for this (there are 20 West Indian students in each of the two final years). There is no pressure to go, but you will learn a lot. You are invited to clinics, where your help is very much appreciated. You're treated as a doctor. Some of the common diseases include type II diabetes and its complications. HIV is quite a major problem here. HTLV-1 is also endemic.

Electives can be done in general medicine, general surgery, orthopaedics, ophthalmology, emergency medicine, pathology, radiology, ENT, child health, psychiatry, family medicine, community health and anaesthesiology. They are all done at the QEH except family medicine (which is conducted in a GP unit) and community health (conducted at the Randel Phillips Polyclinic). You can organize this through the Faculty of Medical Sciences, Queen Elizabeth Hospital, Bridgetown. An administration fee of US$50 is requested. Write VERY EARLY to the administrative assistant (or fax/call on the above number). There is then a further fee of US$150 on commencement of the elective. Electives longer than eight to ten weeks may have a further charge.

Dress code comprises no jeans and no bare shoulders (so be careful with sundresses). Dresses to the knees for the girls and shirt and tie for the boys. No white coats.
Accommodation: Although not actually provided, the electives coordinator can arrange it for you; it tends to be a cosy cartel of ex-secretaries' houses, some of which charge a lot and are not in great areas of town. There can be 20–30 elective students there at any one time so the coordinator may get con-

fused over where you are sent. Try to get confirmation before you go. The best is reported to be Mrs Carter (Interlaken, Worthing, Christchurch). B$500 (£157) gets you a nice double room, or you can share for B$375 (£117) each. Note: If you apply to Bayview (private hospital on Barbados), they give lovely accommodation in a plantation house for free.

WARNING: Insects are very common. Malaria is not a problem, although dengue fever outbreaks do occur. Most places will provide a net, but take some insect repellent. Food is not cheap in supermarkets, but eating out is.

Language: English, but you may need a translator to decipher the accent!

OTHER HOSPITALS:

Bay View Hospital, St Paul's Avenue, Bayville, St Michael. Tel: +1 246 436 5446.
Psychiatric Hospital, Black Rock, St Michael. Tel: +1 246 425 8680.

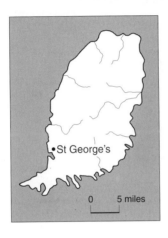
Grenada

Population: 92 000
Language: English
Capital: St George's
Currency: Eastern Caribbean dollar
Int Code: +1 473

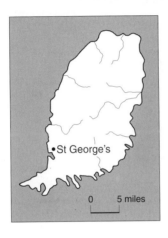

Grenada is one of the most southern islands and has close ties with Cuba. Previously, many Cubans worked in Grenada's hospitals. The country has an offshore American preclinical medical school.

USEFUL ADDRESSES:

Ministry of Health and Environment,
The Carenage, St George's. Tel: +1 473 440 2279.
Fax: +1 473 440 6637.
E-mail: min-healthgrenada@caribsurf.com.
Grenada Medical Association, PO Box 1959,
St George's. Tel: +1 473 440 0633.

Grenada General Hospital

St George's. Tel: +1 473 440 2051.
The hospital: A friendly, medium-sized hospital overlooking the harbour entrance to St George's. Departments include general medicine and surgery, orthopaedics, O&G, anaesthetic and paeds. Hypertension, diabetes and pre-eclampsia are relatively common, with TB, dengue fever, rheumatic fever and leptospirosis also being seen. It is pretty overcrowded with limited facilities. There is a busy psychiatry department that has close links with Mount Gay Psychiatric Hospital and many parishes. Not surprisingly, the unit is very stretched with only relatively basic treatments. The preclinical medical school and library are here.

O Elective notes: The junior doctors do a 1:2 and are therefore grateful for any help, although there is no pressure to help out. There's good teaching with formal lectures. It is popular with Australian students. Lots of sun-bathing and beer-drinking. If you're female, you may find that the local men show a lot of interest. It's a safe place so this shouldn't worry you. Tip: Hang around the yacht club as there are often rich people looking for extra hands. Dive the 'Bianca C' wreck.

Mount Gay Hospital

St George's.

The hospital: Built for 80, this psychiatric hospital has 120 beds/mattresses. It's busy, cramped, and has poor facilities.

OTHER HOSPITALS ON GRENADA AND NEIGHBOURING ISLANDS:

Princess Alice Hospital, Mirabeau, St Andrew's. Tel: +1 473 442 7251. (This is a small public hospital based in the St Andrew's district of the main island.)

Princess Royal Hospital, Carriacou. Tel: +1 473 443 7100. (Another small public hospital.)

St Augustine's Medical Services, St Paul's, St George's. www.staugustinehospital.com. (This is a small private hospital.)

In addition, the islands have a number of district medical centres (small clinics). Contact the Ministry of Health and Environment for more details.

OFFSHORE AMERICAN SCHOOL:

St George's University, School of Medicine, University Centre, PO Box 7, St George's. Tel: +473 444 4357. Fax: +473 444 4823. www.sgu.edu.

Trinidad and Tobago

Population: 1.3 million
Language: English
Capital: Port of Spain
Currency: Trinidad and Tobago dollar
Int Code: + 1 868/809

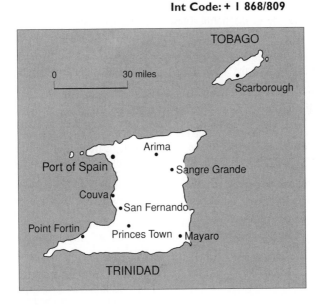

Trinidad, 11 km off the coast of Venezuela, is one of the least-visited Caribbean islands. The language is English (so if you want developing world medicine without a language barrier, this is a good choice). Its sister island, Tobago, gets all the tourism, whereas Trinidad is more industrial, sugar being a major income source. It is, however, still a beautiful island and the people are probably more genuine because of the lack of tourism.

January and February are good times to go as they build up towards carnival time (which takes place on the days before Ash Wednesday), but book accommodation well in advance. There are big parties every night, steel bands fill the evenings with their practice, and everyone has a smile on their face (although, not surprisingly, this is also a busy trauma time in the emergency department). The people are friendly, fun-loving and from a diverse cultural descent (African, Indian and, more recently, Chinese). Crime is increasing, so be wary of wandering streets at night, especially if you are a lone female. There is the idyllic beach on Trinidad (Marcus Bay) as well as mountain ranges covered in forests. However, for the real beauty visit Tobago (approximately £30 for a

*flight or £10 for a ferry). You can go on a
scuba course (£180) or just lie on the beach.*

✪ Medicine:

The healthcare system consists of both a
public and a smaller private sector. The
public sector uses a three-tier system.
Primary care is provided by 102 health
centres with doctors, nurses and midwives across the country. Delivery units
are attached to a number of these. There
is secondary care through three county
and four district hospitals. Tertiary care
comes from two general hospitals, one in
the south and one in the north. These
have specialists in all fields. Primary
care in the private sector is via 600 GPs.
The two teaching hospitals on Trinidad
(for the University of the West Indies)
are the **Port of Spain** and **Mount Hope**.

Type II diabetes is very common, as
are its complications. HIV is also very
prevalent (reports say as high as 70% in
young people in some areas) on both
islands. Leptospirosis is common on
Trinidad due to the number of rats.

➲ Visas and work permits:

No visa is required for EU, British
Commonwealth or US citizens to visit.
Work permits are not required if working
for less than 30 days, otherwise you must
apply to the embassy.

USEFUL ADDRESSES:

Ministry of Health, General Administration, IDC
Building, 10–12 Independence Square, Port of
Spain. Tel: +1 868 627 0010. Fax: +1 868 623 9528.
www.healthsectorreform.gov.tt\.
Trinidad and Tobago Medical Association,
115, Abercromby Street, Port of Spain.
Tel: +1 868 627 8526. Fax: +1 868 623 7246.
www.tntmedical.com.

The University of the West Indies also
has a campus here:

St Augustine Campus

Faculty of Medical Sciences, Eric Williams
Medical Sciences Complex, Champs
Fleurs. Tel: +1 868 645 2640.
Fax: +1 868 663 9836. www.uwi.tt/fms.

Port of Spain General Hospital

Charlotte Street, Port of Spain.
Tel: +1 809 623 2951.

The hospital: Port of Spain General
Hospital is a very large (900-bed), busy
hospital admitting for the whole of the
Port of Spain, the capital of Trinidad. It
is a public hospital and only those
Trinidadians not rich enough to afford
private healthcare (about 95% of the
population) come here. Conditions on
the wards are pretty basic and there are
few advanced facilities (no CT/MRI, for
example). Each team on the medical unit
admits on a 1:6; about 40–50 patients
normally come in.

✪ **Elective notes:** The emergency
department is either fairly or very busy,
but the hours are very flexible (which is
important around carnival time).
There's plenty of practical experience
(stitching, putting on plasters, basic
medical management). All drugs pre-
scribed are by their trade names ... so
take a *BNF*. There's plenty of advanced
pathology, tropical diseases and trauma.
HIV and drug abuse are common. This,
along with the poverty, makes psychiatry an interesting speciality. The doctors
and staff are very friendly and helpful.
The local students are a pretty keen
bunch, but they get plenty of teaching
that you are more than welcome to
attend.

Note: State on application whether
you want the Port of Spain or Mount
Hope hospital as some people have
arrived and been attached to students at
Mount Hope. You can arrange this
through either the University of the West
Indies or the hospital; the latter is recommended.

Accommodation: Make sure you confirm your accommodation and price
before you go as some people have been
ripped off. A list of guesthouses is provided. La Maison Rustique (16 Rust
Street, St Clair) is in a safe area and recommended. Another is Miss May
Cherrie (22 Stone St, Port of Spain).
Accommodation is also available at
Mount Hope Hospital.

Note: There are usually many elective students … this is socially very good, especially since some areas of Trinidad are not particularly safe and you tend to stick together. Also think about getting a Hilton Pool pass as Port of Spain has no beach within walking distance. Beer costs around 37p (supermarket) or 70p (bar).

Mount Hope Hospital
Eric Williams Medical Sciences Complex, Uriah Butler Highway, Champs Fleurs.
Tel: +1 809 645 2640.
The hospital: Built in the early 1980s to solve Trinidad's health problems. It has equipment and facilities similar to those of most Western hospitals, however, people have to pay for their care. So few people can afford it that only 10% of the beds may be occupied. People don't turn up for outpatients and even for operations as they can't pay. Therefore it is not a busy place. The staff are friendly and keen to teach, but not much is seen. Students have in the past felt they have seen more at the Port of Spain General, although there are plenty of lumps and bumps if you are doing surgery (good for short case practice). The hospital is about 16 km out of the city centre, although it can take up to an hour to get there.
Accommodation: A list of guesthouses is provided. Accommodation has occasionally been available in the hospital.

San Fernando General Hospital
Lady Hailes Avenue, Harris Promenade, San Fernando. Tel: +1 809 652 3581.
The hospital: Has the major specialities. There is a wide range of diseases, and 'hands on' experience is encouraged.

Tobago Regional Hospital
Fort Street, Scarborough, Tobago.
Tel: +1 868 639 2551.
The hospital: The small hospital (30 medical beds) for Tobago. It is friendly but has relatively poor facilities. There's medicine, surgery and O&G and a busy emergency department. Diabetes, hypertension and HIV are all common.
O Elective notes: The teaching is good and Tobago is more beautiful than Trinidad. You must learn to dive.
Accommodation: Stay at the Hope Cottage Guest House, Calde Hall Road, The Fort, Scarborough, Tobago.

OTHER HOSPITALS IN TRINIDAD AND TOBAGO:

Arima District Hospital, Queen Mary Avenue, Arima, Trinidad. Tel: +1 809 667 3503.
Caura Chest Hospital, Couva, Central Trinidad. Tel: +1 809 662 2211.
Couva District Hospital, Couva, Central Trinidad. Tel: +1 809 636 2411.
Mayaro District Hospital, Mayaro, East Trinidad. Tel: +1 809 630 4346.
Point Fortin District Hospital, Point Fortin, South Trinidad. Tel: +1 809 48 3281.
Princes Town District Hospital, Princes Town, Trinidad. Tel: +1 809 655 2255.
St Ann's Hospital, St Ann's Road, Port of Spain, Trinidad. Tel: +1 809 624 1151.
St James Medical Complex, St James, Port of Spain, Trinidad. Tel: +1 809 622 4173.
Sangre Grande County Hospital, Sangre Grande, East Trinidad. Tel: +1 809 668 2273.

PRIVATE HOSPITALS:

Adventist Hospital, Western Main Road, Cocorite, Port of Spain, Trinidad. Tel: +1 809 622 1191.
Langmore Health Foundation, Palmyra Village, San Fernando, Trinidad. Tel: +1 809 652 2244.
Nicoll Nursing Home, 44 Coblentz Avenue, Port of Spain, Trinidad. Tel: +1 809 624 7566.
Southern Medical Clinic, 26–24 Quenca and St Vincent Streets, San Fernando, Trinidad. Tel: +1 809 652 2078.

Trinidad and Tobago

Aruba

Population: 81 600
Language: English
Capital: Orajestad
Currency: Dutch guilder
Int Code: + 297

Aruba is the smallest island of the Leeward group, about 24 km (15 miles) off the coast of Venezuela. It is a member of the Kingdom of the Netherlands and its main industry is currently tourism. Note: The two neighbouring islands (Curaçao and Bonaire) comprise the Netherlands Antilles. They have two offshore medical schools as well.

✪ Medicine:

Tropical diseases, including Chagas disease and dengue fever, are present. As of 1995, there had been 117 AIDS cases.

USEFUL ADDRESSES:

Ministry of Health, LG Smith Boulevard 76, Orangestad. Tel: +297 8 39079. Fax: +297 8 39693.

Aruba Dental Association, PO Box 1212, Oranjestad.

HOSPITALS:

Dr Horacio Oduber Hospital, LG Smith Boulevard, Orangestad. Tel: +297 8 74300.
Medical Centre San Nicholas, Bernardstraat 75, San Nicolaas. Tel: +297 8 48833.

MEDICAL SCHOOL:

University of Aruba Medical School

z/n Dr Schaepman Street, Sint Nicolaas. Tel: +297 8 45287. Fax: +297 8 47274. This is very new.

Netherlands Antilles

**Population: 144 000 (Curaçao),
10 000 (Bonaire)
Language: Dutch and Papiamento
(a Spanish–Portuguese–Dutch–
English dialect!)
Capital: Willemstad (Curaçao),
Kralendijk (Bonaire)
Currency: Netherlands Antillean
guilder
Int Code:+599**

*Located 56 km north of the coast of
Venezuela, the Netherland Antilles comprise
Curaçao, Bonaire and the southern part of
Sint Maarten (Saint Martin). These were once
the centre of the slave trade, but with its
abolition in 1863 they turned to oil refining.
They are flat rocky lands and the weather is
hot all year round, although cooled by trade
winds.*

○ Medicine:

Some tropical diseases such as dengue
fever occur. Healthcare is pretty good
overall.

USEFUL ADDRESS:

Ministry of Public Health, Heelsumstraat,
Willemstad. Tel: +599 9 63 0466.
Fax: +599 9 65 3444.

HOSPITALS ON CURAÇAO:

Saint Elisabeth Hospital
193 Breedestraat, Willemstad.
Tel: +599 9 62 4900. Fax: +599 9 62 4739.
The hospital: This is the largest on the
island with 540 beds. It is generally well
equipped.

Antillean Adventist Hospital
1 Groot Davelaarweg, Willemstad.
Tel: +599 9 37 0611. Fax: +599 9 37 0627.

HOSPITALS ON BONAIRE:

San Francisco Hospital
Kaya Souer Bartola 2, Kralendijk.
Tel: +599 7 8900.
The hospital: Has 60 beds, a minor
operating theatre and a recompression
chamber. The island has around eight
doctors, including two surgeons and a
paediatrician. Serious cases are flown to
Curaçao (10 minutes' flying time)

ANGUILLA:

Princess Alexandra Hospital, Stoney Ground, Anguilla. Tel: +264 497 2552. Fax: +264 497 5745.

BRITISH VIRGIN ISLANDS:

Bougainvillea Clinic, PO Box 378, Russell Hill, Road Town, Tortola, BVI. Tel: +284 494 2181. Fax: +284 494 6609.
Peebles Hospital, PO Box 439, Road Town, Tortola, BVI. Tel: +284 494 3497 Fax: +284 494 3833.

GRAND TURK:

Grand Turk Hospital, Hospital Road, Grand Turk. Tel +649 946 2040. (This sounds impressive but is actually a cottage hospital with 24 beds!)

SABA:

A.M. Edwards Medical Centre, The Bottom, Saba. Tel: +599 4 63288.

ST EUSTATIUS:

Queen Beatrix Medical Center, Princessweg, Oranjestad, St Eustatius. Tel: +599 3 82211. Fax: +599 3 82606.

ST MAARTEN:

St Maarten Medical Centre, Cayhill, St Maarten. Tel: +599 5 31111. Fax: +599 5 30116. (Netherland Antilles.)

US VIRGIN ISLANDS:

Roy L. Schneider Hospital, 48 Sugar Estate, St Thomas, USVI 00802. Tel: +1 340 776 8311.
Juan Luis Hospital, 4007 Estate Diamond Ruby, St Croix, USVI 00820-4421. Tel: +1 340 778 6311.

EUROPE

Europe is becoming an increasingly popular destination with the travelling medic. This may in part be due to agreements between European countries making movement and employment easier. Language is not formally tested in transfers between countries, but you are unlikely to get a job if your potential employer realizes that you don't speak the local language.

Since 1975, legislation has been in place that allows doctors within certain European countries to move freely. This system of 'mutual recognition of qualifications' covers Austria, Belgium, Denmark, Finland, France, Germany, Greece, Iceland, Ireland, Liechtenstein, Luxembourg, The Netherlands, Norway, Portugal, Spain, Sweden and the UK. Under this agreement, doctors are entitled to full registration in any European Union (EU) country if they (1) are both citizens of a member state, and (2) have completed their primary training in a member state providing them with a recognized qualification.

Those who trained outside the EU but now live inside the EU do not therefore have automatic recognition of their qualifications. Individual cases can, however, be assessed by the relevant authorities. These 'relevant authorities' are technically known as *competent authorities*. In the UK, for example, the competent authority is the General Medical Council (GMC). Specialists (who have completed certificates of specialized training) and GPs who have completed a minimum period of specific vocational training can also usually have their speciality/GP training recognized. Contact the relevant body in your destination country to confirm this. Note: In many European countries GPs work independently rather than in group practices as they do in the UK.

Most authorities/councils confirming registration will require: your medical degree certificate; a certificate of registration in your own country; your CCST/VT (Certificate of Completion of Specialist Training/Vocational Training) certificate if appropriate; your passport; a 'certificate of good standing' (available from the GMC or equivalent); a CV; and possibly a certificate concerning your 'good health/medical fitness' to practise. Many countries will require these to be translated into their own language (so ask the embassy in your destination country who are recognized as official translators). Registration should take no longer than three months, but allow a lot longer since European bureaucracy can be a nightmare. Other healthcare professionals can also arrange work throughout Europe. Individual councils/associations within your destination country will advise on how to go about getting registered.

The Socrates/Erasmus Programme (*see* Section 1) offers students and researchers of all disciplines the opportunity to work in an affiliated country for periods ranging from three months to one year. The scheme also helps to fund moving and accommodation.

Austria

Population: 8 million
Language: German
Capital: Vienna
Currency: Euro
Int Code: +43

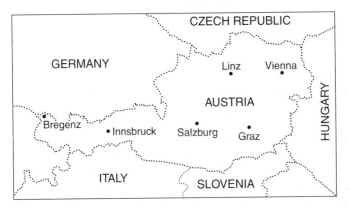

Austria is a landlocked country in central Europe that has a great deal to offer the visiting medic. You can ski in the Alps or sample some of the culture in one of its cities. Despite this, and probably because of language difficulties, Austria is not a popular destination with English-speaking students or doctors.

✛ Medicine:

The healthcare system is funded by a mixture of taxation, compulsory insurance and direct charging, and is controlled seperately in the nine different provines or *Länder* (addresses below). Nearly all the population (those who are employed, their dependents and pensioners) have 'compulsory insurance' (*Krankenkassenscheck*) with one of 24 compulsory sickness funds. This insurance tends to cover outpatient treatment while the taxation covers inpatient treatment. Some people have an additional private health insurance. People can self-refer to specialists without seeing their GP if they wish. Western diseases are the norm, although Lyme disease (transmitted by tick bites) is occasionally seen (about 25 000 people in Austria being affected annually).

⟳ Visas and work permits:

No visa is required to visit or do an elective in Austria of up to six months if you are from the EU. Work permits are only required for non-EU nationals. If you are staying for longer than three months, an identity card must be obtained from the *Bezirkshautptmannschaft*, allowing five years' residence. Note: If working as a GP (usually in a single rather than a group practice), you will have to obtain a contract with an insurance fund provider or patients will have to pay as if they are private patients. You will have to join the medical association of the area you want to work in (each of the *Länder* has its own association).

O **Elective notes:**
There is an exchange programme for medical students within the **International Federation of Medical Students** (IFMSA). The programme offers medical students the possibility of working in a medical institution (e.g. a hospital). In Austria, the exchange programme is organized by the **Austrian Medical Students Association** (AMSA; National Exchange Office, AMSA, c/o Liechtensteinstrasse 13, A–1090 Vienna. www.amsa.at). Students coming to Austria are assigned to a university hospital in Graz, Innsbruck or Vienna. Free board and lodging are provided. The working languages are German and English, although German is obviously needed to communicate with patients. July to September are AMSA's preferred times of exchange as this is when most elective students are present.

The IFMSA exchange is operated on a two-way basis ... for each student they accept, they send one out to the applicant country. This can be a problem in the UK since, as there is no medical students' association, there is no one to organize this. For this reason, direct exchanges between hospitals in the UK and Austria are proposed. Another address to contact is the **Austrian Academic Exchange Service OAD** (Zentrale Geschäftsstelle, Universität Wien, 1/Stiege 9, A-1010 Wien. Tel: +43 1 426742).

USEFUL ADDRESSES:

Federal Ministry of Labour, Health and Social Affairs: Bundesministerium für Arbeit, Gesundheit und Soziales, Stubenring 1, A-1011 Vienna, Austria. Tel: +43 171 1000. www.bmags.gv.at.
Austrian Medical Association: Österreichische Ärztekammer, Weihburggasse 10-12, A-1011 Vienna. Tel: +43 1 5150 1253. Fax: +43 1 5150 1410. www.aek.or.at.
Austrian Nurses Association: Österreichischer Krankenpflegeverband, Mollgasse 3a, A-1180 Vienna. Tel: +43 1 478 6387. Fax: +43 1 478 2710. www.oegkv.at.

Austrian Dental Board: Österreichische Dentistenkammer, Kohlmarkt 11, A-1010 Vienna. Tel: +43 1 5337 0640. Fax: +43 1 533 0758. www.oedk.at.
Austrian Physiotherapists Association, Koestlergasse 1/29, A-1060 Vienna. Tel: +43 1 5879 5130. www.physio.at/physio.
Austrian Association of Dieticians, Raaber Bahngasse 3/2/8, A-1100 Vienna. Tel: +43 222 6269 984.
Austrian Occupational Therapy Association: Verband der Diplomierten Ergotherapeuten Österreichs, Sperrgasse 8-10, A-1150 Vienna. Tel: +43 222 892 9380.
Austrian Radiographers Association: Verband der Diplomierten, Radiologisch-Technischen, Assistentinnen und Assistenten Österreichs, Simmeringer Hauptstrasse 34-40/1/1/VI, A-1110 Vienna.

MEDICAL SCHOOLS:

Karl-Franzens-Universität Graz, Faculty of Medicine, Universitätsplatz 3, Parterre, Zimmer E, A-8010 Graz. Tel: +43 316 380 4101. Fax: +43 316 380 9400.
www.kfunigraz.ac.at/E/fak-inst/medizin.html.
Leopold-Franzens-Universität Innsbruck, Faculty of Medicine, Christoph Probst-Platz 1, A-6020 Innsbruck. Tel: +43 512 507 3004. Fax: +43 512 507 2995. www.uibk.ac.at.
University of Vienna, Faculty of Medicine, Dr Karl Lueger Ring 1, A-1010 Vienna. Tel: +43 142 776 0001. Fax: +43 142 779 600. www.univie.ac.at/medicus.

SOME OF THE MAIN HOSPITALS:

Allgemeines Krankenhaus, 18-20 Währinger Gürtel, A-1090 Vienna. Tel: +43 140 400 4390. Fax: +43 140 400 4392.
Allgemeines Öffentliches Landeskrankenhaus Innsbruck, 35 Anichstrasse, Innsbruck A-6020. Tel: +43 512 504 2000. Fax: +43 512 504 2011.
Allgemeines Öffentliches Krankenhaus der Stadt Linz, 9 Krankenhausstrasse, A-4020 Linz. Tel: +43 7 327 8060.
Kliniken d' Universität, Abteilung für Notfallmedizin, Währinger Gürtel 18-20, A-1090 Wien. Tel: +43 1 402 5777.
Landeskrankenanstalten, 48 Müllner Hauptstrasse, A-5020 Salzburg. Tel: +43 662 431.
Landeskrankenhaus Bregenz, 2 Karl Pedenz-Strasse, Bregenz A-6900. Tel: +435 574 4010. Fax: +43 5 5744 0180.
Landeskrankenhaus–Universitätskliniken Graz, Auenbruggerplatz 1, A-8036 Graz. Tel: +43 316 385 2242. Fax: +43 316 385 3422.

ADDRESSES OF THE *LÄNDER*:

Burgenland: Permayerstrasse 3, 7000 Eissenstadt.
Tel: +43 2 6826 2521.
Kärnten: St Veiterstrasse 34, 9020 Klagenfurt.
Tel: +43 463 5856.
Niederösterreich: Wipplingerstrasse 2, 1010
Wien. Tel: +43 7 3277 8371.
Oberösterreich: Dinghoferstrasse 4, 4010 Linz.
Tel: +43 7 3277 8371.

Salzburg: Bergstrasse 14, 5024 Salzburg.
Tel: +43 7 3277 8371.
Steiermark: Kaiserfeldgasse 29, 8011 Graz.
Tel: +43 316 8044.
Tirol: Anichstrasses 7/IV 6010 Innsbruck.
Tel: +43 5125 2058.
Vorarlberg: Schulgasse 17, 6850 Dornbirn.
Tel: +43 5 5722 1900.
Wien: Beihburggase 10–12, 1010 Wien. Tel: +43
2225 1501.

Belarus

Population: 10.1 million
Language: Belorussian
Capital: Minsk
Currency: Belorussian rouble
Int Code: +375

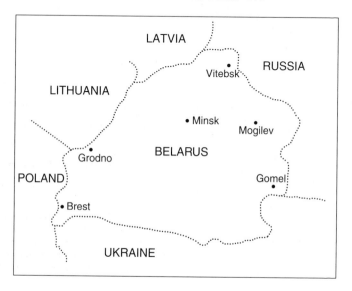

Belarus is a landlocked country bordered by Latvia, Lithuania, Poland, Russia and the Ukraine. Since its split from Moscow in 1991, Belarus has had only agriculture as a viable resource. Since the Chernobyl nuclear disaster in 1986 in next-door Ukraine, many Belorussians have suffered severe ill health.

○ Medicine:
Belarus had a relatively good healthcare system but has been under increasing strain since the Chernobyl disaster. The rates of cancer and leukaemia have risen dramatically, resulting in the need for many new specialist wards. Belorussian doctors, via the 'Know-How Fund', are being trained in specialist techniques such as bone marrow transplantation to try to cure these conditions. (There is one doctor per 246 people.) Diphtheria has recently become an increasing problem. The prevalence of HIV is around 0.3%. The big killers include heart disease and cancer.

◎ Climate and crime:
It varies from warm (20°C) in the summer to very cold (−10°C) in the winter. Because of the poverty, crime has increased greatly since independence.

⊃ Visas and work permits:
Applications for a visa can be made in person or by post. Fill in an application

form from the embassy and send or take it with a valid passport, a passport photo, a formal invitation from the individual or corporate body (government, company or organization) on their letter-headed notepaper or alternatively a letter of support, and finally the appropriate fee, payable only in the local currency, to the Embassy of the Republic of Belarus. (Fees are currently £40 for a visitor visa, £40 for a business one and £10 for a student visa). You may need a short interview, but it's the consular officer's assessment of your intentions that carries weight in the decision. The visas take five to ten working days to process. (*See* Section 4 for the embassy's address.)

Once in the country, you should, within three days of your arrival, register your passport with the **Ministry of Foreign Affairs of the Republic of Belarus** or the **Ministry of Internal Affairs**. If you are staying in a hotel, they will register you at the reception. Contact the Ministry of Health for registration details.

Note: Very few people (including the doctors) speak English so some knowledge of Belorussian is essential.

USEFUL ADDRESS:

Ministry of Health, Myasnikova 39, Minsk 220010. Tel: +375 172 296 095. Fax: +375 172 296 297.

MEDICAL SCHOOLS:

Gomel State Medical Institute, Lange Street 5, Gomel 246000. Tel: +375 232 534 121. Fax: +375 232 539 831. www.gsu.unibel.by/vframes.asp.
Grodno State Medical Institute, Ulica Gorkogo 80, Grodno 230015.
Tel: +375 152 233 0365. Fax: +375 152 233 5341.
www.grsmi.unibel.by/english.
Minsk State Medical Institute, Prospekt Dzerzinskogo 83, Minsk 220116. Tel: +375 172 719 424. Fax: +375 172 726 197. www.msmi.minsk.by.
Vitebsk State Medical Institute, 27 Frunze Avenue, Vitebsk 210602. Tel: +375 212 369 539. Fax: +375 212 242 240. www.vgmu.vitebsk.net.

SOME OF THE MAIN HOSPITALS:

Brest Oblast Hospital, Moscow Road, Brest.
Tel: +375 162 420 061/127.
Gomel Oblast Hospital, 5 Lizukovykh, St Gomel.
Tel: +375 232 485 562.
Grodno Oblast Hospital, 52 Lenin Komsomol Boulevard, Grodno. Tel: +375 152 336 230.
Minsk Clinic No 10, 73 Uborevich St, Minsk.
Tel: +375 172 419 811.
Mogilev Oblast Hospital, 12 Biruli Street, Mogilev. Tel: +375 222 263 097.
Vitebskoblast Hospital, PO Nikropolye, Vitebsk.
Tel: +375 212 221 201.

If you would like to get involved in helping children in Belarus, try the Chernobyl Children's Project or Playcom (www.playcom.org.uk), a charity that transforms old hospital rooms in Minsk into playrooms.

Belgium

Population: 10.3 million
Languages: Dutch, French and German
Capital: Brussels
Currency: Euro
Int Code: +32

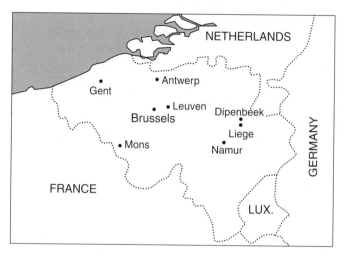

Belgium (bordered by France, Germany, the Netherlands and Luxembourg) has become almost the capital of Europe. It is not commonly visited by UK students. Since it is also on the Socrates/Erasmus programme, only a brief list of medical schools is given below. There is quite a difference between the more well-off Flemish and poorer French communities within Belgium. This has led to diagreements over the contribution each community should make to healthcare provision.

✪ Medicine:

Belgium has some of the best healthcare in the world, but it is costly and quite complex. Most Belgians belong to a compulsory insurance scheme (*une mutelle*) entitling them to an average 75% rebate on cost. There are five non-profit-making insurance funds (run by political or religious institutions) and one public fund. Around two-thirds of hospitals are non-profit-making private hospitals. The other third consists of public hospitals. Belgians can choose their GP/specialist, and pay up front. They can then be reimbursed from their *mutelle*. Their ambulance service consists of many private companies that really operate fast taxis! They are not paramedics. In medical emergencies, a team of doctors goes out, treats and stabilizes patients at the scene and then brings them back in an ambulance. Belgium is particularly renowned for fertility treatment and organ transplantation.

Note: Prior to getting into medical school, Belgians have to do three years of medical science. Only the successful students go on to medical school.

◎ Climate and crime:

A typical maritime climate, it is warmest between June and August. The crime rate is pretty low.

➲ Visas and work permits:

Neither are required for entry by EU members, although you should obtain from your local town hall a 'mauve card' if staying for up to a year or a 'blue card' if staying for up to five years. Contact your local embassy if you're coming in from outside the EU as you will probably need a work permit. If you want to work as a doctor, you should first contact the **Fédération Belge des Chambres Syndicales de Médecins** (address below). Specialists should contact the Belgian Specialist Association (address below) to ensure that their certification is valid. You have to register to be able to obtain an Institut National d'Assurance Maladie-Invalidaté number, which is required for prescribing and charging. Note: There is no equivalent to the MRCP/MRCS, etc.

Adverts for jobs are often placed in the journals *Promotion Médicale*, *Bulletin Syndical* and *Syndikale Berichten*.

USEFUL ADDRESSES

Ministry of Health, 33 Boulevard Bschoffshiem, B-1000 Brussels. Tel: +32 220 2011. Fax: +32 2 220 2067.
Fédération Belge des Chambres Syndicales de Médecins, Rue de Château 15, B-1420 Braine-L'Alleud. Tel: +32 2 384 3930.
Belgian Specialists Association: Groupment des Unions Professionelles Belges de Médecins Spécialistes, Avenue de la Couronne 20, B 1050 Brussels.
Belgian Medical Association: Association Belge des Syndicats Médicaux, Chaussée de Boondael 6 bte 4, B-1050 Brussels. Tel: +32 644 1288. Fax: +32 2 644 1527.
Belgian Medical Council: Ordre des Médecins, Conseil National, Place de Jamblinne de Meux 32, 1040 Brussels. Tel: +32 2 736 8291. Fax: +32 2 735 3563.

Belgian Nurses Association: Fédération Nationale Neutre des Infirmier(ière)s de Belgique, Rue de la Source 18, B-1060 Brussels. Tel: +32 537 0193. Fax: +32 2 143 3453.
Begian Dental Association: Association: Dentaire Belge, 40 rue Washington bte 22, B-1050 Brussels.
Belgian Physiotherapy Association: Association des Kinesitherapeutes de belgique, H H enneaulaan 69, B-1930 Zavrentum. Tel: +32 725 2777. Fax: +32 2 725 3076.
Belgian Occupational Therapy Association: Nationale Belgishe Federation von Ergotherapeuten, 87 rue de Percke, B-1180 Brussels.

UNIVERSITIES:

Facultés universitares Notre-Dame de la Paix, Faculté de Médecine, Rue de Bruxelles 61, B-5000 Namur. www.fundp.ac.be/medecine/gener/genfacf.html. Preclinical only. Clinical students are transferred to:
Universitair Instelling Antwerpen, Faculteit voor Geneeskunde en Farmacie, Universiteitsplein 1, B-2610 Wilruk. www.ua.ac.be. (Clinical only.)
Katholieke Universiteit Leuven, Faculteit der Geneeskunde, Minderbroedersstraat 17, B-3999 Leuven.
Limburgs Universitair Centrum, Universitarie Campus, Faculteit voor Geneeskunde, B-3590 Dipenbeek. www.luc.ac.be.
Rijksuniversitair Centrum Antwerpen, Faculteit voor Geneeskunde en Farmacie, Groenenborgerlaan 171, B-2020 Antwerpen.
Rijksuniversiteit Gent, Caculteit der Geneeskunde, Akademisch Ziekenhuis, De Pintelaan 185, B-9000 Gent.
Université Catholique de Louvain, UCL 5020, Avenue Emmanuel Mounier 5010 (or 10 avenue Hippocrate for the hospital), B-1200 Brussels. www.md.ucl.ac.be. (This is one of the oldest and largest medical schools in Belgium with around 800 beds.)
Université libre de Bruxelles, Faculté de Médecine et de Pharmacie, Bâtiment J, Route de Lennik, 808 Cp 610, Route de Lennik, B-1070 Brussels. www.ulb.ac.be/ulb/fac_inst_ec/medecine.html.
Université de l'Etat á Liége, Faculté de Médecine, Place du 20 août 7, B-4000 Liege. www.ulg.ac.be/facmed.
Université de Mons-Hainaut, 24 avenue du Champ de Mars, B-7000 Mons.
Vrije Universiteit Brussel, Faculteit van de Geneeskunde en de Farmacie, Laarbeeklaan 103, B-1090 Brussels. www.vub.vub.ac.be.

Université libre de Bruxelles, Université Catholique de Louvain and Université de l'Etat á Liége have departments of general practice.

Belgium

Languages:

Dutch is spoken at Antwerp, Vrije Universiteit Brussel, Diepenbeek, Ghent, Katholieke Universiteit Leuven and Wilrijk; French at Université Catholique de Louvain, Université libre de Bruxelles, Brussels, Mons, Liége and Namur.

SOME OF THE MAIN HOSPITALS:

Academisch Ziekenhuis, Vrije Universiteit Brussel, Laarbeeklaan 101, 1090 Brussels. Tel: +32 2 477 4111. Fax: +32 2 477 5362.

AZ Gasthuisberg, Indwendige Genceskunde, Herestraat 46, 3000 Leuven. Tel: +32 1 634 4259. Fax: +32 1 634 4397.

Clinique Universitaire St Luc, Avenue Hippocrate 10, 1200 Brussels. Tel: +32 764 1111. Fax: +32 2 764 3703.

Hôpital Erasme, Clinique Universitaire de Bruxelles, Route de Lennik 808, Anderlecht. Tel: +32 555 3111.

Hôpital Molière Longchamp, Rue Marconi 142, 1180 Brussels. Tel: +32 348 5111.

Hôpital Universitaire Brugmann, Place van Gehuchten, 1020 Brussels. Tel: +32 477 2111.

Hôpital Universitaire St Pierre, Rue Haute 322, 100 Brussels. Tel: +32 535 3111.

Croatia

Population: 4.5 million
Language: Croatian
Capital: Zagreb
Currency: Kuna
Int Code: +385

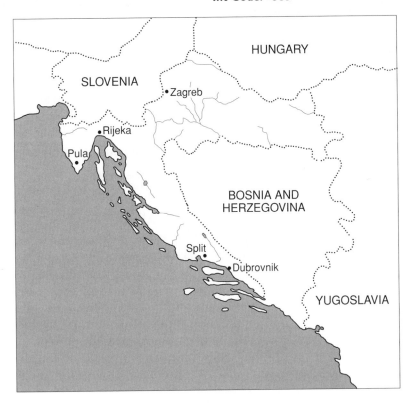

Croatia was involved in heavy conflicts with the break-up of Yugoslavia and the war with Bosnia. Tourism is now returning and the country is once again becoming a place to do an elective.

✛ Medicine:

Although most people are covered by a health insurance scheme, the war put a great deal of pressure on resources. Western diseases are still the big killers.

⊃ Visas and work permits:

Because of the small number of students who go here, no accurate information can be gained regarding the need for student visas. Contact the embassy for up-to-date details.

USEFUL ADDRESSES:

Ministry of Health, 6 Baruna Trenka, 10000 Zagreb. Tel: +385 14 591 333. Fax: +385 1 431 067.
Croatian Medical Association, Subiceva Ulica 9, 41000 Zagreb. Tel: +385 41 416 820.
Croatian Nurses' Association, Kispaticeva 12, Zagreb. Tel: +385 41 233 233.
Croatian Dental Society, University of Zagreb, Gunduliceva 5, 4100 Zagreb.

University of Zagreb Medical School

10 000 Zagreb, p.p. 1026. Tel: +385 14 566 909. Fax: +385 14 566 724. www.mef.hr.
Founded in 1917, Croatia's first medical school now uses many clinics and institutes. These include the Clinical Hospital Center Zagreb (providing all major medical and surgical specialities, as well as O&G, and paeds, **Sestre Milodsrdnice Clinical Hospital, Merkur Clinical Hospital, Sveti Duh General Hospital, Fran Mihaljevic Clinical Hospital for Infectious Diseases, Vuk Vrhovac University Clinic for Diabetes, Endocrinology and Metabolic Diseases, Jordanovac Clinical Hospital for Pulmonary Diseases and Thoracic Surgery, University Clinic for Traumatology, Paediatric Clinic, University Clinic for Tumors, Rehabilitation and Orthopaedic Institute** and **Vapee Psychiatric Hospital**.

Sveti Duh General Hospital

Sveti Duh 64, 10000 Zagreb.
The hospital: Has 800 beds and offers most specialities except paeds and dermatology. There is a six-bed coronary care unit and a specialized cardiology ward. It's an incredibly busy, understaffed hospital where the juniors have few responsibilities (the consultants do all the prescribing). The teaching, however, is excellent. There are very few other students.
Accommodation: Not provided.

University of Rijeka School of Medicine

Bracé Branchetta 20, 51000 Rijeka.
Tel: +385 51 651 111. Fax: +385 51 675 806. www.medri.hr.

University of Split Medical School

Soltanska 2, 21000 Split. Tel: +385 21 565 073. Fax: +385 21 365 389. www.mefst.hr.

MAIN HOSPITALS IN EACH CITY:

KB Split, Spiniceva 1, 21000 Split.
Tel: +385 1 515 055.
KBC Zagreb, Salata 2, 10000 Zagreb.
Tel: +385 1 273 457.
KBC Rijeka, Kresimirova 42, 51000 Rijeka.
Tel: +385 51 212 100.
OB Dubrovnik, Roka Misetica, 20000 Dubrovnik.
Tel: +385 20 411.076.
OB Pula, Zagrebacka 34, 52100 Pula.
Tel: +38 552 214 433.

Cyprus

Population: 700 000
Language: Greek, Turkish, English
Capital: Nicosia
Currency: Cyprus pound
(Turkish Lira in the north)
Int Code: +30

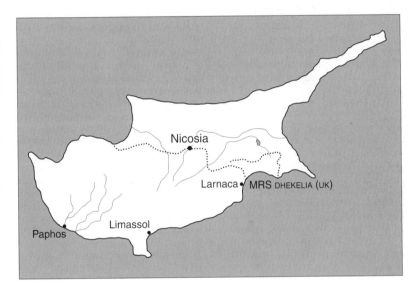

Lying in the eastern Mediterranean, Cyprus became divided in 1974 following an invasion by the Turkish military. This has left the Greek Cypriot Republic of Cyprus in the south and the Republic of Northern Cyprus, which is recognized only by the Turks. There's plenty of history and things to see, for example Aphrodite's birthplace and many beaches. Egypt is not too far. The people know some English, but fluent Greek is ideal.

✪ Medicine:

Healthcare is advanced, more so in the south. Western diseases (heart disease, cancer and accidents) are the common causes of mortality. If you're wanting medicine half-way between European and middle-eastern, this is the place! There is no GP service so everything turns up in hospital.

◎ Climate and crime:

It can get very hot in the summer (up to 35°C), and the winters are mild. Crime is not a major problem. Lone girls get a great deal of male attention but not threatening.

Nicosia General Hospital

Nicosia. Tel: +30 2280 1400.
The hospital: The tertiary referral centre for Cyprus. It carries out some sophisticated surgery.

Archbishop Makarios III Hospital

Acropolis, Nicosia. Tel: +30 22493600.

The hospital: Was built ten years ago principally as a specialist paeds hospital with departments in thalassaemia, cardiology, oncology, endocrinology, metabolic disorders, surgery and neonatal intensive care. It also has some O&G, and ENT.

O Elective notes: There are many clinics to attend and interesting pathologies to see; not much 'hands on' work though.

Accommodation: Not provided.

Paphos General Hospital

Paphos. Tel: +30 2694 0111/6240 1000.

The hospital: Serves a population of 25 000 Cypriots and in the holiday season 50 000 tourists.

O Elective notes: The staff are friendly and tend to speak very good English so don't worry if your Greek isn't great. The working day is 8 am to 2 pm so there's plenty of time for exploring. Surgery is recommended.

Limassol General Hospital

Limassol. Tel: +30 2533 0333.

The hospital: This is a well-set out new building just north-west of Limassol. It is a very busy hospital made busier by the fact that there is no GP service. There is quite a lot of thalassaemia and other things to see, including, kala-azar, scarlet fever and metabolic diseases.

O Elective notes: It's busy but has very friendly staff who go out of their way to teach.

Accommodation: Not provided. Castle Hotel Apartments (2 Prophitis Elias Street, Potamos Yernasoyias) is recommended.

Larnaca General Hospital
Archbishop Makarios III

Larnaca. Tel: +30 0463 0300
Fax: +30 0463 0222.

The hospital: Built in 1986 and offers all the basic specialities. It serves the local population of whom half are true inhabitants and half are refugees who have fled the Turkish invasion of the north. The population doubles in the summer with tourists.

MRS Dhekelia

Dhekelia Garrison, BFPO 58. (Only if you are British; it is best to be involved in the army too.)

Army general practice: This is an excellent opportunity to see general practice in an army setting. The typical day consists of an early (5.30 am) start with compulsory physical training such as basketball, circuits or running. Ward rounds start at 7.30 am with usually only one or two patients to see (children with asthma, post-epileptic fits or squaddies with sore backs). Clinic at 8 am sees a wide range of problems (the GPs see families as well as soldiers) finishing about 1pm. Advanced life support or trauma training occurs most weeks. There's plenty of opportunity to get involved in other aspects of general practice, such as nursing, midwifery, physiotherapy, speech therapy and social work. You can also take part in the military exercises. There's plenty of spare time ... learn to water-ski or kneeboard; take the opportunity to have helicopter or gliding lessons. The weather, even in December, is excellent.

Accommodation: And food are in the garrison's Officers' Mess.

Czech Republic

Population: 10.3 million
Official Language: Czech
Capital: Prague
Currency: Czech koruna
Int Code: +420

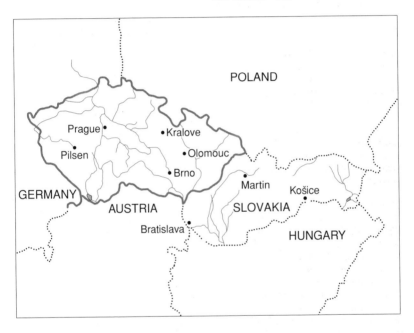

The Czech Republic comprises Bohemia and Moravia and was formally part of Czechoslovakia. Czechoslovakia separated from the former Soviet Union in 1989, since then free elections have taken place, and in 1993 a peaceful split of the country into the Czech Republic and Slovakia was agreed. It's a great country if you're interested in music, architecture, history or the arts as all can be found in abundance in Prague. Book as many concerts as you can at the Rudolfinum as they are popular and very cheap. Although a few people speak English, knowing some Czech is a huge advantage for coming here. It is not a popular destination for electives or work.

✛ Medicine:

Medicine is improving, however, rich Czechs still travel to Germany to have complex operations. Most people rely on the state-run public insurance scheme. Infant mortality has been high. Cancers, heart and cerebrovascular disease are common causes of mortality. The doctor:population ratio is 1:270.

⊃ **Visas and work permits:**

British and US passport holders can stay for 30 days without a visa. As a foreign student studying in the Czech Republic, you may be required to obtain a Long Term Residence Permit (contact the embassy). This is obtained by filling out the appropriate form and sending a letter (in Czech) from the institution offering you a place. You should do this at least eight to ten weeks before departure. A small charge (about £4) is made.

If working, you will require a work permit from the District Labour Office in the area of your work in the Czech Republic. Ask your employer to get in touch with them. They have to prove that the job cannot be given to a Czech national. You will then need a Long-Term Residence Permit as well.

USEFUL ADDRESSES:

Ministry of Health, Palackého nám 4, 128 01, Prague 2. Tel: +420 2497 1111.
Fax: +420 2 29 0092, 2497 2111.
National Institute of Public Health: Státní zdravotní ústav, Šrobárova 48, 100 42, Prague 10. Tel: +420 2 6731 0578. Fax: +420 2 6731 1188.
Czech Medical Association, PO Box 88, Sokolská 31, 120 26 Prague 2.
Tel: +420 2 2491 5195. Fax: +420 2 2421 6836.
Czech National Association of Nurses, I interní Klinika, U nemocnice 2, 12808 Prague. Tel: +420 229 0065. Fax: +420 229 7932.
Czech Physiotherapy Association: Unie Fyzioterapeutu Ceske Republiky, Antala Staska 167/80, CZ 140 46 Prague 4.
Tel: +420 2 6100 6441. Fax: +420 2 6100 6446.

MEDICAL SCHOOLS:

Charles University has three faculties in Prague and two outside:

Charles University in Prague, First Faculty of Medicine, Katerinská 32, 120 00 Prague 2. Tel: +420 2 9615 1315. Fax: +420 2 2491 5413. www.lf1.cuni.cz.
Charles University in Prague, Second Faculty of Medicine, V Úvalu 84, 150 06 Prague 5. Tel: +420 2 2443 1111. Fax: +420 2 2443 5820. www.lf2.cuni.cz.
Charles University in Prague, Third Faculty of Medicine, Ruská 87, 100 00 Prague 10. Tel: +420 2 6731 1812. Fax: +420 2 6731 1812. www.lf3.cuni.cz.

Charles University, Faculty of Medicine in Kralove, Simkova 870, 500 01 Hradec Kralove. Tel: +420 4 9581 6487. Fax: +420 4 9551 3597. www.lfhk.cuni.cz.
Charles University, Faculty of Medicine in Pilsen, Husova 13, 306 05 Pilsen. Tel: +420 1 9722 1200. Fax: +420 1 9722 1460. www.lfp.cuni.cz.

Charles University was founded in the 13th century in Prague, and each faculty has its own speciality. An example is the Third Faculty Hospital:

University Hospital Karlovy Vinohrady

Šrobárová 50, 10034 Prague 10. Tel: +420 2 6716 3010. Fax: +420 2 6731 2664.
The hospital: Is large and has a very prestigious plastic surgery and burns unit. There is also a new cardiac surgery unit. Despite this, there is an atmosphere of decay and general underfunding.
Accommodation: Depends on which department and at which faculty you are based. For the Third Medical Faculty, accommodation is in a nurses' flat opposite the hospital and costs £1 a day.

III Chirurgick Klinika

Londynska 15, 12808, Prague 2.
The hospital: The Third Surgical Clinic is in a converted apartment block away from the main medical faculties in the upmarket area of Prague known as Vinohrady. The ground floor accepts emergencies and has an outpatient department. The next three floors comprise 76 beds and two intensive care units as well as the three theatres. The surgery department covers general surgery for Postal Area 3 in Prague but also thoracic surgery for the whole of the Czech Republic.
O Elective notes: There are ward rounds to attend (other doctors will whisper translations to you) and plenty of investigations and surgery (e.g. cardiac catheterization, ECHOs and bypasses) to see.
Accommodation: Has been free previously.

OTHER MEDICAL SCHOOLS:

Masaryk University, Faculty of Medicine, Komenskeho Nam. 2, 662 43 Brno. Tel: +420 5 4212 6490. Fax: +420 542 1262. www.med.muni.cz.
Palacký University, Faculty of Medicine, Olomouc, tr. Svobody 8, P0 Box 159, 771 00 Olomouc I. Tel: +420 6 8522 3907. Fax: +420 6 8522 3907. www.upol.cz/UP/Struktura/Lf/sidlo.htm.

Foreigners also visit the following hospitals in Prague:

First Medical Clinic of Prague Ltd, Vyšehradská Str, 120 00 Prague 2. Tel/Fax: +420 229 2286. Tel: +420 229 8978/9000 0686. (This is the largest medical clinic catering for foreigners in Prague.)
Hospital Homolka, Roentgenova 2, 150 00 Prague 5. Tel: +420 2 5292 2144 (department for foreigners), +420 2529 3048 (public relations). Fax: +420 2 5721 0689.
Hospital Motol, Vúvalu 84, 150 00 Prague 5. Tel: +420 2 2443 3690 (department for foreigners). Fax: +420 2 2443 1020.

HOSPITALS IN PRAGUE AND NEARBY AREA:

Note: *Nemocnice* = Hospital.

Chirurgická nemocnice u Sv Klementa, Nábr L Svobody 2, 110 00 Prague I. Tel: +420 2 2481 0226.
Fakultní nemocnice Bulovka, Budínova 2, 18000 Prague 8. Tel: +420 2 6608 2963.
Fakultní nemocnice Královské Vihohrady, Šrobárová 50, 100 00 Prague 10. Tel: +420 2 6716 2200.
Fakultní nemocnice v Motole, Vúvalu 84, 150 00 Prague 5. Tel: +420 2 2443 1010.
Fakultní Thomayerova nemocnice, Videnlská 800, 140 00 Prague 4. Tel: +420 2472 1634.

Interní nemocnice v Bubenci, Chittussiho I, 160 00 Prague 6. Tel: +420 2 2431 0194.
Mestská nemocnice v Roztokách, Tiché údolí 376, 252 63 Roztoky U Prahy. Tel: +420 239 7738.
Nemocnice Beroun, Profesora Veselého 490, 266 01 Beroun. Tel: +420 3112 3006.
Nemocnice Kolín, Zizkova 146, 280 02 Kolín. Tel: +420 3212 8414.
Nemocnice Mestec Kráhlové, E Benese 343, 289 03 Městec Králové. Tel: +420 3249 3271.
Nemocnice milosrdn´ych sester Sv K Boromejského v Praze Vlasská 36, 110 00 Prague I. Tel: +420 2 2451 0904.
Nemocnice Mladá Boleslav, V Klementa 147/II, 293 01 Mladá Boleslav. Tel: +420 326/227 23.
Nemocnice na Františku, Na Františku 8, 110 00 Prague I. Tel: +420 2 2481 0502.
Nemocnice na Homolce, Roentgenova 2, 150 00 Prague 5. Tel: +420 2 5292 2531.
Nemocnice na Zizkové, Kubelíkova 16, 130 00 Praha 3. Tel: +420 2627 2002.
Nemocnice Nymburk, Boleslavská 425, 288 00 Nymburk. Tel: +420 325 2601.
Nemocnice s poliklinikou, Brázdínská 1000, 250 01 Brandys nad Labem/Stará Boleslav. Tel: +420 202 3400.
Nemocnice s poliklinikou Kladno, Vancurova 1548, 272 01 Kladno. Tel: +420 312 2277.
Nemocnice s poliklinikou Mělník, Prazská 528, 276 01 Mělník. Tel: +420 2 0662 3146.
Nemocnice s poliklinikou Sedlcany, Tyršova 160, 264 01 Sedlcany. Tel: +420 3042 2055.
Nemocnice s poliklinikou Slany, Polit veznu 576, 274 01 Slany. Tel: +420 314 2554.
Nemocnice Rakovník, Dukelskych hrdinu 200, 269 00 Rakovník. Tel: +420 313 2245.
Nemocnice svaté Alzbety, Na slupi 6, 12000 Prague 2. Tel: +420 2 2491 5694.
Nemocnice ve Vysocanech, Sokolovská 304, 190 00 Prague 9. Tel: +420 2 6631 2011.
Ústřední vojenská nemocnice, U Vojenské nemocnice 1200, 160 00 Prague 6. Tel: +420 2 3800 2203.
Všeobecná fakultní nemocnice v Praze, U nemocnice 2, 120 00 Prague 2. Tel: +420 2 2491 0377.
Zeleznicní nemocnice Praha, Italská 37, 120 00 Prague 2. Tel: +420 2 2421 1534.

Denmark

Population: 5.4 million
Language: Danish
Capital: Copenhagen
Currency: Danish krone
Int Code: +45

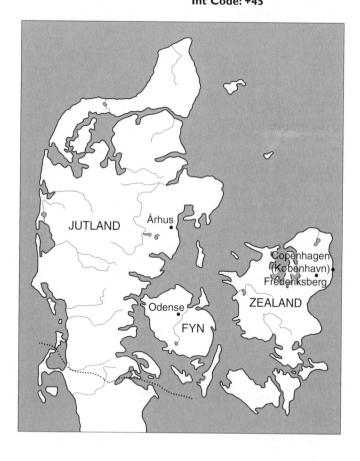

Denmark is made up of 500 islands of which only 100 are inhabited. The largest are Zealand (on which Copenhagen lies), Funen and Jutland. This fragmented nature of Denmark means that nowhere is more than 51 km from the sea. Denmark has a population of just over 5 million, 70% of whom are concentrated in the cities. The capital, Copenhagen, has 1.4 million inhabitants. Most Danes speak English.

✪ Medicine:

Denmark was one of the first countries to establish a national health service and it is still in place today, providing free healthcare to all paid for by taxes. It is well run, and the range of conditions seen is typical of a developed country. Fewer than 1% of beds are private. Most referals to specialists come through GPs. Note: They try to care for the elderly at home for as long as possible. This relies on a network of visiting nurses.

There are three medical schools. Training takes a total of six-and-a-half years (three years preclinical and three-and-a-half clinical). Most of the clinical teaching of students from the University of Copenhagen occurs at a number of teaching hospitals in the Greater Copenhagen area. The teaching hospitals are all publicly funded and controlled. For clinical rotations, students are assigned to one of three *Klinikudvalg*, comprising one or more teaching hospitals.

➲ Visas and work permits:

US, EU, New Zealand and Australian citizens do not need a visa to visit Denmark. Under the EU scheme, EU citizens can stay for up to three months without a visa to search for work. Beyond that, you need a residence permit. Registration for doctors is through the Danish National Board of Health.

USEFUL ADDRESSES:

Ministry of Health, Herluf Trolles Gade 11, DK-1052 Copenhagen K. Tel: +45 33 92 22 60. Fax: +45 33 93 15 63.
Danish National Board of Health, Amaligade 13, Postboks 2020, DK-1012 Copenhagen K. Tel: +45 33 93 16 36.
Danish Medical Association: Dan Almindelige Danske Laegeforening, Trondhjemsgade 9, DK-2100 Copenhagen Ø. Tel: +45 35 44 85 00. Fax: +45 35 44 85 05. www.dadl.dk.
Danish Nurses Organization, Postboks 1084, DK-1008 Copenhagen K. Tel: +45 33 15 15 55. Fax: +45 33 15 24 55.
Danish Dental Association: Dansk Tandlaegeforening, Amaliegade 17, DK-1256 Copenhagen K. Tel: +45 70 25 77 11. www.dtf-dk.dk.

Danish Physiotherapy Association: Danske Fysioterapeuter, Norre Voldgade 90, DK-1358 Copenhagen K. Tel: +45 33 13 82 11. Fax: +45 33 93 82 14. www.fysio.dk.
Danish Occupational Therapy Association, Norre Voldgade 90, DK-1358 Copenhagen K.

COPENHAGEN MEDICAL SCHOOL AND HOSPITALS:

University of Copenhagen

Faculty of Health Sciences, Panum Instituttet, Blegdamsvej 3, DK-2200 Copenhagen N. Tel: +45 35 32 79 00. Fax: +45 35 32 70 70. www.sund.ku.dk/Engelsk.

The University of Copenhagen uses the following hospitals:

Bispebjerg Hospital, Bispebjerg Bakke 23, 2400 Copenhagen NV. Tel: +45 35 31 35 31. Fax: +45 35 31 39 99.
Frederiksberg Hospital, Norde Fasanvej 59, 200 Frederiksberg. Tel: +45 38 34 77 11. Fax: +45 39 34 77 55.
Københavns Amts Sygehus, Sct Elisabeth, Hans Bgbinders Alle 3, 2300 Copenhagen S. Tel: +45 31 55 45 00. Fax: +45 32 84 56 54.
Københavns Amts Sygehus, I Glostrup, Ndr Ringvej, 2600 Glostrup. Tel: +45 43 96 43 33. Fax: +43 96 06 16 (see below).
Københavns Amts Sygehus, I Herlev, Herlev Ringvej, 2730 Herlev. Tel: +45 44 53 53 00. Fax: +45 44 53 53 32.
Københavns Amts Sygehus, I Gentofte Niels Andersensvej 65, 2900 Hellerup. Tel: +45 31 65 12 00. Fax: +45 39 77 76 77 10.
Københavns Universitet, Det Laegevidenskabelige Fakultet, Panum Instituttet, Blegdamsvej 36, DK-2200 Copenhagen.
Kommunehospitalet, Øster Farimgsgade 5, 1399 Copenhagen. Tel: +45 33 38 33 38. Fax: +45 33 38 39 99.
Rigshospitalet (including Finsen) Administrationen, afsnit 522, Blegdamsvej 9 2100 Copenhagen Ø. Tel: +45 35 45 35 45. (This is the main hospital.)
Sundby Hospital, Italiensvej 1, 2300 Copenhagen S. Tel: +45 32 34 32 34. Fax: +45 32 34 39 99.

Copenhagen County Hospital (Glostrup Hospital)

Sdr Ringvej, Glostrup 2600.
The hospital: Glostrup Hospital is owned and run by the county of Greater Copenhagen, along with **Herlev** and **Gentotfe Hospitals**. The Copenhagen County Hospital at Glostrup was built in 1953. It has all major specialities. There

are 25 bed units of 23 beds each – 575 beds in total. Each ward has ten bedrooms, interviewing rooms, living room, toilets and bathrooms as well as offices for staff. It employs around 400 doctors.

ÅRHUS MEDICAL SCHOOL AND HOSPITALS:

Åarhus University

Faculty of Health Sciences, Vennelyst Boulevard 9, DK-8000 Åarhus C. Tel: +45 89 42 41 06. Fax: +45 86 12 83 16. www.health.au.dk.

The University of Åarhus uses the following hospitals:

Århus Amtssygehus, Tage Hansens Gade 2, 8000 Århus C. Tel: +45 89 49 75 75. Fax: +45 89 49 72 49.

Århus Kommunehospital, Norrebrogade 44, 8000 Århus C. Tel: +45 89 49 33 33. Fax: +45 86 18 52 39.
Marselisborg Hospital, PP Ørumsgade 11, 8000 Århus C. Tel: +45 89 49 33 33.
Skejby Sygehus, Brendstrupgårdsvej, 8200 Århus N. Tel: +45 89 49 55 66. Fax: +45 89 49 60 00.

ODENSE MEDICAL SCHOOL AND HOSPITAL:

Syddansk University

Faculty of Health Sciences, Winsløwparken 17/1, DK-5000 Odense C.
Tel: +45 65 50 29 32. Fax: +45 65 91 89 14. www.sdu.dk/health/index.html.

Syddansk uses:
Odense Universitets Hospital, Sdr Boulevard 29, 5000 Odense C. Tel: +45 66 11 33 33. Fax: +45 66 13 28 54. www.ouh.dk.

Finland

Population: 5 million
Languages: Finnish and Swedish
Capital: Helsinki
Currency: Euro
Int Code: +358

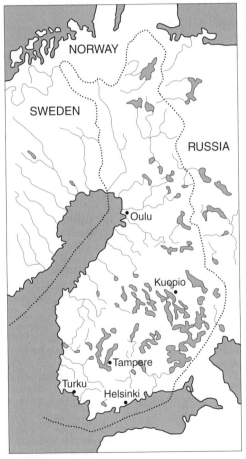

Situated right in the north of Europe, Finland reaches up into the Arctic Circle. It has some beautiful countryside – great if you like walking. There are five provinces (Lääni), each of which has its own medical school.

✪ Medicine:

Finland has a sound healthcare policy aiming to improve both the standard and distribution of healthcare even further. Despite this, cardio- and cerebrovascular diseases are the big causes of mortality, and male life expectancy is low for European standards. Women, however, live longer than the European average. Violent deaths (suicides, traffic accidents, etc.) are very common compared with the rest of Europe, whereas cancer is less common than expected. The healthcare system is run by health authorities through 21 hospital districts. Healthcare costs are met 75% by taxes, 21% by direct payment from patients and 4% from the state sickness insurance (funded by local employers).

➲ Visas and work permits:

For EU nationals, no visa is required for a three-month stay. Technically speaking, students should obtain a residence permit, although some elective students have not found this necessary. Residence permits are easy to obtain if you have a contract for work. Visit: http://virtual.finland.fi. The **National Board of Medicolegal Affairs** (Terveydenhuollon oikeusturvakeskus) is the competent body that recognizes the qualifications of all healthcare professionals. They have a great deal of information on their website (address below).

USEFUL ADDRESSES:

Ministry of Social Affairs and Health, PO Box 267, 4-6 Snellmaninkatu, FIN-0017 Helsinki.
National Board of Medicolegal Affairs (TEO), Lintulahdenkatu 10, PO Box 265, FIN-00531 Helsinki. Tel: +358 9 772 920. Fax: +358 9 772 921. www.teo.fi.
Finnish Medical Association: Suomen Lääkäriliitto PL 49, FIN-00501 Helsinki. Tel: +358 90 393 091. Fax: +358 90 393 0794. www.laakariliitto.fi.
Finnish Nurses Federation: Tervetden-ja sosiaali-huoltoalan ammattijärjestä They ry, Asemamiehenkatu 4, FIN-00520 Helsinki. Tel +358 90 229 0020. Fax: +358 90 148 1840.
Finnish Dental Association: Suomen Hammaslääkäriliitto, Fabianinkatu 9B, FIN-00130 Helsinki. Tel: +358 96 220 250. Fax: +358 96 223 050. www.hammasll.fi.
Finnish Association of Physiotherapists, Asemamiehenkatu 4, FIN-00520 Helsinki. Tel: +358 90 149 6817. Fax: +358 90 148 3054.
Finnish Association of Occupational Therapists: Suomen Toimintaterapeuttiliitto ry, Pautatielaisenkatu 6, FIN-00520 Helsinki. Tel: +358 9 144 360.

MEDICAL SCHOOLS AND THE MAIN HOSPITALS:

There are five universities with medical schools that tend to deal with the more specialized treatments:

University of Helsinki

PO Box 33 (Yliopistonkatu 4), FIN-00014 University of Helsinki. Tel: +358 91 912 2177. Fax: +358 91 912 2176.
www.helsinki.fi.
This uses Helsinki University Central Hospital (Stenbackinpratu 9, Helsinki).

University of Kuopio

PO Box 1627, FIN-70211 Kuopio. Tel: +358 17 162 042. Fax: +358 17 163 496.
www.uku.fi.
This uses Kuopio University Hospital (Puijon Laaksontie 2, FIN-70210 Kuopio. Tel: +358 71 173 311. Fax: +358 71 172 611). This is one of the largest providers of healthcare in Finland, having 1000 beds. It has specialist burns, heart and hand surgery units.

University of Oulu

PO Box 191 (Kirkkokatu 11A), FIN-90101 Oulu. Tel: +358 85 531 011.
Fax: +358 85 534 040. www.oulu.fi/.
This uses **Oulu Hospital** (50 Kajaaintie, FIN-9220 Oulu. Tel: +358 81 315 2011. Fax: +358 81 315 4499).

University of Tampere

PO Box 607. FIN-33101 Tampere. Tel: +358 32 156 549. Fax: +358 32 156 503.
www.uta.fi.
This uses **Tampere University Hospital** (PI 2000, 35 Teiskontie, Tampere 335. Tel: +358 31 247 5111. Fax: +358 31 247 5314).

University of Turku

FIN-20014 Turku. Tel: +358 23 336 582. Fax: +358 23 336 370. www.utu.fi.
This uses **Turku University Hospital** (Kinamyllynkatu 4-6, FIN-20520, Turku. Tel: +358 21 261 1611. Fax: +358 21 261 1164).

Finland

France

Population: 58 million
Language: French
Capital: Paris
Currency: Euro
Int Code: +33

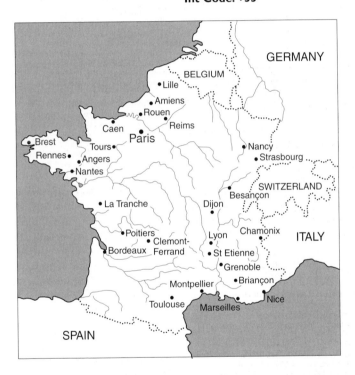

Famed for its fine food, wine and fashion, France offers a great deal for the visiting medic. Paris has its well-known attractions, but the south has other attractions, such as skiing and beaches. That said, France is not a popular elective destination for English-speaking students or doctors, possibly because of its close proximity to the UK. It is also very easy to arrange exchange programmes through the Socrates/Erasmus programme. For these reasons, only a brief list of a few medical schools is given below. If you are interested in the skiing more than the medical aspect, try approaching one of the many ski patrols. Pretty fluent French is obviously needed to get the most out of an elective or work here.

✪ Medicine:

Medical care is run on both a state (compulsory national health insurance) and private healthcare system. Access in both public and private services does not usually require referral. The public services tend to cater for inpatients, whereas the private sector (e.g. GPs) tend to cater for outpatient services.

◎ **Climate and crime:**
The climate varies from mild to almost Mediterranean in the south. The Pyrenees and Alps can obviously get very cold but usually have clear blue skies.

➲ **Visas and work permits:**
Like most of the EU, no visas or work permits are required for visiting EU nationals. Medical training is highly competitive in France and, once qualified, you can either go down the specialist route (sitting the *concours d'internat* exams) or train as a GP. All doctors who practise in the EU can apply to sit the specialist exams (after three years' postgraduate experience), but it is very competitive. For more information, visit www.rhone-poulenc-rorer.fr/guidmed/accueil.htm. Doctors need to register with the **Ordre Nationale des Médecins** (address below).

USEFUL ADDRESSES:

Ministry of Social Affairs, Health and Urban Affairs, 8 Avenue de Ségur, 75700 Paris.
Tel: +33 I 40 56 60 00. Fax: +33 I 40 56 47 92.
Counseil National de l'ordre des Médicins, 180 Boulevard Haussman, 75389 Paris Cedex 08.
Tel: +33 I 53 89 32 00. Fax: +33 I 53 89 32 01.
French Medical Association: Association Médicale Française, 37 rue de Bellefond, F-75441 Paris Cedex 09. Tel: +33 I 45 96 34 52. Fax: +33 I 45 96 34 50.
French Nursing Association: Association Nationale Francaise des Infirmières et Infirmiers Diplômes ou Etudiants (ANFIIDE), I I Boulevard Montmartre, 75002 Paris. Tel: +33 I 47 36 34 60. Fax: +33 I 45 17 56 85.
http://anfiide.infirmiers.com/.
French Dental Association: Association Dentaire Française, 7 rue Mariotte, F-75017 Paris. Tel: +33 I 58 22 17 10. Fax: +33 I 58 22 17 40. www.adf.asso.fr.
French Physiotherapy Association: Fédération Française des Masseurs Kinesithérapeutes Rééducateurs, 24 rue des Petits Hotels, F-75010 Paris. Tel: +33 I 44 83 46 00. Fax: +33 I 44 83 46 01. www.ffmkr.com.

French Occupational Therapy Association: Association Nationale Française des Ergothérapeutes, rue Eugè Oudine, F-75013 Paris. Tel: +33 I 45 83 50 38. Fax: +33 I 45 86 81 71. www.anfe.asso.fr.

MEDICAL SCHOOLS IN PARIS:

Université de Paris, UFR de Médecine Necker-Enfants malades, 156 rue de Vaugirard, F-75015 Paris. www.necker.fr/.
Université de Paris, UFR de Médecine Saint-Antoine, 184 rue Faubourg-Saint-Antoine, F-75012 Paris. www.chusa.jussieu.fr/.
Université de Paris VII, UFR de Médecine Lariboisière-Saint-Louis, 10 Avenue de Verdun, F-75010 Paris.
Université de Paris VII, UFR de Médecine Xavier Bichat, 16 Rue Henri Huchard, F-75018 Paris. www.sigu7.jussieu.fr.
Université de Paris Sud, UFR de Médecine Fremlin-Bicêtre, 63 rue Gabriel Péri, F-75006 Paris. www.kb.u-psud.fr/kb/.
Université de Pierre et Marie Curie (Paris VI), UFR Broussais-Hôtel-Dieu, 15 rue de l'Ecole de Médecine, F-75006 Paris.
Université Pierre et Marie Curie (Paris VI), UFR de Médecine Pitié-Salpêtrière, 91 Boulevard de l'Hôpital, F-75634 Paris Cedex 13. www.chups.jussieu.fr.
Université René Descartes (Paris V), UFR de Médecine Cochin-Port Royal, 24 Rue du Faubourg Saint-Jacques, F-75014 Paris Cedex 14. www.cochin.univ-paris5.fr.

Some hospitals occasionally used for electives:

Cochin Hospital
27 Rue du Faubourg Saint-Jacques, 75679 Paris. Tel: +33 I 42 34 12 12.
The hospital: A very large hospital in the south of the Paris with wards covering all the medical and surgical specialities.

Centre Medico-Chirurical Foch
40 rue Worth, 92151 Suresnes. Tel: +33 I 46 25 20 00. Fax: +33 I 42 04 59 23.
The hospital: This is a medium-sized hospital in Suresnes on the outskirts of Paris. It has a good reputation for general medicine.

Hôpital de Cimez
4 Avenue Reine Victoria, Cimiez, Nice.
The hospital: Serves a large population (about 1.5 million) from Monaco to Fréjus. It has most specialist fields and is a teaching hospital affiliated to the

University of Nice. There are a number of subdivisions, however (e.g. maternity) that are on a different site.

L'Archet II Centre Hospitalier Universitaire de Nice
151 Route de St Antoine de Ginestiere, BP79 06202, Nice Cedex 03.

The hospital: Is the new section of one of the major hospitals serving Nice and most of the Cote d'Azur. It has superb facilities and is on a hilltop with beautiful views of Nice below.

O **Elective notes:** Medical students are treated as house officers and do on calls. For electives, the timetable is free so you can go to theatre, the emergency department or outpatients. There aren't many procedures as senior staff do them and blood taking is done by nurses. Florence is a mere three hours' drive away.

Accommodation: You have to find your own accommodation, but the government organization le Crous can help.

Hôpital Charles Nicolle
Rue de Germont, Rouen 76 00.

The hospital: A very large regional teaching hospital. Rouen is a large industrial city in Normandy, on the Seine. The hospital is on the right bank on the edge of the old red light district. Paris is one hour by train.

For the skiers out there:

Centre Hospitalier
05105 Briançon, Alps.

The hospital: A friendly district hospital in the French Alps. Lots of skiing pathology and its own helicopter rescue service. You need good French to make this worthwhile. There are many Italian tourists so Italian is a plus.

Mountain Medicine and Traumatology Department of Chamonix Hospital
509 route des Pélerins, PO Box 30, Les Bossons, 74400 Chamonix. Tel: +33 4 50 53 84 00. Fax: +33 4 50 53 84 74. www.perso.wanadoo.fr/dmtmcham/ dmtm uk.htm.

The hospital: This is the helicopter rescue service covering the Alps around Chamonix. The hospital also has general and orthopaedic surgical facilities.

Grenoble

Grenoble is surrounded by ski resorts and is hence a place to consider going to if you are really after a skiing holiday.

Contact **Faculté du Médicine de Grenoble** (Domaine de la Merci, 38706 La Tronche). There are two hospitals in Grenoble (population 400 000); one (in the south near the Olympic village) deals with acute trauma. The larger, hospital **Albert Michallon** (near the university campus), is huge and houses most fields of medicine. Write to Le Chef de Service Scolarité at the Bureau Relations Internationales at the above address.

OTHER MEDICAL SCHOOLS:

École Libre de Médicine, 56 Rue du Port, F-59046 Lille Cedex.
Université d'Aix-Marseille, UFR de Médecine, 27 Boulevard Jean Moulin, F-13005 Marseille.
Université d'Angers, UFR des Science médicales et pharmaceutiques, rue Haute de Reculée, F-49045 Angers Cedex. fac.med.univ-angers.fr.
Université de Besançon, UFR de Médecine, 4 place Saint Jacques, F-25030 Besançon Cedex. (Founded in 1806.)
Université de Bordeaux, UFR de Médecine, 146 Rue Léo Saignat, F-33076 Bordeaux. www.u-bordeaux2.fr.
Université de Brest, UFR de Médecine, 22 Avenue Camille Desmoulins, F-29279 Brest Cedex.
Université de Caen, UFR de Médecine, Avenue de la Côte de Nacre, F-10432 Caen Cedex.
Université Claude Bernard, UFR de Médecine Grange Blanche, 8 Avenue Rockefeller, F-69373 Lyon Cedex 08.
Université de Clermont-Ferrand, UFR de Médecine, Boulevard Churchill, F-63000 Clermont-Ferrand.
Université de Dijon, UFR de Médecine, 7 Boulevard Jeanne d'Arc, F-21033 Dijon.
Université François-Rabelais, UFR de Médecine de Tours, 2 bis Boulevard Tonnellé, F-37032 Tours Cedex.
Université de Lille II, UFR de Médecine, 1 place de Verdun, F-59045 Lille. www.univ-lille2.fr/medecine.

France

Université de Louis Pasteur, UFR de Sciences médicales, 4 Rue Kirschleger, F-67085 Strasbourg Cedex.

Université de Montpellier, UFR de Médecine, 2 Rue Ecole de Médecine, F-34060 Montpellier Cedex.

Université de Nancy I, UFR A et B de Médecine, 9 avenue de la Forêt de Haye, BP 184, F-54506 Vandoeuvre-les-Nancy Cedex.

Université de Nantes, UFR de Médecine et Techniques médicales, I Rue Gaston Veil, F-44000 Nantes.

Université de Nice, UFR de Médecine, Chemin de Valombrose, F-06034 Nice. www.unice.fr.

Université de Paris, UFR de Médecine et de Biologie humaine, 74 rue Marcel Cachin, F-93000 Bobigny.

Université Paris Val-de-Marne, UFR de Créyeil, 51 Avenue de Lattre de Tassigny, F-94000 Créteil.

Université Paul Sabatier, UFR de Médecine Toulouse-Rangeuil, 133 route de Narbonne, F-31062 Toulouse Cedex.

Université de Picardie, UFR de Médicine, 12 Rue Frédéric Petit, F-80000 Amiens.

Université de Poitiers, UFR Mixte de Médecine et de Pharmacie, 34 Rue de jardin des Plantes, F-86034 Poitiers Cedex.

Université de Reims, UFR de Médecine, 57 Rue Cognacq-Jay, F-51097 Reims.

Université René Descartes, UFR de Médecine Paris-Ouest, 104 Boulevard Raymond-Poincaré, F-92380 Garches.

Université de Rennes, UFR Clinique et Thérapeutique médicales, Avenue Professeur Léon-Bernard, F-35043 Rennes.

Université de Rouen, UFR de Médecine et de Pharmacie, Avenue de l'Université, BP 97, F-76800 Saint-Etienne-Du-Rouvray. www.univ-rouen.fr/medecine.

Université de Saint-Etienne, UFR de Médecine, F-42100 Saint-Etienne.

Université scientifique et médicale de Grenoble, UFR de Médecine, Domaine de La merci, F-8700 La Tranche.

SOME OTHER LARGE HOSPITALS:

Bichat-Beaujon Hospital, 100 Boulevard de Général Leclerc, Cichy sur seine 92118 Cedex. Tel: +33 1 40 87 50 00.

CHU d'Angers, 4 Rue Larrey, Angers 49033 Cedex 1. Tel: +33 41 35 36 37. www.chu-angers.fr

CHU de Brest, 5 Avenue Foch, Brest 29609 Cedex. Tel: +33 98 22 33 33. www.chu-brest.fr

CHU de Grenoble, BP 127, Grenoble 38043 Cedex 9. Tel: +33 76 76 75 75. www.chu-grenoble.fr

CHU de Nancy, 29 Avenue du Marechal de Lattre de Tassigny, Nancy 54035 Cedex. Tel: +33 83 85 85 85. www.chu-nancy.fr

CHU de Nimes, BP 26, 5 Rue Hoche, Nimes 30029 Cedex. Tel: +33 66 68 68 68. www.chu-nimes.fr

CHU de Reims, 23 Rue Des Moulins, Reims 51092 Cedex. Tel: +33 26 78 78 78. www.chu-reims.fr

Paris-Ouest Hospital, 2 Avenue Charles de Gaulle, Boulogne, Billancourt 92100 Cedex. Tel: +33 1 49 09 50 00.

Saint-Antoine Hospital, 184 rue du Faubourg St Antoine, 75012 Paris. Tel: +33 1 49 28 20 00.

Germany

Population 81.6 million
Capital: Berlin
Language: German
Currency: Euro
Int Code: +49

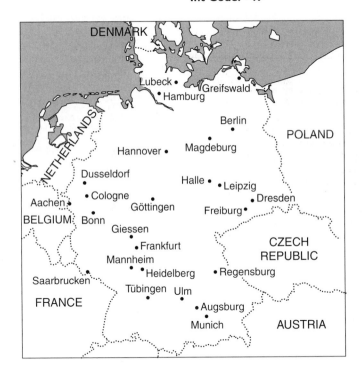

Germany, lying in the heart of Europe, has enjoyed economic growth even while having to support the newly reunited East. It has some vibrant cities and beautiful countryside. Many people are fluent in English and most of the medical terminology is very similar. The European Medical Students' Association frequently runs 'eurotalks' in which you learn medical vocabulary and culture over two to seven days. These are advertised in the Student BMJ.

✪ Medicine:

A very comprehensive social security system is in operation in Germany, compulsory health insurance being paid for by both employer and employee. Most hospitals are state run, but some are run by Christian organizations. There are 313 people per doctor, and the killers of the West (cardiovascular disease, cancers and accidents) are the big causes of mortality. Germany provides free healthcare for all via a statutory sickness fund (which receives money from employers and employees who earn over a certain wage). Ninety per cent of people opt to use this scheme, although there are private systems for those who opt out. As in France, most specialists can be accessed directly without the need for referral.

In the early 1960s it was decided that there needed to be an expansion in the number of doctors being trained; hence there were proposals for seven new medical schools. For this reason, there are a number of relatively new institutions, whereas others date back to the early 15th century. Most medical schools are listed below, although, like much of Europe, exchanges can easily be arranged through Socrates/Erasmus. Germany is currently oversupplied by doctors, around 10 000 actually being unemployed. Some jobs (e.g. anaesthetics) are regarded as a 'service' industry – many of those who give anaesthetics are not doctors.

Hospitals can be grouped into public hospitals (government run), voluntary hospitals (run by non-governmental organizations/churches) and private hospitals.

◎ Climate and crime:

Typically, there are warm summers and wet winters. Germany is a very safe country.

➲ Visas and work permits:

If from the EU, Australia, USA, Canada or New Zealand no visa is needed to visit. Like most of the EU, EU nationals do not need a work permit either, but you will have to obtain a residence permit if staying for more than three months. Doctors need to register with the regional authority and the German Regional Medical Association in the area (*Bundesland*) in which they want to work. Specialists have to get their CCST or equivalent checked by the relevant *Landesärztekammer*. To work independently, you will also need to register with the Regional Statutory Health Insurance Association.

Journals that advertise jobs include *Ärztekammer* and *Deutsches Ärzteverlag* (www.aerzteblatt.de). Also take a look at the Central Placements Office's website at www.arbeitsamt.de.

USEFUL ADDRESSES:

Ministry of Health, Bonn 53108. Tel: +49 228 9410. Fax: +49 228 9414900.
German Medical Association:
Bundesärztekammer, Herbert-Lewin-Strasse 1, D 50931 Cologne Tel: +49 221 4003 209/221 40 04 0. Fax: +49 221 4004 380/388.
www.bundesaerztekammer.de.
German Nurses Association: Deutscher Berufsverband für Pflegeberufe, Hauptsrasse 392, D 65760 Eschborn. Tel: +49 6173 65086. Fax: +49 6173 61644. www.dbfk.de.
German Dental Association:
Bundeszahnärztekammer, Postfach 410168, D 50861 Cologne. www.bzaek.de.
German Physiotherapy Association: Deutzer Freiheit 72–74, D 50679 Cologne. Tel: +49 221 9810270. Fax: +49 221 98102725. www.zvk.org\.
German Occupational Therapy Association: Deutscher Verband der Ergotherapeuten, Postfach 2208, D 76303 Karlsbad.

SOME HOSPITALS AND MEDICAL SCHOOLS:

Aachen

Rheinisch-Westfälische Technische Hochschule Aachen

Medizinische Fakultät, Pauwelsstrasse 30, 52062 Aachen. Tel: +49 241 808 9168. Fax: +49 241 888 8470. www.ukaachen.de.

Berlin

Medizinische Fakultät Charité der Humboldt-Universität zu Berlin

Augustenburger Platz 1, 13353 Berlin
Tel: +49 30 450 70011. Fax: +49 30 450 70911. www.rz.hu-berlin.de/ or www.charite.de/home.
Charité, established in the early 18th century, gets its name from its humble beginnings as a pest house during the Plague. The medical college, mainly for military personnel, was incorporated into

Berlin University in 1806. The new medical college was initially separate from the Charité and hence built new hospitals (such as the **Surgical University Clinic**), which are still in use. Today, this huge institution is spread over three campuses: **Charité Mitte, Virchow-Clinic, Berlin-Buch**.

Freie Universität Berlin
Universitätsklinikum Benjamin Franklin, Fachbereich Humanmedizin
Hindenburgdamm 30, 12200 Berlin.
Tel: +49 8445 3321. Fax: +49 8445 4451.
www.medizin.fu-berlin.de/.

Bonn

Rheinische Friedrich-Wilhelms-Universität Bonn
Medizinische Fakultät, Am Hof 1b, 53113 Bonn. Tel: +49 228 737 246. Fax: +49 228 737 077. www.meb.uni-bonn.de/institute/institute.html.
Founded in 1818, this large university uses 12 different hospitals with a total of 1500 beds.

Cologne

Universität zu Köln
Medizinische Fakultät, Joseph-Stelzmann-Strasse 9, Lindenburg, Cologne 41.
Tel: +49 221 478 0. Fax: 221 478 4095.
www.medizin.uni-koeln.de.
Founded in 1901, the medical college uses 12 hospitals in Cologne and the surrounding areas, one of which is:

Kliniken der Stadt Köln
Kinderkrankenhaus, Amsterdamer Strasse 59, 50735 Cologne.
The hospital: Cologne is one of the largest cities in Germany, with a population of about a million. The hospital is outside the city centre but is well served by the underground. Although it's a large hospital, very complicated cases get referred to the city's Uniklinik, the main academic teaching hospital. Teaching, at least in paeds, is good, with afternoon teaching sessions and seminars. As an elective student, the ward work is pretty much that of helping the house officer ... taking blood, siting venflons, etc.

Dresden

Medizinische Fakultät Carl Gustav Carus der Technischen Universität Dresden
Fiedlerstrasse 27, Dresden. Tel: +49 0351 4580. www.tu-dresden.de/medf/.
Originally founded as a military training institute in 1748, it was refounded in 1954 as a medical school. New building work is trying to locate everything on to one site.

Düsseldorf

Heinrich-Heine-Universität Düsseldorf
Medizinische Fakultät, Universitätsstrasse 1, 40225 Düsseldorf. Tel: +49 211 81 12242. Fax: +49 21181 12285.
www.uni-duesseldorf.de.
The university (founded in the early 20th century) uses a number of specialist hospitals, including a neurology hospital. In total it has around 2000 beds.

Frankfurt

Klinikum der Johann-Wolfgang-Goethe-Universität Frankfurt am Main
Theodor-Stern-Kai 7, 60590 Frankfurt.
Tel: +49 69 6301 62 89. Fax: 69 630 159 22.
www.uni-frankfurt.de.
The hospital: This huge medical centre (founded in 1914) has 1465 beds with 60 buildings. The medical college also uses another 13 hospitals in Frankfurt itself.

Freiburg im Breisgau

Albert-Ludwigs-Universität Freiburg

Medizinische Fakultät, Werthmannplatz, 79098 Freiburg im Breisgau. Tel: +49 761 203 5033. Fax: +49 761 203 5039. www.uni-freiburg.de.

The school's main hospital is **Klinikum der Albert-Ludwigs Universität** (Innere Medezin I, Hugstetter Strasse 55, 79106 Freiburg im Breisgau). It's a friendly place where students are given reasonable responsibility and procedures (central lines, bone marrow aspirates) to do. In the oncology/ haematology department, everyone (from consultants to domestics) has breakfast together to discuss patients. A good knowledge of German is obviously necessary.

Giessen

Justus-Liebig-Universität Giessen

Rudolf-Buchheim-Strasse 8, 35392 Giessen. Tel: +49 641 99 40000. Fax: +49 641 99 40009. www.med.uni-giessen.de.

Founded in 1607, Giessen University has had an interesting history, including famous scientists such as Roentgen, inventor of the X-ray. The new medical/surgical centre is on campus hill, with good views of the Taunus foothills and Lahn valley. It has all major specialities, including cardiothoracic surgery, trauma and neurosurgery. The university is also affiliated with hospitals in nearby towns. It has a forensic medicine department.

Göttingen

Universität Göttingen

Medizinische Fakultät, Robert Cook Srasse 40, 37075 Göttingen. Tel: +49 551 39 6988. www.uni-gottingen.de.

Greifswald

Ernst-Moritz-Arndt-Universität Greifswald

Bereich Medizin, Fleischmannstrasse 8, 17487 Greifswald. Tel: +49 3834 86 5000. Fax: +49 3834 86 5002. www.medizin.uni-greifswald.de.

Greifswald (founded in 1456) provides all major departments, including three medical departments and forensic medicine (**Insitut für Rechtsmedizin**. Tel: +49 86 5743. Fax: +49 86 5752).

Halle/Saale

Martin-Luther-Universität Halle-Wittenberg

Bereich Medizin, Leninallee 5, Halle/Saale. Tel: +49 345 557 1893. Fax: +49 345 557 1493. www.halle.de.

Halle (founded in the early 18th century) has everything from paediatric cardiology to trauma surgery. Full addresses and contacts are on their website.

Hamburg

Universität Hamburg, Fachbereich Medizin

Universitätsklinikum Hamburg-Eppendorf Martinistrasse 52, 20246 Hamburg. Tel: +49 40 42803 6509. www.uke.uni-hamburg.de.

Hannover

Medizinische Hochschule Hannover

30623 Hannover. Tel: +49 511 532 1. Fax: +49 511 532 5550. www.mh-hannover.de.

Although new (1965), the medical school has grown rapidly and now has 1350 beds in its main clinic on campus as well as 18 other medical centres over Hannover. All major departments, as well as sports and forensic departments, are here. Specialist research includes that into inflammatory bowel disease, cystic fibrosis and traffic accidents.

Heidelberg

Ruprecht-Karls-Universität Heidelberg

Medizinische Gesamtfakultät im Neuenheimer Feld 346, 69120 Heidelberg. Tel: +49 6221 562 702. Fax: +49 6221 564 365. http://med.uni-hd.de/.

Although founded in 1386, the university and medical school had a slow start: in 1523, the entire university had 14 pupils. Today, there are seven departments of internal medicine (including sports medicine), and the school uses 15 hospitals, providing over 4000 beds in Heidelberg.

Homburg

Universitätskliniken des Saarlandes

Fachbereich Medizin, 66421 Homburg/Saar. Tel: +49 6841 16 6002. Fax: +49 6841 16 6003. www.med-rz.uni-sb.de.

Homburg (in the far south-west of Germany, near France) has its hospital in the south of the town centre, situated in 200 hectares of woodland. Originally founded in 1947, the hospital has 1500 beds and all specialities, including forensic psychology and medicine.

Leipzig

Universität Leipzig

Medizinische Fakultät, Liebigstrasse 27, 04103 Leipzig. Tel: +49 341 971 5930. Fax: +49 341 971 5939. www.uni-leipzig.

Founded in 1414, this is the oldest medical school in Germany. It has recently built a new heart centre with Europe's largest ITU. Leipzig is a beautiful city (population 700 000), and there is a good student life.

Lübeck

Medizinische Universität Lübeck

Ratzeburger Allee 160, 23538 Lübeck, Schleswig-Holstein. Tel: +49 451 5000. Fax: +49 451 500 2999. www.mu-luebeck.de.

Approximately 20 hospitals provide over 1000 beds to the medical school, which was founded in 1964.

Magdeburg

Otto-von-Guericke-Universität Magdeburg

Medizinische Fakultät, Leipziger Strasse 44, 39120 Magdeburg. Tel: +49 391 6701. Fax: +49 391 67 13440. www.med.uni-magdeburg.de/fme.

This relatively new (1954) medical college only became part of a university in 1993. It uses 29 hospitals and 22 institutes, and enrols 180 students a year. It has specific interests in neuroscience and immunology research.

Mannheim

Fakultät für Klinische Medizin Mannheim der Universität Heidelberg

Theodor Kutzer Ufer, 68167 Mannheim. Tel: +49 621 3 83 25 27. Fax: +49 621 3 83 38 02. www.klinikum-mannheim.de.

Mannheim got its own medical school (part of the University of Heidelberg) in 1964. The university hospital is the major teaching facility. Specialist interests include transplant and minimally invasive surgery, psychiatry, imaging and oncology. It has 2600 beds.

Munich

Ludwig-Maximilians-Universität München

Fachbereich Medizin, Goethestrasse 29/III, 8000 München 15. www.med.uni-muenchen.de.

This very large faculty was founded in 1826. A large cancer centre is associated with it. One of its peripheral hospitals is Zentralklinikum (86009 Augsburg). This is a massive hospital on the outskirts of Augsburg, a medium-sized city in the south of Germany. Here, previous elective students have joined in with Munich student's teaching. There are some excellent pubs and plenty to do in the old town. If you want to get out, Munich and the Bavarian Alps (good weekend skiing) are very close.

Accommodation: Has previously been provided.

Regensburg

Universität Regensburg

Medizin Fakultät, Franz Josef-Strasse-Allee 11, 93042 Regensburg. Tel: +49 941 944 6084. Fax: +49 941 944 6079.
www.uni-regensburg.de.
This new medical college (1970) uses a large clinical centre just outside the city.

Tübingen

Eberhard-Karls-Universität Tübingen

Medizinische Fakultät, Geissweg 5, 72076 Tübingen. Tel: +49 7071 297 3663. Fax: +49 7071 296 864.
www.medizin.uni-tuebingen.de.
Founded in the late 15th century, it has nearly 2000 beds.

Ulm

Universität Ulm

Medizinische Fakultät, Pavillon II, Albert-Einstein Allee 7, D89069 Ulm. Tel: +49 500 22027. Fax: +49 500 22028. www.uni-ulm.de/medizin.
This new medical college (1969) uses large modern hospitals, including the Medical University Clinic. In total it has access to 1500 beds.

ARMY WORK:

Medical Reception Station, Imphal Barracks

Osnabrück, Germany BFPO 36.

General practice: This is an opportunity to see general practice in an army setting, although reports suggest not a particularly good one. You will be expected to be at the station between 8 am and 6 pm, and they like you to spend as little time as possible with the doctors and as much with 'the other services'. So if you fancy spending days going around as a health visitor's 'young trainee' and being allowed to read off a baby's weight from a set of scales … this is the elective for you. You will get some time with the GPs, but again the experience gained has been very limited.

Accommodation: And food are both provided and are excellent.

Gibraltar

Population: 27 000
Language: English and Spanish
Capital: Gibraltar
Currency: Pound
Int Code: +350

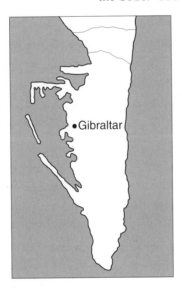

●Gibraltar

Gibraltar is a 3 km by 5 km rock in the southern part of Spain guarding the entrance to the Mediterranean. Its military use has dwindled in recent years, however, it is still very much a British colony, with British shops and banks in its main street. There's a National Health Service-type system of care given by an 11-man GP practice and St Bernard's Hospital. Although English is the official language, some people can only speak Spanish so a little knowledge does help. Medical work here is often advertised in the BMJ and Nursing Times. There's a great deal of concern at present regarding the possibility of joint sovereignty with Spain. A new state-of-the-art hospital is being built.

USEFUL ADDRESS:

Gibraltar Health Authority, 17 Johnstone's Passage, Gibraltar. Tel: +350 76881. Fax: +350 41661. www.gha.gov.gi. (Visit the website for up-to-date information.)

Casemated Health Centre
Gibraltar.

The practice: An 11-man, well-run, busy GP service. Most conditions are similar to those seen in Western Europe.

O Elective notes: A welcoming friendly practice, with a great willingness to teach.

St Bernard's Hospital

Gibraltar.

The hospital: The public hospital for Gibraltar. It has the major specialities (medicine, surgery, paeds, O&G, ENT and care of the elderly), but complicated cases have to be transferred to the UK or Spain. There is one surgeon here.

Elective notes: Due to the rarity of students the staff are keen to teach. A wide range of conditions is seen.

Greece

Population: 10 million
Language: Greek
Capital: Athens
Currency: Euro
Int Code: +30

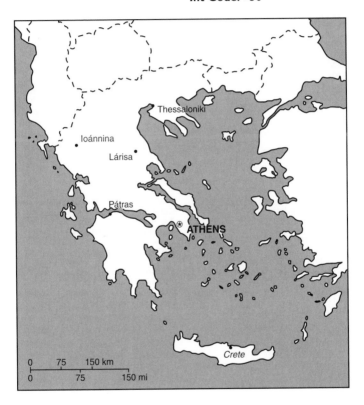

Greece is well known for its beautiful islands and for the hustle and bustle of Athens. If you speak Greek it has quite a lot to offer the visiting medic, however, it is not a popular elective or work destination for overseas visitors.

✪ Medicine:

Greece is one of the less well-off members of the EU, and this is sometimes reflected in the healthcare. There is a state-run system (the ESY, established in 1983) providing free care to all. It is paid for by compulsory insurance and taxation. Because of dissatisfaction with the ESY, private insurance is becoming more popular. Greece produces too many doctors, although there is a problem recruiting to rural areas.

⊃ Visas and work permits:

Like the rest of the EU, no visa is required for up to three months if you are a EU citizen. For longer than this, you will need a residence permit. Registration for doctors is through the Panhellenic Medical Association (which also advertises posts).

USEFUL ADDRESS:

Ministry of Health, Odos Aristotelous 17, 10433 Athens. Tel: +30 1 523 2820. Fax: +30 1 523 1707.

PROFESSIONAL ORGANIZATIONS:

Panhellenic Medical Association, Ploutarchou 3, 10675 Athens. Tel: +30 1 725 8660. Fax: +30 1 725 8663.
Greek Medical Association, Stadiou Street 29, Athens. www.pis.gr.
Athens Medical Association, Themistokleous 34, GR 10678 Athens. Tel: +30 1 384 1234. www.isathens.gr.
Hellenic Nurses Association, Athens Tower, GR 11527 Athens. Tel: +30 1 770 2861. Fax: +30 1 779 0360. www.esdne.gr.
Hellenic Dental Association, Themistokkleous 38, GR 10678 Athens. www.osth.gr.
Hellenic Physiotherapy Association, Gilforodou 12, GR 104 Athens. Tel: +30 1 821 3905. Fax: +30 1 771 1821.
Hellenic Occupational Therapy Association, Aristidou Street 8, GR 10559 Athens. Tel: +30 1 322 8979. Fax: +30 1 323 9776.

There are seven medical schools:

Athens: National and Kapodistrian University of Athens, School of Health Sciences, Faculty of Medicine, 75 Mikras Asias Street (2nd floor), 11527 Goudi, Athens. Tel: +30 7 781 331. Fax: +30 7 706 642. www.uoa.gr.
Crete: University of Crete, School of Health Sciences, Elefterias Square, 71409 Heraklion. Tel: +30 81 393 000. www.uch.gr.
Ioannina: University of Ioannina, School of Medicine, University Campus, Ioannina 45110. Tel: +30 651 97198. Fax: +30 651 97182. www.uoi.gr.
Larisa: University of Thessaly, School of Health Sciences, 22 Papakiriazi, Larissa 41222. Tel: +30 41 259 974. Fax: +30 41 255 420. www.med.uth.gr/en.
Patras: University of Patras, School of Medicine, Patras 26500. Tel: +30 61 992 942. Fax: +30 61 996 103. www.med.upatras.gr.
Thessaloniki: Aristotle University of Thessaloniki, Medical School, Thessaloniki 54006. Tel: +30 31 999 283. Fax: +30 31 999 293. www.med.auth.gr.
Thrace: Democritus University of Thrace Medical School, Alexandroupolis, Thrace. Tel: +30 53 139 104. Fax: +30 53 139 035. www.duth.gr.

SOME HOSPITALS IN THE CITIES:

Asklipion Hospital, Voula, Athens. Tel +30 1 895 8301.
General Regional Hospital Ippokrateo, Constantinopoles 49, 54642 Thessaloniki. Tel: +30 81 837 921.
General Hospital AG Andreas, 118 Girokomeiou, Patras. Tel: +30 61 22 2812.
KAT Accident Hospital, Nikis 2, 14561 Athens. Tel: +30 1 801 4411.
Regional General Hospital Evangelismos, Ypsilantou 45, 11521 Athens. Tel: +30 1 722 0101.

Hungary

Population: 10 million
Language: Hungarian
Capital: Budapest
Currency: Forint
Int Code: +36

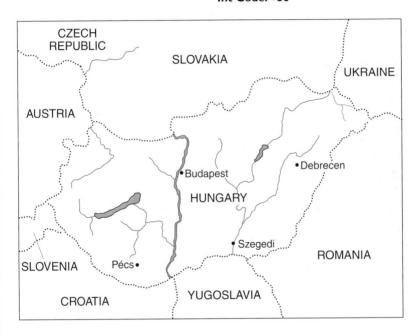

Hungary, a landlocked country in central Europe, has outperformed other Eastern Block countries, receiving a great deal of overseas investment. It is moving closer to the EU. There is a fair bit to see and do. The capital has baths from the Ottoman period, and Lake Balaton is popular with tourists.

✚ Medicine:
A state health system provides free care to everyone, although a 15% charge on prescriptions is made. Like many state systems, however, it is underfunded, hence waiting lists are long. Western diseases are the order of the day.

◎ Climate and crime:
Hungary is warmest between May and August and has a fairly constant level of rainfall. It's a pretty safe country for tourists.

➲ Visas and work permits:
Students from most Western countries (including the UK, USA, Canada and most of Europe) do not need a visa to travel or shadow in a hospital. Australian and New Zealand citizens are exceptions. Contact your local embassy where a visa is easily obtained for a small fee, an application form and a few

photos. To work in Hungary, a permit is required.

USEFUL ADDRESSES:

Ministry of Welfare, 6-8 Arany János Ucta, 1051 Budapest. Tel: +36 1 332 3100. Fax: +36 1 311 8054.
Federation of Hungarian Medical Societies (MOTESZ), Nádor u. 36 - POB 145, 1443 Budapest. Tel: +36 1 269 4391. Fax: +36 1 183 79 18. www.motesz.hu.

Budapest

Semmelweis University of Medical Sciences

Orvostudományi Egyetem, Üllöi út 26, 2nd Floor, H-1085 Budapest VIII. Tel: +36 12 660 120. Fax: +36 11 172 220. www.sote.hu.
Founded in the 18th century, Semmelweis has had a long and interesting history. It now has 3100 beds in its affiliated hospital. Most instruction is in English.

Debrecen

University Medical School of Debrecen

4012 Debrecen, PO Box 48 Nagyerdei krt., 98 Debrecen. Tel: +36 52 417 571. Fax: +36 52 419 807. www.dote.hu.
Established in 1918, the medical school separated from the university in 1951. Most teaching is in Hungarian (and this is obviously what the patients speak), however, 15% of students are taught in English. Most specialities, including traumatology, are catered for.

Debrecen has a population of 250 000 and a number of interesting sites, such as the great forest and thermal baths.
Accommodation: Costs US$200–300 a month.

Pécs

University Medical School of Pécs

Szigeti ut 12, H-7600 Pécs Tel: +36 72 326 222, Fax:72 314 083. www.pote.hu.
This is one of Hungary's oldest medical schools (founded in 1367), although it was rebuilt after World War I. It admits 175 students per year, and all the teaching and clinical activities are in one area.

Szegedi

Albert Szent-Györgyi Medical University

Dugonics tér 13, PO Box 479, H-6701 Szegedi. Tel: +36 62 455 007. Fax: +36 62 455 005. www.szote.u-szeged.hu/.
Established in 1921, the university uses a number of hospitals situated between the cathedral and the River Tisza. It has all major specialities and preclinical departments, including forensics. Students are required to be able to speak English.

Szegedi is situated on the banks of the River Tisza of the southern edge of the Great Hungarian Plains. It has 200 000 people and a very pleasant climate.

Iceland

Population: 300 000
Language: Icelandic
Capital: Reykjavík
Currency: New Icelandic króna
Int code: +354

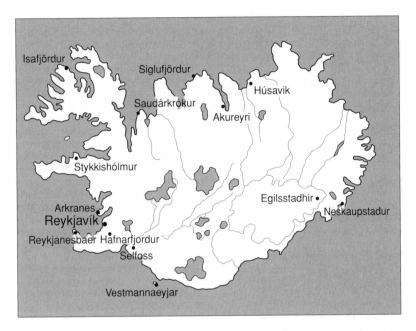

Iceland, just south of the Arctic Circle, is situated between the American and European continental plates, which accounts for its numerous volcanoes and geysers. It has some spectacular scenery although obviously gets very cold. There are plenty of natural interest spots such as the 'Golden Waterfall' and the Geysir Geothermal Area near Reykjavik. In the north go to Myvatn with old and new volcanoes, lava fields, boiling mud pots and steam vents on the North Atlantic Ridge. Organized tours cost about £40, but if you're there in the summer (June to September), public transport is good. Although the official language is Icelandic, most people can speak English very well.

✚ Medicine:

Iceland has an excellent record on health, with a free healthcare service for all and one of the longest life expectancies and lowest infant mortalities anywhere. It has one medical school and a number of hospitals across the island.

➲ Visas and work permits:

No visa is required for elective students. EU citizens can spend up to three months looking for work without a visa, but once they find work, they need one. Doctors must apply to one of the hospitals below. Before being allowed to practise medicine in Iceland, confirmation from the Ministry of Health and Social Security has to be obtained. The hospitals are very helpful with that.

USEFUL ADDRESSES:

Ministry of Health, 116 Laugavegour, 150 Reykjavik. Tel: +354 560 9700. Fax: +354 551 9165.
Icelandic Medical Association, Hlioasmara 8, 200 Kópavogur. Tel: +354 564 4100. Fax: +354 564 4106. www.icemed.is.
Icelandic Nurses Association, Sudurlandsbraut 22, IS-108 Reykjavik. Tel: +354 568 7575. Fax: +354 568 0727.
Icelandic Dental Association, Tanaeknafélag Islands, PO Box 8596, IS-128 Reykjavik.
Icelandic Physiotherapy Association: Felag Islenkra Sjukrapjalfara, Box 5023, IS-125 Reykjavik. Tel: +354 568 7661. Fax: +354 588 9239. www.physio.is.
Icelandic Occupational Therapy Association, Postholf 8845, IS-128 Reykjavik.

Reykjavík

MEDICAL SCHOOL AND MAIN HOSPITAL:

Landspitalinn, National University Hospital

Baronstigur, 101-Reyjavík or Thverholt 18, IS-105 Reykjavík. Tel: +354 560 2360. Fax: +354 560 2359.
Medical school address: Læknagarður, Vatnsmýrarvegur 16, 101 Reykjavík.
Tel: +354 525 4881. Fax: +354 525 4884. www.hi.is/facu.
The best way to obtain information about medical students' exchange programmes is to contact the extremely friendly and well-run **Icelandic Medical Students International Committee** (IMSIC) via e-mail on imsic@rhi.hi.is, or the **University of Iceland Office of International Education** (Neshagi, IS-107 Reykjavík. Tel: +354 525 4311. Fax: +354 525 5850). They can help to organize placements and board and lodging. They even arrange weekend outings. The main hospital used is:

Sjúkrahús Reykjavíkur (Reykjavík Hospital)

Landakot 5.haed, IS-108 Reykavík. Tel: +354 525 1800. Fax: +354 525 1959. Mark all correspondence 'Starfsmannathjonusta'.
The hospital: The main teaching hospital in Iceland. It is so big that it uses 22% of the health sector budget. It offers most specialities but particularly prides itself on its use of laparoscopic surgery, *in vitro* fertilization, paeds and maternity services, and cardiac surgery. It has 11 operating theatres and an emergency department that sees 10 000 patients a year.
O Elective notes: The staff are very friendly. In the summer, there are no other students around so there's plenty of teaching. The surgeons are heavily into laproscopic surgery. There's a great deal of gastric surgery as Iceland has the second-highest incidence of gastric cancer in the world. The 'general surgeon' really is doing mastectomies and aortic aneurysms on the same list.
Accommodation: Iceland is an expensive place, but the medical student association is well organized, and since they can arrange accommodation and board in the hospital as well as sightseeing trips, the cost is actually very reasonable.

OTHER HOSPITALS IN ICELAND:

Fjórdungssjúkrahúsid Akureyri

IS-600 Akureyri. Tel: +354 463 0101. Fax: +354 462 4621.
The hospital: A quiet, friendly place in Iceland's second-largest town (population 15 000). The day starts at 7.45 am with X-ray meetings and a ward round. There's plenty of elective surgery, and the days tend to finish about 4 pm. They are quite happy for you to disappear for a bit.

Heilbrigdisstofnunin, Egilstödum, IS-700 Egilstadhir. Tel: +354 471 1400. Fax: +354 471 1971.
Heilbrigdisstofnunin Sudurnesja, Mánagata 9, IS-230 Reykjanesbaer. Tel: +354 422 0580. Fax: +354 421 3471.
Heilbrigdisstofnunin í Vestmannaeeyjum, Sólhlíd 10, IS-900 Vestmannaeyjar.
Tel: +354 481 1955. Fax: +354 481 1072.

Iceland

St Fransiskusspítalinn, Austurgata 7,
IS-340 Stykkishólmur. Tel: +354 438 1128.
Fax: +354 438 1628.
St Jósefsspítali, Sudurgata 41, IS-220
Hafnarfjördur, Iceland Tel: +354 555 0000.
Fax: +354 565 3255.
Sjúkrahús Akraness, Merkigerdi 9, IS-300
Akranes. Tel: +354 431 2311. Fax: +354 431 2319.
Sjúkrahús Húsavíkur, Audbrekku 4, IS-640
Húsavík. Tel: +354 464 0500. Fax: +354 464 0575.
Sjúkrahús Ísafjardar, IS-400 Ísafjödur. Tel: +354
450 4500. Fax: +354 450 4522.

Sjúkrahúsid Neskaupstad, Myrargata 20,
IS-740 Neskaupstadur. Tel: +354 477 1402.
Fax: +354 477 1879.
Sjúkrahús Saudárkróki, IS-551 Saudárkrókur.
Tel: +354 455 4000. Fax: +354 455 4010.
Sjúkrahús Siglufjardar, Hvanneyrarbraut,
IS-580 Siglufjördur. Tel: +354 467 2172.
Fax: +354 467 1551.
Sjúkrahús Sudurlands, Árvegi, IS-800 Selfoss.
Tel: +354 482 1300. Fax: +354 482 2534.

Ireland

Population: 3.8 million
Language: Irish and English
Capital: Dublin
Currency: Euro
Int Code: +353

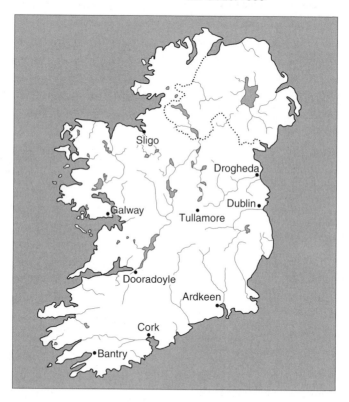

Ireland is a beautiful, friendly country with coastal hills, charming bays in the west and some lovely people. The vast majority simply want peace (so do not let the conflict in the north put you off going). It's a superb place for those who are easily sunburned!

✛ Medicine:

Most people rely on the 'public' health service. Some people (of low income) receive all health services free of charge. Others of higher income have care provided by private insurance or they have to pay directly. There are three types of hospital: health board (government run), voluntary (often run by religious organizations) and private. Typical Western pathologies (heart disease and cancer) are the order of the day, and there is a good doctor:patient ratio (1:588). Ireland claims to have the lowest consumption of alcohol in the EU (surely they lost count!).

⮕ **Visas and work permits:**
British citizens do not require a visa to enter Ireland. However, if enrolling in study or actually practising medicine, permits are required. British students doing electives have not reported any need for a visa. Contact the embassy for more details. Doctors need to register with the **General Register of Medical Practitioners of the Irish Medical Council** (address below). EEC qualifications give full registration and others usually grant temporary registration. Note: Irish doctors swap around on 1st July so it can get chaotic around then. Many doctors also take their holidays in the first two weeks of August; therefore you can get busy as a student. If you're going from the UK, why not take a car if you have one?

PROFESSIONAL ORGANIZATIONS:

Irish Medical Organisation, 10 Fitzwilliam Place, Dublin 2. Tel: +353 1 676 7273. Fax: +353 1 661 2758. www.imo.ie.
Irish Medical Council, Lynn House, Portobello Court, Lower Rathmines Road, Dublin 6.
Tel: +353 1 496 5588 Fax: +353 1 496 5972.
www.medicalcouncil.ie.
Royal College of Surgeons of Ireland, 123 St Stephen's Green, Dublin 2. Tel: +353 1 402 2100.
E-mail: info@rcsi.ie. www.rcsi.ie.
Royal College of Physicians of Ireland, 6 Kildare Street, Dublin 2. Tel: +353 1 661 667.
Fax: +353 1 676 3989. www.rcpi.ie.
Irish Nurses' Organisation, 11 Fitzwilliam Place, Dublin 2. Tel: +353 1 676 0137.
Fax: +353 1 661 0466. www.ino.ie.
Irish Dental Association, 'Boyne', 10 Richview Office Park, Clonskeagh Road, Dublin 14.
www.dentist.ie.
Irish Society of Charted Physiotherapists:
Address as Royal College of Surgeons. Tel +353 1 402 2148. Fax: +353 1 402 2160. www.iscp.ie.

Association of Occupational Therapists of Ireland, 29 Gardiner Place, Dublin 1.
Tel: +353 1 878 0247. www.aoti.ie.
Irish Association of Speech Therapists, PO Box 1344, Dublin.

Dublin

A vibrant, lively city, Dublin is probably most famous for its Guinness brewery. There's plenty to do and some beautiful countryside nearby. You won't get bored in the evenings.

MEDICAL SCHOOLS:

Royal College of Surgeons of Ireland, 123 St Stephen's Green, Dublin 2. Tel: +353 1 402 2100. Fax +353 1 402 2460. E-mail: info@rcsi.ie. www.rcsi.ie. (Since 1784, the college has had its own medical school. It also has a school of physiotherapy.)
University College of Dublin, Faculty of Medicine, Bellfield Capmus, Dublin 4. Tel: +353 1 706 7440. Fax: +353 1 475 3655. www.ucd.ie.
University of Dublin, School of Physic, Trinty College, Dublin 2. Tel: +353 1 608 1727. Fax: +353 1 671 3956. www2.tcd.ie. (The oldest medical school in Ireland, it is now based at St James's Hospital.)

If applying to do an elective, enquire whether accommodation can be arranged as it can be expensive in Dublin.

TEACHING HOSPITALS IN DUBLIN:

Beaumont Hospital
Beaumont Road, Dublin 9.
Tel: +353 1 837 7755. Fax: +353 1 837 6982.
www.beaumont.ie.
The hospital: A big (620-bed), busy teaching hospital affiliated to the medical school of the Royal College of Surgeons of Ireland and situated on the north side of the city. It has all major specialities and houses the **National Neurology and Neurosurgery Unit**. It is also the national centre for renal transplants, pancreatic disorders and cochlear implantation. It has an emergency department for its catchment of 250 000.
O Elective notes: There are usually around 50 students from the Royal College of Surgeons of Ireland. They

Ireland

have comprehensive daily tutorials and lectures, as well as their weekly departmental meetings. It's a friendly hospital and great for a cheap, fun elective.

Accommodation: No hospital accommodation is available, however, it has previously been arranged through the College. Lodgings cost about £100 (130 Euros) a week.

St James's Hospital

PO Box 580, James's Street, Dublin 8. Tel: +353 1 453 7941. Fax +353 1 454 4494. www.stjames.ie.

The hospital: Although only built in 1971, St James's is now the largest university teaching hospital in the Republic of Ireland. It is the hospital for Trinity College, Dublin, and accordingly has nearly all medical and surgical specialities.

O **Elective notes:** The teaching and clinical experience are usually very good. It's a very friendly hospital.

Accommodation: Not provided.

Mater Misericordiae Hospital

Eccles Street, Dublin 7. www.mater.ie.

The hospital: An acute tertiary referral university teaching hospital with many specialist services. It is the national centre for cardiothoracic surgery and spinal injuries and has the major emergency department serving Dublin's inner city. It is associated with University College Dublin.

Coombe Women's Hospital

Dolphins Barn, Dublin 8. Tel: +353 1 453 756. Fax: +353 2 453 6033. E-mail: info@coombe.ie. www.coombe.ie.

The hospital: Established in 1826, this is the busiest women's hospital in Ireland, delivering over 6000 babies a year. It is a centre of excellence, with a low Caesarean section rate because of their very successful active management of labour. It has a busy ultrasound department, a modern homely delivery suite and a state-of-the art SCBU. It is affiliated to University College Dublin, Trinity College and the Royal College of Surgeons in Ireland. It has its own midwifery school.

National Children's Hospital

Temple Street, Dublin 1. Tel +353 1 874 8763. Fax +353 1 874 8355.

The hospital: This is the main paediatric hospital.

Central Mental Hospital

Dundrum, Dublin.

The hospital: This is the only centre for forensic psychiatry in Ireland. Of the 80 or so patients, half are admitted on a short-term basis from the prison system for acute psychiatric crises. The others are long-stay chronic patients who are detained as they are judged unfit to plead. They have usually committed very serious crimes.

O **Elective notes:** The elective consists of shadowing a registrar, assessing patients and going to court. If you're into this, it has been a highly recommended elective.

Cork

Cork is a lively city in the south of Ireland, with plenty of festivals in the summer. It's great if you like hill walking.

MEDICAL SCHOOL:

University College, Cork, Faculty of Medicine, National University of Ireland, Cork, Co Cork. **University Hospital**, Wilton, Cork, Co Cork. Tel: +353 21 490 2809. Fax: +353 21 427 0339. www.ucc.ie.

HOSPITALS:

Cork University Hospital

Wilton, Cork, Co Cork. Tel: +353 2 154 6400. Fax: +353 2 134 3307.

The hospital: Is the main university hospital and has all major specialities. Apply through the university to do an elective here.

Mercy Hospital

Cork, Co Cork.

The hospital: This is in central Cork and is smaller than the University Hospital

(City Hospital). It is still used by Cork medical students and students from elsewhere in Europe, but its smaller size makes it that bit more friendly. The teaching has been reported to be excellent.

Accommodation: Not provided but available nearby for approximately £30 (40 Euros) a week.

Bantry General Hospital
Bantry, Co Cork.

The hospital: Bantry General has a medical ward (29 beds), a surgical ward, an ITU and a psychiatric department. The catchment area is West Cork and South Kerry. Bantry itself is a small town right on the Atlantic coast. Outside Bantry, there is plenty to do for the outdoors type with a car (mountain biking, hill walking, golf). However, some have found it too isolated for their liking.

O **Elective notes:** Despite the hospital's small size, there is usually quite a variety of cases and the staff are very friendly and keen to teach and let students do procedures.

Accommodation: Not provided, although there is an independent hospital in Bantry.

Galway

MEDICAL SCHOOL:

University College, Galway
Faculty of Medicine, National University of Ireland, Clinical Sciences Institute, Galway, Co Galway. Tel: +353 9 152 4268. Fax: +353 9 175 0519. www.nuigalway.ie/med/.

It uses:

University College Hospital
Galway, Co Galway. Tel: +353 9 152 4222. Fax: +353 9 152 6588.

OTHER MAJOR HOSPITALS IN IRELAND:

Limerick Regional Hospital, Dooradoyle, Co Limerick. Tel: +353 6 130 1111. Fax: +353 6 130 1165.
Our Lady of Lourdes Hospital, Drogheda, Co Louth. Tel: +353 4 137 601. Fax: +353 4 133 868.
Sligo General Hospital, The Mall, Sligo, Co Sligo. Tel: +353 7 171 111. Fax: +353 7 145 520.
Tullamore General Hospital, Tullamore, Co Offaly. Tel: +353 5 062 1601. Fax: +353 5 065 1204.
Waterford Regional Hospital, Dunmore Road, Ardkeen, Co Waterford. Tel: +353 5 173 321. Fax: +353 5 179 495.

Italy

Population: 58 million
Language: Italian
Capital: Rome
Currency: Euro
Int Code: +39

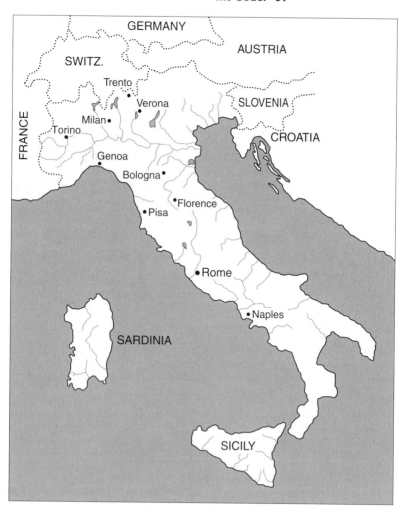

GERMANY

AUSTRIA

SWITZ.

Trento

Verona

SLOVENIA

FRANCE

Milan

Torino

CROATIA

Genoa

Bologna

Florence

Pisa

Rome

Naples

SARDINIA

SICILY

Italy has a great deal to offer, from excellent skiing in the Alps to beautiful sun-drenched Mediterranean beaches. There are many cosmopolitan cities and many sights to see. Italian culture and food are yet more reasons to visit this country. One major drawback, however, is the real need to have fluent Italian in a hospital setting. For this reason (and because it is expensive), Italy is not a popular elective destination. Because of this and the fact that many schools are on the Erasmus/Socrates programme, only a few medical schools and hospitals are listed here. If you can speak Italian, there are a number of great resources on the web. Try a Google search or go to www.iime.org.

In total, Italy has 33 medical schools.

○ Medicine:

The relaxed lifestyle, daily glass of red wine and Mediterranean food are supposed to make Italians very healthy, and indeed they are. They have one of the highest life expectancies. Nonetheless, typical Western diseases get them in the end. There is a state-run healthcare system (Servizio Sanitario Nazionale, or SSN) that's run by 650 local health groups. Although the service was originally free, patients now have to pay a proportion of prescription and investigation charges. The state hospitals have been described as pretty poor. This is a reason why they are not popular with elective students and also why the private sector (catering for 20% of the population) is growing. GP services are free (funded by the local health unit), and a referal is required to access specialist care.

The system for medical training is also is a bit odd. Once qualified, you get a job. You then (if you want) never have to apply for another job. You just progress up through the ranks in that job. It can make people a bit lazy. Undergraduate medicine has been described as a bit of a spectator sport and hence is a further deterrent. Italy vastly overproduces doctors – around 70 000 are currently unemployed so getting a job from outside is virtually impossible.

○ Visas and work permits:

Citizens of the EU, USA, New Zealand and Australia don't need a visa to stay in Italy for up to 90 days. Note: Australian, US and a few other citizens may require a Schengen visa if they intend to visit some other European countries as well. For work permits, contact the embassy. Registration as a doctor is a lengthy process. Even though they should recognize an EU graduate (as the rest of the EU does), you have to have your qualification checked by the Italian Consulate General, who in turn has to consult the Italian Cultural Institute. The Italian Health Ministry can then officially validate you. You next have to register with the **Federazione Nazionale degli Ordini dei Medici Chirurghe e degli Odontoiatri** (addresss below). Finally, you have to register in the region in which you wish to practise.

USEFUL ADDRESSES:

Ministry of Health, 20 Viale del'I Industria, Rome 00144. Tel: +39 6 59944/59941. Fax: +39 6 964 7687.
Italian Medical Association: Società Italiana di Medicina Generale, via II Prato 66, I 50123 Firenze. www.simg.it.
Italian Medical Organization: Federazione Nazionale Ordine dei Medici. www.fnomceo.it.
Federazione Nazionale degli Ordini dei Medici Chirurghe e degli Odontoiatri, Piazza Cola de Rienzo 80/A, 00192 Roma. Tel: +39 6 362 031. Fax: +39 6 322 2429.
Italian Nurses Association: Consociazione Nazionale delle Associazioni Infermieri ed altri Operatori Sanitario-Sociali, via Arno 62, I 00198 Rome. Tel: +39 6 884 0654. www.cnai.info.
Italian Dental Association: Associazione Nazionale Dentisti Italiani, Via Savoia, I 00198 Rome. www.andi.it.
Itailain Physiotherapy Association: Associazione Italiana Terapisti della Rehabilitazione, Via Claterna 18, I 00183 Rome. Tel: +39 6 7720 1020. www.aifi.net.
Italian Occupational Therapy Association: Associazione Italiana di Terapia Occupazionale, via Peralba 9, I 00141 Rome. www.aita-onlus.it.

SOME MEDICAL SCHOOLS:

Instituto Scientifico H san Raffaele
Fondazione Centro San Raffaele del Monte Tabor, Milano, Via Olgettina 60. Tel: +39 2 26431. www.fondazionesanraffaele.it.

The hospital: This huge private institution has a worldwide reputation and is claimed to be *the* place in Italy to do virtually any speciality (coming very highly recommended for electives). It is the only private medical school in Italy. The main Institute (in Olgettina Street), with 1300 beds, has everything from the emergency room to gamma knife neurosurgery. Also associated is the **Centro San Luigi**, an HIV treatment and research centre with 35 beds, a resuscitation unit to assist terminal cases and a dedicated operating theatre. The **Department of Neuropsychic Science** is a 280-bed centre for the treatment of mental disorders. There is also a department of biological and technological research.

O **Elective notes:** If you can't speak Italian, they can organize electives in molecular biology, cellular biology, neuroscience, immunology and radiology. They are on the Socrates/Erasmus system. Write to Ufficio Socrates/Erasmus, Universita Vita-Salute San Raffaele (via Olgettina 58, 20132 Milano. Tel: +39 2 2643 3813. Fax: +39 2 2643 4704).

Note: There is a second San Raffaele in Rome, with 500 beds providing general services and a spinal unit.

MAIN MEDICAL SCHOOLS IN ROME:

Università Campus Bio-Medico di Roma, Facoltà di Medicina e Chirurgia, Via Emilio Longoni, 83, I-00155 Roma. Tel: +39 6225 411. Fax: +39 6 225 417. www.unicampus.it.
Università Cattolica de Sacro Cuore, Facoltà di Medicina e Chirurgia Agostino Gemelli, Via della Pineta Sacchetti 644, I-00168 Roma.
Università di Roma-La Sapienza, Facoltà di Medicina e Chirurgia, Città Universitaria, Piazzale Aldo Moro 5, I-00185 Roma. (This was founded in 1303, making it Rome's oldest medical school.)

OTHER MEDICAL SCHOOLS:

Università di Bologna, Facoltà di Medicina e Chirurgia, Via San Vitale 59, I-40138 Bologna.

Tel: +39 51 232 468. Fax: +39 51 233 062. (Founded in the 13th century.)
Università di Milano, Facoltà di Medicina e Chirurgia, Via Festo del Perdonon 7, I-20122 Milan. www.unimi.it.
Università di Napoli, Facoltà di Medicina e Chirurgia II, Via Sergio Pansini 5, I-80131 Naples. www.unina.it.
Università di Pisa, Facoltà di Medicina e Chirurgia, Via Roma 55, I-56100 Pisa.
Tel: +39 50 555 434. Fax: +39 50 551 369.
www.med.unipi.it. (This is an old medical school, also founded in the 13th century.)
Università di Roma-Tor Vergata, Facoltà di Medicina e Chirurgia, Via A Raimondo, I-00173 Rome.
Università degli Studi di Torino, Facoltà di Medicina e Chirurgia, Cso Bramante 88/90, I-10126 Torino. Tel: +39 11 663 5814. Fax: +39 11 696 3737. www.molinette.unito.it.
Università di Verona, Facoltà di Medicina e Chirurgia, Via dell'Artigliere, 8, I-37129 Verona.
Tel: +39 45 807 4466. Fax: +39 45 820 222.
www.medicina.univr.it.

NON-TEACHING HOSPITALS PREVIOUSLY USED FOR ELECTIVES:

Ospedale Santa Chiara
L'Go Medaglie D'Oro, 838100 Trento.
The hospital: Santa Chiara is a large general hospital serving the city of Trento and the surrounding areas in Trentino, north Italy. The general medical and dermatology departments are at least relaxed and friendly. There is no medical school here so although the doctors are very friendly, it lacks something in social life. The surrounding areas are beautiful, with the lakes and Verona nearby.

Istituto G. Gaslini
167147 Genoa.
The hospital: The largest paediatric hospital in Italy and a specialist referral centre for the entire country. It is very friendly.
O **Elective notes:** Teaching is informal. Genoa is a small city on the coast of north-west Italy. It is very pretty.

Luxembourg

Population: 400 000
Language: Letzeburgish
Capital: Luxembourg
Curency: Euro
Int Code: +352

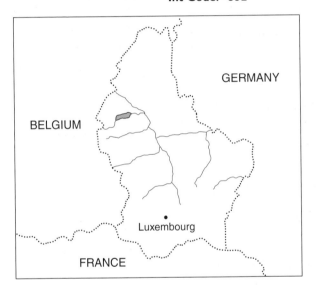

Despite its small size and population, Luxembourg has the highest income per capita in the EU. It borders the industrial regions of France, Belgium and Germany, but today it is its tax haven status and banking that generate its prosperity. The countryside consists of rolling hills and forests.

✛ Medicine:

There are no private hospitals in Luxembourg. They are run either by the state or by nuns. All nationals are covered by the *Caisse de Maladie* (the state sickness fund), from which any expenses can be reclaimed. Everybody contributes to this fund via one of nine insurance funds. The contributions to this are roughly one-third employee, one third-employer and one-third government. All doctors therefore work in this public system, and patients can directly visit a specialist without the need for GP referral. Doctors are paid not by hospitals but directly from the *Caisses de Maladie*, hence they need to be approved by the Ministry of Health. The big killers are Western: heart and cerebrovascular disease and cancer. The doctor:patient ratio is 1:476.

◎ Climate:

It's warmest (20°C) between June and August. The winter in the Ardennes (south) can get cold and snowy.

⮑ Visas and work permits:

Like most of the EU, no visa is required for EU nationals staying less than three months, longer than this and you'll need to get an identity card. Non-EU nationals will need to obtain a work permit from the **Ministry of Justice** (16 Boulevard Royal, L-2934 Luxembourg). As Luxembourg has no medical schools, it relies on doctors coming in from outside.

USEFUL ADDRESSES:

Ministère de la Santé, Boulevard de la Pétrusse 57, L-2320 Luxembourg. Tel: +352 4781. Fax: +352 491 337/472 614. www.santel.lu.
Luxembourg Medical and Dental Association: Association des Médecins et Médecins Dentistes du Grand-Duché de Luxembourg, 29 rue de Vianden, L-2680 Luxembourg. Tel: +352 444 033. Fax: +352 458 349.

Physicians, Dentists and Pharmacists Institute of Luxembourg, Collège Médical, 90 boulvard de la Pétrusse, L-2320 Luxembourg. Tel: +352 478 5514.
Luxembourg Nurses Association: Association nationale des Infirmiers Luxembourgeois, Boîte Postale 1184, L 1011 Luxenbourg. Tel: +352 495 809. Fax: +352 408 585.
Luxembourg Physiotherapy Association: Association Luxembourgeoise des Kinesthérapeutes Diplomes, Boîte Postale 645, L-2016 Luxembourg. Tel: +352 448 039. Fax: +352 333 904.
Luxembourg Association of Occupational Therapists: Association Luxembourgeoise des Ergothérapeutes Diplomes, Boîte Postale 1176, L-1011 Luxembourg.

MAIN HOSPITALS:

Centre Hôpitalier, 4 rue Barblé, Luxembourg-ville L-1210. Tel: +352 441 111. Fax: +352 458 762.
Hôpital de la Ville d'Esch, Rue E Mayrisch, Esch-sur-Alzette, L-4005 Luxembourg. Tel: +352 571 111. Fax: +352 571 139.

Macedonia

Population: 2.2 million
Language: Macedonian/Albanian
Capital: Skophe
Currency: Macedonian denar
Int Code: +389

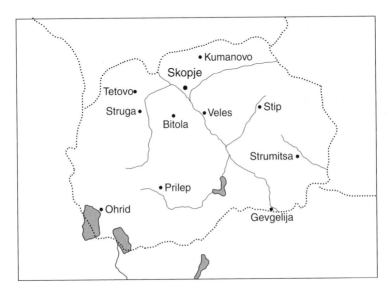

The Former Yugoslav Republic of Macedonia (FYRM) had its economic blockade of Serbia and Montenegro lifted in 1996. Greece, however, is still hostile as it worries that the FYRM may try to take over an area also called Macedonia in northern Greece. This is certainly not a popular elective destination at present, although the Sara Mountains offer good skiing.

✿ Medicine:
The state guarantees universal health-care. However, for quick and reliable treatment people have to go privately.

➲ Visas and work permits:
Contact the embassy of the Republic of Macedonia. No clear information is available.

USEFUL ADDRESSES:

Macedonia Ministry of Health, 50 dud, bb Vodnjanska, 91000 Skopje. Tel: +389 91 231 128. Fax: +389 91 220 163.
Chamber of Doctors of the Republic of Macedonia, Ul 'Naroden Front', BR 21 91009 Skopje. Tel/Fax: +389 91 124 066.
Macedonian Medical Association, Dame Gruev Br. 3, PO Box 174, 91000 Skopje. Tel/Fax: +389 91 232 577.

MEDICAL SCHOOL:

SS Cyril and Methodius University

Faculty of Medicine, Bul Krste Misirkov bb, 91000 Skopje. Tel: +389 91 118 155. Fax: +389 91 116 370. www.ukim.edu.mk.

The main hospital in Skopje is:

Clinical Center of the Republic of Macedonia

17 Vodnjanska St, Skopje. Tel: +389 91 114 244. Fax: +389 91 122 130.

HOSPITALS IN SKOPJE:

Army Hospital, Ilindenska BB, Skopje. Tel: +389 91 362 622. Fax: +389 91 250 340.
Bucharest Polyclinic, Bul Partizanski odredi BB, Skopje. Tel: +389 91 364 088.
City Hospital, 11 Oktomvri 53, Skopje. Tel: +389 91 221 133. Fax: +389 91 128 097.
Main Hospital, Vodnjanska BB Skopje. Tel: +389 91 114 244.

MEDICAL CENTRES OUTSIDE SKOPJE:

Bitola Medical center, bb Partizanka, St Bitola. Tel: +389 97 31 211. Fax: +389 97 33 435.
Dr Trifun Panovski Medical Centre, Partizanska BB, Bitola. Tel: +389 251 211/252 448. Fax: +389 253 435.
Gevgelia Medical Centre, Slobodan Mitros-Danko BB, Gevgelija. Tel: +389 89 710/351. Fax: +389 89 693.
Kumanovo Medical Centre, Boris Kidrich 11, Kumanovo. Tel: +389 901 23 621. Fax: +389 20 334.
Medical Centre Borka Taleski, Borka Taleski BB, Prilep. Tel: +389 22 450/430. Fax: +389 22 457.
Ohrid Medical Centre, Sirma Vojvoda BB, Ohrid. Tel: +389 96 34 144. Fax: +389 96 22 749.
Stip Medical Centre, Ljuben Ivanov 25, Shtip. Tel: +389 92 33 666/34 099. Fax: +389 31 357.
Struga Medical Centre, 8 Noemvri BB, Struga. Tel: +389 71 464. Fax: +389 72 142.
Strumitsa Medical Centre, Mladinska BB, Strumitsa. Tel: +389 24 888. Fax: +389 26 448.
Tetovo Medical Centre, 29 Noemvri 16, Tetovo. Tel: +389 32 861/24 988/24 419. Fax: +389 20 148.
Veles Medical Centre, Shefki Sali 5, Veles. Tel: +389 33 322. Fax: +389 33 322/102.

Malta

Population: 400 000
Languages: Maltese and English
Capital: Valletta
Currency: Maltese lira
Int Code: +356

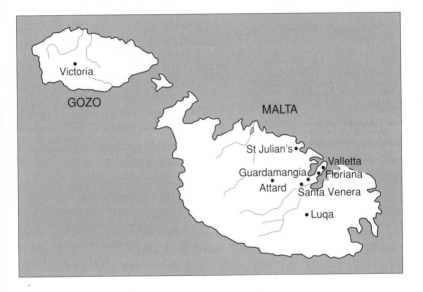

Lying midway between Europe and North Africa, Malta was controlled by a number of colonial powers until its independence from the UK in 1964. A number of islands belong to Malta, but only Gozo and Kemmuna are inhabited. The economy is based mainly around the tourists who visit for the warm climate and beaches. Most people (bar the elderly) can speak both Maltese and English. All doctors' communications are in English.

✪ Medicine:

The Maltese government provides a comprehensive free health service to all Maltese residents. Government health centres and hospitals provide preventa-tive (both education and vaccinations), investigative, curative and rehabilitative services. Those on a low income or with a chronic condition are also entitled to free pharmaceuticals. Private healthcare also exists and is becoming more popu-lar. In total, there are eight healthcare centres providing primary care and a number of hospitals providing secondary and tertiary care. The main teaching hos-pital is St Luke's with 850 beds. This is being replaced with a new (800-bed) hospital next to the university. In total Malta has about 2000 acute beds. There is a shortage of nurses but they have plenty of doctors.

◎ **Climate and crime:**

The climate is similar to Greece, being warmest between July and September (reaching 30°C). The crime rate is pretty low.

➲ **Visas and work permits:**

EU nationals do not require a visa to do an elective. Contact the Maltese embassy for work permits as Malta is not yet part of the EU.

USEFUL ADDRESSES:

Ministry of Health, St Joseph High Road, St Venera. Tel: +356 485 1000. Fax: +356 443 595. www.health.gov.mt.
Maltese Medical Council, Castellania Place, 15 Merchants Street, Valletta. Tel: +356 224 071.
Malta Medical Association, Medisle Village, St Andrews STJ 14. Tel: +356 338 851.
Fax: +356 235 638. www.synapse.net.mt.
Malta Nurses Association, PO Box 63, Hamrun.
Malta Dental Association, Federation of Professional Bodies, Alamein Road, Medisle Village, St Andrews STJ 07.
Malta Association of Physiotherapists, Marwin, Carob Street, Msida MSD 03.
Tel: +356 312 367.
Malta Association of Occupational Therapists, OT Department, St Luke's Hospital, G'Mangia MSD 07. Tel: +356 241 251.
Fax: +356 240 176.

MEDICAL SCHOOL AND HOSPITALS:

Medical School, St Luke's Hospital

MSIDA, Guardamangia 06.
Tel: +356 3290 2224. www.um.edu.mt.
This is the only Maltese medical school and is very well set up for arranging electives (and Socrates/Erasmus programmes). Write to the **Maltese Medical Students Association Exchange Committee** at the above address or look at their website (www.mmsa.org.mt). They operate an 'exchange' programme whereby they try to tie in one of their students going to your country. This is not a problem. If you arrange an exchange, your accommodation is free, if not, it costs £3.75 a night. Elective fees work out at £1.50 a day. The medical

school provides the following specialities: medicine, neurology, O&G, paeds, cardiology, geriatrics, pathology, community medicine, public health, surgery, radiology, ENT, ophthalmology, psychiatry, health information, dermatology, oncology, orthopaedics, dentistry and emergency medicine. These can be arranged in St Luke's or in one of the other hospitals.

St Luke's Hospital

Guardamangia. Tel: +356 241 251/247 860/234 101.
The hospital: St Luke's, the teaching hospital (850 beds) of Malta, is at the top of a very large hill, 1.5 km out of the capital, Valletta. Life is very relaxed and you can join in with this and that as you please. Teaching is good although there is little 'hands on' for students. The beaches nearby are not brilliant, but the water sports are good. The working day usually lasts from 8 am until 2 pm.
Accommodation: See above.

OTHER HOSPITALS:

Boffa Hospital, Floriana. Tel: +356 224 581. Fax: +356 225 705.
Gozo General Hospital, Victoria, Gozo. Tel: +356 561 600. Fax: +356 560 881. (This is a general hospital for those on the island of Gozo. It has 159 beds.)
Mount Carmel Hospital, Attard. Tel: +356 415 183. Fax: +356 415 009. (Malta's main psychiatric hospital, with 625 beds.)
St Philip's Hospital, Psaila St, Santa Venera. Tel: +356 442 211. Fax: +356 446 030.
St Vincent de Paule Residence, Luqa. Tel: +356 224 461/462/463. (A residence for the elderly with over 1000 beds.)
Sir Paul Boffa Hospital, Floriana. Tel: +356 224 491/224 581/245 019/245 091. (A skin cancer, convalescence and fever hospital, it has 110 beds.)
Ta'L-Ibragg Hospital, Gozo. (This is the psychiatric and geriatric hospital for the island of Gozo. It has 100 beds.)
Zammit Clapp Hospital, St Julian's. Tel: +356 344 950. Fax: +356 344 914. (This is a specialized geriatric hospital with 60 beds.)

HEALTH CENTRES:

For primary healthcare contact Dr Ray Busuttil (7 Harper Lane, Floriana VLT

14. Tel: +356 233 393. Fax: +356 233.393). There are eight health centres:

Centru Civiku, Mosta. Tel: +356 433 256/432 062/411 065.
Centru Civiku, Paola. Tel: +356 691 314/315.
Centru Civiku, Rabat. Tel: +356 459 082/083.
Dr Enrico, Mizzi Street, Victoria VCT 107. Tel: +356 561 600.

Pjazza M Scicluna, Gzira GZR 05. Tel: +356 337 245/344 766.
Triq FS Fenech, Florina VLT 14. Tel: +356 243 314/243 315/244 340.
Triq iL-Vitorja/Triq San Dwardu, Qormi. Tel: +356 484 450/451/452/453.
I Triq Sofia, Cospicua CSP 02. Tel: +356 675 492/673 292/673 293.

Monaco

Population: 31 000
Language: French
Capital: Monaco
Currency: French franc
Int Code: +377

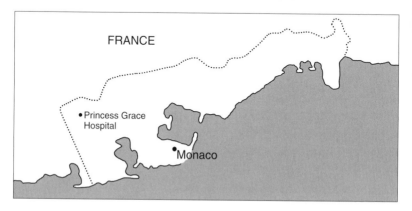

Monaco, on the Côte d'Azur in south-eastern France, is a centre for the international jet-setter. It has a lucrative banking and tourist industry. With this in mind, the healthcare provides for not only its 31 000 citizens but many overseas as well.

⊕ Medicine:

A private healthcare system operates to provide a costly but effective health service. There are no establishments for training doctors. Most come from France. Heart and cerebrovascular diseases with cancers are the big causes of mortality.

⊃ Visas and work permits:

Since 1998, no members of the EU state have needed to obtain a settlement visa to enter Monaco. You will, however, need a *Carte de Séjour Monegasque*. Write directly to the Police Directorate

(Direction de la Sûreté Publique, Section des étrangers, 3 Rue Louis Notari, Monaco-Cedex. Tel: +377 93 15 30 17). Contact the embassy in your country for more details.

HOSPITALS:

Princess Grace Hospital

Avenue Pasteur BP 489, MC 98012. Tel: +377 93 25 99 00. Fax: +377 92 05 91 75.
The hospital: The main hospital in Monaco. Officially founded in 1958, it has been at the forefront of medical advances. There's a maternity unit, good surgical facilities, a nursing school, a geriatric and psychiatric unit and a good radiology department. There are many other units but remember this is a private hospital and the facilities reflect this.

Monaco Cardio-thoracic Centre
CCM 11 bis av D'Ostende-BP 223,
MC 98004. Tel: +377 92 16 80 00.
Fax: +377 92 16 82 99.
E-mail: info@com.mc. www.ccm.mc.

The hospital: Is renowned for its diagnosis and treatment of cardiac disease of all ages, from neonatal to the oldest of patients. Each year, about 800 open heart operations and more than 2000 investigations are performed. In nine years, it has operated on 800 children with congenital heart disease. The permanent team has a particular interest in the reconstruction of the left ventricle after myocardial infarction. Again, this is very much in a private setting. Quoting from the brochure 'All types of accommodation [for patients] are available ... from the adaptable suite, a private room with lounge or office area fitted with a fax to the standard room for two patients.'

The Netherlands

Population: 15.5 million
Language: Dutch
Capital: Amsterdam
Currency: Euro
Int Code: +31

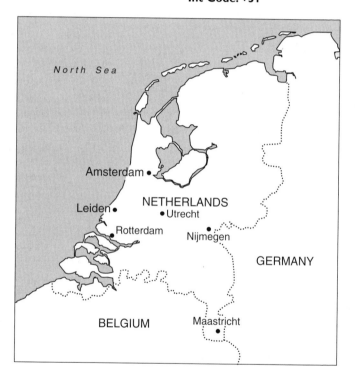

Situated in the north-west of Europe, the Netherlands is best known for its tulips, clogs and flat reclaimed land. It is not a popular elective destination, which is surprising since most Dutch speak English extremely well. In total there are 152 hospitals. A number of these are on the Socrates/Erasmus programme.

☧ Medicine:

The Dutch are covered by three types of insurance-based health system: Exceptional Medical Expenses Compensation is compulsory for everyone and covers acute and long-term expenses. Social Care covers GP care and care of the elderly expenses. Finally, there is a general medical insurance that two-thirds of the population pay into via a compulsory Social Insurance. The other third have to take out private insurance. The public health system requires GP referral to access a specialist.

Hospital consultants get a 'fee for service' directly from the insurance fund. GPs can work in groups or individually and form contracts with the Social Insurance fund.

➲ Visas and work permits:

EU citizens do not need a visa or work permit to go to or work in the Netherlands. They have signed up to the EU agreement on the recognition of EU qualifications, and registration is via the BIG (address below). You should then register with the **Landelijke Huisartsen Vereniging** (National Association of GPs) or **Landelijke van Artsen in Dienstverband** (Association of Hospital Doctors) as appropriate. At present there is no real shortage of doctors or nurses. Medical jobs are sometimes advertised in *Medisch Contact* (via www.knmg.nl) and *Nederlands Tijdschrift voor Geneeskunde*.

USEFUL ADDRESSES:

Ministry of Health, Welfare and Sports:
Ministerie voor Volksgesondheid, Welzijn en Sport, Algemen Gezondheidszorg en Opleidingen, t.a.v. Bureau Buitenslandse Diplomahouders, Postbus 20350, NL-2500 EJ, Den Haag. Tel: +31 70 340 6954/7409/7188. Fax: +31 70 340 7834.
Royal Dutch Medical Association: Koninklijke Nederlandche Maatschaapij tot Bevordering der Geneeskunst (KNMG), Somus Medica, Postbus 20051, NL-2501 LB Utrecht 3526XD.
Tel: +31 30 282 3911. Fax: +31 30 282 3326. www.knmg.nl.
BIG, Postbus 16114, NL-2500 BC Den Haag.
Dutch Nurses Association: Nieuwe Unie '91, Leideseweg 83, Postbus 6001, NL-3503 PA Utrecht. Tel: +31 30 964 144. Fax: +31 30 963 904. www.nu91.nl.
Dutch Dental Association: Nederlandsche Maatschappij tot Bevordering der Tandheelkunde, Geelgors 1, Postbus 2000, NL-3430 CA Nieuwegein. Tel: +31 30 607 6276. Fax: +31 30 604 8994. www.nmt.nl.
Dutch Physiotherapy Association: Koninklijk Nederlands Genootschap Fysiotherapie, Postbus 248, Van Hogendorplan 8, NL-3800 AE Amersfoort. Tel: +31 33 467 2900. Fax: +31 33 467 2999. www.kngf.nl.
Dutch Association of Occupational Therapists: Nederlandse Vereniging van Ergotherapie, Kaap Hoorndreef 48B, NL-3536 AV Utrecht. www.ergotherapie.nl.

Amsterdam

Universiteit van Amsterdam
Faculteit der Geneeskunde, Meibergdreef 15, NL-1105 AZ Amsterdam.
Tel: +31 20 525 9111. www.uva.nl..
This is the oldest medical school in Holland and uses:

Academisch Medisch Centrum
Universiteit van Amsterdam, Meibergdreef 9, Amsterdam, NL-1105 AZ Amsterdam.
Tel: +31 20 566 9111.
The hospital: The Academic Medical Centre is a new hospital, built in the 1970s, and serves a wider catchment population than the older hospital in town. It lies on the metro line about 15 minutes out of town. It is a very pleasant hospital to work in and has a well-known intensive care unit.

Free University (Vrije Universiteit)
Faculteit der Geneeskunde, Van der Boechorststraat 7, NL-1081 BT Amsterdam. www.med.vu.nl.
It uses:

Academisch Ziekenhuis der Vrije Universiteit
Postbus 7057, NL-1007 MB Amsterdam.
Tel: +31 20 444 4444. Fax: +31 20 444 4645. www.azvu.nl.
The hospital: This has 733 beds and provides most specialities. It has a trauma centre and provides Helicopter Emergency Medicine Service (HEMS).

Leiden

Rijksuniversiteit Leiden
Faculteit der Geneeskunde, Wassenaarseweg 62, NL-2333 AL Leiden.
Tel: +31 71 526 4487. Fax: +31 71 526 6882. www.medfac.leidenuniv.nl.
It uses:

Academisch Ziekenhuis Leiden
PO Box 9600, NL-2300 RC Leiden. Tel: +31 71 526 9111.

Maastricht

Universiteit Maastricht/ Rijksuniversiteit Limburg

Faculteit Der Medische Wetenschappen, Medical Education Office, Postbus 616, Dr Tanslaan 10, NL-6200 MD Maastricht. Tel: +31 43 881 448. Fax: +31 43 884 145. www.unimaas.nl.
It uses:

Academische Ziekenhuis Maastricht

PO Box 5800, NL-6202 AZ Maastricht. Tel: +31 43 387 543.

Nijmegen

Katholieke Universiteit Nijmegen – Universitair Medisch Centrum St Radboud

Faculteit Medische Wetenschappen, Geert Grooteplein Noord 9, Postbus 9101, NL-6500 HB Nijmegen.
Tel: +31 24 361 9203. Fax: +31 24 354 0529. www.umcstradboud.nl.
It uses:

Academische Ziekenhuis Radboud

PO Box 9101, NL-6500 HB Nijmegen. Tel: +31 24 361 111.

Rotterdam

Erasmus Universiteit

Faculteit der Geneeskunde, Postbus 1738, Dr Molewaterplein 50, NL-3015 CN Rotterdam. www.eur.nl.
It uses:

Academisch Ziekenhuis Rotterdam

PO Box 70029, Rotterdam. Tel: +31 10 463 9222. Fax: +31 10 463 5306.
The hospital: Has 1304 beds.

Utrecht

Universiteit Utrecht

Faculteit Geneeskunde, Universiteitsweg 100, Postbus 80030, NL-3508 TA Utrecht. Tel: +31 30 253 8888. Fax: +31 30 253 9025. www.med.uu.nl.
It uses:

Academische Ziekenhuis Utrecht

PO Box 8500, NL-3508 GA Utrecht. Tel: +31 30 250 9111.

Norway

Population: 4.5 million
Language: Norwegian
Capital: Oslo
Currency: Norwegian krone
Int code: +47

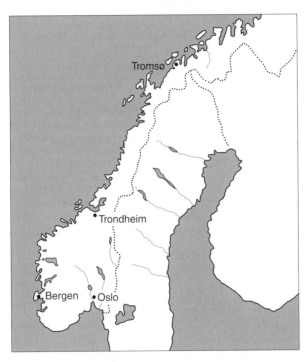

Tromsø

Trondheim

Bergen • Oslo

Norway, the furthest west of the Scandinavian countries, is a beautiful land of fjords and dramatic coastline. Fishing and oil are the mainstays. All doctors can speak English as there are few Norwegian textbooks. Most patients can also speak at least a little.

✛ Medicine:

Norway has an excellent healthcare system. It is very efficient and, even though only 8% of the GDP is spent on it, Norway has one of the lowest infant mortalities and highest life expectancies of any country. Telemedicine has recently been introduced so that people in the far north do not have to travel to receive specialist consultations (working in the north is not that popular). Nearly all care is public although there are five private hospitals. Most GPs work in groups and there is usually a small fee to be seen. Specialists (who are free at the point of need) can only be seen via a GP referral.

Information on working in Norway can be found at www.aetat.no.

⊃ Visas and work permits:

EU, US, Canadian, Australian and New Zealand passport holders can enter without a visa. EU passport holders will need a work/residence permit after three months. Non-EU citizens will need to arrange a work permit in their home country first. Norway has signed up to the reciprocal acceptance of medical qualifications agreed within the EU, and registration is via the Ministry of Health (*Helsetilsynet*; address below). Speicalist qualifications are checked by the Norwegian Medical Association (*Den norske Lægerforening*; address below). They also produce a journal that advertises jobs.

USEFUL ADDRESSES:

Ministry of Health: Helsetilsynet, Postboks 8128, Dep N-0032 Oslo. Tel: +47 22 24 88 88. Fax: +47 22 24 95 75. www.odin.dep.no.
Norwegian Medical Association: Norske Laegeforening, Postboks 1152, Sentrum N-0107 Oslo. Tel: +47 23 10 90 00. Fax: +47 23 10 90 10. www.legeforeningen.no.
Norwegian Nurses Association: Norsk Sykepleierforbund, Postboks 2633, St Hanshaugen N-0131 Oslo. Tel: +47 22 04 33 04. Fax: +47 22 71 60 96.
Norwegian Dental Association: Norske Tannlaegeforening, Frederik Stangs gt 20, N-0264 Oslo. Tel: +47 22 54 74 00. Fax: +47 22 55 11 09. www.tannlegeforeningen.no.
Norwegian Association of Physiotherapists: Norske Fysioterapeutes Forbund, Postboks 7009, Majorstua N-0306 Oslo. Tel: +47 22 69 78 00. Fax: +47 22 56 58 25.
Norwegian Association of Occupational Therapists: Norsk Ergoterapeut Forbund, Lakkegaten 19-21 N-0187 Oslo.

UNIVERSITIES:

There are four universities that teach medicine in Norway. All bar the Norwegian University of Science and Technology also teach nursing.

University of Bergen

Harald Hårfagres gt, N-5020 Bergen.
Tel: +47 55 58 90 22. Fax: +47 55 58 90 25.
www.uib.no/med.
Situated in Norway's second-largest city (population 220 000). This seaport is surrounded by mountains. The school uses:

Haukeland Sykehus
N-5021 Bergen. Tel: +47 55 29 80 60.
Fax: +47 55 97 47 85.
(A modern hospital near the centre of Bergen. There's lots to do with a very busy procedures unit. The elective comes recommended.)

University of Oslo

Postboks 1078, Blindern N-0316 Oslo.
Tel: +47 22 85 50 50. Fax: +47 22 85 44 42.
www.uio.no.
The capital of Norway (population 500 000) is surrounded by hills and forests. Write to the medical faculty at the above address for elective details. It uses:

National Hospital (Rikshospitalet)
Pilestredet 32, N-0027 Oslo. Tel: +47 22 86 70 10.
Fax: +47 22 86 75 80.
(A state-run hospital acting as both a regional and a national referral centre. The hospital encompasses the 'old' National Hospital, the Oslo Rheumatism Hospital (Akersbakken, Oslo) and the National Centre for Orthopaedics (Carl Berners plass, Oslo). It provides a national centre for transplantation, epilepsy surgery, bone marrow transplantation, haemophilia and trans-sexualism. The only things it doesn't do are geriatrics, psychiatry and a few cancer treatments.)
Radiumhospitalet Montello
Ullernchausséen 70, N-0310 Oslo.
Tel: +47 22 93 40 00.
Ullevål University Hospital
Ullevål University Hospital, Kirkeveien 166, N-0407 Oslo. Tel: +47 22 11 80 80. www.ulleval.no. (This is the largest hospital in the country, with over 1200 beds and 60 professors.)
Aker University Hospital
Trondheimsveien 235, N-0514 Oslo. Tel: +47 22 89 40 00. Fax: +47 22 89 41 55. www.aker.uio.no. (This 806-bed hospital serves the north-east portion of Oslo and includes Gaustad Hospital, Norway's oldest psychiatric hospital.)
Akershus University Hospital
Sykehusveien 27, N-1474 Nordbyhagen. Tel: +47 67 92 88 00. Fax: +47 67 90 21 40.

Norway

University of Tromsø

N-9037 Tromsø. Tel: +47 77 64 46 10.
Fax: +47 77 64 53 00. www.uit.no.
The world's most northern university is in Tromsø (population 50 000) and was founded in 1972. It uses:

Regionsykehuset I Tromø
N-9038 Tromsø. Tel: +47 77 62 60 00.
Fax: +47 77 62 60 42.

Norwegian University of Science and Technology

NTNU, N-7034 Trondheim. Tel: +47 73 59 88 59. Fax: +47 73 59 88 65. www.unit.no.
Trondheim is Norway's third-largest city. The university uses:

Regionsykehuset I Trondheim
17 Olav Kyrres gt, N-7006 Trondheim.
Tel: +47 73 99 80 00. Fax: +47 73 99 80 44.

Romania

Population: 23 million
Language: Romanian
Capital: Bucharest
Currency: Leu
Int Code: +40

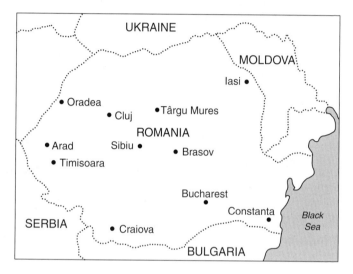

Romania left Communism in 1989 after a coup and has slowly developed a free market economy. It is, however, still very poor. It has some beautiful countryside – the Danube, the Carpathian Mountains – and lies on the Black Sea. Like most of Eastern Europe and Russia it is not a common elective destination.

✛ Medicine:
Romania's health is probably the worst in Europe, TB being highly prevalent. Developed country diseases are also common. HIV has become a real problem, leaving many HIV-positive orphans. Despite a lack of resources, there is no shortage of doctors. This means that an elective here is not really the same as in a deprived country in Africa: you don't get to do as much as you're actually not needed.

◎ Climate:
Romania has a continental climate in the summer but can get bitterly cold with snow in the winter.

➲ Visas and work permits:
A visa is required to enter Romania (contact the embassy), but the fee can be reduced if there is an official exchange. Work permits can only be obtained in Romania.

USEFUL ADDRESSES:

Ministry of Health, 1–3 Strada Ministerului, Bucharest 70109. Tel: +40 1 614 1526.

Romanian Medical Association, Str Progresului 10, Sect. 1, Bucarest 70754. Tel: +40 614 1071. Fax:+40 1 312 1357.

MEDICAL SCHOOLS:

Brasov-Universitatea Transilvania (Transilvania University), Bd Eroilor 29. Tel: +40 6 814 2343. Fax: +40 6 815 0274. www.unitbv.ro.
Bucharest-Universitatea de Medicină si Farmacie Carol Davila (Carol Davila University of Medicine and Pharmacy), 70183 Bucharest, Str Dionisic Lupu 37. Tel: +40 1 210 3108. Fax: +40 1 211 0276. www.univermed-cdgm.ro.
Cluj-Napoca-Universitatea de Medicină si Farmacie Iuliu Hateaganu (Iuliu Hateganu University of Medicine and Pharmacy), Str Emil Isac 13. Tel: +40 6 419 6585. Fax: +40 6 411 7257. www.umfcluj.ro.
Constanta-Universitatea Ovius (Ovidus University), Bd Mamaia 124. Tel: +40 4 161 4576. Fax: +40 4 161 8372.
Craiova-Universitatea Craiova (University of Craiova), Str Al.1, Cuza 13. Tel: +40 5 141 4548. Fax: +40 5 141 1688. www.umfcv.ro.
Iasi-Universitatea de Medicină si Farmacie Grigore T Popa (Griore T Popa University of Medicine and Pharmacy), Str Universitătii 16. Tel: +40 3 211 6104. Fax: +40 3 221 3573. www.edu.ro/umfis.
Oradea-Universitatea Oradea (Oradea University), Str Armatci Romane 5. Tel: +40 5 913 2830. Fax: +40 5 943 2789. www.uoradea.ro.
Sibiu-Universitatea Lucian Blaga (Lucian Blaga University), Bd Victorici 10, R2400. Tel: +40 6 942 2005 Fax: +40 6 921 0512. www.sibiu.ro.
Târgu Mures-Universitatea de Medicină si Farmacie (University of Medicine and Pharmacy), Str Gh Marinesu 38. Tel: +40 6 521 3127. Fax: +40 6 521 0407. www.umftgm.ro.

Timisoara-Universitatea de Medicină si Farmacie (University of Medicien and Pharmacy), Piata Etimie Murgu 2. Tel: +40 5 622 0484. Fax: +40 5 622 0479. www.umft.ro.
Universitatea de Vest (Western University), Facultatea de Medicina, Bulvardul Revolutiei 81, R-2900 Arad. Tel: +40 5 728 0335. Fax: +40 5 728 0810.

SOME SPECIALIST HOSPITALS:

Children's Hospital, Maria Sklodowska Centre, 20 Bdul C Brincoveanu, Bucharest. Tel: +40 1 682 4160.
Colentina Infectious Hospital, Sos Panteliomon, Bucharest. Tel +40 1 201 5070.
Emergency Hospital, 10 Sos Berceni, Sector 4, Bucharest. Tel: +40 1 683 6895.
Municipal University Hospital, 169 Splaiul Independentei, Sector 1, Bucharest. Tel: +40 1 637 2190.

A couple of hospitals in Bucharest that take elective students directly:

Fundeni Hospital
258 Fundeni Road, Bucharest – Z.

Spitalul de Copii Victor Gowoiv
Bd Basarabrei ur 21, Bucharest.
The hospital: A paediatric hospital with a great deal of poverty and very limited resources (no gloves and few drugs). Children get dumped here by parents who don't come back to pick them up. It is the hospital commonly featured on the news.

Russia

Population: 150 million
Language: Russian
Capital: Moscow
Currency: Rouble
Int Code: +7

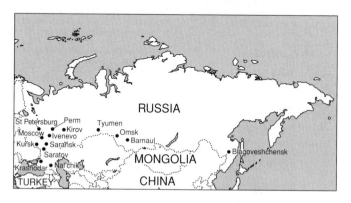

Russia is huge – nearly twice as large as China or the USA. Despite this, it is not a popular destination for Western doctors, nurses or medical students. This is probably mainly because of the language barrier, but the country's economic and political problems (and climate!) don't really help its appeal. That said, there is a desperate need within the healthcare system, and reports from those who have worked with organizations and hospitals have found it very worthwhile.

✪ Medicine:

With Communism a comprehensive healthcare system was provided by employers; however, since its collapse, the now-privatized companies do not have to provide such cover. This is just one way in which Russian people have suffered as they attempt to leave their Communist past. The state itself simply doesn't have the resources to provide an adequate national health service and the cost of private healthcare is way beyond the pocket of most Russians. For that reason, bribery within the profession has become common. There is a shortage of all bar the very basic medications. Patients keep the cost down by supplying their own food and relatives often act as nurses. There is not, as you might imagine, a shortage of doctors (1:220 people). An unusual combination of medical conditions is relatively common. On the one hand, Western diseases (cardiovascular disease and accidents) are prevalent but so are infectious diseases (TB, tick-borne encephalitis and diphtheria). With the Chernobyl disaster, oncological pathology has increased.

Medical students choose at the outset whether they want to do adult, paeds or preventative medicine and are trained in it specifically.

◎ **Climate:**

It is cold, falling to –15°C in winter. The summers can get up to 20°C. The climate obviously varies across such a huge country.

➲ **Visas and work permits:**

You will need to contact the embassy. They have so few elective students that they don't really understand what an elective is. Regarding paid work, no one goes to do that except through an aid agency.

USEFUL ADDRESSES:

Ministry of Health, 8 Rakhmanovsky per, Moscow 101431. Tel: +7 95 923 84 06. Fax: +7 95 292 41 53.
Russian Dental Association, Office 202, 34 Novly Arbat Str, Moscow 121099. Tel: +7 95 205 03 40. Fax: +7 95 205 03 40.

MAIN MEDICAL SCHOOLS:

There are nearly 60 medical schools in Russia and, until recently, virtually no one visited them for electives. With the advent of the Internet and the opening up of Russia, more is known about them. Many now have their own websites. Rather than list all the addresses, some of the medical schools with websites are listed below – for lists of other medical schools and their addresses, check www.medicstravel.com.

Arkhangelsk: Arkhangelsk State Medical Academy, www.asma.ru.
Barnaul: Altai State Medical University, www.medlink.ru/asmu/.
Blagovestchensk: Amur State Medical Academy, www.amursu.ru:8101\.
Chelyabinsk: Chelyabinsk State Medical Academy, Institute of Medical Education, www.vita.chel.su.
Ekaterinburg: Ural State Medical Academy, www.usma.ru.
Ivanovo: Ivanovo State Medical Academy, www.isma.indi.ru.
Kirov: Kirov State Medical Institute, www.ksmi.chat.ru.
Krasnodar: Kuban State Medical Academy, www.ksma.ru.

Kursk: Kursk State Medical University, www.ksmu.kursknet.ru.
Moscow: I.M. Sechenov Moscow Medical Academy, www.mma.ru.
Jewish State Academy (Moscow), Faculty of Medicine, Ulica B. Bronnaja 6, Moscow 103104. Tel: +7 95 122 33 36.
Moscow State University (M.V. Lomonosov), www.fbm.msu.ru.
People's Friendship University of Russia, Faculty of Medicine, www.med.pfu.edu.ru.
Russian State Medical University (RSMU), Medical Faculty, www.chat.ru/~ussrgmu.
Nal'chik: Kabardino-Balkarian State University, Medical Faculty, www.kbsu.ru.
Novgorod: Nizhny Novgorod State Medical Academy, Faculty of Medicine, www.n-nov.mednet.com.
Novgorod State University (Jaroslav the Wise), Faculty of Medicine, www.novsu.ac.ru.
Novosibirsk: Novosibirsk Medical Institute, www.nsu.ru.
Omsk: Omsk State Medical Academy, www.omsk.net.ru/education/vuz/med/fr_eng.htm.
Orenburg: Orenburg State Medical Academy, www.osma.ru.
Perm: Perm State Medical Academy, www.psma.ru.
Ryzan: Ryazan State Medical University, Medical Faculty, www.ttc.ryazan.ru.
St Petersburg: Military Medical Academy, www.mma.spb.ru.
St Petersburg State, Pavlov Medical University, www.spmu.runnet.ru.
Saransk: Mordovian N.P. Ogarev State University, www.mrsu.ru.
Saratov: Saratov State Medical University, www.med.sgu.ru.
Smolensk: Smolensk State Medical Academy, www.smolensk.ru/user/sgma.
Tyumen: Tyumen State Medical Academy (TSMA), www.tsu.tmn.ru.
UFA: Bashkiran State Medical University, www.bsmu.anrb.ru.
Volograd: Volgograd State Medical Academy, www.avtlg.ru/~vlgmed.
Voronezh: Voronezh N.N. Burdenko State Medical Academy, www.vsma.ac.ru.
West Siberia: Siberian State Medical University, www.ssmu.ru/ofice/kaf/mo.html.
Yaroslacl: Yaroslavl State Medical Academy, Medical Faculty, www.gw.yma.ac.ru.

An institution that has previously taken Western volunteers is:

New Life Drug Rehabilitation Centre
47 Karl Marx St, 188450 Kingisepp, St Petersburg.
This is a very friendly group who go into the community to aid drug rehabilitation.

Russia

Slovak Republic

Population: 5.5 million
Language: Slovak
Capital: Bratislava
Currency: Slovak koruna
Int Code: +421

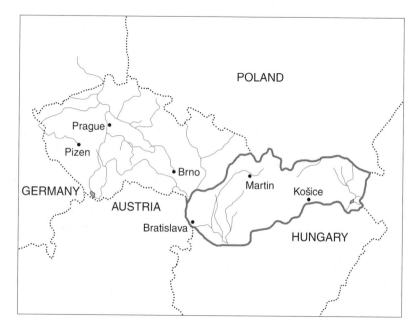

In 1918, Slovakia joined the Czechs to form Czechoslovakia, which then became a Communist nation following World War II. In 1993, the two countries split peacefully. Because of historical, geographical and political factors, it has been slower to Westernize than the Czech republic.

✚ Medicine:

Despite the relative poverty, healthcare is fairly good and Western diseases are the most common causes of death. It has three well-organized medical schools. Possibly because of the language barrier, Slovakia is not commonly visited.

➲ Visas and work permits:

Visas are not required for many countries if you are visiting for fewer than 30 days. Most EU and Canadian citizens can stay for 90 days. US and Italian citizens have a 30-day upper limit, whereas UK citizens have a 180-day maximum. For official study or work, you need a residence permit. For this, you need confirmation of work or place of study, a medical (including HIV test), confirmation of accommodation and a criminal record check in both your home country and Slovakia. All this has to be in Slovak and can take up to 60 days.

Slovak Republic

USEFUL ADDRESS FOR ELECTIVES:

Slovak Medical Students Association (Slovenská asociácia študentov medicíny (SloMSA))

c/o BSM, Sasinkova 2, 813 72 Bratislava. Tel: +421 7 593 57 458. www.slomsa.sk. SloMSA, as well as representing their own students, can help to arrange exchanges in Bratisvala, Martin or Košice. They offer a vast array of electives in each place.

Accommodation: Shared accommodation in a student hostel can usually be provided. Full details are on the web.

USEFUL ADRESSESS:

Ministry of Health, 2 Limbová, 83 341 Bratislama. Tel: +421 7 377 940. Fax: +421 7 377 659.
Slovak Medical Association, Legionarska 4, 81 322 Bratislava. Tel. +421 7 554 24 015. Fax: +421 7 554 23 63.
Slovakian Dental Association, Fibichova 14, 821 05 Bratislava. Tel: +421 2 432 93 122. Fax: +421 2 434 10 518. www.internet.sk/skzl.

MEDICAL SCHOOLS/MAIN HOSPITALS:

Comenius University

Faculty of Medicine (Universita Komenskeho, Lékarská Fakulta), špitálska 24, 811 08 Bratislava. Tel: +421 7 593 57 111. Fax +421 7 593 57 201. E-mail: sd@fmed.uniba.sk. www.fmed.uniba.sk.

The medical faculty was founded in 1919 and has 1500 students, making it the largest and oldest in Slovakia. It uses the Faculty Hospital in Miciewiczova Street, the Faculty Hospital of Academian L. Derer and Paediatric Hospital in Limbova Street, Ruzinov Hospital in Ruzinovska Street and the Hospital of St Cyril and Metod and the Oncological Institute of Al Beta in Heydukova Street.

P.J. Safarik University

(Universita P.J. Safarika) Lékarská Fakulta, Dekanát LFUPJS Košice, Tr SNP è1, PO Box 38, 041 80 Košice. Tel: +421 95 64 28 151. Fax: +421 95 64 28 151. www.upjs.sk. The second-largest medical school in Slovakia has a new large University Hospital as well an old one (L. Pasteur S. Faculty Hospital, 43 Rastislavna, 040 00 Košice. Tel: +421 95 62 25 251).

Comenius University

(Universita Komenskeho) Jesenius Medical Faculty, MaláHora C4, 036 01 Martin. Tel: +421 842 333 05. Fax: +421 842 363 32. The university uses the teaching hospital in Martin (Faculty Hospital, 2 Kollárová, 036 59 Martin. Tel: +421 842 341 31), a town in central Slovakia below the Low Fatra Mountains, 40 minutes from excellent skiing and tourist facilities.

Spain

Population: 40 million
Languages: Spanish, Galician,
Basque and Catalan
Capital: Madrid
Currency: Euro
Int Code: +34

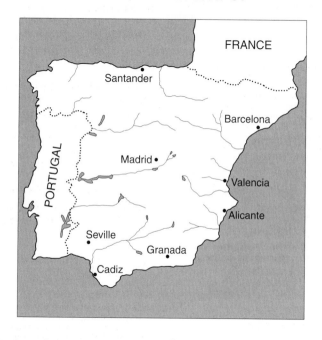

Situated in the south-west corner of Europe, Spain has a beautiful Mediterranean coast and the Pyrenees in the north. There is plenty to see and do as it has a very rich history. However, because it is not a popular elective destination and because the Socrates/Erasmus exchange programme makes it easy to organize electives here, this chapter will not go into much detail. A comprehensive list of hospitals is available from the Spanish embassy or by looking on the Yahoo Spain home page. Fluent Spanish is needed to work or do an elective in most parts of Spain.

✪ Medicine:

The public health service is good and the Spanish tend to be a healthy population. HIV has, however, crept in, and Spain has the second-highest rate in Europe. Spain itself is divided into 17 regions, of which seven (e.g. the Canary Islands and Andalucia) have complete control over their health services. The other ten are run by the National Institute of Health (INSALUD). This is funded by taxes. Around 20% of the population have private insurance. To enter specialist training in Spain (to be either a hospital specialist or a GP), you have to sit the Medico Interno Residente examination (in Spanish). All doctors (even if setting up as a private GP) need to register with the **Colegio de Medicos de la Provincia** (the provincial medical college) they wish to work near, as well as the **Spanish Medical Association**.

➲ **Visas and work permits:**
No visa is required for other EU nationals to enter Spain. Contact the Spanish consulate if you require a work permit.

USEFUL ADDRESSES:

Ministry of Health: Ministerio de Sanidad y Consumo, Paseo del Prado 18–20, 28071 Madrid. Tel: +34 1 596 1000. Fax: +34 1 596 1547.
Spanish Medical Association: Consejo General de Colegios Oficiales de Médicos, Villanueva 11, 28001 Madrid. Tel: +34 91 431 7780.
Fax: +34 91 576 4388. www.cgccom.org.
Spanish Nurses Association: Organización Colegial de Enfermería, Consejo general, c/Don Ramón de la Cruz 67 , E 28001 Madrid.
Tel: +34 91 401 1200. Fax: +34 91 309 3049.
Spanish Dental Association: Alcalá, 79-2, 28009 Madrid. Tel: +34 91 426 4410. Fax: +34 91 577 0639. E-mail: consejo@infomed.es.
Spanish Physiotherapy Association: Asociacion Espanola de Fisioterapeutas, Conde de Penalver 38-2, E 28006 Madrid. Tel: +34 91 401 1136. Fax: +34 91 401 2749.
Spanish Occupational Therapy Association: Asociacion Professional Espanola de terapia Ocupacional, c/o Modesto Lafuente 63 3C, E 28002 Madrid.

MAIN MEDICAL SCHOOLS AND THEIR HOSPITALS:

There are 31 medical schools in Spain. Only those in the main cities will be listed here. A full list can be found on www.medicstravel.org.

Madrid

La Fundacion Universitaria San Pablo (CEU)
Faculdad de Medicina, Paseo Juan XXIII, 3, 28040 Madrid. Tel: +34 15 536 518. Fax: +34 15 336 888. www.ceu.es.

Universidad Autónoma de Madrid
Facultad de Medicina, Arzobispo Morcillo, No. 2, 28029 Madrid. Tel: +34 913 397 5473. Fax: +34 913 397 5353. www.uam.es.
Its affiliated hospitals include:

Fundacion Jimenez Diaz, Clinica de la Concepcion, Avda De Los Reyes Católicos No 2, 28040 Madrid. Tel/fax: +34 543 1071.
Hospital del Niño Jesús, Avda/ Medéddz Pelayo No 65, 28009 Madrid. Tel: +34 504 6193. Fax: +34 504 4612.
Hospital de la Princesa, C/Diego de León No 62, 28006 Madrid. Tel: +34 520 2220. Fax: +34 520 2344.
Hospital Puerta de Hierro, 28040 Madrid. Tel: +34 316 2340.
Hospital Universitario la Paz, C/ Arzobispo Morcillo No 2 y 4, Facultad de Medicina, 28029 Madrid. Tel: +34 397 5495. Fax: +34 91 729 2280.

Universidad Complutense de Madrid
Facultad de Medicina, Ciudad Universitaria, 28040 Madrid.
Tel: +34 91 394 1325. Fax: +34 91 394 1235.
www.ucm.es/info/fmed.
Its associated hospitals include:

Clínica Puerta de Hierro (Hospital Universitario)
C/San Martín de Porred, 4/ 28035 Madrid. Tel: +34 91 316 2240 Fax: 91 316 0535. www.cph.es.

Alicante

Universitat d'Alicante Facultad de Medicina, Carretera San Vicente del Raspeig s/n, 03690 San Vicente del Raspeig, Alicante. Tel: +34 96 565 8529. Fax: +34 96 565 8513. www.enfenet.ua.es.
Universidad Miguel Hernández de Elche, Facultad de Medicina, Carr. Alicante-Valencia, KM. 87, 03550 San Juan, Alicante. Tel: +34 965 919 526. Fax: +34 965 919 528. www.medicina.umh.es.

Barcelona

Universitat de Barcelona
Facultad de Medicina, Calle Casanova, 143, 08036 Barcelona. Tel: +34 93 403 5250. Fax: +34 93 403 5254. www.ub.es/medicina.
As well as the university hospital, the University of Barcelona also uses:

Spain

Vall d'Hebron Hospitals
119–129 08035 Barcelona. Tel: +34 93 489 3000. www.ar.vhebron.es.
The hospitals: The Vall d'Hebron hospitals are a group of four large centres in Catalonia: the **General Hospital**, the **Maternity and Children's Hospital**, the **Traumatology and Rehab Hospital** and the **Adrià Surgical Clinic**, totalling 1400 beds.

Universitat Pompeu Fabra
Facultat de Ciències de la Salut i de la Vida, Doctor Aiguader 80, 08003 Barcelona. Tel: +34 93 542 2801. Fax: +34 93 542 2802. www.upf.es.

Cadiz

Universidad de Cádiz, Facultad de Medicina, Plaza Fragela, 9, 11003 Cadiz. Tel: +34 956 213 923. Fax: +34 956 223 139. www.uca.es/facultad/medicina.

Granada

Universidad de Granada, Facultad de Medicina, Avenida de Madrid 11, 18071 Granada. Tel: +34 958 243 503. Fax: +34 958 291 834. www.ugr.es.

Seville

Universidad de Sevilla, Facultad de Medicina, Avda. Dr. Fedriani, s/n, 41009 Seville. Tel: +34 954 559 826. Fax: +34 954 559 825. www.us.es.

Santander

Universidad de Cantabria
Facultad de Medicina, Edificio Escuela de Enfermería, Avenida de Valdecilla s/n, 39008 Santander. Tel: +34 942 201 990. Fax: +34 942 201 695. www.unican.es.
This uses:

Hospital Universitario Marques De Valdecilla
39008 Santander, Cantabria.

The hospital: The Marques de Valdecilla is the major teaching hospital in Santander, a town on Spain's north-west Atlantic coast. Santander is a compact city with an abundance of good cafes and bars, and a superb night-life. There are good beaches and occasional good surf. The nearby Picos de Europa offer superb walking and climbing.

Valencia

Universidad de Valencia
Facultad de Medicina y Odontologia, Avenida Blasco Ibañez, 17, 46010 Valencia. Tel: +34 96 386 4151. www.uv.es.
One of their hospitals is:

Hospital de Sagunto
Avenida Ramón y Cajal, s/n-46520 Puerto de Sagunto, Valencia. Tel: +34 96 265 9400. Fax: 96 265 9420.
The hospital: Provides general medical and surgical services to part of Valencia.

MEDICAL SCHOOLS ON SOME OF SPAIN'S ISLANDS:

Canary Islands:
Colegio Oficial de Médicos de la Provincia de Santa Cruz de Tenerife, C/ Horacio Nelson 17, 38006 Santa Cruz de Tenerife. Tel: +34 922 271 431. www.comtf.es. (This use the Hospital Universitario de Canarias, Carretera Cuest-Taco s/n, Santa Cruz de Tenerife. Tel: +34 922 645 411.)
Universidad de la Laguna, Facultad de Medicina, Campus de Ofra s/n, Ctra. Gral. La Cuesta-Taco, s/n, 38071 La Laguna de Tenerife. Tel: +34 922 319 277. Fax: +34 922 319 279. www.ull.es.
Universidad de Las Palmas de Gran Canaria, Facultad de Medicina, Campus Universitario de San Cristóba, c/ Doctor Pasteur s/n, 35016 Las Palmas de Gran Canaria. Tel: +34 928 452 701. Fax: +34 928 452 784.

Malaga:
Universidad de Málaga, Facultad de Medicina Málaga, Campus de Teatinos, Colonia de Santa Ives, 29071 Malaga. Tel: +34 95 213 1542. Fax: +34 95 213 3442. www.medicina.uma.es.

Mallorca:

Hospital Son Durota, 55 Andrea Doria, 07014 Palma de Mallorca. Tel: +34 71 175 000. Fax: +34 71 175 500.

Complejo Hospitalario de Mallorca, Plaçe de la Sang, 07012 Palma de Mallorca. Tel: +34 71 728 484. Fax: +34 71 717 140.

Menorca:

Hospital Vergo del Toro, Barcelona 3 07701 Mao, Menorca. Tel: +34 71 157 700. Fax: +34 71 378 338.

Ibiza:

Hospital Can Misses, Barrio Can Misses, 07800 Ibiza. Tel: +34 71 312 412.

Sweden

Population: 8.8 million
Language: Swedish
Capital: Stockholm
Currency: Krona
Int Code: +46

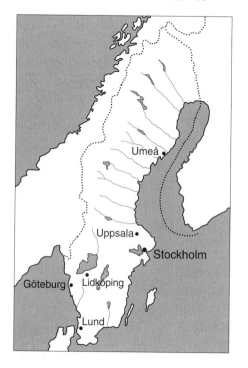

Sweden (a member of the EU since 1995) reaches high into the Arctic Circle and is situated between Finland and Norway. Most of the country is dense forest. Many people can speak English, but despite that it is not a common elective destination. Electives can be arranged through the Socrates/Erasmus programme.

✪ Medicine:

Sweden spends less of its GNP (8.8%) on healthcare than nearly every other country in Europe and is trying to reduce it still further. Despite this, it manages to have the second-lowest infant mortality and fifth-highest life expectancy in the world. This says a great deal about their well-run comprehensive healthcare system. A GP consultation costs 100SEK (£10), but hospital care is free. For chronic disorders, there is a ceiling of 1500SEK (£150). Private practice has only recently become available.

◎ Climate:

It's pretty cold all the time but really cold in winter and extremely cold in the north, where the Baltic Sea often freezes.

➲ Visas and work permits:

EU passport holders do not require a visa to stay or work in Sweden for up to three months. If staying or working for longer, a residence permit and working permit are required. Other nationals, including those from Australia, New Zealand and the USA, also do not require a visa to visit. The **National Board of Health and Welfare** will register general and specialist medical qualifications, but do contact the **Swedish Medical Association** as they can provide futher information. There is currently a surplus of doctors. Posts are advertised in the Swedish Medical Journal (*Läkartidningen*).

USEFUL ADDRESSES:

Ministry of Health, 26 Jakobsgt, S-103 33 Stockholm. Tel: +46 8 405 1000. Fax: 8 723 11 91.
National Board of Health and Welfare, S-106 30 Stockholm. Tel: +46 8 555 530 00.
Fax: +46 8 555 532 52.
Swedish Medical Association: Sveriges Läkarförbund Villagatan, 5 PO Box 5610, S-114 86 Stockholm. Tel: +46 8 790 3300.
Fax: +46 8 20 5718. www.slf.se.
Swedish Nurses Association: Östermalmsgatan 19, S-114 26 Stockholm. Tel: +46 8 412 2400.
Fax: +46 8 412 2424. www.swenurse.se. (Note: There is a Swedish Association of Trauma Nurses; visit www.trauma.c.se.)
Swedish Dental Association: Svierges Tandläkarförbund, Box 5843, S-102 48 Stckholm.
Tel: +46 8 666 1500 Fax: +46 8 662 5842.
www.tandlakarforbundet.se.
Swedish Physiotherapy Association: Legitimerade Sjukgymnasters Riksförbund, PO Box 3196, S-10363 Stockholm. Tel +46 8 696 9745.
Fax: +46 8 696 9754. www.lsr.se.
Swedish Occupational Therapy Association, PO Box 760, S-13 124 Nacka.

MEDICAL SCHOOLS AND HOSPITALS:

Karolinska Institutet

SE-171 77 Stockholm. Tel: +46 8 728 6400.
Fax: +46 8 310 343. www.ki.se.
Founded in 1810, the capital's medical school has a good reputation for research. The university only does medicine and uses:
Södersjukhuset Hospital, 118 83 Stockholm.

Lund University

Medicinska Fackulteten, Box 117, S-221 01 Lund. Tel: +46 222 7219. Fax: +46 222 4170. www.medfak.lu.se.
Founded in 1666, Lund University uses:

Lund University Hospital

S-22100 Lund. Tel: +46 46 17 7502.
Fax: +46 46 14 7327.
The hospital: The medical school and hospital (built in 1968) are large institutions with a great deal of history. Most diseases are typical of the West. There are no general medical wards. Patients are admitted to an acute ward and then transferred to the relevant speciality. Write to the elective committee to do an elective here. Lund can arrange electives in more peripheral hospitals as well and also sort out accommodation.

Göteborg University

Medicinaregatan 16, SE-413 90 Göteborg.
Tel: +46 31 773 1000. Fax: +46 31 773 3866. www.medfak.gu.se.
This uses:

Sahlgrenska University Hospital

(Sahlgrenska Universtetssjukhuset), S-413 45 Göteborg. Tel: +46 31 342 1000).
The hospital: This is one of the biggest hospitals in Europe and has been created by the fusion of six smaller hospitals. You'll be hard pushed to find a speciality not catered for.

Universitetet I Uppsala

Medicinska Fakulteten, Box 256, S-751 05 Uppsala. Tel: +46 18 471 0000. Fax: +46 18 471 1600. www.medfak.uu.se.
For detailed information on their participation in the Socrates/Erasmus programme, visit www.inter.uadm.uu.se.
Uppsala uses:

Uppsala University Hospital

S-751 85 Uppsala. Tel: +46 18 663 000.
Fax: 18 508 127. www.uas.se.
The hospital: This is a large, 924-bed hospital with a vast array of specialities.

Sweden

Umeå University

Faculty of Medicine, SE-901 87 Umeå.
Tel: +46 90 165 000. Fax: +46 90 167 660.
www.umu.se.

Linköping University

Faculty of Health Sciences,
Hälsouniversitetet, Universitetssjukhuset,
SE-581 85 Linköping. Tel: +46 13 222 000.
www.hu.liu.se.

Switzerland

Population: 7.2 million
Official Languages: German,
French and Italian
Capital: Bern
Currency: Swiss franc
Int Code: +41

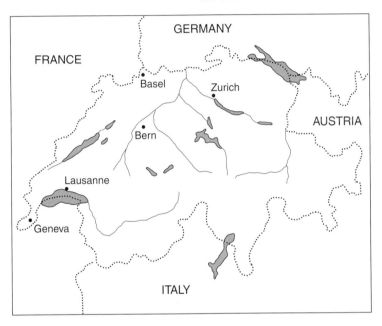

Despite being right in the middle of Europe, Switzerland has managed to avoid European politics and remained neutral in all conflicts. It has many rivers and the Alps in the south, with some excellent ski resorts. Like much of Europe, it is surprisingly not a popular elective destination. The universities and many of the hospitals are, however, on the web.

✚ Medicine:

The healthcare costs of Switzerland are covered by compulsory insurance schemes (amounting to 8% of the GNP). From this, the Swiss have built up a very efficient and advanced health service.

◎ Climate:

This obviously depends on altitude. The Alps can get extremely cold, but away from them it is considerably warmer.

➲ Visas and work permits:

The embassy states that full-time students require a residence permit. Send a CV, proof of acceptance by the university, proof of finances and three photographs to the Swiss Embassy. To work in Switzerland as a medical practitioner, you need the Swiss qualifications and a work permit.

USEFUL ADDRESSES:

Federation of Swiss Medical Doctors:
Verbindung der Schweizer Aerzte/Fédération des
médecins Suisses, Elfenstrasse 18, CH-3000 Bern
16. Tel: +41 31 359 1111. Fax: +41 31 359 1112.
Swiss Nurses Association: Association Suisse
des Infirmières et Infirmiers, Cade Postale,
CH-3001 Bern. Tel: +41 31 388 3636.
Fax: +41 31 388 3635.
Swiss Dental Association: Société Suisse
d'Odonto-Stomatologue, Münzagraben 2, CH-3000
Bern 7. Tel: +41 31 311 7628. Fax: +41 31 311 7470.
Swiss Association of Physiotherapists:
Fédération Suisse des Physiothérapeutes,
Oberstadt 8, CH-6204 Sempach-Stadt.
Tel: +41 41 462 7050. Fax: +41 41 462 7061.
www.physioswiss.ch.
Swiss Association of Occupational Therapists:
Association Suisse des Ergothérapeutes,
Stauffacherstrasse 96, Postfach, CH-8026 Suricj.
Tel: +41 1 242 5464. Fax: +41 1 291 5440.

MEDICAL SCHOOLS:

Universität Basel, Medizinische Fakultät,
Hebelstrasse 25, CH-4031 Basel. Tel: +41 61 267
3029. Fax: +41 61 267 3003. www.unibasel.ch.

Universität Bern, Medizinische Fakultät,
Murtenstrasse 11, CH-3010 Bern. Tel: +41 31 632
3553. Fax: +41 31 632 4994. www.unib.ch.
Université de Genève, Faculté de Médecine,
Anée d'Etudes à Option, CMU, I rue Michel
Servet, CH-1211 Geneva. Tel: +41 22 702 5111.
Fax: +41 22 347 3334. www.medecine.unige.ch.
(They use Cantonal Universitaire Hopital, Rue
Micheli du Crest 24, Geneva 14. Tel: +41 22 372
3311. Fax: +41 22 347 6486.)
Université de Lausanne, Faculté de Médecine,
CH-1005 Lausanne. Tel: +41 21 692 1111.
Fax: +41 21 692 2015. www.unil.ch/med.
Universität Zürich, Medizinische Fakultät
Rämistrasse, CH-8091 Zurich. Tel: +41 1 634 1063.
Fax: +41 1 634 1079. www.med.unizh.ch. (They use
Universitätsspital Zürich, Rämistrasse 100,
CH-8091 Zurich. Tel: +41 1 255 1111.
Fax: +41 1 255 4444.)

HOSPITAL ASSOCIATIONS:

**H+ Schweizerische Vereinigung der Privat-
kliniken/Association Suisse des Cliniques
privées,** Moosstrasse 2, CH-3073 Gümligen.
Die Spitäler der Schweiz/H+ les Hôpitaux de
Suisse, Rain 32, 5001 Aarau.

Turkey

Population: 62 million
Language: Turkish
Capital: Ankara
Currency: Turkish lira
Int Code: +90

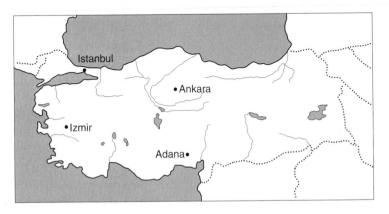

Turkey is in an unusual situation. It is 'nearly Europe' (and trying to join the European community), but its Islamic status pulls it eastwards. Most people live in the west, whereas the east and south-east are Kurdish areas. Work and electives here are relatively unusual, hence only major institutions are listed below. Turkey has recently suffered terrorist attacks. Check with the Foreign Office (www.fco.gov.uk) before arranging work or electives here.

✛ Medicine:

A national health service provides care for all; however, it is underequipped. There are 35 medical schools.

USEFUL ADDRESSES:

Ministry of Health, Saglik Bakanligi, Yenisehir, Ankara. Tel: +90 312 431 2486. Fax: +90 312 433 9885.
Turkish Medical Association: GMK Bulvari Sehit Danis Tunaligil Sok. No:2 Kat: 4, Maltepe 06570, Ankara. Tel:+90 312 231 3179. Fax: +90 312 231 1952.

Turkish Dental Association, Ziya Gökalp Caddesi Bo:37/11, Kizilay, Ankara 06410. Tel: +90 312 435 9394. Fax: +90 312 430 2959.

SOME MEDICAL SCHOOLS:

Adana

Çukurova Üniversitesi
Tip Fakültesi, Balcaly´ 01330, Adana.
Tel: +90 322 338 6084 Fax: +90 322 338 6945. www.cu.edu.tr.

Ankara

Gazi Üniversitesi
Tip Fakültesi, Balgat, Ankara. Tel: +90 312 223 7467. Fax: +90 312 212 4647.
www.med.gazi.edu.tr.
This uses:

Ankara Numune Hospital
Ankara. Tel: +90 312 310 3545.
The hospital: Founded in 1881, the Ankara University Hospital is the biggest postgraduate service hospital (1250–1700 beds) and offers a full range of specialities. The emergency department sees 20 000 patients a year.

Istanbul

Istanbul Üniversitesi
Tip Fakültesi, Kocamustafa Pasa Caddesi, Aksaray 34303, Istanbul.
Tel: +90 212 588 4800. Fax: 212 632 0050.
www.ctf.istanbul.edu.tr.
It uses:

University of Istanbul Faculty of Medicine Hospital
Gapa, Istanbul. Tel: +90 212 534 0000.
Fax: +90 212 532 6066.

Marmara Üniversitesi
Tip Fakültesi, Tibbiye Caddesi, Haydarpasa, 81010 Istanbul. Tel: +90 216 336 0212.
Fax: +90 216 414 4731.
www.marun.edu.tr.

This uses Haydarpap Numune Hospital, which was established in 1903 and has grown to house 700 beds and level 1 trauma and tertiary referral centres.

Izmir

Ege Üniversitesi
Medical School, 35100 Bornova, Izmir. Tel: +90 232 388 1023. Fax: +90 232 342 2142. http://medicine.ege.edu.tr.
Founded in 1955, it uses the 1733 bed hospital of Ege University (Bornova, Izmir. Tel: +90 232 388 1920. Fax: +90 232 388 2852).

Dokuz Eylul Üniversitesi
Tip Fakültesi, Mithatpasa, Incirati, Izmir.
Tel: +90 232 277 7777. Fax: +90 232 259 0541. www.deu.edu.tr.
This is a relatively modern medical school founded in 1982. It uses:

Dokuz Eylul University Hospital
Dokuz Eylul Üniversitesi Tip Fakültesi, Arastrima Ve Uygulama, Hastanesi, Bilgi Islem Merkezi Izmir.

United Kingdom

Population: 58 million
Language: English
Capital: London
Currency: Pound
Int Code: +44

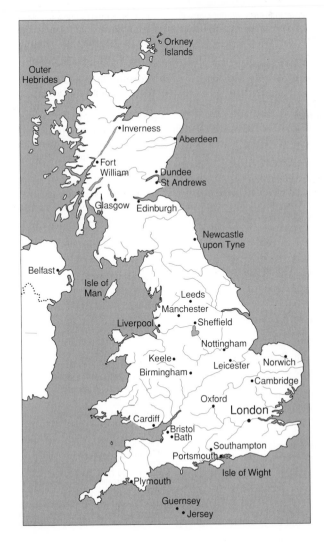

Orkney
Islands

Outer
Hebrides

•Inverness

•Aberdeen

•Fort
William

•Dundee
St Andrews

Glasgow Edinburgh

Newcastle
upon Tyne

Belfast•

Isle of
Man

•Leeds
•Manchester
Liverpool• •Sheffield

Nottingham•

Keele•
Birmingham• Leicester• Norwich

•Cambridge

Oxford
• London

Cardiff

•Bristol
•Bath
Southampton
Portsmouth
Isle of Wight

•Plymouth

Guernsey
• Jersey

The UK (England, Wales, Scotland and Northern Ireland) to many people reading this is 'home', a land in, but slightly separated from, the rest of Europe. Many medics from overseas spend some time here, and many students stay here for their elective period. Why? In the UK, there are no safaris, no sun-drenched beaches and no natural wonders. There's also little risk of heat stroke, no risk of rabies or malaria, and you're unlikely to break any bones skiing. It is however, a great place to see some historic institutions and experience one of the many vibrant cities. If it's home and you are broke, staying here can keep things cheap. It can also be a safety net if other plans fall through. If you're visiting, however, it can be expensive. Always enquire about the cost of accommodation when applying.

✪ Medicine:

The UK uses the National Health Service, a system whereby the state provides (nearly) all healthcare needs for everyone. This includes both GP and hospital treatment, although patients have to pay a modest charge for prescriptions. Because of the increasing demand on hospital services, waiting times for non-urgent cases are getting very long. This is encouraging more and more people to turn to private medicine. Common conditions are those of any developed nation – cardiovascular disease and cancer.

◎ Climate and crime:

It doesn't rain all year – just the winter mainly. There is quite a variation between north Scotland and the south coast. Crime is mainly confined to inner-city areas. Because of the paucity of guns, penetrating trauma is comparatively rare compared with many other countries.

➲ Visas and work permits:

Requirements vary greatly depending on nationality. Those coming from New Zealand and Australia to work can easily obtain a two-year working holiday visa if they are under 26. Most hospitals, however, would rather you had a training permit. The conversion is usually not a problem once you're in the UK. The UK recognizes medical qualifications from the EU countries listed at the beginning of this chapter. For other medical qualification enquiries, contact the **General Medical Council** (address below). If you are coming from a non-English-speaking country, you may well have to sit the PLAB (a language test) before you can do much else.

Full details of how to arrange work in the UK for all types of medical professional is available from the Department of Health website at www.doh.gov.uk/international-recruitment.

Working in the UK:

There are currently fantastic opportunities for all health professionals. The government is actively trying to recruit overseas doctors and nurses (since most of theirs seem to have gone to Australia!). This means that things are being made much easier and relocation packages are available. Full details are on the **Department of Health** website (see below). UK hospitals vary widely, often depending on the area they are in. For details on training as a doctor in the UK, visit www.doh.gov.uk/medicaltrainingintheuk.

USEFUL ADDRESS:

Department of Health, Richmond House, 79 Whitehall, London SW1A 2NS. Tel: +44 20 7210 4850. www.doh.gov.uk.

PROFESSIONAL ORGANIZATIONS:

Doctors:

British Medical Association, BMA House, Tavistock Square, London WC1H 9LP, Tel: +44 20 7383 6177. Fax: +44 20 7383 6220. www.bma.org.uk.
General Medical Council, 44 Hallam Street, London W1N 6AE. Tel: +44 20 7580 7642. Fax: +44 20 7915 3641. www.gmc-uk.org.
Royal College of Physicians of Edinburgh, 9 Queen Street, Edinburgh EH2 1JQ. Tel: +44 131 225 7324. Fax: +44 131 225 2053. www.rcpe.ac.uk.
Royal College of Surgeons of Edinburgh, Nicholson Street, Edinburgh EH8 9DW.

Tel: +44 131 527 1600. Fax: +44 131 557 646. www.rcsed.ac.uk.
Royal College of Physicians and Surgeons of Glasgow, 242 St Vincent Street, Glasgow G2 5RJ. Tel: +44 141 221 6072. Fax: +44 141 248 3414. www.rcpsglasg.ac.uk.
Royal College of Physicians of London, 11 St Andrew Place, Regent's Park, London NW1 4LE. Tel: +44 20 7935 1174. Fax: +44 20 7486 4514. www.rcplondon.ac.uk.
Royal College of Surgeons of England, 35/43 Lincoln's Inn Fields, London WC2A 3PN. Tel: +44 20 7405 3474. Fax: +44 20 7973 2179. www.rcseng.ac.uk.
Royal College of Anaesthetists, 48–49 Russell Square, London WC1B 4JY. www.rcoa.ac.uk.
Royal College of Obstetricians and Gynaecologists, 27 Sussex Place, Regents Park, London NW1 4RG. Tel: +44 20 7772 6263. Fax: +44 20 7772 6359. www.rcog.org.uk.
Royal College of Ophthalmologists, 17 Cornwall Terrace, Regents Park, London NW1 4QW. Tel: +44 20 7935 0702. Fax: +44 20 7935 9838. www.rcophth.ac.uk.
Royal College of Pathologists, 2 Carlton House Terrace, London SW1Y 5AF. Tel: +44 20 7930 5863. Fax: +44 20 7321 0523. www.rcpath.org.
Royal College of Psychiatrists, 17 Belgrave Square, London SW1X 8PG. Tel: +44 20 7235 2351. Fax: +44 20 7245 1231. www.rcpsych.ac.uk.
Royal College of Radiologists, 38 Portland Place, London W1N 4JQ. Tel: +44 20 7636 4432. Fax: +44 20 7323 3100. www.rcr.ac.uk.

Nurses:
Royal College of Nursing,20 Cavendish Square, London W1M 0AB. Tel: +44 20 7409 3333. Fax: +44 20 7355 1379. www.rcn.org.

Midwives:
Royal College of Midwives, 15 Mansfield Street, London W1M 0BE. Tel: +44 20 7312 3535. Fax: +44 20 7312 3536. www.rcm.org.uk.

Dentists:
British Dental Association, 64 Wimpole Street, London W1M 8AL. Tel: +44 20 7935 0875. Fax: +44 20 7487 5232. www.bda-dentistry.org.uk.
General Dental Council, 37 Wimpole Street, London W1M 8DQ. Tel: +44 20 7887 3800. Fax: +44 20 7224 3294. www.gdc-uk.org.

Physiotherapists:
Charted Society of Physiotherapy, 106–114 Borough High Street, London SE1 1LB. Tel: +44 20 7357 6480. Fax: +44 20 7450 2299. www.csphysio.org.uk.

Occupational therapists:
British Association of Occupational Therapists, 6–8 Marchalsea Road, London SE1 1HL. Tel: +44 20 7357 6480. Fax: +44 20 7378 1353. www.cot.org.uk.

Speech and language therapists:
Royal College of Speech and Language Therapists, 2/3 White Hart Yard, London SE1 1NX. Tel: +44 20 7378 1200. Fax: +44 20 7403 7254. www.rcslt.org.

Pharmacists:
Royal Pharmaceutical Society of Great Britain, 1 Lambeth High Street, London SE1 1NX. Tel: +44 20 7735 9141. Fax: +44 20 7735 7629. www.rpsgb.org.uk.

Radiographers:
Society of Radiographers, 2 Carriage Row, 183 Eversholt Street, London NW1 1BU. Tel: +44 20 7391 4500. Fax: +44 20 7391 4504.

Northern Ireland Council for Postgraduate Medical Education, 5 Annadale Avenue, Belfast BT7 3JH. Tel: +44 1232 491731. Fax: +44 1232 642279.

Note: The UK is a very popular destination for overseas elective students. Apply VERY EARLY (a year in advance is often necessary). Most places will only take you for a maximum of eight weeks and only if you are in your final year. Some places charge, whereas others don't and provide free accommodation.

ENGLAND

Birmingham University Medical School
Edgbaston, Birmingham B15 2TT.
Tel: +44 121 414 3344 Fax: +44 121 414036.
www.bham.ac.uk.
The university and medical school are about 10 km (6 miles) from the centre of Birmingham. **Queen Elizabeth Hospital** (Edgbaston, Birmingham. Tel: +44 121 472 1311) is the main teaching hospital, although others, both in and around Birmingham, are also used. These include **Birmingham Women's/Maternity Hospital** (Edgbaston, Birmingham. Tel: +44 121 472 1377), **City Hospital** (Dudley Road, Birmingham B18. Tel: +44 121 554 3801), the **Children's Hospital** (Steelhouse Lane, Birmingham B4. Tel: +44 121 333 9999) and the **Royal Orthopaedic Hospital** (The Woodlands,

Bristol Rd, Birmingham. Tel: +44 121 685 4000).

There is not a great deal to do in the centre (shops and a few theatres), but around the hospital there's a good young social life. Outside you can explore the Midlands. Electives can be arranged in any department. There is an administration charge of £100. Some hospitals provide free accommodation; others charge around £35 a week.

Bristol University Medical School
Clinical Dean's Office, Dolphin House, BRI, Bristol BS2 8HW. Tel: +44 117 928 8333. Fax: +44 117 934 9854. www.bris.ac.uk.

Bristol is a fairly compact town, and the medical school and its hospitals have some pioneering departments. The main teaching hospital is the **Bristol Royal Infirmary** (Marlborough Street, Bristol BS2. Tel: +44 117 923 0000), but there are a couple of others (including **Bristol General**, Guinea Street, Bristol BS3. Tel: +44 117 926 5001) in the city and many DGHs outside that are also used. Electives can be arranged in most subjects depending on availability (the school has to see whether any consultants are able to take you). There are no elective fees and accommodation is provided free. This is a popular elective destination. Apply at least a year in advance.

University of Cambridge
Addenbrooke's Hospital, Faculty of Medicine, Hills Road, Cambridge CB2 2QQ. Tel: +44 1223 336700. Fax: +44 1223 336709. www.cam.ac.uk.

Cambridge has a reputation for academic excellence. **Addenbrooke's Hospital** (address as above. Tel: +44 1223 245151) reflects this, being a large (900-bed), well-run hospital with nearly all specialities provided on-site. It is particularly well known for its liver and kidney transplant services, but other specialities, including paeds, neurology and neurosurgery, are also very highly regarded. Cardiothoracic surgery is done at **Papworth Hospital** (Papworth Everard. Tel: +44 1480 830541), about

30 minutes away by car. The town itself (two miles from the hospital) is very much a university town. There's an excellent college social life so get involved with the local students. Other hospitals include **Hinchingbrooke Hospital** (Hinchingbrooke Park, Huntingdon. Tel: +44 1480 416416) and the **West Suffolk Hospital** (Hardwick Lane, Bury St Edmunds. Tel: +44 1284 713000). Electives can be arranged in most subjects. There is an administration charge of £150, and accommodation can be provided on the Addenbrooke's hospital site for £25 a week.

Peninsula Medical School, University of Exeter and Plymouth
Tamar Science Park, Davy Road, Plymouth PL6 8BX. Tel: +44 1752 764261. Fax: +44 1752 764226. www.pms.ac.uk.

This is the new medical school for the south-west of England, a beautiful area with a great deal to offer. Hospitals used include those run by Plymouth, Royal Devon and Exeter, and North and South Devon NHS Trusts.

Keele University, School of Medicine
60 The Covert, Keele, Staffordshire ST5 5BG. Tel: +44 1782 583937. Fax: +44 1782 583903. www.keele.ac.uk.

This is a new medical school that has only just started taking students for the full five years. Check their website for further details.

Leeds University School of Medicine
Worsley Medical and Dental Building, University of Leeds, Leeds LS2 9JT. Tel: +44 113 233 4361. Fax: +44 113 233 4373. www.leeds.ac.uk/medicine/home.html.

Leeds is a hilly city in the north of England. The main hospital, **St James' University Hospital** (Beckett Street, Leeds LS9 7TF. Tel: +44 113 243 3144), has found fame through the long-running TV series *Jimmy's*. This hospital has every speciality under the sun. The other main hospital is **Leeds General**

Infirmary (Great George Street, Leeds LS1. Tel: +44 113 243 2799).

The University of Leeds will only permit visiting students between June and October, and attachments outside this will not be considered. They will, however, try to provide hospital accommodation free of charge. A £50 non-refundable fee is charged to cover the cost of a blood test on arrival to ensure hepatitis B status. Applications should be made six months in advance and no later than February. The minimum stay is four weeks, the maximum ten.

Leicester University Medical School
Morris Shock Building, PO Box 138, Leicester. Tel: +44 116 252 2295/2969. Fax: +44 116 252 3013. www.lwmc.ac.uk.
This is one of the UK's youngest medical schools, situated just a few minutes' walk from the city centre. Its main hospital is **Leicester Royal Infirmary** (Infirmary Close, Leicester LE1 5WW. Tel: +44 116 254 1414. www.lri.org.uk), but others used include **Leicester General** (Gwendolen Road, Leicester. Tel: +44 116 249 0490), the **Glenfield** (Groby Road, Leicester LE3 9QP. Tel: +44 116 287 1471) and a number of DGHs. Leicester itself is a fairly small town but has plenty of pubs and restaurants. Electives can be done in most subjects. There is no elective charge, and accommodation is provided free.

University of Liverpool
Faculty of Medicine, 1st Floor, Duncan Building, Daulby Street, Liverpool L69 3GA. Tel: +44 151 706 2000/4263. Fax: +44 151 709 2601/5667. www.liv.ac.uk.
This is very large, with nearly 1000 students. It is part of the **Royal Liverpool University Hospital** (Prescot Street, Liverpool. Tel: +44 151 706 2000). This hospital offers most specialities and has a very busy emergency department (possibly the largest in Europe).

There are a number of specialist hospitals within Liverpool. The **Broadgreen** (Thomas Drive, Liverpool L14. Tel: +44 151 282 6000) and **Alder Hey**

Children's Hospital (Eaton Rd, Liverpool L12 2AP. Tel: +44 151 228 4811) are in the suburbs. The Alder Hey is a very large paediatric hospital with 25 wards catering for everything from medicine and surgery to intensive care, psychiatry and emergency medicine. There are many specialized clinics. Other specialist hospitals include the **Liverpool School of Tropical Medicine** (Pembroke Place, Liverpool L3. Tel: +44 151 708 9393), the **Liverpool Women's Hospital** (Crown Street, Liverpool L8. Tel +44 151 708 9988) and the **Walton Centre for Neurology and Neurosurgery** (Rice Lane, Liverpool L9. Tel: +44 151 525 3611).

The university is a keen player on the Socrates/Erasmus exchange programme, but unfortunately says that this restricts it to only accepting elective students from the UK and the rest of the EU. It is still worth asking if you are from outside this area, but if they can't take you, try applying to the hospital/NHS trust directly. Some hospitals (such as the Alder Hey) have previously been able to provide free accommodation.

Liverpool is a vibrant city with plenty of night-life (home to the Beatles) and a world-famous football team. The people are genuine and friendly. There is, however, quite a bit of crime about. Just be careful with your valuables.

London

London, the capital of the UK, has everything to offer a visiting medic. There are some world-class institutions set in a vibrant, busy city. There are many attractions, from the usual tourist traps to the many and varied bars and clubs. London is known for being expensive and with good reason. However, if you budget carefully, there's no reason why it need be any more expensive than anywhere else. Accommodation can be costly, so try and arrange this as early as possible. London is home to a very diverse range of people and this has a big impact on the type of medicine seen. The West End tends to be relatively well off, whereas the East End has areas of real poverty and many immigrants. Only a few years ago there were ten medical schools that were principally affiliated to one hospital each (e.g. Bart's Medical School was at Bart's Hospital). For better or worse, it was decided that all the medical schools should merge and join multifaculty universities. Today, this means that there are technically only five medical schools in London. However, the original hospitals are all still present. It has been worked so that there is a north, south, east and west school. St George's is a little further out in south London. Whichever you visit they are all on the tube and hence give easy access to the night-life and attractions of central London.

Royal Free and University College Medical School

Gower Street, London WC1E 6BT. Tel: +44 20 7679 2000. Fax: +44 20 7383 2462. www.ucl.ac.uk.
Royal Free site: Rowland Hill Street, London NW3 2PF. Tel: +44 20 7830 2686. Fax: +44 20 7435 4359.

In the early 1990s, University College Hospital (UCH) Medical School merged with the Middlesex Hospital Medical School. More recently, the Royal Free has also been engulfed. The new medical school is based in the heart of the London's West End, near Oxford Street. It is now huge, using smaller hospitals such as the **Whittington**, many specialist hospitals such as **Great Ormond Street** and the **National Hospital for Neurology and Neurosurgery** as well as its original teaching hospitals. Because of the merger, the situation regarding electives is currently a bit up in the air. Apply to one of the above addresses. If you have no luck, write directly to one of the hospitals. Affiliated hospitals include:

University College Hospital

Grafton Way, London WC1E 6AU. Tel: +44 20 7387 9300.
The hospital: This is the acute admitting hospital for the UCH/Middlesex partnership. It has a busy emergency department

that gets a variety of customers from businessmen and media types to down and outs and intravenous drug users.

Middlesex Hospital

Mortimer Street, London W1N 8AA. Tel: +44 ,20 7636 8333.
The hospital: Once admitted from UCH, patients are transferred to the Middlesex. It has many medical and surgical specialities, but O&G, paeds and neuro go to the relevant specialist centres (*see* below).

Royal Free Hospital

Rowland Hill Street, London NW3 2PF. Tel: +44 20 7794 1876 Fax: +44 20 7435 5803.
The hospital: The Royal Free has only recently joined the huge University College jungle. It is situated in Hampstead, which sets it a little bit out of the hustle and bustle of the rest of UCH. It has many highly regarded departments and areas of research.

The Obstetric Hospital

Huntley Street, London WC1E 6AU. Tel: +44 20 7387 9300.
The hospital: This is the main obstetric hospital for north and central London.

Great Ormond Street Hospital for Children

Great Ormond Street, London WC1N 3JH. Tel: +44 20 7405 9200. Fax: +44 20 7829 8643.
www.ich.bpmf.ac.uk/center.htm.
The hospital: Probably the most famous paediatric hospital in the UK, Great Ormond Street has all specialities and many research areas in paediatrics. It has very large cardiac and oncology departments. Accommodation for students has previously been provided but is expensive.

Hospital for Tropical Diseases

4 St Pancras Way, London NW1 0PE. Tel: +44 20 7387 4411.
The hospital: Its history extends back to the Seaman's Hospital Society wanting to care for returning sailors. They

first set up hospital on board *HMS Grampus* on the River Thames. The medical conditions were obviously orientated towards diseases brought in from the tropics and subtropics. In 1899, the London School of Tropical Medicine was founded, and in 1929 the London School of Hygiene and Tropical Medicine in Keppel Street was established. It was in 1951 that the Hospital for Tropical Diseases was built.

This has an 18-bed inpatient facility, travel clinic, outpatients and an emergency department for people who are ill having just returned from abroad. Note: Tropical diseases include typhoid, cholera and typhus, all of which were in Britain in the 19th century so it may see more than what you simply imagine to be tropical. The hospital is at the forefront of research against new strains of drug-resistant malaria.

O **Elective notes:** The hospital charges £200 for a four-week elective. There is no student teaching, but you join the SHO teaching and teaching for the tropical medicine diploma. Ward rounds are very good learning experiences. The wards often have chloroquine-resistant malaria, and schistosomiasis and leishmaniasis may be seen in outpatients.

National Hospital for Neurology and Neurosurgery

Queen's Square, London WC1N 3BG.
Tel: +44 20 7837 3611.
Fax: +44 20 7278 5069.

The hospital: This is an international centre of excellence for neurology and neurosurgery. Every aspect is catered for, with very good teaching from people who are passionate about this subject. It's popular with American, German and Australian students, so there's a good social life. Contact the student office at the above address.

Elizabeth Garrett Anderson Hospital and Hospital for Women, Soho

144, Euston Road, London NW1 2AP.
Tel: +44 20 7387 2501.

Eastman Dental Hospital

256 Gray's Inn Road, London WC1X 8LD.
Tel: +44 20 7915 1000.

Imperial College School of Medicine

London SW7 2AZ. Tel: +44 20 7594 3598/8014. Fax: +44 20 7594 8004/9833. www.med.ic.ac.uk.

The Imperial College School of Medicine was formed in 1995 by the merger of St Mary's Medical School and the National Heart and Lung Institute. It then increased further, absorbing the Charing Cross and Westminster Medical Schools and the Royal Postgraduate Medical School in 1997. Each of these original institutions still has its own hospital in various parts of west London. Each has a long history of its own. All this merging has now made this one of the largest medical schools in the UK. It has the following campuses:

St Mary's Hospital, Praed Street, Paddington, London W2. Tel: +44 20 7530 3500. (This is a large teaching hospital providing most specialities.)
Charing Cross Hospital, Fulham Palace Road, London W6. Tel: +44 20 8846 1234. (Again, a large teaching hospital.)
Chelsea and Westminster Hospital, 369 Fulham Rd, London SW10. Tel: +44 20 8746 8000. (This is a very plush hospital in a very nice area of London. It has a new state-of-the-art emergency department.)
Hammersmith Hospital, 150 DuCane Rd, London W12. Tel: +44 20 8743 2030. (The Hammersmith is a postgraduate teaching hospital. It is highly regarded for its academic and clinical excellence.)
Royal Brompton Hospital, Sydney Street, London SW3 6NP. Tel: +44 20 7352 8121. Fax: +44 20 7351 8473. www.rbh.nthames.nhs.uk. (The Royal Brompton is a large cardiothoracic unit in the West End.)

Hospitals throughout Middlesex and Surrey are also associated. Because of the recent merger, they are not, at the time of writing, accepting elective students. This will change. Electives have previously been possible at all hospitals free of charge. Write to the elective coordinator at the above addresses.

St Bartholomew's and the Royal London School of Medicine and Dentistry

Queen Mary and Westfield College, Turner Street, London E1 2AD. Tel: +44 20 7377 7611/7603. Fax: +44 20 7377 7612. www.mds.qmw.ac.uk.

St Bartholomew's and the Royal London hospital merged with Queen Mary and Westfield in 1993. Bart's is situated within the Square Mile of the city of London in an attractive court-yard setting. 'The London' is in Whitechapel, a pretty deprived area of London with many Asian and Muslim immigrants. The hospitals therefore span the full breadth of social classes. Hospitals in Hackney (the **Homerton**), Whipp's Cross, Newham and Southend in Essex are also used, as are a number of specialist units, including the **London Chest** (Bonner Road, London E2).

A well-organized elective package in subjects from ITU to cardiothoracic surgery is available. Dental electives are also possible. There is no elective fee, and you should apply 6–18 months before your intended date. A list of sources of accommodation is provided.

Royal London Hospital

Mile End Road, Whitechapel, London E1 1BB. Tel: +44 20 7377 7000.

The hospital: 'The London' is a busy teaching hospital in the rough East End of London. Nearly all specialities are catered for. The emergency department (level 1 trauma unit) is highly regard-ed. It has a Helicopter Emergency Medical Service on the roof that deals with all major trauma within the area enclosed by the M25 motorway. The emergency department has a five-bed resuscitation area and a paediatric emergency department. There is plenty for students to see and do. In addition, students get to spend time on the heli-pad and at the '999' ambulance control centre (unfortunately students are not allowed on the helicopter for insurance reasons).

St Bartholomew's Hospital

West Smithfield, London EC1A 7BE. Tel: +44 20 7601 8888.

The hospital: Bart's is a beautiful hospital in the heart of London. It has a great history and many famous old boys. Today, most acute care (emergency medicine) has been transferred to 'The London'. Bart's has now become a specialist centre for cancer, endocrine and a number of other specialities.

Guy's, King's and St Thomas' Medical School

Guy's Campus, London Bridge, St Thomas Street, London SE1 9RT. Tel: +44 20 7955 4127/7848 6971. Fax: +44 20 7955 4425/7848 6969. www.kcl.ac.uk.

'Guy's' and 'Tommy's' merged a number of years ago to form UMDS. In the past couple of years, they have merged with the other big south-east London medical school, King's College. All have retained their original hospitals, but organization has been centralized. A number of hospi-tals throughout south-east England are associated. The **Maudsley Hospital** in Lewisham is a specialist psychiatry centre.

St Thomas's Hospital

Lambeth Palace Rd, London SE1. Tel: +44 20 7928 9292.

The hospital: Situated on the River Thames right opposite the Houses of Parliament, Tommy's has a busy emer-gency department and many specialities. It's in an excellent location for getting into the West End.

Guy's Hospital

St Thomas St, London SE1. Tel: +44 20 7955 5000.

The hospital: Situated nearer the finan-cial city at London Bridge, Guy's has a number of medical and surgical speciali-ties as well as a minor injuries unit. Some departments are moving over to St Thomas'.

King's College Hospital and School of Medicine and Dentistry

Bessemer Road, Denmark Hill, London SE5 9PJ. Fax: +44 20 7346 3589.

The hospital: King's is a large hospital with a busy emergency department. It is also the regional liver unit for the whole of London and the south of England. It has an affiliated hospital in Dulwich.

St George's Medical School
Crammer Terrace, London SW17 ORE.
Tel: +44 20 8725 5992/8672 9944.
Fax: +44 20 8725 5919/8672 6940.
www.sghms.ac.uk.
This is the last London medical school not to have been engulfed. It is in Tooting, South London. Although away from the city, it has an interesting range of patients with diverse needs. Central London is a few stops away on the northern line.

St George's Hospital (Blackshaw Road, London SW17. Tel: +44 20 8672 1255) is the main teaching hospital. The **Atkinson Morley Neurosurgical Unit** has just moved to the main campus. There is a forensic medicine unit on the main site (Tel: +44 20 8725 0015), which has previously been popular with visiting (UK) students. Electives can be arranged in most departments. Accommodation is provided cheaply. German students must apply under the DAAD scheme. Write to the electives coordinator for more details.

Other speciality hospitals:

Moorfield's Eye Hospital
City Road, London EC1V 2PD. Tel: +44 20 7253 3411. www.moorfields.org.uk.
The hospital: Moorfield's was founded in 1805 as a postgraduate teaching hospital and national centre for ophthalmic care. It is a centre of quality care, research and teaching. It has eight outreach centres and a mobile unit.

Royal National Ear, Nose and Throat Hospital
330 Gray's Inn Rd, London WC1.
Tel: +44 20 7837 8855.

University of Manchester
Faculty of Medicine, Stopford Building, Oxford Road, Manchester M13 9PT.

Tel: +44 161 275 5025/2077. Fax: +44 161 275 5697/5584. www.medicine.man.ac.uk.
Manchester has a large medical school. The principal hospital is the **Manchester Royal Infirmary** (Oxford Road, Manchester M13 Tel: +44 161 276 1234); however, it also uses hospitals in an 80km (50 mile) radius around Manchester. These include **St Mary's** (Whitworth Park, Manchester M13. Tel: +44 161 276 1234 – O&G and paeds), the **Hope**, **Withington** (Nell Lane, Manchester M20. Tel: +44 161 445 8111), **Wythenshawe**, (Southmoor Road, Manchester M23, Tel: +44 161 998 7070), **North Manchester General** (Tel: +44 161 740 1444), **Stepping Hill** and **Tameside General Hospitals**. **Booth Hall Children's Hospital** (Charlestown Road, Manchester. Tel: +44 161 795 7000) and the **Royal Manchester Children's Hospitals** (Pendlebury, Manchester. Tel: +44 161 794 4696) are the specialist paediatric centres. There is also the **Christie Hospital** (Wilmslow Road, Manchester M20. Tel: +44 161 446 3000) which is a specialist cancer hospital.

The city itself has 50000 students, hence there are always places to go. There are many pubs, clubs and curry houses. Ask people where to go as some areas aren't all that safe for wandering around at night. There is no formal procedure for electives. You need to write to the undergraduate tutor in the postgraduate department of the subject you wish to do. They can sometimes arrange accommodation. If you need a form signed by the Dean of the medical school, you must enrol as a Manchester medical student and pay fees.

Newcastle University Medical School
Framlington Place, Newcastle upon Tyne NE2 4HH. Tel: +44 191 222 7034/6138.
Fax: +44 191 222 6139 /6521.
www.ncl.ac.uk.
Situated right at the north end of England, Newcastle is a medium-sized, friendly city. The medical school is situated in the centre and is on the same

site as its principal teaching hospital, the **Royal Victoria Infirmary** (Victoria Road, Newcastle. Tel: +44 191 232 5131). The school also uses a number of other hospitals in and around Newcastle. Write to the elective coordinator. All subjects except dermatology, O&G and radiology can be catered for. There is currently no fee, and accommodation can be provided for approximately £120 a month in the doctors' residence.

University of East Anglia Norwich School of Medicine

Norwich Campus, University of East Anglia, Norwich, NR4 7TJ. Tel: + 44 1603 593061. Fax: +44 1603 593752. www.med.uea.ac.uk.

Norwich is a new medical school, founded in 2001 and taking 110 students a year. It uses hospitals throughout East Anglia, but principally the **Norfolk and Norwich University Hospital** (Colney Lane, Norwich, NR4 7UY. Tel: +44 1603 286286. www.norfolk-norwich-hospitals.net).

Nottingham University

Medical School Faculty Office, Queen's Medical Centre, Nottingham NG7 2UH. Tel: +44 115 970 9379. Fax: +44 115 970 9922. www.nott.ac.uk.

Nottingham is a pleasant city towards the north of England. It uses **University Hospital** (**Queen's Medical Centre**) on campus as well as **City Hospital** and **Derby Hospital**. Queen's Medical Centre has most specialities and is highly regarded for paediatric surgery.

Oxford University

Medical School Offices, John Radcliffe Hospital, Headington, Oxford OX3 9DU. Tel: +44 1865 221689/270207. Fax: +44 1865 750750. www.ox.ac.uk.

Oxford, renowned for its academic excellence, has more to offer than just highbrow clinicians. The main teaching hospital, the **John Radcliffe** (Headley Way, Headington, Oxford. Tel: +44 1865 741166) is huge and caters for most needs. The **Churchill** (Old Road, Headington, Oxford. Tel: +44 1865 741

841) and **Radcliffe Infirmary** (Woodstock Road, Oxford. Tel: +44 1865 311188) are older hospitals that are also used. The city has a pleasant centre, and there is abundant student life. It's not just a university town though. London is only an hour away by train. Electives can be arranged in most subjects. The school has limited accommodation for a reasonable rent. There is no elective fee.

University of Sheffield Medical School

Faculty of Medicine, Medical School, Beech Hill Road, Sheffield S10 2RX Tel: +44 114 271 1910/3349. Fax: +44 114 271 3960. www.shef.ac.uk.

Sheffield conjures up images of mining, steel works and unemployed male strippers. The reality is very different. The hospitals are in a nice part of town, and the surrounding countryside is great if you like hill walking or rock climbing. The university has two main hospitals: the **Royal Hallamshire** (Glossop Road, Sheffield S10 2JF. Tel: +44 114 271 1900. Fax: +44 114 271 1901), where the school is situated, and the **Northern General** on the other side of town (about 20 minutes away). Together with the **Jessop Hospital for Women** (Leavygreave Road, Sheffield S3 7RE. Tel: 0114 226 8000), these cover all specialities. A number of DGHs in Humberside and South Yorkshire are also affiliated. There is a well-known forensic pathology department on the main site.

University of Southampton Medical School

Southampton General Hospital, Tremona Road, Bassett Crescent East, Southampton SO16 6YD. Tel: +44 238059 5000. www.medschool.soton.ac.uk.

Southampton is situated in the middle of the south coast of England. It has better weather than the north of England and there's a beach on which to appreciate it. There's pleasant countryside to see and a trip to the Isle of Wight to make. The school is modern, and students get patient contact from day one of the course. **Southampton General** (Tremona Road, Southampton. Tel: +44 1703 777222) and the **Royal South Hampshire** (Brintons Terrace, Southampton. Tel: +44 1703 634288) are the main teaching hospitals, but hospitals in Bournemouth and Portsmouth are also used.

Royal United Hospitals Bath

Conbe Park, Bath. Tel: +44 1225 428331.
This is also a popular elective destination although not attached to a specific medical school.

ISLANDS NEAR ENGLAND:

Guernsey:

Guernsey has a population of 66 000, 50 km (30 miles) of coastline and beautiful beaches. Healthcare is private, and there is no national health service. There are no junior doctors either, only consultants, specialists and GPs. Primary care is provided by GPs, and islanders have to pay (£16) to see them. The GPs also run the emergency departments, and patients have to pay (around £40 depending on treatment) to be seen there. The people of Guernsey pay a compulsory premium giving access to secondary healthcare (specialists) for free. The specialists run wards in **Princess Elizabeth Hospital** and clinics in **Alexandra House**. If a treatment is not available, patients are transferred to the mainland, usually to Southampton. Consultants sometimes visit.

Princess Elizabeth Hospital

Le Vanquiedor, St Martins, Guernsey GY4 6UU, Channel Islands. Tel: +44 1481 725241. Fax: +44 1481 359065.
The hospital: Has all major specialities and an emergency department. There are five physicians with speciality interests who rotate on a 1:5 on-call rota. To arrange an elective here, write to the postgraduate tutor at the above address. There is a £25 administration cost and they need a CV. Tour all the specialities, meet some GPs and go out to their practice.

Accommodation: Available, but may cost around £12 a night.

Two other hospitals on the island are the **King Edward VII Hospital** (geriatrics) and **Câtel Psychiatric Hospital**.

Jersey:

General Hospital

Gloucester Street, St Helier, Jersey JE2 3QS, Channel Islands. Tel: +44 1534 59000. Fax: +44 1534 59805.
The hospital: A system similar to that in Guernsey exists, although junior doctors are present (a popular job). Again, write to the postgraduate tutor at the above address.

Alderney:

Mignot Memorial Hospital

Route de Crabby, Alderney GY9 3XY.
Tel: +44 1481 822 822.
Fax: +44 1481 823 087.

Isle of Wight:

St Mary's Hospital

Newport, Isle of Wight PO30 5TG.
Tel: +44 1983 524081.
The hospital: This is the main acute hospital on the Isle of Wight. It caters for all basic and some advanced specialities.

Isle of Man:

Noble's Isle of Man Hospital

Westmoreland Road, Douglas, Isle of Man. Tel: +44 1624 642642.
The hospital: This is actually a teaching hospital for Manchester University but also takes elective students in medicine or surgery for a maximum of four to six weeks. There is a relaxed atmosphere, and you are not expected to be on call, although there is a bleep if you want one. Accommodation is free in the nurses' home directly opposite the hospital. There is a lively mess for doctors and nurses. Douglas is a short walk away and has a few shops. The island has beautiful scenery and ancient heritage.

Ramsey Cottage Hospital
Cumberland Rd, Ramsey, Isle of Man. Tel:
+44 1624 811811.

SCOTLAND

Aberdeen University
Faculty of Medicine, Aberdeen Royal
Infirmary, Foresterhill, Aberdeen AB29
2ZB. Tel: +44 1224 681818. Fax: +44 1224
840 708. www.bms.abdn.ac.uk.
On the east coast of Scotland, Aberdeen
has a great deal of history but now plays
a major role in the oil industry. Although
cold, the city is friendly, and there's
plenty to do. The multifaculty university
is about 3 km from the hospital. The
medical school and infirmary are on the
same site. The teaching hospital
(**Aberdeen Royal Infirmary**, Fosterhill)
is large hospital with a busy emergency
department that admits from a large area,
including the Shetland and Orkney Isles
as well as the oil rigs and shipping in real
emergencies. All major specialities,
including neurosurgery, are on-site.
Elective students have reported good
practical experience in the emergency
department.

Dundee University
Medical School, Level 10, Ninewells
Hospital, Dundee DD1 9SY. Tel: +44 1382
344160. Fax: +44 1382 664267.
www.dundee.ac.uk.
Three hospitals in Dundee – **Ninewells**,
a very large purpose-built teaching
hospital, **Dundee Royal Infirmary**
(Barrack Road) and **Kings Cross
Hospital** (Clepington Road), all on Tel:
+44 1382 660111 – and a number of
hospitals outside the city are used.
Dundee itself may not have the best
weather, and there may not be much to
do in the centre, but there is easy access
for skiing and hill walking. Electives can
be arranged for a £100 administration fee
in any subject depending on availability.
Rotations are available all year. There's a
£25 per week compulsory hospital
accommodation fee. Contact the electives coordinator.

University of Edinburgh
Faculty of Medicine, Teviot Place,
Edinburgh EH8 9AG. Tel: +44 131 650
1000. Fax: +44 131 650 6525.
www.med.ed.ac.uk.
Edinburgh University itself has a great
history and very well-known medical
school. Although you can apply to
departments directly, the faculty much
prefers that you apply through them
(with a £25 administration charge). They
have a quota system so apply early. They
can arrange electives at central and
peripheral hospitals. If you apply
through a department, the school may
not recognize you as a student and therefore will not provide a certificate of
attendance (so you'll need to get the consultant to do it).
    Affiliated hospitals include the **Royal
Infirmary of Edinburgh**, the **Royal
Hospital for Sick Children**, the
Western General, the **Eastern
General**, **Princess Margaret Rose**, **City
Hospital** (Greenbank Drive, Edinburgh)
and **St John's** (Livingston, Howden
Road, West Livingston EH54 6PP).
Accommodation is not provided by the
school, although it may be available in
peripheral hospitals. There is also a
Community Drug Problem Service
(Spittal Street Centre, 22–24 Spittal
Street, Edinburgh EH3 9DU), which has
previously taken students.

The New Royal Infirmary of Edinburgh
51, Little Frances Crescent, Old Dalkeith
Road, Edinburgh, EH16 4SA.
This is a brand-new hospital housing all
the major specialities. It is situated four
miles from the city centre, about 25 minutes by bike. Although it has had
teething problems, facilities are excellent. The staff are friendly and usually
very good at teaching. The orthopaedics
and surgical departments (it is the
Scottish Liver Transplant Centre) are
world-renowned.

Western General Hospital

Crewe Road, Edinburgh EH4 2XU.

The hospital: The Western is a busy hospital with many specialities and the neurosurgical centre. A large HIV unit has just moved here from **City Hospital**. It also has the **National Surveillance Unit for Creutzfeldt–Jakob disease**. There is a limited supply of accommodation in the nurses' home.

Law Hospital

Carluke, Lanarkshire ML8 5ER.

The hospital: Law is a rural hospital used by Edinburgh, Glasgow and Dundee students. It is a friendly DGH with some good teaching.

University of Glasgow

Faculty of Medicine, Glasgow G12 8OO. Tel: +44 141 330 4424/5921. Fax: +44 141 330 5440/233 4373. www.gla.ac.uk.

Glasgow is a very lively, cultural city with plenty to do both day and night. It also has some very poor areas, affecting the population's health (drug abuse and TB being relatively common). The medical school is based in the West End of the city and uses six large hospitals and 13 DGHs in the region.

Its main teaching hospitals include **Glasgow Royal Infirmary** (84 Castle Street, Glasgow G4. Tel: +44 141 211 4000), the **Western Infirmary** (Dumbarton Road, Glasgow G11. Tel: +44 141 211 2000), **Gartnavel General** (1053 Great Western Road, Glasgow G12 0YN. Tel: +44 141 211 3600) and **Stobhill** (Balornock Road, Glasgow G21. Tel: +44 141 201 3000) hospitals. All tend to be very friendly and welcoming. The **Royal Hospital for Sick Children** (Yorkhill, Glasgow G3 8SJ) is the main paediatric hospital in Glasgow, with many specialists and a dedicated emergency department. It has previously provided free accommodation to students.

Electives can be arranged in most subjects for six weeks in term time. There is a £20 admininstration fee and no elective charge. Electives of eight weeks are only available in the summer holidays, and, because of the length of time, you have to enrol as a Glasgow student (for £357). The university requires proof of certain vaccinations to do an elective in one of its hospitals. You have to arrange accommodation with the accommodation officer at whichever hospital you are placed in. Those in Glasgow itself often do not provide accommodation, which then has to be arranged through the university (costing up to £100 a week). Those on the outskirts can sometimes provide it free.

When you have 'done' Glasgow, there is plenty of beautiful countryside to the north, such as Loch Lomond and the highlands. Skiing is about two hours away.

University of St Andrews

Faculty of Medicine, Old Union Building, St Andrews, Fife KYL6 9AJ. Tel: +44 1334 476 161. Fax: +44 1334 462 144. www.st-andrews.ac.uk.

OTHER INTERESTING HOSPITALS IN SCOTLAND:

Glasgow Homeopathic Hospital

1000 Great Western Road, Glasgow G12 0NR.

The hospital: This is an NHS hospital that treats with conventional as well as alternative medicines. It has 16 beds and an extensive outpatients department. It is very friendly, and the reasons for doing things are explained. It has a very holistic approach –'Which side of the bed do you sleep on?' is not a question many of us normally ask. The results are apparently 'astounding'. This is recommended as an elective for both homeopathy fans and total sceptics.

Raigmore Hospital

Perth Road, Inverness IV2 3UJ. Tel: +44 1463 704000. Fax: +44 1463 711322.

The hospital: Raigmore is the main trauma centre for the region. It is a busy hospital and used by Aberdeen students. It provides good teaching and a very friendly setting.

Belford Hospital
Fort William, PH33 6BS.

The hospital: A friendly hospital with a medical and surgical ward, emergency department and maternity unit. It is excellent for mountain-climbers (Ben Nevis is just around the corner). All the doctors are outdoor types. There's good skiing nearby (when it snows), and the emergency department and ski patrols get busy as a result.

SCOTTISH ISLANDS:

Western Isles Hospital
Macaulay Road, Stornoway, Isle of Lewis HS1 2AF. Tel: +44 1851 704704.

The hospital: This hospital is in Stornoway in the Outer Hebrides. It has general and orthopaedic surgery, medicine, O&G, geriatrics and psychiatric services. There is a high-dependency unit but no ITU. CT scanners, MRI, neuro/cardiothoracic surgery are all on the mainland.

This is an incredibly friendly hospital in a beautiful area. There are outreach clinics to other islands. An elective here has been highly recommended, although it's not for high-powered city types. On Sunday, the only things open are the hospital and the churches. There's no cinema, just some quiet pubs. However, the hospital is great and there's plenty of wildlife and places to see. This is an excellent cheap elective. If you have a car, take the ferry from Ullapool.

Accommodation: On-site (very good) accommodation has previously been available.

GP work/electives in the Outer Hebrides
GP work on the islands is also popular. Rather than writing a great list of GPs (who will be bombarded with letters), contact the Primary Care Manager, **Western Isles Health Board** (Health Board Offices, 37 South Beach Street, Stornoway, Isle of Lewis, Western Isles HS1 2BN). They have previously contacted GPs to arrange electives.

A small GP/minor ops unit is the **Griminish Surgery** (Griminish, Benbecula, Western Isles HS7 5QA), which has two GP/anaesthetists and one locum surgeon, allowing them to do one elective list a week and also emergency surgery. Anything that can't be done is transferred by helicopter to the mainland. Hospitals in the Outer Hebrides are:

Balfour and Eastbank Hospitals, Orkney. Tel: +44 1856 885400.
Gilbert Bain General Hospital, Shetland Isles. Tel: +44 1595 695678.

NORTHERN IRELAND

Queen's University Belfast
Faculty of Medicine and Health Sciences, Ground Floor, Whitla Medical Building, 97 Lisburn Road, Belfast BT9 7BL.
Tel: +44 1232 245133. Fax: +44 1232 330571.
www.qub.ac.uk.

Queen's Universtiy Belfast is situated in the heart of Belfast and uses the **Royal Victoria** and **Belfast City** (Lisburn Rd, L9 Belfast, Northern Ireland. Tel: +44 1232 329241) hospitals as well as a number of smaller peripheral sites. Despite its reputation, Belfast is a safe, friendly city, and there is certainly plenty to do, both within and outside it. Dublin is only two hours away, and there is beautiful countryside nearby. Electives can be arranged here in any subject between June and December. There is no charge and accommodation is provided free (and is fine). Write to the electives coordinator at the above address.

The Royal Hospitals
Grosvenor Road, Belfast BT12 6BA.
Tel: +44 1232 894702.

The hospitals: The group comprises the **Royal Victoria** (Grosvenor Road, Belfast BT12. Tel: +44 1232 240503), the **Royal Maternity** (Grosvenor Road, Belfast BT12. Tel: +44 1232 240503), the **Royal Belfast Hospital for Sick Children** (Falls Road, Belfast BT12.

Tel: +44 1232 240503) and a dental hospital. Almost two-thirds of Northern Ireland's population lives within 40 minutes of these hospitals, which are a few minutes out of Belfast centre.

The Royal Victoria is a large, busy, central teaching hospital with all specialities. The A&E is the trauma centre for Northern Ireland, seeing 118 000 patients a year, some affected by the conflict. It has a worldwide reputation. The cardiology department set up the world's first mobile coronary care unit and played a major role in the development of the defibrillator. There is the opportunity to see patients first and do minor procedures. Electives here come thoroughly recommended. The Royal Belfast Hospital for Sick Children is the only dedicated paediatric hospital in Northern Ireland.

OTHER INTERESTING HOSPITALS IN NORTHERN IRELAND:

Ulster Hospital
Dundonald, Belfast BT16 0RH.
The hospital: This is a general hospital on the outskirts of Belfast. It can get very busy. Belfast students are also present so visitors may not always get into theatre or specialist clinics. Orthopaedic trauma can be very interesting.

Tyrone County Hospital
Hospital Road, Omagh, Co Tyrone.
The hospital: Tyrone County is very friendly, 200-bed hospital. Elective reports show students are a bit of a rarity, hence teaching is enthusiastic and good. A few Queen's University Belfast students are around.

Colerane Hospital
Mount Sandle Road, Colerane, Co Londonderry.
The hospital: Colerane has three medical, two surgical and one geriatric ward and an emergency department. It is popular with students from Dundee so apply early. It's a friendly place and you are fairly free to do as much or as little as desired.

Antrim Area Hospital
45 Bush Road, Antrim, Co Antrim.
The hospital: This is a relatively new district general hospital providing care for a large area of Co Antrim. It has a friendly emergency department, and the staff are very helpful. It is used as a teaching hospital by Queen's University Belfast so there are quite a few other students around. Apply early. There's a good bus and train service into Belfast. Accommodation is available.

WALES

University of Wales
College of Medicine, Heath Park, Cardiff CF14 4XN. Tel: +44 1222 743436.
www.uwcm.ac.uk.
This is the only medical school in Wales and is situated in the capital. The **University Hospital of Wales** is the principle teaching hospital, but the faculty has links with many hospitals throughout Wales. With a student population of over 20 000, Cardiff is great for young people. There are lovely pubs and theatres. Outside there are the Brecon Beacons and some beautiful coastal sites to explore. Electives here can be arranged in most subjects. There is a £200 administration fee per eight weeks and a charge for accommodation.

SOMETHING DIFFERENT:

Motor racing

Medical Centre, Silverstone Circuit
Silverstone, Towcester, Northamptonshire NN12 8TN.
The centre: Arranges the provision of medical support for motorsport events. Learn how to get drivers out and the priorities after a crash.

Diving

Diving Diseases Research Centre
Deriford Hospital, Plymouth, Devon.

PACIFIC
ISLANDS

The Cook Islands

Population: 20 000
Languages: English and Maori
Capital: Avarua
Currency: New Zealand dollar
Int Code: +682

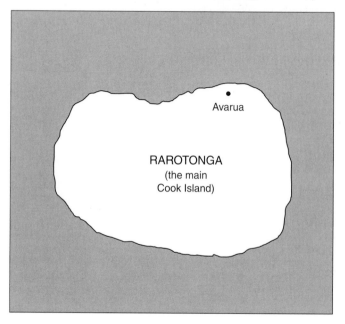

Avarua

RAROTONGA
(the main
Cook Island)

*The Cook Islands are over 3000 km
(2000 miles) into the Pacific from the coast of
New Zealand and consist of 24 volcanic and
coral islands. Tourism and banking are now
their main economy, although clam and pearl
farming are still very important. The capital is
Avarua on Rarotonga in the south. In total,
there are 13 government-run hospitals.*

USEFUL ADDRESS:

Ministry of Health, Box 109, Rarotonga.
Tel: +682 22664.

Rarotonga

**Avarua Hospital/Rarotonga
General Hospital**
PO Box 109, Avarua.
Tel: +682 22664.
The hospital: This is the main hospital
for the Cook Islands. It offers all major
specialities and can also arrange attach-
ments in other hospitals.

Mauke

Mauke is a small Island (population 639) in the middle of the South Pacific, one hour's flight from Rarotonga.

Mauke Hospital

Mauke. Tel: +682 35664.

The hospital: The hospital has one doctor, two nurses and three beds, and supplies all the healthcare needs for the island!

O **Elective notes:** In 1998, the doctor on the island was allegedly dismissed for negligence and general drunkenness. Since then, there has been the odd newly qualified doctor from Bulgaria but nothing particularly well organized. An elective here may well result in your being the island doctor. With a population of 639, you are unlikely to be wildly busy, but organizing the hospital and basic child care is very much needed. Any emergencies are very worrying. This is the perfect remote elective! Write to the hospital in Rarotonga for more details.

HOSPITALS ON OTHER ISLANDS:

Aitutaki Hospital, Ministry of Health, Aitutaki. Tel: +682 31041. Fax: +682 31002.
Atiu Hospital, Ministry of Health, Atiu. Tel: +682 33664.
Mangaia Hospital, Ministry of Health, Mangaia. Tel: +682 34027.

Fiji

Population: 800 000
Language: English
Capital: Suva
Currency: Fiji dollar
Int Code +679

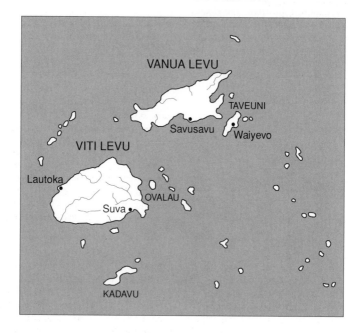

Fiji comprises a number of volcanic islands in the South Pacific, the two largest being Viti Levu and Vanua Levu. There are 880 smaller islands. Indians were brought in as slaves by the British, and now the numbers of natives and Indians are about equal (although there was a mass exodus of Indians after the 1987 coup). The islands, especially the smaller ones, are beautiful and offer a host of water sports, including scuba diving. The Fijians (including the local medical students) are very friendly and keen to feed visitors and make sure you get kava (the national drink, a mild opiate!). Elective students normally get into the country by saying they are tourists. *Note: In recent years there has been political unrest with violent clashes. Check with the Foreign Office before going.*

✪ Medicine:

The Fiji health service is pretty poor. Although it covers most things, some drugs have to be paid for by the patients and anyone needing a major operation (such as a transplant) has to raise funds (or have private insurance) to get themselves to Australia or New Zealand. Rural areas have a number of nursing stations. Despite what you may imagine, there are actually few tropical diseases on the islands and there is no malaria. Dengue fever outbreaks (especially on Melansia) do, however, occur, and typhoid and helminthic infections are not uncommon. Leading causes of death include cardiovascular disease, cancers and accidents. The doctor to patient ratio is 1:2000.

◎ **Climate and crime:**
New Year and Christmas are good times to visit as it is warm and sunny every day. The east side of the islands gets more rain than the west. Hurricanes and cyclones are not uncommon.

USEFUL ADDRESS:

Ministry of Health, PO Box 2223, Ports Authority Building, Flagstaff, Suva, Viti Levu. Tel: +679 306177. Fax: +679 306163.

VITI LEVU

Suva

MEDICAL SCHOOL:

Fiji School of Medicine
Private Mail Bag Suva, Viti Levu. Tel: +679 311700. Fax: +679 303469. www.fsm.ac.fj. There is also a dental and nursing school within the health sciences complex. To arrange electives on Fiji, write either to the hospital itself or the electives coordinator at this address. It takes about two months to get an application form, but it's relatively well organized. The main teaching hospital is:

Colonial War Memorial Hospital
GPO Box 115 Suva, Viti Levu. Tel: +679 313444. Fax: +679 303232.
The hospital: A very well-equipped hospital. The largest and most high-tech hospital in Fiji. Excellent for training as it has good facilities and a wide range of pathologies. It is friendly and relaxed.

'Mercy missions' to outlying islands are occasionally carried out in emergencies.
O **Elective notes:** This provides an excellent opportunity for experience and some responsibility. If applying through the university, ask to do some community medicine in Taveuni and/or Savusavu so you can get some touring at the same time.
Accommodation: Not provided but the South Seas motel is 9.8 FJD (£3) a night.

The other hospital in Suva is:

Tamavua Hospital, Private Mail Bag, Suva, Viti Levu. Tel: +679 321066.

Lautoka

Lautoka is a port for many of the small boats that visit the nearby islands. This makes it easy to get off the mainland, go to the Yasawa Islands and to Abaca to trek in the rainforest. Scuba diving, windsurfing, etc. are a must. Lautoka is not touristy, but there's a cinema and an Internet café. There are wonderful beaches once you get out of Lautoka (which is otherwise quite a sleepy and not an attractive town).

Lautoka Hospital
PO Box 65, Lautoka, Viti Levu. Tel: +679 660399. Fax: +679 665423.
The hospital: A 400-bed, 1970s hospital in a city on the west coast of Viti Levu. Lautoka is the second-largest city (after the capital Suva), and is populated by Fijians and Indians in equal number. The languages are therefore English, Fijian and Hindi. The hospital is funded largely by voluntary aid and is relatively primitive by Western standards. Diabetes (1:5 prevalence), TB, rheumatic fever (and its heart complications) and SLE are fairly common. The hospital has general medical and surgical wards (divided into male and female), a paeds, O&G and TB ward.
O **Elective notes:** The medical staff's teaching has had good reports (you can move around to find the best), with many opportunities for performing lumbar

punctures, aspirations, etc. Those who have done emergency medicine and orthopaedics have found it busy (TB, many traffic accidents and the occasional shark bite!) but interesting and well worthwhile. Paeds tends to have diseases of deprivation: malnutrition, gastroenteritis and infectious diseases. The two medical house officers work a 1:2 rota and are grateful for any help you can give. The attendance requirement is low but you need to be in at 8 am. Spending some time in the outpatients is good experience as you get to see and treat people on your own. People present late, often because they may have to pay for treatment but also because they are a very uncomplaining race.

The hospital also runs 'mercy missions' in a helicopter to rescue people from neighbouring islands. Try to get to any clinics on other islands. The staff are very keen that you get out and see more of the main island as well as some of the smaller islands. Take long weekends to do this.

Accommodation: An accommodation block is being built, but the Cathay Hotel (PO Box 239) is a ten-minute stroll away and comes highly recommended. Prices vary from $9 (dormitory with fan) to $22 (single room), with negotiable reductions for three sharing a room. Across from the Cathay is the Northern Club, a colonial establishment serving good (cheap) food, with tennis and squash courts, a swimming pool and snooker tables. Membership is a mere $10 (£5) a month. There are usually many elective students here.

VANUA LEVU

Savusavu Hospital

PO Box 230, Savusavu, Vanua Levu. Tel: +679 850444.

The hospital: A small district hospital with very limited resources. There are only three doctors so they are grateful for any help they can get. There's not much to do in the town (as it's not really on the

tourist route), although there's a local dive centre. They are very friendly, but it can get lonely. You may also have language problems, although there's often a Fijian medical student to help.

TAVEUNI

Taveuni is Fiji's third-largest island, but having said that, there are no roads, mains electricity or (more importantly) bars. It does have three shops!

Taveuni Hospital

PO Box 28, Waiyevo, Taveuni. Tel: +679 880444. Fax: +679 880744.

The hospital: This is a collection of wooden huts (built in the 1920s) run by a husband and wife team. It has four wards (female, male, O&G, and paeds) each with eight beds. The lack of staff means that you will get heavily involved in running your own clinics. The main problems on the island are hypertension and diabetes. There are also many antenatal clinics. Take comfort if you have any fears of running clinics by the fact that there are very few facilities and so it's pretty difficult to kill anyone. Days start early (8 am) but finish by 1 pm so there's plenty of time for swimming and sunbathing (there's not a lot else to do!). Repeatedly highly recommended as an elective.

OVALAU

Levuka Hospital

Levuka, Ovalau.

The hospital: A small, almost cottage, hospital, this has male, female and 'paying' wards, and an outpatients department that acts as a general practice. It covers the villages of Ovalau and some of the surrounding islands.

O Elective notes: They are very grateful for the extra pair of hands so this is actually a hard-working elective. They may well be relying on you to turn up and do your own clinics and ward rounds. Throw yourself into it and you'll be rewarded with the Fijians' great kindness. You will meet the chiefs and be considered a guest of honour at dinners. It can get lonely if you're on your own but it is a beautiful country and the beaches are amazing.

KADAVU

Kadavu Hospital
Kadavu.
The hospital: Another small cottage hospital on an island about 65 km

(40 miles) long catering for the scattered population of around 4000.

HOSPITALS ON OTHER ISLANDS:

Ba Hospital, PO Box 162, Ba. Tel: +679 674022. Fax: +679 670248.
Labasa Hospital, PO Box 577, Labasa. Tel: +679 811444. Fax: +679 813444.
Nadi Hospital, PO Box 214, Nadi. Tel: +679 701109. Fax: +679 700563.
Rakiraki Hospital, PO Box 34, Rakiraki. Tel: +679 694368. Fax: +679 694610.

Kiribati

Population: 79 000
Languages: English and Gilbertese
Capital: Bairiki
Currency: Australian dollar
Int Code: + 686

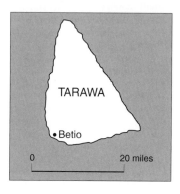

The Republic of Kiribati is a collection of 33 very isolated islands in the South Pacific. It gained independence from the UK in 1979. Most of the 79 000 Gilbertese population live in thatched huts. Previously, the British had extensively phosphate-mined the island of Banaba. Now the islands are very poor, and coconut growing and fishing are the main livelihoods. Most of the islands are coral reefs and surround a lagoon. Due to their remoteness, it may not rain for months and droughts have occurred.

✚ Medicine:
Until recently the locals had a healthy diet, although this has changed as canned food has been imported. There is an incredibly high death rate. Of the 192 countries in the world, it comes in at 154 for poor life expectancy. TB, measles, diabetes and heart conditions are all very common. Dengue fever outbreaks can occur, and diarrhoeal and helminthic infections are not uncommon.

◎ Climate and crime:
It is hot all year round (30°C) with variable rainfall. Apart from the odd pub brawl, there's not much for the police to do (with only around 70 prisoners in total!).

USEFUL ADDRESS:

Ministry of Health, PO Box 69, Bairiki, Tarawa. Tel: +686 28100. Fax: +686 28152.

Tungaru Central Hospital
Nawerewere, Tarawa. Tel: +686 28100. Fax: +686 28152.
The hospital: Tarawa is 80 km north of the equator and next to the international date line. The Japanese built the hospital in 1989 to care for all the central Pacific islands that were too far from Papua New Guinea or Australia. It's a modern, 120-bed hospital with medicine, surgical, paeds, O&G, TB

and private wards as well as an emergency department.

○ **Elective notes:** It is a friendly hospital but a real pain to get to (fly Air Marshall or Air Nauru from Fiji). Accommodation is not provided and can be a real problem. You need someone to put you up or it'll cost more than £30 a night in a guesthouse. It's not all palm trees – some of the island is very polluted – but the elective comes highly recommended if you can get there.

OTHER HOSPITALS:

Betio Hospital, Tarawa Tel: +686 26444
Christmas Hospital, Christmas Island. Tel: +686 81242.

Samoa

Population: 10 000
Languages: Samoan and English
Capital: Apia
Currency: Tala
Int Code: +685

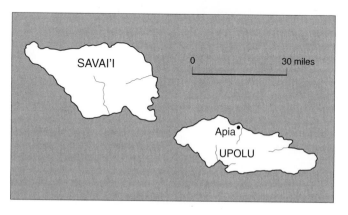

SAVAI'I

0   30 miles

Apia
UPOLU

The nine islands that make up Samoa lie in the middle of the South Pacific between Fiji and the Cook Islands. Only four of the volcanic islands are inhabited, most of the population living on Upolu. There are beautiful beaches, rainforests and coconut plantations. The people are very welcoming and hospitable. It is now officially Samoa since the east (formally US-controlled) and the west (formally governed by New Zealand) became fully independent in 1962.

✪ Medicine:

Just take a look at their rugby team. Samoans are big. This was fine when on the natural diet, but now that it has become heavily Westernized, diabetes, hypertension and cardiovascular disease are common. Tropical diseases such as dengue fever and filiariasis also occur.

◎ Climate:

It is hot all year round (30°C) but rains most around Christmas time.

USEFUL ADDRESS:

Department of Health, Private Bag, Apia. Tel: +685 21212.

Western Samoa National Hospital

Moto'otua, Apia, Upolu, Western Samoa. Tel: +685 21212.

The hospital: The national hospital is 15 minutes' walk from the centre of the capital. All the major specialities (medicine, surgery, O&G, orthopaedics and paeds) are present. Facilities are pretty basic, with very few laboratory resources. There's only a limited amount of drugs and no crash trolley. The medical staff are enthusiastic and work very hard. Diabetes is a major problem here.

○ Elective notes: Students have found this a wonderful elective, with lots of 'hands on' experience and the opportunity to run clinics. It's a beautiful and very friendly place. The work is not too strenuous and the weekends are always free. There are lots of Australian and New Zealand students. Thoroughly recommended.

Note: There is also the opportunity to go to small hospitals on other islands. Savai'i (the next main one) has only two doctors so there's an opportunity to do a bit more.

Accommodation: Sometimes provided, however, previous students have stayed with Samoan families and had a wonderful time.

OTHER HOSPITALS ON UPOLU AND SAVAI'I:

Leulumoga District Hospital, Upolu. Tel: +685 42210.
Lalomanu District Hospital, Upolu Island. (No phone – only radio!)
Malietoa Tanumafili II Hospital, Savai'i. Tel: +685 53510.
Sataua Hospital, Savai'i. Tel: +685 58086.

Solomon Islands

Population: 400 000
Language: English
Capital: Honiara
Currency: Solomon Islands dollar
Int Code: +677

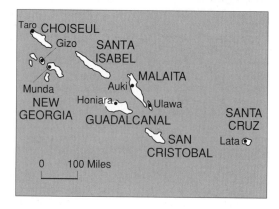

The 922 Solomon Islands form an archipelago in the south-west Pacific. They have been independent from the UK since 1978. The six main islands are Choiseul, Guadalcanal, Malaita, New Georgia, San Cristobal and Santa Isabel. The capital is Honiara on the island of Guadalcanal. There are 80 languages, but most inhabitants speak Pidgin (a variant of English) in addition to their local language. Ninety-three per cent of the population are of Malaysian origin. There are many beautiful beaches and sites for the best in diving. Note: There has been civil unrest. Check with the Foreign Office before you go.

✛ Medicine:

It's tropical medicine in a developing country. There are many infectious diseases: masses of TB, malaria and many pyrexias of unknown origin. Dengue fever, filariasis and Japanese encephalitis occur. In addition to the six government hospitals (listed below), there are also church missions that visit the islands.

To find out what it's really like to work on the Solomon Islands, *see* www.hermannoberli.ch.

◎ Climate:

It has a tropical climate, the temperature averaging 28°C with 70% humidity. January and February comprise the rainy season.

➲ Visas and work permits:

No visa is required for Solomon Island electives. Ask the embassy about the need for a work permit.

USEFUL ADDRESS:

Ministry of Health and Medical Services, PO Box 349, Honiara. Tel: +677 23600. Fax: +677 24243. (The ministry is based in the main hospital. The Director of Medical Services is also based at this address.)

Guadalcanal

Guadalcanal makes an excellent base from which to explore the other islands.

Central Hospital (Numbaneen)/ National Referral Hospital

Box 349, Honiara. Tel: +677 23600.
Fax: +677 24243.

The hospital: The main hospital for the islands and has 280 beds. Originally known as 'Number 9', it was built as a military hospital by the US army during World War II. Mainly tropical diseases (malaria, TB, pyrexia of unknown origin, tropical splenomegaly) are seen. It is very busy.

O **Elective notes:** There are friendly staff and excellent teaching. It comes very highly recommended for medicine and surgery. There's plenty of assisting in theatre and the opportunity to perform procedures under supervision (although this can vary depending on the number of doctors around). O&G has a similar story.

Accommodation: Can be provided in 'Kiwi House' (approximately SI$15 (£30) for as long as you want), but can get fully booked and is not great.

New Georgia

Munda is the name given to the largest settlement on the island of New Georgia. It comprises six villages in the Roviana lagoon. The largest village, Lambete, has three grocery stores, a baker and a bank that changes travellers' cheques. There is also Agnes Lodge, a pub/restaurant. Most people live in leaf huts. There is a Japanese-built railway, a remnant from the war. There was a great deal of heavy fighting here during World War II, which now provides some sites for excellent diving and snorkel opportunities.

Helena Goldie Hospital

PO Box 82, Munda. Tel: +677 61121.

The hospital: A 55-bed general hospital, in the village of Kokkngolo in Munda. It serves a population of 25 000 spread over 10 000 km² of ocean. It is a mission hospital financed by the United Church and overseas donations. It has male, female, maternity and paeds wards and an air-conditioned operating theatre. There's a nurse aide training school on-site, taking 20 self-funding nurses a year. The hospital is run by two doctors, seven registered nurses, a radiographer/ pharmacist and two lab technicians. The most common cause of admission and death is malaria. TB, abscesses and obstetric problems are also common. The surrounding islands are visited by motorized canoe to run clinics (giving immunizations and weighing children).

O **Elective notes:** After prayers at 7.30 am, there is a ward round and and a (very busy) outpatient clinic at 9.00 am. Then there may be theatre. Student on call is 1:3. The medical student is often the anaesthetist (mostly using ketamine). You can do clinics in the hospital and are often sent out on the remote clinics with a nurse. Swimming and diving are excellent (sunken ships and planes). Traditional dancing, bush walks and crocodile spotting are other pastimes.

Accommodation: A student flat is available for around SI$159 (£20) a week.

Gizo

Gizo Hospital

PO Box 36, Gizo, Gizo Province.
Tel: +677 60224.

The hospital: Opened by the Duke of Edinburgh in 1959, Gizo has 55 beds and around four doctors. The four wards are male, female, paeds and maternity, and there's an outpatient/emergency service. All are well run. Many patients travel a great distance by canoe to get here. Nurses see patients first and can prescribe. If concerned, they can then refer to the doctor. Malaria and TB are common, as are bush-knife injuries. There is a well-equipped theatre.

O **Elective notes:** There are very few students so less teaching but lots more opportunity to do practical procedures. There's excellent scuba diving nearby.

Accommodation: Not available so stay at Paradise Lodge (SI$40 (£5) a night).

Santa Cruz Island

Lata Hospital
Lata, Santa Cruz, Temotu Province.
Tel: +677 53044/53045. Fax: +677 53044.
The hospital: This is a 40-bed hospital with eight antenatal (one delivery room), eight male, eight female and eight paediatric beds, one TB ward (four beds), one isolation bed, an operating theatre and a minor ops room. There are about 20 minor cases a month. There's lots of paeds, TB, STDs (though not HIV), malaria and scrub typhus. It's good for general medicine and minor surgery (most major surgery taking place at the central hospital).

O **Elective notes:** The doctors and nurses are friendly and speak English. The patients speak Pidgin. Every two to three months, a coconut ship tours surrounding islands for a week from which staff do clinics. You may have to canoe to some clinics. There's excellent snorkelling from here. Temotu is very remote and can be very hot (35°C). Electricity and water are in short supply.

Accommodation: Has to be arranged on arrival.

Malaita Island

Kilu'ufi Hospital
Auki, Malaita Island. Tel: +677 40272.
The hospital: This is the hospital for a large island just north of Guadalcanal.

Ulawa

Kira Kira Hospital
Kira Kira, Ulawa. Tel: +677 50100.

Choiseul

Taro Hospital, Choiseul
E-mail: kirisi@solomon.com.sb
The hospital: Taro Hospital is a small, 22-bed hospital in the Western Province of the Solomon Islands. It acts as the referral hospital for all of Choiseul (population 23 000). It is in the process of being upgraded to a 54-bed hospital to provide TB, male, female, O&G, paeds, X-ray, dental and outpatient facilities. Currently Taro is run single-handedly by a very enthusiastic doctor who would appreciate some help! This really is a paradise island, unspoilt by tourism. It certainly sounds like a fantastic place for an elective or short period of voluntary work.

Accommodation: Can be arranged.

Tonga

Population: 98 000
Language: Tongan
Capital: Nuku'alofa
Currency: Pa'anga
Int Code: +676

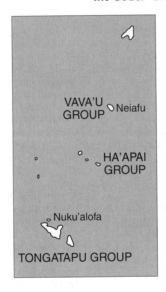

The Kingdom of Tonga consists of 170 islands in an idyllic location in the South Pacific. Only 39 are inhabited. Tongatapu is the main island with Nuku'alofa as its capital. The main language is Tongan but nearly all Tongans speak some English. Tonga has never been colonized by a European power and hence has maintained its own identity. It is also not yet a tourist destination. The people are very sincere and hospitable. There is no TV, a negligible crime rate and no deadlines. Its royal family has one of the world's oldest dynasties and Tonga is probably the smallest kingdom in the world. Although the main island is only 18 m (60 feet) above sea level, the seabed around Tonga is up to 10 km (6 miles) deep. Things to do include kava drinking (a brew made from mixing the dried and powdered root of the pepper plant Pipermethysticum). It has many medicinal properties, from antifungal to anticonvulsive! See the flying foxes in Kolovai, blow holes in Houma and go to the Royal Palace, the national centre, the beaches (Keleti and Oholei), the churches and the temples. Definitely snorkel, but wear something on your feet (to prevent coral cuts).

✪ Medicine:

All medical care in Tonga is free except small private clinics and the Tongan witchdoctors. It's pretty modern, but specialist services are available only in New Zealand or Australia. Diabetes, from the westernization of their diet, and infectious diseases are common. Dengue

Tonga

fever and filariasis are present, and Japanese encephalitis outbreaks occur sporadically. Serious cases get flown to Pago Pago (in American Samoa).

➲ **Visas and work permits:**
The procedure for medical students taking their electives in Tonga is as follows. Medical students apply to the Director of Health, Nuku'alofa, Tonga to ask about the possibility of undertaking an elective in Tonga (allow months for a reply). They will then be sent a letter of approval from the Director of Health that is handed to the immigration officer at the point of entry in Tonga for endorsement of the appropriate visa. Medical students usually make their accommodation reservation in Tonga with the help of the Ministry of Health, Tonga Visitors' Bureau and Sela's guesthouse. Where possible, the Ministry of Health assists with the medical student's transportation.

USEFUL ADDRESSES:

Ministry of Health, Nuku'alofa. Tel: +676 23 200. Fax: +676 24 291.
Tonga Visitors' Bureau, Vuna Road, Nuku'alofa. Tel: +676 25 334. Fax: +676 23 507.
Sela's Guest House, Pahu Kolofo'ou, Nuku'alofa. Tel: +676 21 430. Fax: +676 22 755.

Nuku'alofa

The city can be a bit of a disappointment if you're expecting a tropical paradise and it can be quite hard to get to some of the islands. It does, however, make a good base.

Vaiola Hospital
PO Box 59, Nuku'alofa. Tel: +676 23 200. Fax: +676 24 291.
The hospital: This is the main hospital (200 beds) and is situated in the capital city of Nuku'alofa. It has medical and surgical, paeds, O&G, ophthalmological, psychiatric and emergency services run by ten consultants and a similar number of junior staff. The medicine is pretty

basic, but the hospital is very clean and well run. The outpatients also functions as a GP service. X-ray and ultrasound facilities are available. Major problems include diabetes (and subsequent wound sepsis), rheumatic fever, hepatitis A and B, dengue fever, STDs, asthma (increasing) and gastroenteritis. HIV is not yet a major problem.

O **Elective notes:** Medical students are encouraged as much as possible, and there's the opportunity to do minor procedures such as lumbar punctures and assisting in theatre. Because of limited resources, there is no complex surgery, but there is good surgical teaching. There are also clinics to do. Attendance is occasionally discouraged, offering ample opportunity to explore. It's very popular with the Australian students. There are three other hospitals (which are more like clinics) in Tonga, but attachment to these can be arranged once in Vaiola. You won't see much at these, but they give a good excuse for visiting other islands.

Accommodation: Not provided but not a problem to get (around £5 a night). Tonga is not yet a well-known tourist spot; while this has advantages, it does mean there aren't many leisure activities. Toni's Guesthouse in Nuku'alofa comes recommended, as does the Beach House (PO Box 18, Nuku'alofa). The food may not be that good. One month here may be enough.

Ngu Wellington Hospital
Neiafu, Talau, Vava'u. Tel: +676 702 01.
The hospital: Has around 60 beds and is situated on Vava'u, 200 km north of Tongatapu. It caters for the northern islands and is run by about five doctors. The waters around here are especially beautiful. Anything major gets sent to Tongatapu.

Niu'ui Hospital
Hihifo, Ha'apai. Tel: +676 60 201.
The hospital: A 28-bed hospital with one doctor and very limited resources.

Vanuatu

Population: 160 000
Languages: Bislama and English
Capital: Efaté
Currency: Vatu
Int Code: +678

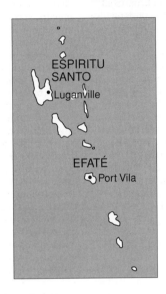

ESPIRITU
SANTO
Luganville

EFATÉ
Port Vila

Vanuatu is a cluster of 80 small islands in the South Pacific. They lie between a triangle formed by the Solomon Islands, Fiji and New Caledonia. The islands were originally populated in around 3000 BC and christened as the New Hebrides by Captain James Cook in 1774. Until 1980, they were governed jointly by the French and English, but now they are independent. Most people speak English, some speak French as well, but the most widely spoken is Bislama, a creole based on English (e.g. Hed blong yu i goroan = Does your head go round?, Taem yo slip wetem wuman kok blong yu i go slak = are you impotent!). It is pretty easy to learn and within a couple of weeks you'll be able to take a good history. The main island (the third-largest) is Efaté. The others have mainly

small villages with leaf huts. Vanuatu is a developing nation that has preserved its traditional heritage and is largely unspoilt by Western tourism (although the capital is a port for Australian cruise ships). The Vanuatu people are very warm and welcoming. Unfortunately since independence, the government has mismanaged the economy and there's a great deal of poverty (although a number of Westerners have settled here as it is a tax haven). As alcohol has become commonplace so has the abuse of women. There's plenty of spectacular diving and snorkelling. The sister ship of the Titanic, the Star of Russia, which sank in Vila harbour, is a popular dive, as are the USS Coolidge and Semle Federson. Some of these are very deep (55 m), hence diving accidents are not uncommon. The nearest recompression chamber is Sydney. Don't have any accidents. Tanna is a nearby island that still has an active volcano. Pentecost has the famous land-diving sport (bungee jumping with linola vines instead of rope). There is also plenty of bush walking.

✪ Medicine:
Like the other Pacific Islands, tropical diseases such as filiariasis, dengue fever and Japanese encephalitis occur. In addition, there are the more common diseases of Westernization.

◉ Climate:
November to April is the wet season, with a temperature of around 30°C and high humidity. May to October (winter) is the best time to go as it's cooler and drier. When it rains, it really rains. The odd hurricane can do a lot of damage.

➲ Visas and work permits:
No visa is required with a Commonwealth passport. You will have to contact the hospital regarding the need for a work permit.

Vila Central Hospital
Private Mail Bag 013, Port Vila, Efaté. Tel: +678 22100. Fax: +678 27618/27621.
The hospital: The hospital is in the city (Port Vila) on the main island of Efaté. It's set on the side of a hill overlooking a lagoon and is ten minutes' walk from the town centre. It has medical, surgical, delivery and paeds wards totalling 150 beds. There are two theatres, a radiology department (with ultrasound) and a very busy outpatients. Lab facilities are mainly for malaria, although basic blood tests are available. There are usually six or seven doctors, but much of the work is done by nurse practitioners. Pathology in outpatients can be somewhat poor as many people just want a sick note, but there is malaria, measles, diabetes, hepatitis B, rheumatic fever and gastrointestinal upsets. Reactive arthritis and trauma (including wife beating) are

relatively common. TB (drug-resistant) is common, and all the rare presentations are seen. Pathology is commonly advanced as people tend to try traditional medicines first.

The nurses and the 60 nursing students here are exceptionally friendly and helpful with language problems. They have a football team and commonly invite students out to play volleyball.

○ Elective notes: In previous years, the doctors have varied from being exceptionally good, very experienced medics and surgeons to very poor with no interest in teaching. Fortunately, the most recent reports have been of very friendly and knowledgeable staff. Students get to run their own clinics. If you want to catch babies, this is the place – 100 deliveries a month and encouragement from the midwives for you to be involved. Medical students also do on calls as the admitting doctor, working from 4.30 pm to 7.30 am on a 1:5 rota. This is very rewarding. As the hospital is relatively well staffed, the doctors tend to encourage students to get out and about the island. Book early as this is becoming a popular destination. Write to the medical student coordinator.
Accommodation: And food are provided but cost around 1000VT (approximately £5.50) a night.

Northern District Hospital
PO Bag 006, Luganville, Espiritu Santo. Tel: +678 36345.
The hospital: This is home to the world's largest accessible recreational diving wreck, the *USS Coolidge* and hence is probably better for diving medicine.

HOSPITALS ON NEIGHBOURING ISLANDS:

Lenakel Hospital, Lenakel, Tanna. Tel: +678 68659.
Lolowai Hospital, Lolowai, East Ambae, Via Longana. Tel: +678 38302.
Norsup Hospital, Norsup, Malekula. Tel: +678 48410.

Other Pacific Islands with Hospitals

AMERICAN SAMOA

Lyndon B. Johnson Tropical Medical Centre, Pago Pago 96799.
Tel: +684 633 1222.
This acts as a referal centre for serious cases from some of the other Pacific Islands.

NAURU

Nauru General Hospital.
Tel: +674 555 4303.
Nauru Phosphate Corporation.
Tel: +674 555 4155.
There are 14 GPs on the island; ten work at Nauru General Hospital and four with the Nauru Phosphate Corporation (which treats employees and locals).

NIUE

Lord Liverpool General Hospital,
Alofi. Tel: +683 4100. Fax: +683 4265.
This is the only hospital, but it also runs three clinics around the island.

PACIFIC ISLANDS OF MICRONESIA

This group of islands comprises four archipelagos, each of which is made up of hundreds of islands. They were all under US control until 1990, but now each group has autonomy. Infectious diseases, including dengue fever, filiariasis, typhoid, Japanese encephalitis, hepatitis B, TB and helminthic infections, are all relatively common.

Marshall Island group:
Ebeye Hospital, PO Box 5219, Ebeye, Kwajelien 96970. Tel: +692 329 3029. Fax: +692 329 3022.
Majuro Clinic, PO Box 79, Majuro MH 96960.
Tel: +692 625 6455.
Majuro Hospital, PO Box 16, Majuro MH 96960.
Tel: +692 625 3355.

Federated Islands of Micronesia:
Chuuk State Hospital, Weno, Chuuk 9694.
Tel: +691 330 2444.
Kosrae State Hospital, Tofal, Kosrae.
Tel: +691 370 3012.
Pohnpei State Hospital, Nett, Pohnpei 96941.
Tel: +691 320 2216.
Yap State Hospital, Colonia, Yap 9694.
Tel: +691 350 3446.

Northern Mariana:
Commonwealth Health Centre, PO Box 409, Navy Hill, Saipan MP 96950. Tel: +670 234 8950.
Rota Health Centre, PO Box 1249, Rota MP 96951. Tel: +670 532 9463.
Saipan Health Centre, As Lito, Saipan MP 969950. Tel: +670 234 2901. Fax: +670 234 2906.
Tinian Health Centre, PO Box 446, Tinian MP 96952. Tel: +670 433 9292.

Palau:
Belau National Hospital, PO Box 6027, Koror, Palau 96940. Tel: +680 488 2552.

TAHITI (AND SURROUNDING ISLANDS):

Tahiti comprises 130 islands. There are nine hospitals with over 300 doctors on the islands.

Clinique Cardella, Papeete. Tel: +689 428190.
Fax: +689 410691.
Clinique Paofai, Papeete. Tel: +689 437700. Fax: +689 419835.
Hôpital Jean Prince, Papeete. Tel: +689 464500.
Fax: +689 464686.
Hôpital Mamao, Papeete. Tel: +689 466262. Fax: +689 466282.

Hôpital de Moorea, PO Box 1, Papao, Moorea.
Tel: +689 562424.
Hôpital de Taravao, Taravao. Tel: +689 571333.
Hôpital de Uturoa, PO Box 40, Uturoa, Raiatea.
Tel: +689 663503.
Ministry of Health, PO Box 2551, Papeete. Fax:
+689 410651.

TUVALU:

Princess Margaret Hospital, Funafuti.
Tel: **+688 20751.**
This is a well-equipped 30-bed hospital
on the main island of nine atolls.

THE MIDDLE
EAST

Israel

Population: 5.6 million
Language: Hebrew
Capital: Jerusalem
Currency: New shekel
Int Code: +972

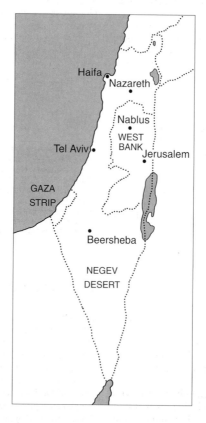

Although Israel has become better known for its Gaza Strip and West Bank disputes, it still offers a great deal of history and mixed cultures. Jerusalem, Nazareth, the Dead Sea and Bethlehem are commonly visited. It is a popular destination for both Christian and Jewish medics. Doctors trained in Israel can speak English as it is taught in school from the age of ten, and many of the textbooks are in English. Many patients also speak English, albeit rarely enough to give a history. It may well be worth doing a basic course in Hebrew before you go. The war with Iraq and the 'Road Map' to peace have made the Middle East anything but peaceful. In Israel, a number of Westerners have been killed by

Israeli defence forces in the West Bank and Gaza. The Foreign Office advise against all travel to these two areas. If you go against this advice, prepare to be interrogated by the Israeli authorities. Access to Gaza is very limited without a diplomatic visa. More terrorist attacks (not targeting foreigners but in public places) have been vowed by Hamas, who have advised all foreigners to leave. You are also advised to stay away from Israel's border with Lebanon because of clashes between the Israeli army and Hizbollah. Also avoid the Israeli side of the Israel–Gaza border because of the risk of stray shots, snipers and mortars. Check www.fco.gov.uk for the latest advice (or, more sensibly, turn to the Pacific Islands section of this book and make other plans!).

✪ Medicine:

Healthcare is available to all people in Israel and is pretty good. Indeed, many hospitals have pioneered new treatments. The conditions of developed countries (cardiovascular disease and cancer) are common.

Note: Israel has the second-highest litigation rate in the world after the US, and medicine is practised with this in mind.

◎ Climate:

Between June and September it can get very hot (30°C) and dry.

⊃ Visas and work permits:

Officially, to study in Israel, you need to apply for a student visa. Once you have a confirmed place of study you can apply, with the help of your destination, to the Ministry of Interior in Israel for one. Despite this, Tel Aviv University say that elective students need only a tourist visa, and many students visiting other institutions also don't bother. It would be worth asking your host institution directly whether they require a study visa; if not, a tourist visa should suffice for an elective. In order to be able to do paid work in Israel you have to have a work permit. This has to be applied for in Israel, directly to the Ministry of Interior, by the person who would be employing you.

SHABBAT AND HOLIDAYS

Shabbat begins at sunset on Friday evening and finishes at sunset on Saturday evening. Many Jewish families attend the synagogue on Friday and Saturday. It is traditionally a time for the family to be together, especially for the Friday night meal. All buses stop running and shops close for the period.

There are several holidays during March and April, including *Pesach* (Passover), Holocaust Memorial Day, Remembrance and Independence Day. All the Jewish holidays begin at sunset. *Pesach* lasts a full week (the medical students have two weeks off), and Moroccan Jews celebrate its end by feasting.

USEFUL ADDRESSES:

Ministry of Health, PO Box 1176, Ben-Tabai Street, Jerusalem 91010.
Israel Medical Association, 2 Twin Towers, 35 Jabotinsky Street, PO Box 3566, Ramat-Gan 52136. Tel: +972 3 610 0444. Fax: +9723 575 1616. www.ima.org.il.
Israel Dental Association: www.ida.org.il.
Israel Medical Association in Britain, c/o Dr David Katz, Secretary, 6 Lawn Road, London NW3 2XS, UK.

Jerusalem

In this capital, with such an extensive religious history, there are plenty of places to visit. If you are on elective, the Jerusalem Society of Medical Students organizes parties and excursions to the local sights. These include Jerusalem's old city (Muslim Quarter, Dome of the Rock, Western Wall, Mosque of Asqa), Zion square and the new city, the Jewish Market (haggle!), the Israel Museum, Knesset and its gardens, Yad Vashem (Holocaust Museum), the Talpiot Promenade, the Hebrew University on Mount Scopus, the Mount of Olives and any of the historical districts (Meah Shearim, Russian Compound, American Hill). Outside Jerusalem you must get to the Dead Sea (get a bus from the central bus station to Ein Gedi), Tel Aviv, Jaffa, *the Golan Heights and Sea of Galilee, the Negev Desert, Eilat and Sinai. That's enough for the first few weeks!*

O **Elective notes:** To do an elective in Jerusalem, you can either write to the hospital or, more easily, contact the Exchange Officer, **Jerusalem Society of Medical Students** (JSMS) (Hebrew University-Hadassah School of Medicine, Ein Kerem, POB 12272, Jerusalem 91120). For this society to find you a place, you have to send a letter 'certifying your good standing as a medical student' from your dean, and $50.

Accommodation: Not provided by the university or hospitals and can often be arranged only on arrival. There are plenty of hostels in Jerusalem but two that come particularly recommended are Ein Kerem Youth Hostel (POB 16091, Jerusalem. Tel: +972 2 416282) and Beit Shmuel Youth Hostel (King David 13, Jerusalem. Tel: +972 2 203466). The one in Ein Kerem is a 15-minute walk from the university and Haddash Hospital in a quiet location (with beautiful views) 20 minutes' bus ride from the city centre. Many medical students stay here as it is near the hospital and cheaper than those nearer the city. Allow $400–600 for eight weeks. The JSMS provides cheap lunchtime food.

A couple of tips:
- Buy a monthly bus pass (£35) but note that it's only valid until the first of the next month rather than the day you bought it (so don't buy it at the end of a month)
- Also change money at the post office in the University Hospital to save commission.

Hebrew University, Hadassah Medical School

PO Box 12272, Jerusalem 91120. Tel: +972 2 675 8137. Fax: +972 2 675 8118.
www.md.huji.ac.il.

Established in 1946, the faculty of medicine has five schools, including medicine and nursing. Based on the Ein Kerem campus, the major hospitals used are the **Ein Kerem** and **Mount Scopus Hadassah University Hospitals** (both run by the Hadassah Medical Organization, Kiryat Hadassah POB 12000, Jerusalem 91120. Tel: +972 2 677 6078. Fax: +972 2 677 7013. www.hadassah. org.il). These provide over 1000 beds. The **Kaplan** hospital in Rehovot and the **Shaare Zedek** and **Bikur Cholim** hospitals in Jerusalem are also affiliated. The university is the oldest in Israel and is world-renowned for its research into brain function, cancer, biotechnology and AIDS.

Hadassah Teaching Hospital

Ein Kerem, POB 12272, Jerusalem 91120.
The hospital: The Hadassah is a 700-bed tertiary referral hospital situated on the south-western side of Jerusalem on the hillside above the village of Ein Kerem. It has departments covering all the major specialities plus the medical school and research laboratories. The emergency department consists of 28 beds, four of which are in the trauma unit and six for high-risk patients. There is also a paediatric emergency facility. Every patient admitted comes through the emergency room. IVF, bone marrow, lung and liver transplantation, laproscopic and cold laser surgery are examples of its advanced specialities. The working week begins on Sunday morning; the working day is 8 am to 4 pm. Hadassah is one of four major hospitals in Jerusalem and takes part in an 'on-duty' rota arranged between them.

O **Elective notes:** This is a friendly teaching hospital. You can join their students' teaching which is usually in Hebrew with English slides. Many lecturers will speak in English for you; if not, the other students are more than happy to translate. In the emergency room, practical procedures of suturing, central lines and chest drains can all be practised. Traffic injuries are very common, but alcoholic injuries are not seen. The neurosurgery department is well recommended, with good teaching that rotates on a two-weekly basis with the new group of students. They also encourage you to go out and explore the country.

Accommodation: *See* above.

Mount Scopus Haddash University Hospital

The hospital: Has 300 beds and serves the Jewish and Arab neighbourhoods of north and eastern Jerusalem. It has most specialities and an emergency department (but neuro goes to Ein Kerem). It also runs a 'hospice on wheels'.

Shaare Zedek Medical Centre

POB 3235, Jerusalem, 91031.
Tel: +972 2 655 5316/655 5111.
Fax: +972 2 654 0744.

The hospital: A large modern hospital affiliated with the Hebrew University. It has a busy emergency department. Patients come from a wide variety of backgrounds and consultations can be in Hebrew, English, Arabic, Russian, Yiddish, French or Spanish. Most major specialities are catered for.

O Elective notes: You should have good command of Hebrew here as all notes and many consultations are in it. If you do, it's a very worthwhile elective, with quite a lot of responsibility and practical skills. Write to the director of the foreign medical student's programme.

Accommodation: Not provided (*see* above).

Also in Jerusalem is the **St John Ophthalmic Hospital** PO Box 19960, Sheikh Jarrah, Jerusalem 97200. Tel: +972 2 582 8325. Fax: +972 2 582 8327. E-mail: stjohn@palnet.com.

Nazareth

Nazareth is the largest Palestinian settlement in Israel, with a population of around 60 000. A great deal of building work has occurred for the new millennium. From Nazareth, excursions to the Golan Heights and Sea of Galilee are relatively easy, and there are good bus connections to Tel Aviv and Jerusalem.

Nazareth Hospital (EMMS)

71501–71502 PO Box 11,16100
Nazareth. Tel: +972 6 657 1501. Fax: +972 6 657 5912. E-mail: nazhosp@rannet.com.

The hospital: Is a Christian mission institution (owned by the Edinburgh Medical Missionary Society) and is the oldest hospital in Israel. It is small (136 beds) but offers medical, surgical, emergency, paediatric, psychiatric, obstetric and gynaecological services. In the past decade it has become integrated into the Israeli State Health Service as a district general hospital. A new wing has recently been constructed, and there are plans for further expansion. The hospital currently has 6000 inpatients and 37 000 outpatients a year. It serves the ever-growing community of Nazareth and the surrounding Gallilean villages. Arab–Israeli relationships in this area are entirely peaceful, but the Jewish communities use other hospitals.

Most staff are local Nazarenes, although a few medics and paramedics are expatriates. There is an unusual mix of cultures – Jewish, Muslim and Christian. Communication is not always easy: the patients speak in Arabic, but the doctors communicate with each other and write notes in Hebrew regardless of their background. Fortunately, many of them also speak English.

O Elective notes: There's no formal teaching, but most doctors (mainly expatriates) are happy to teach on ward rounds and in clinics. O&G is very busy (and some of the staff a bit volatile!), and there is very little time for teaching. There is, however, a 'muck in' approach and you'll get great 'hands on' experience. There are a higher number of congenital defects as there are many first-cousin marriages. If the prognosis is poor, the child is often rejected by its parents. Overall, at least in other departments (emergency, respiratory medicine and paeds), its a fairly relaxed atmosphere (the hospital day is from 8.30 am to 3.30 pm). This elective has been highly recommended by some as an excellent way to see some common conditions, some Arabic culture and some very genuine people.

Accommodation: Can be arranged. There are single-sex flats where many young people stay – carpenters, gardeners, etc. It is important to get involved as otherwise you'll just 'pass through' this experience. There are plenty of evening activities such as sport, cinema and eating out. Regardless of personal belief, attendance at religious ceremonies (although not compulsory) and respect is recommended.

For more details, write to the **Edinburgh Medical Missionary Society** (7 Washington Lane, Edinburgh EH11 2HA, UK. Tel: +44 131 313 3828).

Beersheba

Ben Gurion University of the Negev
School of Medicine, 84 105 Beer-Sheva.
www.medic.bgu.ac.il.
This is part of the **Soroka Medical Centre,** PO Box 151, Beersheba 84101.
Tel: +972 7 640 0909. Fax: +972 7 627 4096.
The hospital: The Negev Desert makes up 60% of Israel (6000 square miles) and is home to a number of different ethnic peoples, many of whom are still semi-nomadic. The hospital (1200 beds) serves the entire population of the Negev. Community medicine is obviously important in this area, and the medical school (founded 1974) takes great pride in the fact that it trains good generalists rather than specialists.

Tel Aviv

Tel Aviv University
Sackler Faculty of Medicine,
PO Box 39040, Tel Aviv 69978.
Tel: +972 3 640 9657. Fax: +972 3 640 9103.
www.tau.ac.il/medicine.
The medical faculty was founded in 1963 to cope with the increasing population. It is now based on the Ranat Aviv

campus and uses 14 hospitals (totalling 6000 beds) in the greater Tel Aviv area, providing care for 40% of Israel's population. All the hospitals are state owned. Hospitals include the **Assaf Harofeh Medical Center** (800 beds, 19 km southeast), which is renowned for its orthopaedics and paediatrics; the **Rabin Medical Center** (1650 beds in two hospitals 10 km east); the **Sapir Medical Center** (672 beds in the Sharon region), with excellent spinal and max-fax departments; the **Schneider Children's Medical Center of Israel** (224 beds), a very advanced paediatrics centre (transplants, MRI); the **Chaim Sheba Medical Center** (1600 beds and a busy emergency department); the **Tel Aviv-Sourasky Medical Center** (the second-largest hospital in Israel, with 1100 beds), with all departments; and the **Dana Paediatric** and **Serlin Maternity** hospitals in the same complex.

O Elective notes: The Tel Aviv **University Medical Students' Organization** sorts out electives. You need your own travel insurance and malpractice insurance is recommended although not obligatory. You only require a tourist visa (check their website).

Haifa

Technion-Israel Institute of Technology
Bruce Rappaport Faculty of Medicine,
PO Box 9649, 31 096 Haifa.
www.technion.ac.il.
Founded in 1969, the newest medical faculty in Israel uses the **Rambam Medical Center** (a 900-bed hospital receiving Jews, Muslims and Christians from northern Israel and southern Lebanon that lies at the base of Mount Carmel on the shores of the Mediterranean); the **Bnai-Zion Medical Center** and **Carmel** hospitals in Haifa; the **Haemek Medical Center** in Afula; the **West Galilee Medical Center** in Naharia; and the **Hillel Yafe Hospital** in Hadera.

There are also two Palestinian Medical Schools (check with the Foreign Office regarding safety):

Al-Quds University
Faculty of Medicine, PO Box 19356, Jerusalem (East). Tel: +972 2 279 9203. Fax: +972 2 279 6110. www.alquds.edu.

An-Najah National University
PO Box 7, Nabulus, West Bank, Palestine. Tel: +972 9 237 6584. Fax: +972 9 238 7982. www.najah.edu.

Jordan

Population: 5.5 million
Language: Arabic
Capital: Amman
Currency: Jordanian dinar
Int Code: +962

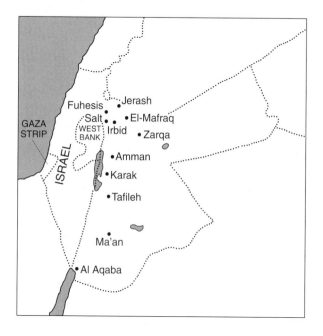

Jordan has some good beaches (with scuba diving in Al Aqaba and the ruins of Petra. It is, sadly, now more famous for the dispute with Israel over the West Bank. It is not a popular destination for elective students (possibly because of the need for fluent Arabic) and information is difficult to come by. For this reason, only the main hospitals (and the medical school) are listed below. As with all countries in the Middle East, the threat to Westerners from terrorist attacks is constantly changing. At the time of writing, the threat is said to be 'high'. Check www.fco.gov.uk for the latest advice.

✪ Medicine:

The government provides a subsidised healthcare system, and reasonable hospitals are widely available. Jordan's healthcare has improved dramatically over the past two decades. The country's 84 hospitals provide 8700 beds, about a third of these being run by the Ministry of Health and another third by the private sector. The rest are run by the armed services and by the **Jordan University Hospital**.

Cardiovascular and respiratory diseases and cancer are common causes of mortality.

Jordan

⊃ Visas and work permits:

A three-month visitors' visa for British, French, German, US, Australian and New Zealand citizens is available, usually within 48 hours, from the embassy, (two weeks by post) by filling in a simple form.

USEFUL ADDRESSES:

Ministry of Health, PO Box 86, Amman, Tel: +962 6 607144.
Jordan Medical Association, PO Box 941070, Amman. Fax: +962 6 5686435.
Jordan Nurses and Midwives Council, PO Box 10076, Amman. Tel: +962 6 689468.
Jordan Dental Association, PO Box 1326, Amman 11118. Tel: +962 6 5665520.
Fax: +962 6 5696479.
Jordan Physiotherapy Society, PO Box 510489, Amman 11151. Tel: +962 6 84084.
Fax: +962 6 682299.
www.jordandrs.com lists all of Jordan's hospitals.

MEDICAL SCHOOLS:

Jordan University of Science and Technology, School of Medicine, PO Box 3030, Irbid 22110. Tel: +962 2 709 5111. Fax: +962 2 709 5010. www.just.edu.jo.
University of Jordan, Faculty of Medicine, University Street, Amman. Tel: +962 6 535 5000. Fax: +962 6 535 6746. www.ju.edu.jo. This uses:
Jordan University Hospital, University Highway, Amman. Tel: +962 6 535 3444.

HOSPITALS IN AMMAN:

Akleh Maternity, Jabal Amman.
Tel: +962 6 464 2441.
Al-Ahli Hospital, Abdali. Tel: +962 6 566 4164.
Al-Amal Maternity Hospital, Jabal Al Hussein.
Tel: +962 6 560 7155.
Al Basheir Hospital, Jabal Ashrafieh.
Tel: +962 6 775 1111/1128.
Alkhalidi Maternity, Jabal Amman.
Tel: +962 6 464 4281/4284.
Al- Muasher Hospital, Jabal Al Hussein.
Tel: +962 6 566 7227/7228/7229.
Al-Rahmeh Hospital, Marka.
Tel: +962 6 586 3855/3856/3857/3858.
Amman Surgical Hospital, Jabal Amman.
Tel: +962 6 464 1260/1261.

Arab Center for Heart and Special Surgery, Jabal Amman, Fifth Circle. Tel: +962 6 586 5199.
Army Hospital, Marka. Tel: +962 6 568 1611.
Dar Al-Shifa Hospital, Jabal Al Hussein.
Tel: +962 6 566 7158.
Farah Maternity, Jabal Amman.
Tel: +962 6 464 4440.
Hussein Medical Center, Amman
Tel: +962 6 585 6856.
Islamic Hospital, Abdali Tel: +962 6 568 0127/0130.
Italian Hospital, Al-Muhajreen. Tel: +962 6 777 101/102/103.
Jabal Amman Maternity, Fourth Circle.
Tel: +962 6 534 2362.
Jordan Red Crescent Hospital, Misdar Street.
Tel: +962 6 779 131/135.
Jordan-Hospital, Queen Nour Street,
PO Box 520248, Amman 11152.
Tel.: +962 6 562 0777/560 7550.
Fax: +962 6 560 7575. www.jordan-hospital.com.
Luzmila Hospital, Jabal El Weibdeh.
Tel: +962 6 462 4345.
Malhas Hospital, Jabal Amman.
Tel: +962 6 463 6140.
Palestine Hospital, Shmeisani
Tel: +962 6 560 7071.
PLO Hospital, Jabal Al Hussein
Tel: +962 6 566 6177/1909.
Queen Alia Military Hospital, Tareq
Municipality Tel: +962 6 515 7100.
Shmeisani Hospital, Shmeisani.
Tel: +962 6 560 7431.
Specialty Hospital, Shmeisani.
Tel: +962 6 569 3693.

SOME HOSPITALS IN ZARAQA, KARAK AND AQABA:

Aqaba Hospital, Aqaba. Tel: +962 6 316 677
Hikmeh Hospital, Zarqa. Tel: +962 990 991.
Islamic Hospital, Aqaba. Tel: +962 6 318 444.
Italian Hospital, Karak. Tel: +962 351 145.
Karak Cov. Hospital, Karak. Tel: +962 386 190.
Prince Ali Hospital, Karak. Tel: +962 386 370.
Princess Haya Hospital, Aqaba.
Tel: +962 6 314 111.
Zarqa Government Hospital, Zarqa.
Tel: +962 983 323.

SOME SMALLER HOSPITALS:

King Hussein Hospital, Salt (100 beds).
Ma'an Surgical Hospital, Ma'an (78 beds).
Princes Basma Hospital, Irbid (168 beds).
Tafileh Hospital, Tafileh (32 beds).

The Lebanon

Population: 3.6 million
Capital: Beirut
Language: Arabic (French and English)
Currency: Lebanese pound
Int Code: +961

Lebanon, situated just above Israel, has progressed well since its 16-year civil war, which ended in 1991. A more liberal political system has developed giving Muslims (who make up 70% of the country) a greater say. It has not been a popular elective destination but that is changing. At the time of writing the threat to Westerners is said to be high owing to reactions over the war with Iraq and the Middle East Peace Process. The Foreign Office advises you to be vigilant in public places and avoid military sites, Palestinian refugee camps, the northern Beka'a Valley and areas of South Lebanon close to the Israeli border fence. Check www.fco.gov.uk before you go.

✛ Medicine:

Prior to the war, the Lebanon was regarded as having the best healthcare in the region. It is now regaining this status, but of the 150 hospitals, only a few are public. People living in and around poor urban areas can have great difficulty in accessing care. There is a national medical insurance programme funded by employers, employees and the government, but a contribution is still required when in hospital. To arrange an elective here, you can either apply directly to one of the addresses below or go through Medsin/IFMSA (www.ifmsa.org).

USEFUL ADDRESS:

Ministry of Health: www.public-health.gov.lb.

MEDICAL SCHOOLS:

American University of Beirut, Bliss Street, Beirut. Tel: +961 1 374374 Fax: +961 1744469. www.aub.edu.lb.
Beirut Arab University, PO Box 11-5020, Beirut. Tel: +961 1 300110. Fax: +96 1 1818402. www.bau.edu.lb.
University of Balamand, Deir El-Balamand El-Koura. Tel: +961 6930 250. Fax: +961 6 930278. www.balamand.edy.lb.
Université Libanaise (Lebanese School of Medicine), Rectorat, BP 14-6573, Place du Musée, Beyrouth, Liban. Tel: +961 1 612618. Fax: +961 1 612621. www.ul.edu.lb.
Université Saint-Joseph, PO Box 11-5076 Riad El Solh, Beirut 1107 2180. Tel: +961 1 614004. Fax: +961 1 614054. www.usj.edu.lb.

SOME HOSPITALS:

There is a complete listing of all Lebanon's hospitals at www.lebanesedoctors.com.

American University of Beirut,
PO Box 11-0236, Beirut 1107 2020.
Tel: +961 1 350000. Fax: +961 1 345325.
(This is the major hospital for the university above.)
Da Al Ajaz Al Islamia Hospital, Sabra Street, East of Sports City, PO Box 14 5795, Beirut 1105 2070. Tel: +961 1 856658.
Sahel General Hospital, Airport Avenue, PO Box 99/25 Ghobeiry, Beirut. Tel: +961 1 858 333 40. Fax: +961 1 840146. www.sahelhospital.com.lb.
(This is a 172-bed hospital serving 700 000 people in South Beirut. It is affiliated to the Lebanese School of Medicine.)

Saudi Arabia

Population: 17 million
Language: Arabic
Capital: Riyadh
Currency: Riyal
Int Code: +966

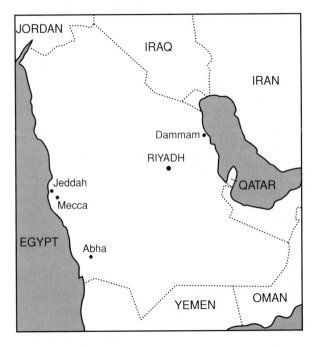

Saudi Arabia occupies four-fifths of the Arabian peninsula and is bordered by Jordan, Iraq, Kuwait, the Gulf of Oman, Qatar, the United Arab Emirates, Yemen and the Red Sea. It is famed for its oil, excellent healthcare and Mecca. It is a common place for experienced medics to work for a while but not a common place for electives. The religion, the culture and the law are Islam. You MUST be aware of this. This means that alcohol is forbidden (hence medical students rarely go there). It also means that women must not drive and that they must dress appropriately. You must also be aware that you should observe daytime fasting during Ramadan. At the time of writing, Westerners have recently been the target of terrorist attacks. The Foreign Office currently advises against all but essential travel to Saudi Arabia. Check www.fco.gov.uk for the latest advice.

✪ Medicine:

Healthcare is provided free to all Saudi citizens and foreign residents via a total of 267 hospitals. The healthcare is of a very high standard. In some centres, up to half the staff are Westerners. The long-term plan was that these Westerners would train up Saudi nationals (by a process called 'Saudisation'). This is happening very slowly, but Western specialists will still be required for some time to come. Jobs can be organized through a number of agencies (*see* www.medicstravel.org for listings).

➲ Visa requirements:

You will need to be sponsored by a hospital or an agency to get an entry visa. This is usually organized for you. Contact the embassy for more details.

USEFUL ADDRESS:

Ministry of Health, Airport Road, Riyadh 11176. Tel: +966 1 401 5555. Fax: +966 1 402 9876.

MEDICAL SCHOOLS:

King Abdul Aziz University, Faculty of Medicine and Allied Health Sciences, Department of Medicine, PO Box 1540, Jeddah 21441. Tel: +966 2 6952035. Fax: +966 2 640 0855. www.kaau.edu.sa.
King Faisal University, College of Medicine, PO Box 2114, Dammam 31451. Tel: +966 3 857 5307. Fax: +966 3 857 5329. www.kfu.edu.sa.
King Khalid University, College of Medicine and Medical Sciences, PO Box 641, Abha. Tel: +966 7 226 0711. Fax: +966 7 224 7570. www.saudimedicine.net/Abha Medicine/main index.shtm.
King Saud University, College of Medicine, PO Box 2925, Riyadh 11461. Tel: +966 1 467 0878. Fax: +966 1 467 2650. www.ksu.edu.sa.
Umm Al-Qura University, College of Medicine, PO Box 715, Mecca. Tel: +966 2 528 1189. Fax: +966 2 528 1189. www.uqu.edu.sa.

SPECIALIST HOSPITALS:

Riyadh Central Hospital, PO Box 2897, Riyadh 11196. Tel: +966 1 435 5555.
King Abdul Aziz University Hospital, PO Box 245, Riyadh 1141. Tel: +966 1 477 4134. Fax: +966 1 477 5766.
King Khaled EyeSpecialist Hospital, PO Box 7191, Riyadh 11462. Tel: +966 482 123. www.kkesh.med.sa.
King Faisal Specialist Hospital and Research Centre, PO Box 3354, Riyadh 11211. Tel: +966 1 477 7272. Fax: +966 1 441 4839. www.kfshrc.edu.sa.
King Khalid National Guard Hospital, PO Box 9515, Jeddah 21423. Tel: +966 2 665 6200. Fax: +966 2 665 3031.
Riyadh Armed Forces Hospital, PO Box 7897 Riyadh 11159. Tel: +966 1 477 7714. Fax: +966 1 476 9250.

United Arab Emirates

Population: 2.3 million
Language: Arabic
Capital: Abu Dhabi
Currency: UAE Dirham
Int Code: +971

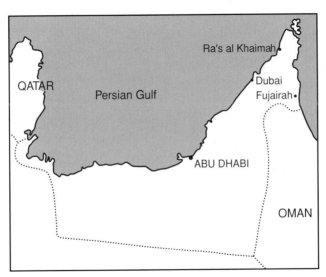

The United Arab Emirates (UAE) comprises seven former sheikdoms, the largest being Abu Dhabi. The land is both mountainous and desert. The discovery of oil has dramatically changed this country since the British pulled out in 1971. As in Saudi Arabia, Islam is the religion and culture (see Saudi Arabia). It is a common place for Westerners to work for a while but not a common elective destination. Because of the war with Iraq and developments in the Middle East Peace Process, local public opinion is in a state of flux. The Foreign Office currently says that the threat to British nationals is high and that terrorist attacks could involve chemical and biological materials – check with www.fco.gov.uk before you go.

☉ Medicine:

Healthcare has advanced dramatically with the rapid increase in prosperity. Many of the staff in the 40 hospitals are Westerners. Emergency treatment is free for all, but non-emergency care is very expensive. Lists of agencies arranging work can be found on www.medicstravel.org. Some hospitals arrange work directly; check their websites for details.

⮑ Visas and work permits:

Most people gain work through an agency, which will normally arrange the necessary paperwork. Contact the embassy directly if you are arranging things yourself.

USEFUL ADDRESS:

Ministry of Health, PO Box 848, Abu Dhabi, Tel: +971 2 214100 Fax: +971 2 212732.

MEDICAL SCHOOLS:

Dubai Medical College for Girls, PO Box 20170. Tel: +971 2 646465. Fax: +971 2 646130. www.dmcg.edu.
United Arab Emirates University, Faculty of Medicine and Health Sciences, PO Box 17666, Al Ain. Tel: +971 3 7678686. Fax: +971 3 7672008. www.fmhs.uaeu.ac.ae.

HOSPITALS:

Al Jazira Hospital, PO Box 2427, Abu Dhabi. Tel: +971 2 214800.

Al Mafraq Hospital, PO Box 233, Abu Dhabi. Tel: +971 2 324300.
Al Tawam Hospital, PO Box 15258, Al Ain, Abu Dhabi. Tel: +971 3 677410. www.aamd.gov.ae. (This is a 300 bed referral hospital for paediatrics, neurosurgery and oncology. They recruit directly.)
Kuwaiti Hospital, PO Box 1853, Dubai. Tel: +971 4 691200.
New Dubai Hospital, PO Box 7272, Dubai. Tel: +971 4 229171.
New Fujarah Hospital, Fujairah. Tel: +971 9 224611.
Saqr Hospital, PO Box 91, Ras Al Khaimah. Tel: + 971 7 223666.
Zaid Military Hospital, PO Box 3755, Abu Dhabi. Tel: +971 2 448100.

SOUTH AND CENTRAL AMERICA

Argentina

Population: 34.6 million
Language: Spanish
Capital: Buenos Aires
Currency: Argentine peso
Int Code: +54

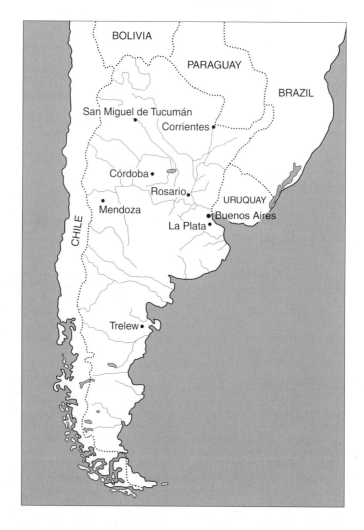

The 3432 km (2145 miles) of Argentina extends from Bolivia to Cape Horn. The Andes separate it from Chile in the west. Farming forms the main source of income and, since 1983, Argentina has had multiparty democracy. To get anything out of and enjoy working here you will have to speak very fluent Spanish. Few people speak English. The only way around it is to go to Patagonia in the south where you'll need to speak fluent Welsh (see below)! This language barrier makes it an unusual place for electives/work.

✪ Medicine:

Access to medical healthcare is available throughout Argentina. Proportionally, there are more doctors than in the USA (one per 330 people). The big killers include heart disease, cancers and accidents. Most nationals rely on health insurance as doctors charge. Indeed, you tend to only see the poor in state hospitals. The Menem administration introduced a Worker's Health Plan system to improve healthcare for the poor. There are 2573 hospitals in total in Argentina and they are not all listed here; a full list (by region) is available on www.hosfio.org.ar/hospitales.

◎ Climate and crime:

Such a great length of the country means that a whole range of climates can be encountered. In the north-east, it is virtually tropical, becoming semi-arid in the Andes. In the south, it can get very cold and snowy. The lowlands in the west are desert; the pampas are mild. South America is not generally regarded as safe; Buenos Aires is, however, one of the safest cities in Latin America. Beware of the small shanty towns where crime is rising.

➲ Visas and work permits:

A visa is required to enter Argentina. Contact the embassy for more details. As a foreign medic, you need to get your degree validated and contact the provincial health authorities or the **Dirección de Control del Ejercicio Profesional y Establecmientos Sanitarios** (Defensa 120, 5 piso, 1345 Buenos Aires), which is attached to the Ministry of Health.

USEFUL ADDRESSES:

Ministry of Health, 9 de Julio 1925, 1332 Buenos Aires. Tel: +54 1 381 8911. Fax: +54 1 381 2182.
Argentine Medical Association: Confederación Médica Argentina, Avenida Belgrano 1235, 1093 Buenos Aires. Tel: +54 11 4383 8414. www.ama-med.com.
Argentine Nurses Association: Federación Argentina de Enfermeria, Avenue Rivadavia 3518, Casilla de Correo 59-Sucursal 53, CP 1204 Buenos Aires. Tel: +54 1 865 1512.
Argentine Dental Association: Asociación Odontológica Argentina, Junin 959, 113 Buenos Aires. Tel: +54 11 4961 6141. Fax: +54 11 4961 1110. www.aoa.org.ar.

MAIN MEDICAL SCHOOLS:

Universidad de Buenos Aires

Facultad de Medicina, Paraguay 2155, 1121, Capital Federal, Buenos Aires. Tel: +54 11 4961 9980. Fax: +54 11 4961 9598. www.fmed.uba.ar.

This, the nation's oldest medical school, is situated in the capital and has links with over 50 hospitals in Argentina (a full list is available on their website). The main hospitals are: **Hospital de Clínicas José de San Martín**, Avenida Córdoba 2351, Buenos Aires. Tel: +54 4 1508 3994. This is a major centre, founded in 1877 with an emergency department and many specialist departments; **Hospital Municipal de San Miguel**, in the north-west of Buenos Aires is a 236-bed general hospital catering for a poor population, of whom only half have running water and 15% don't have a toilet.

Universidad Nacional de Córdoba

Facultad de Ciencias Médicas, Pabellón Argentina-Ciudad Universitaria, 1° Piso a la izquierda, 5000 Córdoba. Tel: +54 35 1433 4040. Fax: +54 35 1433 4036. www.unc.edu.ar.

This is Argentina's second oldest medical school and uses **Hospital Nacional de Clínicas** (Tel: +54 337025/337014) and **Hospital Universitario de Maternidad y Neonatologia** (Tel: +54 331053/ 331050/331052) in Córdoba.

Argentina

SOME OTHER MEDICAL SCHOOLS:

For a full list see www.medicstravel.org.

Universidad Católica de Córdoba, Facultad de Medicina, Jacinto Rios 571, 5000 Córdoba-CBA. Tel: +54 35 1451 7299. Fax: +54 35 1423 1937. www.uccor.edu.ar.

Universidad Nacional de Cuyo, Facultad de Ciencias Médicas, Parque General San Martin, Casilla de Correo 3, 5500 Mendoza-MZA. Tel: +54 26 1449 4046. Fax: +54 26 1449 4047. www.fmed2.uncu.edu.ar.

Universidad Nacional del Nordeste, Facultad de Medicina, Moreno 1240, 3400 Corrientes-CTS. Tel: +54 37 8342 3155. Fax: +54 37 8342 5508. www.med.unne.edu.ar/inicio.htm.

Universidad Nacional de La Plata, Facultad de Ciencias Médicas, Calle 60 y 120, 1900 La Plata, Buenos Aires. Tel: +54 22 1424 1596/3068/2711/6711. Fax: +54 22 1425 8989. www.unlp.edu.ar.

Universidad Nacional de Rosario, Facultad de Medicina, Santa Fe 3100, 2000 Rosario-SF. Tel: +54 34 1480 4558. Fax: +54 34 1251 533. www.fmedic.unr.edu.ar.

Universidad Nacional de Tucumán, Facultad de Medicina, Casilla de Correo 159, Lamadrid 875, 4000 San Miguel De Tucumán. Tel: +54 38 1424 7752, ext. 277. Fax: +54 38 1424 8024. www.fm.unt.edu.ar.

Universidad del Salvador, Facultad de Medicina, Tucumán 1859, 1050 Buenos Aires-CF. Tel: +54 11 4813 2935. Fax: +54 11 4811 8519. www.salvador.edu.ar.

Patagonia

Patagonia is the huge wasteland of southern Argentina. On 28th July 1856, the sailing ship Mimosa *landed on the coast of Patagonia. Aboard were 150 Welsh emigrants who had sailed from Liverpool in search of a new land where their culture would be safe. Between then and 1911, 3000 Welsh men, women and children endured the three-month voyage to Patagonia. For many years, Welsh culture flourished. Even now, there is a lively (though diminishing) Welsh community, and outside the hospital, the language can be pure Welsh. The Welsh community is strongest in the province of Chubut (which is about the size of Spain) and especially in the town of Trelew ('Tre' meaning town in Welsh, 'Lew' after Lewis Jones, one of the community's founders). This is where Trelew's Zonal Hospital lies.*

Hospital Zonal Trelew

9100 Chubut, Patagonia. Tel: +54 2965 42 7542 28.

The hospital: A state-funded hospital with 150 beds serving a population of 80 000. Welsh is the language of the hospital, but it is advisable to take some Spanish lessons before arriving. NO ONE SPEAKS ENGLISH. Lots of the nurses can, however, speak Welsh.

Since it is a state hospital, it tends to only see the poor Chilean immigrants. Treatment is free and so theoretically are all prescriptions (subject to means testing). Expensive drugs are simply not available. Chubut is renowned throughout Argentina for the progress it has made in combating the two major diseases of hydatid disease and TB, and the work has been centred in Trelew. Chubut has the world's highest incidence of hydatid disease (Wales having the highest in Europe!). This is probably because of the many sheep and dogs (known as the 'poor man's blanket') that live in close proximity to the people. The incidence has declined by a programme of public education and the treatment of all dogs with the anti-parasitic prasiquantel.

O Elective notes: You can follow the physicians, neonatologists, paediatricians, neurologists or casualty officers. There are also peripheral clinics and a psychiatric hospital to attend.

Belize

Population: 216 000
Language: English
Capital: Belmopan
Currency: Belizean dollar
Int Code: +501

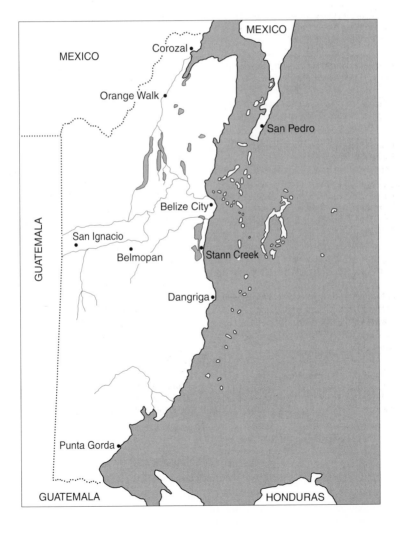

MEXICO

MEXICO

Corozal •

Orange Walk •

San Pedro •

GUATEMALA

Belize City •

San Ignacio •

Belmopan •

Stann Creek •

Dangriga •

Punta Gorda •

GUATEMALA

HONDURAS

Belize

Belize (formerly British Honduras) lies on the eastern shores of the Yuctan Peninsula and is bordered in the west by Guatemala and Mexico. Since its independence in 1981, Belize has slowly increased in prosperity. It is the least populous country in Central America with over half the land still covered in dense forest. The coast has the world's second-largest barrier reef, giving protection from flooding. The population is diverse in nature, but there is still great poverty. Spanish-speaking black Creoles now make up over half the population, the rest being Maya groups, black Caribs and immigrants from Mexico. Because of a successful education system, there is a high literacy rate. This is a good central American country to go to as so many people speak English. There's plenty to do in Belize, with excellent diving and beautiful coastlines. You can trek into the jungle and when finished visit a Caribbean island.

○ Medicine:

There are seven government hospitals and many mobile clinics in Belize, to which around 75% of the population have access. Basic sanitation and water supplies have been a priority, and now over half the houses in Belmopan have both. Respiratory, heart and cerebrovascular diseases are the big killers. The HIV rate in Belize City is pretty high because of drug abuse. The doctor:patient ratio is also rather high, at 1:1809. They'll appreciate any old copies of the *BNF* or textbooks here.

◎ Climate and crime:

Hot and humid weather is normal throughout the year. However, hurricanes often cause havoc in the coastal regions. Belize is a route for Colombian cocaine, and there are a few drugs gangs in Belize City. The city is not a safe place at night. Rural Belize is usually fine.

○ Visas and work permits:

European, American and British Commonwealth citizens (bar those of India and Nigeria) do not need a visa to enter Belize. If gaining employment, you need a temporary employment permit, and certificates confirming you are HIV negative and have no criminal convictions. Application forms can be obtained in any labour department office in Belize. Contact the High Commission for more information.

USEFUL ADDRESSES:

Ministry of Health, East Block, Independence Hill, Belmopan. Tel: +501 8 22325 Fax: +501 8 22942. www.belize.gov.bz.
Belize Dental Association, PO Box 1810, Belize City. Tel: +501 2 71947. Fax: +501 2 75390.

PUBLIC HOSPITALS:

Karl Huesner Memorial Hospital
Princess Margaret Drive, Belize City, Belize, CA. Tel: +501 2 31584.
The hospital: Is the main hospital and brand new. Although it caters for nearly all specialities, it does lack some facilities. There is a very busy emergency department.
○ Elective notes: Students play an active role in the emergency department, with lots of suturing of machete and knife wounds. There's a good supportive staff. O&G and surgery are also highly recommended.

Belize City Hospital, Eyre Street, Belize City, Belize, CA. Tel: +501 2 77251.
Belmopan Hospital, Florina Drive, Belmopan, Belize, CA. Tel: +501 8 22263/22264.
Corozal Hospital, Corozal, Belize, CA. Tel: +501 4 22081.
Dangriga Hospital, Dangriga, Belize, CA. Tel: +501 5 22084.
Orange Walk Hospital, Orange Walk, Belize, CA. Tel: +501 3 22143.
Punta Gorda Hospital, Punta Gorda, Belize, CA. Tel: +501 7 22026.
San Ignacio Hospital, Hospital Street, San Ignacio, Belize, CA. Tel: +501 9 22066. (This is a private hospital.)

SMALL CLINICS:

To do community work in one of the 40 health centres, write to the Chief Medical Officer, Ministry of Health at the above address.

RURAL CLINICS:

San Pedro Health Centre
San Pedro.

It is possible to spend some time doing clinics on one of Belize's cayes (islands), for example Ambergris Caye. You need to get a boat to San Pedro and then, once a week, you can fly in a tiny plane to the neighbouring island. There are no hospitals on these islands so you are the only medical care. There is a new recompression chamber here since it is a popular diving spot.

Independence Health Centre
Independence, Stann Creek.

Mongo Creek, on the edge of the jungle, is a rural village also with a clinic. You do home visits on a bike. This is a great place to go to experience developing medicine in a beautiful country.

Bolivia

Population: 7.4 million
Languages: Spanish, Aymará and Quechua
Official Capital: Sucre
Administrative Capital: La Paz
Currency: Boliviano
Int Code: +591

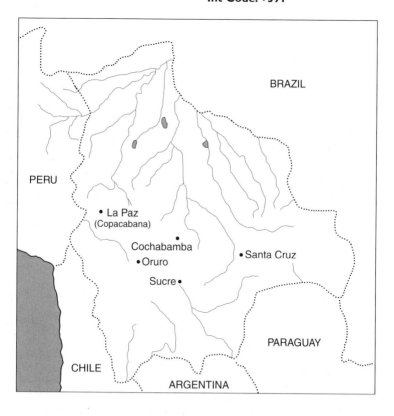

Bolivia, South America's fifth-largest country, is very mountainous. Seventy per cent of the population lives above 11 000 ft on the Altiplano Plateau (which is only 10% of the area of the country). The mountainous areas include La Paz, the world's highest capital city. The lower eastern regions are more tropical and are rapidly becoming populated. Being surrounded by five other South American countries, Bolivia relies on Chile's port facilities. Despite its rich mining resources, Bolivia is the poorest country in South America. The majority of the population rely on agriculture, although many ascend

even higher into the mountains to mine.
Bolivia's third-largest economy is coca leaves.
These have a huge importance in traditional
medicines, but also generate around $1
billion in illegal trafficking. The country has a
great cultural heritage. Things you must see in
Bolivia include the Valle du Luna (the valley of
the moon), Chacaltaya, the 'world's highest ski
area', the ancient ruins at Tiahuanaco
(Tiwanaku), the Yungas, the beginning of the
tropical rainforest, and Lake Titicaca, the
world's highest navigable lake. It's also worth
going to Copacabana, staying the night and
going to the Isla del Sol and Isla de la Luna.
After that, cross the border and see Peru.
Although two-thirds of the population is of
pure Indian descent, many of the remainder
are mestizos (mixed Spanish). The national
languages are Aymará and Quechua, but
Spanish is taught in the schools (although
outside the cities many cannot speak
Spanish). To get on in working out here, you
must have a basic knowledge of Spanish. The
local currency is Boliviano (B$) but US dollars
are used everywhere (B$5 = about US$1).

✪ Medicine:
Because of their isolation, many people do
not have access to Western medicine, and
basic provisions such as clean water and
sanitation are only available to half of the
population. Many children don't receive
immunizations and hence preventable
infectious diseases are a common cause of
death. Big killers are influenza, TB and
malaria. TB vaccination is free, but mothers
don't want it for fear it may do harm. TB
treatment is also free, but TB is still a problem
because the diagnostic test is not free so people
don't find out whether they have it.
Rheumatic fever is also common. Chagas'
disease and its complications are more
confined to South and Central America.
Trypanosoma cruzi is carried by the Reduvid
bug, which lives in the roofs of mud houses.
This makes it difficult to eradicate so this is a
common 'unusual' disease. Its prevalence is as
high as 80% in some populations. Chronic
diseases of the West are not really seen as the
life expectancy is about 60 years. Infant
mortality is also outrageously high, ranging
from 92 to 300 per 1000 in some areas.

Acute mountain sickness (nausea,
vomiting, headache, pulmonary and cerebral
oedema and retinal haemorrhage) is also seen
in natives but more commonly in tourists. For
the treatment, *see* Section 1. In chronic
mountain sickness, polycythaemia (with
complications of thrombosis, haemorrhage and
cardiac failure), drowsiness, cyanosis, clubbing,
right ventricular enlargement, cor pulmonale
and hypertension are seen.

There are three types of hospitals: general,
Caja Nacional de Salud ('house of the nation's
health'; CNS) and private. The general
hospitals are accessible to everyone for a small
fee for all diagnostic tests and treatment. The
facilities are very limited here. The CNS
hospitals, which are for those who pay social
security, give them free treatment. These are
the most common. The third type are private.
Doctors train at either government or private
medical schools. There are three preclinical
years, two clinical years and then an intern
year, after which students sit exams and then
have to complete a year in a rural hospital. The
doctor:patient ratio is 1:1971. Although 95%
of the population are Roman Catholic, they still
have traditional beliefs such as guidance from
witches.

◎ Climate and crime:
The climate varies greatly. The plateau
between the Andes has a tropical highland
climate and is very cold at night. The eastern
regions are lower and therefore tend to be
warmer. Bolivia has had a very good crime
record and it's still a very safe place for
tourists. Drug-related crime is, however, on the
increase, especially in the east and in Santa Cruz.

⊃ Visas and work permits:
Elective students have previously entered on a
tourist visa. The official line from the consulate
is that a student visa can be obtained from them
once the student provides the necessary
documents certifying registration with a
university or any other education institution. Work

visas can only be obtained at the Immigration Office in Bolivia, and the applicant should enter Bolivia with a business visa issued by the consulate. The requirements to obtain a working visa are a passport valid for one year from the date of entry into Bolivia and a working certificate or business contract.

To work in any city here, write to the General Hospital, City Name, Bolivia.

Note: You may well get acute mountain sickness here, especially if you fly straight in. Follow the guidelines at the beginning of this book (rest, no smoking, no drinking, etc.). The locals sell Soroche pills in most pharmacists in La Paz, which allegedly help in the first few days. *Mate de coca* (coca leaf tea) is another remedy the locals swear by.

USEFUL ADDRESSES:

Office of the Secretary of Health, Plaza del Estudiante, La Paz. Tel: +591 2 375471. Fax: +591 2 391590.
Bolivian Medical Association: Colegio Médico de Bolivia, Pastor Sainz 273, Sucre.
Tel: +591 64 41 690. Fax: +591 6 441670.

La Paz

La Paz at 3636 m is the highest capital in the world and is the largest city in Bolivia. It is the centre of commerce and finance, but Sucre remains the judiciary capital. La Paz has more than a million people. The weather is very changeable, even within a single day. The temperature is about 20°C by day and 10°C at night. There's plenty to do: San Francisco Cathedral, four museums and a couple of markets (Mercado de Heciceria, the 'witches market', and Linares market, which sells herbs, seed and llama skeleton remedies). The local cinema shows a number of English films.

UNIVERSITY AND MEDICAL SCHOOLS:

Universidad Iberoamericana, Facultad de Medicina, Avenida 14 de Septiembre 5809, Casilla 3498, La Paz. Tel: +591 2 783177. Fax: +591 2 782431.

Universidad Mayor de San Andres, Facultad de Medicina, Avenida Villason No. 1995, La Paz.
Tel: +591 2 359588. Fax: +591 2 359491.
www.umsanet.edu.bo.
Universidad Nuestra Senora de La Paz, Facultad de Medicina, Calle Presbitero Medina 2412, Casilla 5995, La Paz. Tel: +591 2 418167. Fax: +591 2 410255.
Universidad del Valle, La Paz, Facultad de Medicina, Casilla 13602, La Paz. Tel: +591 2 431112.
Fax: +591 2 433261. www.univalle.edu.

Hospital Obrero

Avenida Brasil, Miraflores, La Paz.
Tel: +591 2 462 1509.
The hospital: Hospital Obrero ('hospital of the workers') is the best CNS hospital in Bolivia. It has good facilities (e.g. a CT scanner), but only few patients are scanned because of the cost. The hospital sees all the diseases listed above. The surgical department performs not only your standard Western list, but also the unusual, such as bowel resection due to megacolon caused by Chagas' diseases. Many cholecystectomies are carried out as the locals have a high-fat diet. Gynae is busy with cancers (because of poor screening) and the complications of illegal abortion.

Hospital du Mujer

La Paz.
The hospital: The 'Hospital of Women' (O&G only) is about five minutes' walk from Hospital Obrero. It is much poorer, and patients' treatment is governed by what they can afford. To the Western eye it can seem brutal. In the delivery suite there are eight beds, no curtains, no relatives and no midwives. The only staff are doctors. The women are given an enema and shaved. In the delivery room, aparous women get an episiotomy. There is no analgesia. When it's all over, they are monitored and get a night on the ward. This costs £10 so, not surprisingly, 80% of women deliver at home.

Cochabamba

Universidad Mayor de San Simón
Facultad de Medicina, Avenida Aniceto Arce 0371, Casilla 3999, Cochabamba.
Tel: +591 4 259833. Fax: +591 4 231690.
This uses:

Hospital Viedma
Avenida Aniceto Arce E-0257,
Cochabamba. Tel: +591 42 20226.
The hospital: Viedma is the main public hospital in Cochabamba (there are many surrounding clinics/small hospitals), serving a population of one million. It's poorly equipped (the only ECG being in ITU). Gloves and needles are resterilized (so take your own). It's a friendly place with a lot of respect for foreigners. Unusual pathologies that are more common here include Chagas' disease, TB, rheumatic heart disease and Fournier's gangrene.
O Elective notes: It's very busy but enjoyable. The final year students work as interns, doing a 96-hour week with an on call of 1:2 or 1:3. They get paid $15 a week for the privilege. The patients and hospital are very poor. They may ask for a blood donation while you are there ... students have said this is fine but just make sure they use a new set. You get a lot of 'hands on' experience. Few patients can afford a plastic surgeon so you'll be dealing with facial lacerations.
Accommodation: There is a dormitory block if you are on call in the emergency department, but accommodation is otherwise not provided. Hotel Elisa (SO 834 Calle Agustin Lopez) is recommended (about B$38 (£4) a night).

Universidad del Valle
Facultad de Medicina, Campus Tiquipaya, Casilla 4742, Cochabamba.
Tel: +591 42 87373. Fax: +591 42 88550.
www.univalle.edu.

Oruro

Universidad del Altiplano, Facultad de Medicina, Calle La Plata Esquina Murgia, Oruro.
Tel: +591 5 254946.

Sucre

Universidad San Francisco Xavier, Facultad de Medicina, Calle Junin Esquina Estudiantes, Casilla 233, Sucre. Tel: +591 64 22402. www.usfx.edu.bo.

Santa Cruz

Universidad Católica Boliviana, Facultad de Medicina, Calle Espana 368, Casilla 3201, Santa Cruz. Tel: +591 3 351 549. Fax: +591 3 332 389. www.bolivar.udo.edu.ve .
Universidad Cristiana Boliviana, Facultad de Medicina, Campus Universitario Km 5, Calle Norte, Avenida Banzer, Casilla 4780, Santa Cruz.
Tel: +591 3 410 472. Fax: +591 3 426 311.

HOSPITALS AND CLINICS IN BOLIVIA:

La Paz:
Clinica Adventista La Paz, C. Carrasco 1405, Miraflores, La Paz.
Clinica Alemana, Avenida 6 de Agosto 2821, La Paz. Tel: +591 612 320 355/323 023.
Clinica del Alto, Urb Boris Banzer, El Alto, La Paz.
Clinica Americana, Avenida 14 de Septiembre, Obrajes, La Paz. Tel: +591 612 783 371/783 372.
Clinica Boston, Avenida Ecuador 2475, La Paz.
Clinica Britanica, Avenida Mscal Santa Cruz, Edif Esperanza, La Paz.
Clinica de Neurocirugia, C. Genaro Amarra 1887, La Paz.
Clinica Radiologica, Avenida Arce 2081, La Paz.
Clinica Rengel, C. Victor Sanjines 2762, La Paz.
Clinica Santa Maria, Avenida 6 de Agosto 2487, La Paz.
Clinica del Sur, Avenida Hernando Siles 5353, Obrajes, La Paz.
Hospital Juan XXIII, Avenida Naciones Unidas, Munaypata, La Paz.
Hospital Metodista, Avenida 14 de Septiembre, Obrajes, La Paz. Tel: +591 612 783 509/510/511.
Hospital Neumologico, Av. Vicente Burgaleta V, Copacabana, La Paz.
Hospital de Psiquiatria, Avenida Villalobos 1477 Miraflores, La Paz.

Cochabamba:
Clinica Boliviano Americano, Avenida San Martin S-1023, Cochabamba. Tel: +591 42 56316.
Clinica Cochabamba, C. Lanza S-0931, Cochabamba. Tel: +591 42 29433.
Clinica Copacabana, Avenida Potosi N-1253, Cochabamba.
Clinica de Especialidades Pediatricas, Avenida Heroinas E-1024, Cochabamba. Tel: +591 42 54133.
Clinica Geriatrica Dorian, C. Felix Del Grando N-1251, Cochabamba. Tel: +591 42 45009.
Clinica Iriarte, C. Victor Cabrera Lozada E-023, Cochabamba. Tel: +591 42 33780.
Clinica La Paz, Plaza Barba de Padilla E-0233, Cochabamba. Tel: +591 42 45998.
Clinica Maternologica Santa Ines, C. La Merced O-1585, Cochabamba. Tel: +591 42 46768.
Clinica del Nino Cochabamba, C. Bolivar E-1113, Cochabamba. Tel: +591 42 31839.
Clinica Policial No 2 Virgen de Copacabana, Plaza Sucre 206, Cochabamba. Tel: +591 42 50374.

Bolivia

Clinica Pronto Socorro de Fracturas Laser C. Pasteur N-0210, Cochabamba. Tel: +591 42 52424.

Clinica Recolete, Avenida Potosi N-1326, Cochabamba. Tel: +591 42 44235.

Clinica Saavedra, C. Calama O-0380, Cochabamba. Tel: +591 42 22776.

Clinica San Francisco Ltda, C. Sucre E-0987, Cochabamba. Tel: +591 42 21379.

Clinica San Joaquin, Avenida Del La Fuerza Aerea 2433, Cochabamba. Tel: +591 42 53875.

Clinica San Pablo, Avenida Simon Lopez O-0375, Cochabamba. Tel: +591 42 46009.

Clinica del Valle, Avenida Tadeo Haenke O-1171, Cochabamba. Tel: +591 42 82228.

Hospital Albina Patino, C. Jordan E-0886, Cochabamba. Tel: +591 42 26161.

Hospital Antituberculoso, Avenida Aniceto Arce E-0257, Cochabamba. Tel: +591 42 21120.

Hospital Clinico Viedma, Avenida Aniceto Arce E-0257, Cochabamba. Tel: +591 42 28106.

Hospital Cuschieri, Plaza 15 de Abril Cocap 17, Cochabamba. Tel: +591 42 61891.

Hospital Elizabeth Seton, Avenida Blanco Galindo Km 5, Cochabamba. Tel: +591 42 41889/40201.

Hospital Militar No. 2, Avenida Ramon Rivero s/n, Cochabamba. Tel: +591 42 21086.

Hospital San Vicente, C. Baptosta N-0541, Cochabamba. Tel: +591 42 54321. Fax: +591 42 54352.

Santa Cruz:

Clinica del Accidentado, 6 C/1 Oeste Pasillo 1, Barrio Hamacas, Santa Cruz. Tel: +591 3 425 988.

Clinica Angel Foianini, Avenida Irala, Chuquisaca, Santa Cruz. Tel: +591 3 62211/66005. Fax: +591 3 65577.

Clinica Baldivieso, 764 Avenida Viedma, Santa Cruz. Tel: +591 3 37868.

Clinica de Cirugia Plastica, 489 C. Junin, Santa Cruz. Tel: +591 3 51915.

Clinica Cristo Rey, Avenida Roca y Coronado, Chilon, Santa Cruz. Tel: +591 3 533914.

Clinica Dr Torres, Km 3 1/2 Carr al Norte, Santa Cruz. Tel: +591 3 426710.

Clinica de Emergencia Cardenal Maurer, 103 Avenida Melchor Pinto, Santa Cruz. Tel: +591 3 35558.

Clinica de Emergencias Bilbao, 482 Avenida Mons Rivero, Santa Cruz. Tel: +591 3 22255.

Clinica Incor, Avenida 26 Febrero/Caranda, Santa Cruz. Tel: +591 3 529236.

Clinica Infantil San Patricio, Libertad/Canoto, Santa Cruz. Tel: +591 3 41190.

Clinica Instituto de Gastroenterologia, 265 Avenida Mons Rivero, Santa Cruz. Tel: +591 3 42385. Fax: +591 3 43430.

Clinica Medica Sirani, 667 Rene Moreno, Santa Cruz. Tel: +591 3 52200.

Clinica Odontogica Integrada, 216 Campero, Santa Cruz. Tel: +591 3 23827.

Clinica de Ojos Santa Cruz, Avenida Centenario, Pasillo Barbery, Santa Cruz. Tel: +591 3 32478. Fax: +591 3 27327.

Clinica Pereira, Radial 26, Final Barr Oriental, Santa Cruz. Tel: +591 3 426368.

Clinica del Reposo Monte Sinai, 3er Anillo Ext/Radial 19, Santa Cruz. Tel: +591 3 520895.

Clinica Saavedra, 382 Avenida Saavedra, Santa Cruz. Tel: +591 3 64688.

Clinica San Prudencio, Km6 Carr a Cochabamba, Santa Cruz. Tel: +591 3 529664.

Clinica Santa Cruz, 140 Avenida Busch, Santa Cruz. Tel: +591 3 66111.

Clinica Santa Maria, 754 Avenida Viedma, Santa Cruz. Tel: +591 3 52001. Fax +591 3 24288.

Clinica Urkupina, 550 Avenida El Trompillo/O Chavez, Santa Cruz. Tel: +591 3 527081.

Clinica Virgen del Carmen, 163 Piriti, Santa Cruz. Tel: +591 3 527502.

Clinica Virgen de Lourdes, 352 Rene Moreno, Santa Cruz. Tel: +591 3 25518.

Hospital, Avenida 3er Anillo Ext 747, Calle Ballivian, Santa Cruz. Tel: +591 3 32516.

Hospital Modelo San Lucas, 747 Ballivian, Santa Cruz. Tel: +591 3 32514.

Hospital de Nino Dr Mario Ortiz, C. Santa Barbara/Buenos Aires, Santa Cruz. Tel: +591 3 36841.

Hospital San Juan de Dios, C. Cuellar/Espana, Santa Cruz. Tel: +591 3 32222.

Hospital Urbari, Calle Igmiri, Santa Cruz. Tel: +591 3 534000.

Brazil

Population: 161.8 million
Language: Portuguese
Capital: Brasília
Currency: Real
Int Code: +55

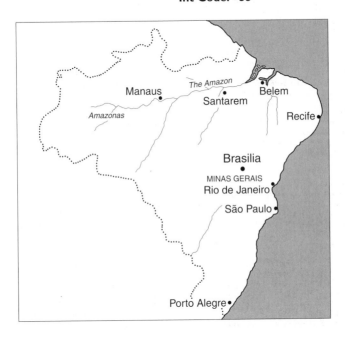

Brazil, the largest country in South America, is famous for its rainforest, the huge Amazon river and its coffee, gold and diamonds. It has 1989 km (1243 miles) of Atlantic coastline and a diverse population based on original Indians, Portuguese colonizers and African slaves brought to work in the sugar plantations. Over the past century, many of the Indian villages have been wiped out by disease or by Western force. The total number of Indians is now only 200 000. The history and the annual Mardi Gras in Rio de Janeiro make it a popular tourist destination; however, probably because of difficulties with the language (which is a variation of European Portuguese), Brazil is not a popular elective destination. It is not a popular work destination either. For this reason, only a brief outline will be given here. Contact the NGOs listed in Section 4 for more ideas.

☉ Medicine:

For Brazil's rich, the private healthcare is good. However, for the vast majority, healthcare is sparse or non-existent. Only 20% of the country's hospitals are state run. Infectious diseases, in particular malaria, leprosy and parasitic skin infections, are on the increase. This is because of the lack of preventative medicine for which Brazil has been strongly criticized.

◉ Climate and crime:

High temperatures and a relatively constant rainfall are usual in the Amazon basin. The north-east of the country has little rainfall and over recent years has suffered episodes of drought. The Brazilian plateau has a wider temperature range and most rainfall between October and April. The south has a temperate climate of warm summers and cool winters.

Over the past couple of decades, crime has risen sharply. This is particularly so in the shanty towns and urban conurbations where street children have been murdered by uncontrolled death squads. Drug-related crime is also on the increase. The displacement of original people and land workers is still occurring.

➲ Visas and work permits:

A visa is required to enter, as is a work permit to work. Consult the embassy for more details.

There are over 100 medical schools in Brazil, and since Brazil is not a common elective or work destination, they are not all listed here. A full list can be obtained through the World Health Organization, at www.iime.org or at www.medicstravel.org. A number of charities and NGOs also do a considerable amount of work in Brazil (*see* Section 4). **Action In International Medicine** (125 High Holborn, London WC1V 6QA, UK. Tel: +44 20 7405 3090. Fax: +44 20 7405 3093) has been particularly recommended for primary care work and arranges work with **Fundação Esperanca** (*see* page 421).

USEFUL ADDRESSES:

Ministry of Health, Esplanda dos Ministérios, Bloco G, 5° andar, Brasília 70.058. Tel: +55 61 223 7340. Fax: +55 61 224 8747.

Brazilian Medical Association: Associação Médica Brasileira, Rua São Carlos do Pinhal 324, Bela Vista, São Paulo SP 01333 903. www.amb.org.br.
Brazilian Nurses' Association: Associação Brasileira de Enfermagem, SGAN Avenida L2 Norte, Quadra 603 Módulo B, CEP 70830-30 Brasília DF. Tel: +55 61 226 0653. Fax: +55 61 225 4473.
Brazilian Dental Association, Rua Thirso Martins 100, Sala 114, São Paulo SP 04120 050. Tel: +55 11 5574 5244. Fax: +55 11 5574 5244. www.abonac.org.br.

SOME MEDICAL SCHOOLS:

Brasília:
Fundação Universidade de Brasília, Faculdade de Ciências da Saúde, Campus Universitário, Asa Norte Residencial 70910-900, Brasília. Tel: +55 61 273 3862. Fax: +55 61 273 0105. www.unb.br/fs.

Minas Gerais:
Universidad Federal de Minas Gerais, Faculdade de Medicina, Avenida Alfredo Balena 190, Belo Horizonte-MG CE: 30.130–100 PO Box 340, Minas Gerais. Tel: +55 31 3248 9300. Fax: +55 31 3248 9664. www.medicina.ufmg.br.

Rio de Janeiro:
Universidade Federal do Rio de Janeiro, Faculdade de Medicina, Avenida Brigadeiro Trompowsky s/n, Ilha do Fundão, CEP: 21941-590, Rio de Janeiro – RJ. Tel: +55 21 260 7386. Fax: +55 21 260 7750. www.ufrj.br/home.php.

São Paulo:
Universidade Federal de São Paulo, Escola Paulista de Medicina, Rua Botucatu 740, 5° andar, Caixa Postal 7144, 02023 São Paulo. Tel: +55 11 5576 4000. www.unifesp.br. (The medical school uses the huge 654 bed São Paulo Hospital. Clinics are also run in rural communities.)

SOME OF THE LARGER HOSPITALS:

Fundação Hospital Felicio Roxo, 9530 Avenue do Contorno, Bairro Prado, Belo Horizonte, Minas Gerais. Tel +55 31 339 7244.
Hospital de Base do Distrito Federal, Area Especial SMHS, Brasilia, Distro Federal. Tel +55 61 325 5050.
Hospital João de Barros Barreto, 4487 End Rua dos Mundurusuc, Bairro Guama-Belém, Para. Tel: +55 91 249 2323.
Hospital Metropolitan, 172 Rua Visconte, Bairro Luz, Rio de Janeiro. Tel: +55 21 281 7452.
Sociedade Portuguesa Beneficente do Amazonas, 1359 Avenue Joaquim Nabuco, Centro Manaus, Amazonas. Tel: +55 92 622 3939.

PRIMARY CARE WORK:

Fundação Esperanca
Rua Coaracy Nunes, 3344, Caixa Postal
222, Santarem, Para CEP 68040–100. Tel:
+55 91 522 2726. Fax: +55 91 522 7878.
E-mail: fesperan@ax.apc.org or
fesperan@ax.ibase.org.br.

The clinic: Fundação Esperança ('Hope
Foundation') is a non-profit-making
organization run largely by North
Americans and is based in Santarem in
the mid-Amazonian basin. It is a primary
healthcare facility that runs clinics.
Santarem is a short flight or a three-day
boat trip down the Amazon from Belem.
The region is poor with very deficient
health services. The Fundação serves the
town's 30 000 inhabitants and rural people scattered through the municipality
(about the size of Belgium).

There is a great deal of tropical medicine (leprosy, leishmaniasis and malaria)
and general medicine (diabetes, hypertension and TB). Paeds and O&G are also
busy. The main doctor in charge is very
friendly, and there are a number of volunteers who work here. The elective
surgery programme brings volunteer
orthopaedic, plastic and ophthalmological teams to the Fundação every three
months.

O Elective notes: This is an excellent
place to see medicine (and dentistry) in a
developing world. It is not the place if
you want loads of trauma and chest
drains. At the education centre (good
library), training is provided at various
levels and in different areas of health
work. It is demanding but rewarding. A
typical day starts at 7.30 am with a
two-hour tutorial and goes through to
5.30 pm, with a two hour lunch break. In
the clinics, students consult patients.
There are very few acute cases but many
tropical diseases, gynae and paeds
problems. Students can also go out with
a health worker on a four-day journey
into the jungle to check on remote
communities and immunize and weigh
children. Being able to speak Portugese
is a big advantage although not necessary due to the American presence.

Accommodation: Provided free to volunteers. Some elective students have had
to pay 17.5 BRL ($10) a day, but this
includes food and laundry. There are
plenty of opportunities at weekends to go
off with the Americans and explore the
beauties of the region.

Good Samaritan Clinic
São Paulo.
This is a 100-bed unit that oversees a
number of projects on the edge of a slum
housing 1200 families.

Porto Alegre

*Porto Alegre, with its 1.5 million inhabitants, is
the capital of Brazil's southernmost states in
the most affluent and developed part of the
country. Many southerners are descended
from Germans and Italians, and take pride in
their 'non-Third-Worldism'. They are famed
throughout Brazil for their 'work ethic'
mentality, their barbeques, their money and
their lack of 'Brazilianess' (carnival and chaos).*

Hospital Nossa SRA da Conceicao
Rua Francisco Trein, 556, Porto Alegre.

The community health service: Has
been in existence for almost 20 years. It is
modelled on the UK GP system and is one
of the only services of its kind in the country. It started from within a public hospital
and gradually, through demand from local
communities, spread outwards so that
today there is the largest and original
'post', with 13 others scattered throughout
the north of the city. Originally financially
independent, it is now government subsidized and offers primary healthcare, free
of charge, to anyone within ill-defined
catchment areas. Working at one of these
posts means that you can get to see the rich
diseases (similar to those of the UK) as
well as those of the terrible conditions in
the shanty towns.

Instituto Matern Infantil de
Pernambuco
Rua Dos Coelhos, 300 Boa Vista, CEP
50070–550, Recife.

Chile

Population: 14.3 million
Language: Spanish
Capital: Santiago
Currency: Chilean peso
Int Code: +56

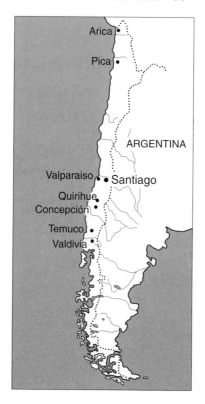

Chile stretches some 4315 km (2697 miles) down the west coast of South America. In the east, it is bordered by the Andes. The length and variation in altitudes gives Chile a wide range of climates. During the Pinochet years, a dramatic decline in tourism occurred. However, since democracy in 1993, tourism to the Andes, the Elqui Valley wine region and Easter Island has increased. Very few doctors and even fewer locals speak English. If you are thinking of going here it is vital that you have at least some basic Spanish. This is especially true in rural hospitals. If you can at least try, most people will be sympathetic and keen to help.

❂ Medicine:
There is a public health service that covers 80% of the population. However, it does not reach the rural areas. The overcrowding of the capital, Santiago, is also a major health problem. The doctor:patient ratio is 1:2150. Heart disease and cancer are the big killers.

◎ Climate:
The climate varies widely from a wet south and the glaciers of the Andes to the pleasant central region.

➲ Visas and work permits:
A visa is required to enter Chile; however, as it is not a popular elective destination, there is no clear information on the need for a visa specifically for electives. You should be OK with a tourist visa, but contact the embassy for more details or if intending to work.

USEFUL ADDRESSES:

Ministry of Health, Enrique MacIver 541, Santiago. Tel: +56 2 639 4001. Fax: +56 2 632 2405.
Chile Medical Association: Colegio Médico de Chile Esmeralda 678, Casilla 639, Santiago. Tel: +56 2 633 0505. Fax: +56 2 633 0940. www.colegiomedico.cl.
Chile Nurses Association: Colegio de Enfermeras de Chile, Miraflores 563, Casilla No 9752 Correo Plaza de Armas, Santiago. Tel: +56 2 639 8556.
Chile Dental Association, Ibieta 070, Rancagua. Tel +56 72 241 170. Fax: 72 236 169. www.colegiodentistas.com.

Santiago

Pontificia Univeridad Católica de Chile, Facultad de Medicina, Avenida Bernardo O'Higgins 340, Santiago. Tel: +56 2 639 6794. Fax: +56 2 633 1457. www.puc.cl.
Universidad de Chile, Facultad de Medicina, Avenida Independencia 1027, Casilla 13898, Santiago. Tel: +56 2 737 6655. Fax: +56 2 777 4890. www.uchile.cl.

Hospital Clinico, Universidad de Chile
Santos Dumont 999, Independencia, Santiago. Tel: +56 2 678 8000\8134. Fax: +56 777 1373.
The hospital: Has 614 beds and all major specialities. It is situated just north of downtown. Although Spanish is the primary language, some staff do speak a little English, French or German. It is privately funded. It has a major trauma centre and is advanced, with cardiothoracic and neurosurgery.

Hospital del Salvador
Avenida Salvador 364, Santiago.
Tel: +56 2 204 7919.
The hospital: One of the main public hospitals in Santiago (and enormous). For such a large hospital, the facilities are pretty basic, but the standard of clinical care is high. Despite poor amenities, renal transplants and other major operations are often carried out.
❂ Elective notes: There's not much 'hands on' work for students as they tend to use their own junior doctors. There are many consultants, but most tend to do private clinics in the afternoons which are therefore quiet. There is a very relaxed atmosphere and they are very keen to teach. Some doctors do speak English but you really must speak Spanish to survive here.

Hospital Clinico, Universidad Catolica de Chile
Marcoleta 367, Santiago. Tel: +56 2 633 205. www.escuela.med.puc.cl.
The hospital: Is a major university hospital in Chile with all the specialities, incorporating ambulatory clinics and a complete health network in geographically distant areas of the Santiago conurbation. The medical school itself (*see* above) is in downtown Santiago.

Valparaiso

Chile's third-largest city is on the coast, just two hours by car from Santiago. It is a picturesque and colourful city.

MEDICAL SCHOOL:

Universidad de Valparaiso
Facultad de Medicina, Avenida Hontaneda 2653, Casilla 92-V, Hontaneda 2653, Valparaiso. Tel: +56 32 507 300. www.uv.cl.

Hospital Carlos van Buren

Servicio de Salud Valparaiso y San Antonio, Valparaiso.

The hospital: Is a large teaching hospital with excellent facilities. The internal medicine department occupies one very large ward on one floor. In it are a number of specialities. There is a much higher staff:patient ratio than is seen in provincial hospitals in north Chile.

O Elective notes: There is good support and teaching. The medical students are very friendly and may well take you out around the city.

Accommodation: Not provided but you can stay in 'pensiones'.

OTHER MEDICAL SCHOOLS:

Universidad de los Andes, Facultad de Medicina, San Carlos de Apoquindo 2200, Las Condes, Santiago. Tel: +56 2 214 1258. Fax: +56 2 214 2014. www.uandes.cl.

Universidad de Antofagasta, Facultad de Ciencias de la Salud, Casilla 170, Campus Coloso, Temuco. Tel: +56 45 637 486. Fax: +56 45 637 802. www.uantof.cl.

Universidad Austral de Chile, Facultad de Medicina, Isla Teja, Casilla 567, Valdivia. Tel: +56 63 221 330. Fax: +56 63 221 331. www.uach.cl.

Universidad de Concepción, Facultad de Medicina, Barrio Universitario s/n, Casilla 60-C, Concepción. Tel: +56 41 204 932. Fax: +56 41 215 478. www.udec.cl.

Universidad de la Frontera, Facultad de Medicina, Casilla 54-D, Temuco. Tel: +56 45 325 701. www.ufro.cl.

Universidad Mayor, Facultad de Medicina, Sede Alameda, Avenida Libertador Bernardo O'Higgins 2013, Santiago Centro. Tel: +56 2 420 5770. www.umayor.cl.

Universidad San Sebastián, Escuela de Medicina, Pedro de Valdivia 1161, Concepción. Tel: +56 41 332 185. www.uss.cl.

Arica

Arica is a large coastal town near the Peruvian border in northern Chile. It is surrounded by desert but does have some beautiful national parks and good beaches. It has one state hospital and numerous private practices.

Hospital de Arica

1 Region de Tarapaca, Arica.

The hospital: This is the main city hospital in Arica, the most northern city in Chile. It serves a large population, including many immigrants from Peru. There's a paeds department run by 12 consultants. There is a lot of TB and childhood leukaemias. Morning clinics cater for a number of specialities, such as respiratory medicine and neurology. Many of the doctors do private clinics in the afternoon. The staff are keen to teach and take you on day trips to the local communities in the mountains.

Accommodation: Not provided.

Hospital Dr Juan Noe

18 de September 1000, Arica.

The hospital: A relatively large state hospital, covering all specialities. The doctors do ward rounds and clinics in the mornings but tend to disappear in the afternoons to their private clinics. The emergency department is often busy but usually with minor complaints (flu) as there is no GP service. Internal medicine has all the subspecialities. TB is common, and there is a surprising amount of SLE, Chagas' disease and gallstones. O&G can be very interesting and different from that in the West: abortion is illegal so most of the workload is dealing with the often sinister complications of back street abortions. The plastic surgeon is the only one in north Chile so if plastics is what you want to see, there's plenty of it mainly skin-grafting for diabetic and deep varicose ulcers. There's no on-call anaesthetist so the nurses step in after hours.

Accommodation: Not provided, but lunch is! There are many cheap hostels and student places.

RURAL HOSPITALS:

Hospital de Quirihue

Quirihue.

The hospital: This is a small, basic public hospital in a rural town located in the north of the Lake District region of Chile. It provides the surrounding area with emergency medicine, paeds, O&G, medical and minor surgical facilities. However, the most serious cases get sent

to nearby cities. It is run by newly qualified doctors (there are only six), the most
senior usually being only a few years out
of medical school. Doctors work in such
hospitals before specializing. There are
often Chilean medical students doing
attachments here; they tend to run the
emergency department.

O **Elective notes:** You can do as much
or as little as you want. There are many
procedures (suturing, plastering and
helping with Caesarian sections) to get
involved in. They are keen to teach and
there is plenty of opportunity to go on
rural clinics. You can also spend a week
with a GP in a nearby coastal village.

Consultorio de Pica

Balmaceda Sin Numero, Pica.

The hospital: Not a hospital but just a
consultorio run by a doctor with a resident dentist. There are also one midwife
and six nurses. It provides medical and
dental services to the town and also a
large area of the Altiplano in the Andes.
Clinics are run daily, and the doctor's role
is very much that of a GP. They also,
however, provide an emergency service
which is run by the paramedics. There are
superb clinics to go on in the Altiplano.

O **Elective notes:** Make sure you're all
right at altitude as these indigenous
Indian villages are above 5500 m and
hence clinics can be physically exhausting. There is an extensive vaccination
campaign (MMR) in the local communities. Back down in Pica, there's plenty of
suturing and minor surgery to be done.
The medicine may not be cutting edge,
but you get to see and do more than at
the major hospitals in Chile. No one will
speak English.

Accommodation: Food has previously
been provided by the *consultorio* in the
local hotel. The doctor and midwife live
in the hospital.

Chile

Colombia

Population: 36 million
Language: Spanish
Capital: Bogotá
Currency: Colombian peso
Int Code: +57

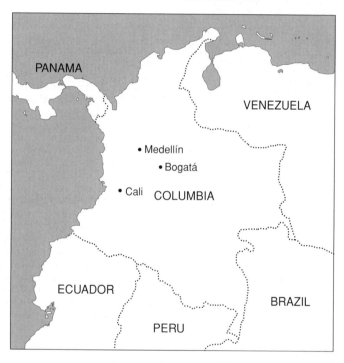

Lying at the top of South America, Columbia is better known for its drug trafficking than its healthcare. All instruction is in Spanish so the hospitals are not commonly visited by English-speaking medics.

✛ Medicine:

Only a small minority, usually in remote areas where it is physically impossible for them to get help, are covered by the state healthcare system. Depending on where you are, trauma, both through deliberate violence and traffic accidents, is common.

◉ Climate and crime:

The Caribbean side tends to be dry and hot while the Pacific side is wet and hot. The Andes are obviously cool, and Bogotá seems to have an everlasting spring. Violent crime and kidnapping are a real problem and a reason for the lack of tourism and lack of interest in overseas medics. These incidences are usually drug related and usually confined to Bogotá, Mendellín and Cali. Be very careful if contemplating trekking in the jungle.

USEFUL ADDRESSES:

Ministry of Health, Calle 16, No 7-39, Sante Fe de Bogotá. Tel: +57 1 282 0047. Fax: +57 1 282 0003.
Colombian Medical Association: Federación Médica Colombiana, Calle 72, No 6-44, Piso 11 Santa Fe de Bogotá, DE. Tel: +57 1 211 0208. Fax: +57 1 212 6082.
Colombian Nurses Association: Asociación Nacional de Enfermeras de Colombia, Carrera 27, No 46 21, Apartado Aéreo No 059871, Bogotá DE. Tel: +57 1 268 3535. Fax: +57 1 269 2095.
Colombian Dental Association: Federación Odontológica Colombiana, Calle 71, No 11-10, Piso 11, Bogotá DE. Tel: +57 1 255 6560. Fax: +57 1 255 4564. www.encolombia/odontologica.

Columbia has 26 medical schools. A full list can be found at www.medicstravel.org. Some of the main ones are included below. If planning work, it is best to approach NGOs (*see* Section 4).

Bogotá

Universidad Nacional de Columbia
Facultad de Medicina, Ciudad Universitaria, Bogotá. Tel: +57 1 316 5514. Fax: +57 1 316 5267.
www.dnic.unal.edu.co.
This is the oldest and largest medical school in the capital.

Centro Medico Cristiano
Avenida Caracas, No 46-26, Santa Fe de Bogotá.
The hospital: The Centro Medico Cristiano is run by a Columbian Christian organization that for the past ten years has been establishing a wide network of services aimed at alleviating the suffering of the city's poorest, especially the large population of drug abusers and street children. The medical arm of the organization involves clinics and education programmes as well as vaccination schemes. There is obviously a great deal of work to be done by the paediatricians; however, investigation and treatment facilities are severely limited. There is a mobile clinic that goes into many of Bogotá's 'no-go' areas where there is a great deal of deprivation pathology.

Cali

Universidad del Valle
División de Ciencias de la Salud, Calle 4B No 36-00, Sede San Fernando, Cali, Valle.
Tel: +57 25 542 475. Fax: +57 25 542 484.
www.salud.univalle.edu.co.
This is Cali's oldest medical school and has its own university teaching hospital. The Central Hospital is the university's main hospital, with 50 admissions a day from the emergency department. There's plenty of violent trauma. There are also associated smaller family heath clinics.
O **Elective notes:** Many procedures can be done in the emergency department as the turnover is so great. It is almost a 'war setting'. Time can also be spent at the smaller clinics. You must speak Spanish ... not necessarily fluently but enough to get by. Write to the **Directora Promocion Academica y Asuntos Internacionales** at the above address.

Antioquia

Universidad de Antioquia
Facultdad de Medicina, Apartado Aéreo 1226, Urabá por Juan del Corral, Medellín, Antioquia. Tel: +57 94 510 6001. Fax: +57 94 263 8282. www.medicina.udea.edu.co.
This is the main medical school in Columbia's second-largest city.

Colombia

Costa Rica

Population: 3.8 million
Language: Spanish
Capital: San José
Currency: Costa Rican colón
Int Code: +506

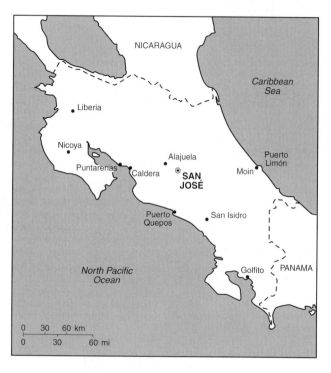

Costa Rica lies between Nicaragua and Panama in Central America, with the Caribbean Sea on its east coast and the North Pacific Ocean on its west. Costa Rica's democratic development over the past century has been healthy compared with that of other countries in Central and South America. The country is unique because a clause in its constitution forbids the formation of a national army. The main sources of income are agriculture (coffee and bananas), electronic exports and, more recently, tourism.

✪ Medicine:

The public health system is one of the best in Latin America. In 1995, the World Health Organization put Costa Rica's life expectancy as the third-highest in the world (behind that of Japan and France and ahead of Great Britain and the USA). People tend to be well educated (95% being literate).

Costa Rica has a government-sponsored network of 29 hospitals and over 250 clinics divided between nine regions. Private healthcare is also wide-spread, and the country is well known for its plastic surgery. Health tourism is becoming more and more popular. Malaria was virtually eradicated but has recently been a problem on the Caribbean coast. Other infectious diseases include dengue, filariasis and Chagas' disease.

⊃ **Visas:**

UK citizens do not need a visa to visit as a tourist. A return ticket and passport will allow you to stay for up to 90 days. The Costa Rican embassy does not issue student visas.

USEFUL ADDRESS:

Ministry of Health: Ministerio de Salud, Apartado 10 123, San José. Tel +506 223 0333. www.netsalud.sa.cr/ms/. (The ministry's website has a number of useful links and gives information on healthcare in Costa Rica, with details of each health region.)

MEDICAL SCHOOLS

Escuela Autonoma de Ciencias Medicas de Centro America, Universidad de Ciencias Medicas (UCIMED), PO Box 638-1007 Centre Colon, San José. Tel: +506 231 4368. Fax: +506 296 3944. www.ucimed.com.
Universidad Autonoma de Centro America, Colegio Clorito Picado, Campus Los Cipreses, 1 KM Norte del Servicentro la Galera Interseccion

Curridabat-Tres rios, Cipreses, Curridabat, San José. Tel: +506 271 2829. Fax: +506 271 3839. www.uaca.ac.cr.
Universidad de Costa Roca, Facultad de Medicine, Ciudad Universitaria Rodrigo Facio, San Pedro de Montes de Oca, San José. Tel: +506 207 4570. Fax: +506 207 5667.
Universidad Hispanoamericana, Barrio Aranjuez, 100M Norte, 200M Ests, Hospital Calderon Guardia, PO Box 408-1002, San José. Tel: +506 256 8197. Fax: +506 223 2349. www.uhispanoamericana.ac.cr.
Universidad Internacional de las Americas, Escuela de Medicine, Apartado Postal 1447-1002, Calle #23, Avenida 7, Frente Fercori, San José. Tel: +506 258 0220. Fax: +506 222 6132. www.uia.ac.cr.

SOME HOSPITALS

For details on hospitals (especially rural ones) take a look at the Ministry of Health's website and contact them for more details.

The main public hospitals in San José are:

Calderon Guardia, calle 17 a 9, San José. Tel: +506 224 4133.
Hospital de Ninos, San José. (The Children's Hospital.)
Paseo Colon, San José. Tel: +506 222 0122.
San Juan de Dios, Paseo Colon Calle 14, San José. Tel: +506 222 0166.

The many private hospitals, with specialties ranging from cardiology to plastic surgery, can easily be found by searching on the Internet for 'Costa Rica' and, for example, 'plastic surgery'.

Costa Rica

Ecuador

Population: 12 million
Language: Spanish
Capital: Quito
Currency: Sucre
Int Code: +593

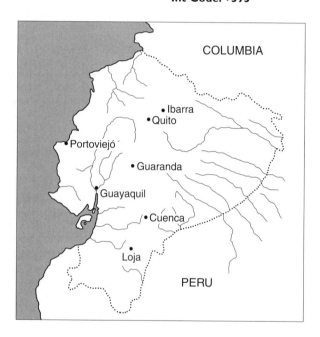

Ecuador is a country with amazing diversity – from coastal mangrove swamps and beaches to the high Andes and the rainforest in the Amazon basin. Flights are relatively cheap and frequent buses mean that no place is more than a day's journey from Quito. Very few people speak English so fluent Spanish is pretty much essential.

☉ Medicine:

Basic healthcare provisions are being established throughout Ecuador with rural clinics. Malaria and other infectious diseases are common, as is stomach cancer.

USEFUL ADDRESSES:

Ministry of Health, 444 Juan Larrea, Quito.
Tel: +593 2 529 163. Fax: +593 2 569 786.
Ecuador Medical Association: Federación Médica Ecuatoriana, V.M. Rendón 923 - 2 do.Piso Of. 201, PO Box 09-01-9848, Guayaquil.
Tel: +593 4 2562 569.
Ecuador Dental Association, Casilla 2046, Luis Saá 118 y Sodiro, Edif.
Cio Daniel Cadena 50, Of. 508, Quito. Tel: +593 2 54 1539. Fax: +593 2 52 0163.

Quito

MEDICAL SCHOOL AND HOSPITALS:

Universidad Central del Ecuador

Escuela de Medicina, Facultad de Ciencias Médicas, Sodiro e Iquique, Sodiro e Iquique s/n, Casilla Postal 17-116120, El Dorado. Tel: +593 2 528 810. Fax: +593 2 526 530. www.ucentral.edu.ec. This is the oldest medical school of Ecuador, founded in the early 19th century. It is situated in the capital and uses a number of hospitals, totalling 3000 beds. These include:

Hospital voz Andes, Desarrollo Comunidad, Villa Lengua 267, Casilla 691, Quito.
Hospital Gineo-Obstetrico, Isiror Ayora, Quito.
Hospital de Niños Baca Oritz, N 6 de diciembre y Colon, Quito.

There is a private hospital that has been thoroughly recommended in Quito:

Hospital Metropolitano

Avenidas Mariana de Jesús y Occidental, Quito. Tel: +593 2 261 520. Fax: +593 2 269 247. www.hospitalmetropolitano.org. **The hospital:** This hospital is ten minutes north of the centre of Quito and has very good facilities for Ecuador.

Cuenca

Cuenca, situated at 2530 m above sea level and with over 300 000 inhabitants, is the third-largest city in Ecuador. It has a compact, central 'old town' area with cobbled streets and colonial buildings. There are plenty of restaurants, bars and cinemas. Nearby there are national parks, Inca ruins and a spa town (Banos).

Cuenca has two medical schools.

MEDICAL SCHOOLS AND HOSPITALS:

Universidad Católica de Cuenca, Facultad de Medicina y Ciencas de la Salud, Car Tomás Ordoñez No 6-41, Casilla 19A, Cuenca. Tel: +593 7 830 752. Fax: +593 7 838 011.
Universidad de Cuenca, Facultad de Ciencas Médicas, Avenida El Paraíso s/n, Casila Letra 'X', Casilla Postal 01-01-1891, Cuenca. Tel: +593 7 811 002. Fax: +593 7 881 406. www.rai.ucenca.edu.ec.

Hospital de IESS (Instituto Ecuaroriano de Seguridad Social)

Avenida Guayna-Capac, Cuenca.
The hospital: This hospital is affiliated to Cuenca university and has over 200 beds and all surgical specialities (bar cardiac surgery). The emergency department is extremely busy and well worth spending time in.
O Elective notes: This offers a wonderful opportunity to observe many procedures, although you may not actually get to do much. Seek out the very friendly colorectal surgeon who will provide excellent one-to-one teaching (and introductions to most people in Cuenca). There are loads of parties and fiestas to go to as well.

Hospital Vicente Corral Moscoso

Casilla 418, Cuenca.
The hospital: This is a regional hospital for Cuenca and surrounding areas that has about 500 beds covering all specialities. It cares for the majority of the population who cannot afford to pay either social security or private health insurance. It is government funded but very poorly equipped compared with the Hospital de IESS.
O Elective notes: There's plenty to see, and cases such as malnutrition and infectious diseases tend to present very late so you often see them at their worst. You will be busy ... ward rounds start at 7 am.

OTHER MEDICAL SCHOOLS:

Pontificia Universidad Católica del Ecuador, Facultad de Medicina, Avenida 12 de Octubre 1076 y Patria, Torre 1, Piso 7, Quito. Tel: +593 2 235 470. Fax: +593 2 509 684. www.puce.edu.ec.
Universidad Católica de Santiago de Guayaquil, Facultad de Ciencias Médicas Dr Alejo Lascano Bahamonde, Avenida Carlos Julio Arosemena, Km. 1 1/5 Vía Daule, Santiago de Guayaquil. Tel/fax: +593 4 281 047. www.ucsg.edu.ec.

Universidad Estatal de Bolívar, Facultad de Medicina, Panamericana Norte, Km 3 1/5 Vía Ambato, Casilla Postal 92, Guaranda. Tel: +593 3 980 122. Fax: +593 3 980 123. www.ueb.isfun.net.

Universidad de Guayaquil, Facultad de Ciencias Medicas, Ciudadela Universitaria Salvador Allende, Casilla Postal 5852, Guayaquil. Tel: +593 4 281 148. Fax: +593 4 281 1481. www.ug.edu.ec.

Universidad Laica Eloy Alfaro de Manabi, Facultad de Medicina, Ciudadela Universitaria, Calle 12 Vía San Mateo, Casilla Postal: 27-32, Manta, Portoviejo. Tel: +593 5 623 051. Fax: +593 5 623 009. www.uleam.edu.ec.

Universidad Nacional de Loja, Facultad de Ciencias Médicas, Avenida Manuel Monteros Valdivieso, Casilla Postal 439, Loja. Tel: +593 7 571 379. Fax: +593 7 573 478. www.unl.edu.ec.

Universidad San Francisco de Quito, Colegio de Ciencias de Salud, PO Box 17-12-841, Quito. Tel: +593 2 895 723. Fax: +593 2 890 070. www.usfq.edu.ec.

Universidad Técnica de Manabí, Escuela de Medicina, Avenida Universitaria entre Calle Che Guevara y 12 de Marzo, Portoviejo, Manabi. Tel: +593 4 632 677. Fax: +593 4 651 569. www.utm.edu.ec.

Universidad Técnica del Norte, Facultad de Medicina, Juan Montalvo y Velasco, Esquina Antiguo Hospital San Vicente de Paul, Casilla Postal 199, Ibarra. Tel: +593 6 955 349. Fax: +593 6 641 511. www.utn.edu.ec.

Falkland Islands

Population: 2000
Language: English
Capital: Stanley
Currency: British pound
Int Code: +500

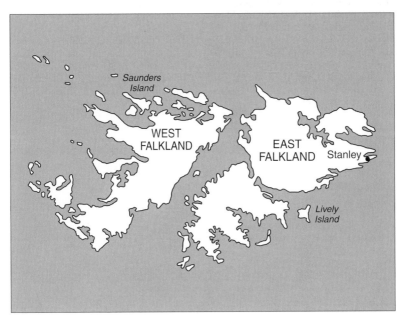

Southernmost in the South Atlantic, the Falkland Islands consist of hundreds of little islands surrounding the main East and West islands. They are famed for the dispute they caused between Argentina and the UK. They have a large agricultural and fishing industry. The recent discovery of oil could transform their economy and may cause further disputes. It's usually pretty damp and windy.

Stanley

King Edward (VII) Memorial Hospital

Stanley, Falkland Islands, South Atlantic.
Tel: +500 27328. Fax: +500 27416.
The hospital: The King Edward Memorial Hospital is a small (28-bed) hospital that caters for the 2000 civil-

ians and 2000 military personnel who live on the Falkland Islands. It is run by four GPs and a military field surgical team (one surgeon and one anaesthetist) providing GP, emergency facilities, medical inpatient, emergency and some elective surgery services. Despite its size, it can get quite busy, especially when there are visiting Antarctic cruise ships and fishermen.

Most of the population lives in Stanley. However, due to the large size of the Falklands, many of the outside settlements can be reached only by a 'flying doctor' service. As a medical student, you can participate in this, setting up surgery in someone's lounge before returning the next day. There may also be the opportunity to join the RAF in their search and rescue helicopter. As there are no medical students around, the doctors are very keen to teach. Most of the medicine is fairly similar to that in the UK and this is a very British elective; however, there's plenty to do with some great scenery, penguins and remnants of the 1982 conflict to visit. There are sports facilities and if you have time, Chile is within reach. The beer is cheap and Stanley has a night-club!

Accommodation and transport: Flights to the Falklands, by RAF TriStar from Brize Norton, can be arranged through the Falkland Islands government in London. A student rate is available. The hospital provides accommodation. Considering the distance, this can be a relatively inexpensive elective.

Guatemala

Population: 10.6 million
Official language: Spanish
Capital: Guatemala City
Currency: Quetzal
Int Code: +502

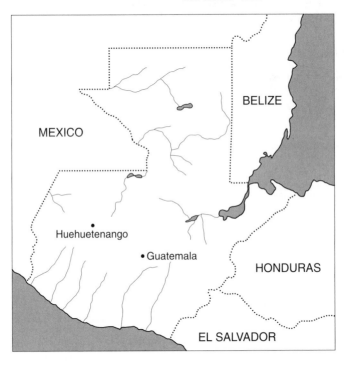

Guatemala is the largest, most populous and poorest of the Central American states. Although it has been independent since 1838, military rule between 1954 and 1986 means that 90% of people are now below the poverty line. This is not a popular destination, presumably because of the need for fluent Spanish.

✛ Medicine:

As a nation, Guatemala spends very little on healthcare, as demonstrated by the small number of hospitals (there are actually quite a few more private than public hospitals). Mortality rates are the highest in Central America. Seventy per cent of health funding goes to the capital, where 80% of the doctors work. Many deaths are linked to poverty, common causes being heart disease, violence, TB and accidents. Infectious diseases include leishmaniasis, filariasis, dengue fever, Chagas' disease and schistosomiasis. There is only one doctor per 2200 people.

⮑ Visas and work permits:
As a British citizen, no visa is required if you are staying less than 90 days and your passport is valid for six months from the time of entry. If you wish to stay longer or work in Guatemala, contact the **Direction General de Migracion** (41C–17–36, Zona 8, Ciudad de Guatemala. Tel: +502 475 1390/1302). To work, you also need to register with the **Colegio de Médicas y Cirujanos de Guatemala** (17 Calle 1–61, Zona 1, Guatemala City).

USEFUL ADDRESSES:

Ministry of Health, Palacio Nacional, 6a Calle y 7a Avda, Zona 1, Guatemala City.
Tel: +502 251 6816.
Gutemala Medical Association: Colegio de Médicos y Cirujanos de Guatemala, O Calle 15-46, Zona 15 Colonia El maestro, 01015 Ciudad de Guatemala City.
Gutemala Nurses Association: Asociación Guatemalteca de Enfermeras Profesionales, 14 Calle 1-15, Zona 3, Apto 6 Guatemala City.
Gutemala Dental Association, 17 Calle 14-20, Zona 13, Cuidad de Guatemala.
Tel: +502 11 502 2 34 1093.

UNIVERSITIES:

There are three universities teaching medicine in Guatemala:

Universidad Francisco Marroquin
Facultad de Medicina, 6a Avenida 7–55, Zona 10, Guatemala. Tel: +502 334 8327. Fax: +502 334 8329. www.ufm.edu.gt.
The university: This private university, based in Guatemala City, uses, among others, the **Esperanza** (Hospital Universitario Esperanza 6a Avenida 7-55, Zona 10, Guatemala. Tel +502 393 2457) in the city. For rural healthcare, the medical students run clinics on their own. San Juan Sacatepequez is a market town 24 km outside Guatemala City and clinics are also held here. There are next to no facilities, but it gives a superb insight into how the locals live. Most consultations are related to antenatal care or paeds. You will need good Spanish in the clinics but most of the

medical students will translate if you get stuck.

Universidad de San Carlos
Facultad de Ciencias Médicas, Edifico M-2, Ciudad Universitaria, Zona 12, Guatemala City. Tel: +502 476 7370 Fax: 476 9639 www.usac.edu.gt.

Universidad Mariano Gálvez de Guatemala
Facultad de Medicina, 3ra Avenida 9-00, Zona 2, Interior Finca El Zapote, Guatemala City. Tel: +502 288 7589. www.umg.edu.gt.

MAIN PUBLIC HOSPITALS:

Hermeroteca Nacional, Lic Clemente Marroquin Rojas, 5 Avenida 7-26 Z-1 Niv 2, Guatemala City. Tel/fax: +502 232 7625.
Hospital General de Accidentes, 13 Avenida y Calz, San Juan Z-4 Mixco, Guatemala City. Tel: +502 597 9626.
Hospital General del Igss, 9 C 7-55 Z-9, Guatemala City. Tel: +502 332 1009.
Hospital General San Juan de Dios, Avenida Elena 9 y 10 C Z-1, Zacapa, Guatemala City. Tel: +502 232 3741/3744/0423/3764. Fax: +502 253 6604. (The main hospital.)
Hospital de Gineco-Obstetrica, 14 Av y 4 C Z-12 Col Colinas de Pamplona, Planta Telefónica, Guatemala City. Tel: +502 471 0249.
Hospital Infantil de Infectologia y Rehabilitacion, 9 Avenida 7-01 Z-11, Guatemala City. Tel: +502 472 3532.
Hospital de Infectologia, Z-7 Fca La Verbena, Guatemala City. Tel: +502 471 2790.
Hospital de la Polcia Nacional, 11 Avenida 4-49 Z-1, Guatemala City. Tel: +502 232 6467/7633.
Hospital de Rehabilitacion, 14 Avenida y 4 C Z-12 Col Colinas de Pamplona, Guatemala City. Tel: +502 472 1678.
Hospital Roosevelt, Calz Roosevelt Z-11, Guatemala. Tel: +502 471 1441/6380/3384/6390. Fax: +502 471 5074.
Hospital de Salud Mental, Z-18 Col Atlántida, Guatemala City. Tel: +502 256 1486.

There are also a number of private hospitals. Enquire with the embassy for a list.

RURAL HOSPITAL:

Hospital de Jacal Tenango
Jacaltenango, Huehuetenango.
The hospital: Jacal Tenango is a rural town in the Chucumantes mountains. It

is a very beautiful area. The hospital is a 50-bed mission hospital run by Mexican nuns. The three doctors (a medic, surgeon and obstetrician) who work there cover a vast population and are generalists in themselves since they do a 1:3 rota (i.e. the medic does appendectomies, etc.). It's a friendly place and has a residential nutrition centre for malnourished children. You will definitely need to speak Spanish.

Guyana

Population: 800 000
Official language: English
Capital: Georgetown
Currency: Guyana dollar
Int Code: +592

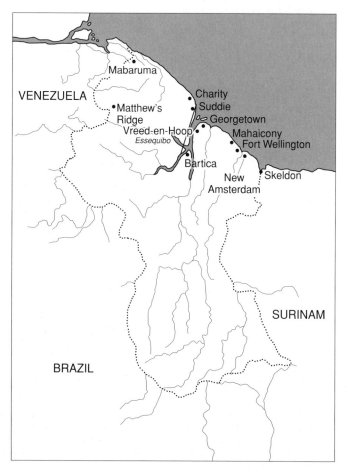

VENEZUELA

Mabaruma

Charity
Suddie
Matthew's
Ridge
Georgetown
Vreed-en-Hoop
Essequibo
Mahaicony
Fort Wellington
Bartica
New
Amsterdam
Skeldon

SURINAM

BRAZIL

Eighty-five per cent of Guyana's 83 000 square miles consists of its dense rainforest interior and hence virtually all of its population (90%) lives on the coast (which is itself partially reclaimed land). Guyana gained independence from the UK in 1966 and since then its economy has relied on the export of bauxite, gold, rice and sugar. There are still border disputes with Surinam and Venezuela. In the north-east (the coastal belt), sugar and rice are grown. In the inner forest, bauxite, diamonds, gold and manganese are found. 'Guyana' means 'land of many waters' – with the rivers Demerara, Berbice, Essequibo and Potaro, and the Kaieteur falls (222 m high = five times Niagara), you can see where it gets its name. The country is currently ruled by the People's Progressive Party, supported in the main by the East Indian community. The Afro-Guyanese tend to support the People's National Congress Party.

Georgetown is famous for its Dutch-inspired wooden architecture, street layouts and drainage canals. Fifty-one per cent of people are East Indian, 30% African and the rest European, Chinese and Amerindians (living in the west, south or on the reserves). Note: Be sensible in Georgetown as it is not all that safe. Girls get chatted up, but it's non-threatening. Guyana is still a developing country with poor transport facilities. If you are on for an adventure, it has some of the world's most unexplored rainforests and largest waterfalls.

✛ Medicine:

The Guyana state-run health system (on a national insurance scheme) is actually pretty good and covers 95% of the population. Life expectancy is over 70 years. The main causes of death include heart disease, violence, accidents, cancer and TB. The doctor:population ratio is around 1:3000 and the nurse:population ratio 1:500. There is a desperate shortage of doctors, many being supplied by Cuba. The average wage for a doctor is £300 a month.

◎ Climate and crime:

It is hot all year round (20–30°C), most rain falling between April and August and again over December and January. The Highlands are cooler. Crime is rife in the poorer areas so care should be taken not to enter these at night. The police are pretty ineffectual.

➲ Visas and work permits:

British nationals and nationals of other EU countries do not require a visa to visit Guyana, just a passport valid for six months and a return ticket. Since no doctors are trained in Guyana, they have to accept those from a recognized medical school outside. Contact the **Guyana Medical Board**. For work permits, contact the **Guyana High Commission** (www.guyana.org). Also visit Guyana on the web (www.guyana.org).

USEFUL ADDRESSES:

Ministry of Health, Lot 1, Brickdam, Georgetown. Tel: +592 2 65861. Fax: +592 2 56985. www.sdnp.org.gy/moh/.
Guyana Medical Association, 77 Lamaha St, Alberttown, Georgetown. Tel: +592 272 019.
Guyana Dental Association, National Dental Centre, Thomas and Guamina Streets, Georgetown. Tel: +592 2 601194. Fax: +592 2 74648.

UNIVERSITIES:

University of Guyana

Admission Office, Turkeyen Campus, East Coast Demerara, PO Box 101110, Georgetown. Tel: +592 2 223586. Fax: +592 2 224181. www.sdnp.org.gy/uog
Although this has some health-related subjects, medicine itself is not taught anywhere in Guyana.

HOSPITALS

Public Hospital Georgetown

New Market Street, Georgetown.
Tel: +592 2 56900/62687/59673/78224.
The hospital: Tries to provide most major specialities. The hospital has recently been rebuilt, and although it looks brand spanking new, there's an obvious lack of facilities (drugs and nursing staff). TB and cardiovascular disease are relatively common. AIDS is also a major problem. You'll see a great deal of violent trauma in the emergency department.
O Elective notes: There is loads to see and do in the emergency department (although few practical procedures on the wards).

Bartica Hospital

Second Road, Bartica, Essequibo.
Tel: +592 5 2339.

The hospital: The hospital is reached by
forest track or boat. It has 40 beds and
poor facilities. Rural clinics are run.

(P) = Private.
Best Hospital, Best, West Coast Demerara.
Tel: +592 64 702.
Charity Hospital, Charity, Essequibo.
Tel: +592 71 204.
Davis Memorial Hospital, 121 Durban
Backlands Lodge, Georgetown.
Tel: +592 2 72041. (P)
Fort Wellington Hospital, Public Road, New
Amsterdam, Berbice. Tel: +592 3 2396.
Jesus Rescue Mission Children's Hospital,
67 Croal Street, Stabroek, Georgetown.
Tel: +592 2 54090. (P)
Leonora Hospital, Leonora, West Coast
Demerara. Tel: +592 61 2502.
Mabaruma Hospital, Mabaruma Compound,
North West District. Tel: +592 77 205.
Mahaica Hospital, Mahaica Village, East Coast
Demerara. Tel: +592 28 211.

Matthew's Ridge Hospital, Matthew's Ridge,
North West District. Tel: +592 75 205.
Medical Arts Centre, 265 Thomas Street, North
Cummingsburg, Georgetown. Tel: +592 2 57402
Fax: +592 2 65220. (P)
New Amsterdam Hospital, New Amsterdam,
Berbice. Tel: +592 3 2266.
Port Mourant Hospital, Corentyne, Berbice.
Tel: +592 37 2883.
Prashad's Hospital Ltd, 258–9 Middle and
Thomas Streets, North Cummingsburg,
Geogetown. Tel: +592 2 67214
Fax: +592 2 67213. (P)
St Joseph's Mercy Hospital, 130–2 Parade
Street, Kingston, Georgetown. Tel: +592 2 72070.
Fax: +592 2 502260. www.mercy.hospital.org.gy. (P)
Skeldon Hospital, Corriverton, Berbice.
Tel: +592 39 2211.
Suddie Hospital, Suddie, Essequibo. Tel: +592 74
227. (A small (50–100 bed) rural hospital on the
coast. Rural outreach clinics go into the remote
interior.)
West Demerara General Hospital, Best
Village, Vreed-en-Hoop, West Coast Demerara.
Tel: +592 64 271.
Woodlands Hospital, 110–11 Carmichael Street,
North Cummingsburg, Georgetown. Tel: +592 2
54050 Fax: +592 2 55865. (P)

Honduras

Population: 6 million
Language: Spanish
Capital: Tegucigalpa
Currency: Lemipra
Int Code: +504

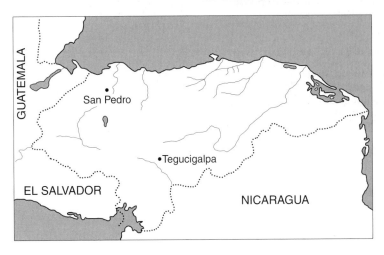

Despite being one of the world's biggest banana exporters, Honduras is undoubtedly poor. It has been independent from Spain since 1821 but military dictatorships prevented democracy until 1984. Natural disasters, including Hurricane Mitch, have also contributed to Honduras's problems. The land itself spans Central America and has some beautiful, virtually uninhabited coasts and a mountainous interior. A knowledge of Spanish is essential, but the experience makes the effort to learn it well worthwhile.

✪ Medicine:

The healthcare system is by no means comprehensive: only two-thirds of the population live in areas with access to hospitals and clinics. Infectious diseases are rampant. Malaria, cholera, dengue fever (which has recently had severe outbreaks) and visceral leishmaniasis are common and everything from infective diarrhoea to Venezuelan equine encephalitis occurs. There is only one doctor per 2000 people. The prevalance of HIV varies from area to area, but the national average is estimated to be 2%.

➲ Visa and work permits

British citizens do not need a visa if staying for less than 90 days. However, if gaining employment, work visas through the Embassy can take up to six months to obtain. For more information, contact the Ministry of Health.

USEFUL ADDRESSES:

Ministry of Health, 3 Calle, 4 Avenida Tegucigalpa MDC. Tel: +504 222 8518. Fax: +504 238 4141. www.paho-who.hn/ssalud.htm.
Honduran Dental Association, Apartado Postal 274, Tegucigalpa DC. Tel: +504 37 5297. Fax: +504 37 5297.

MEDICAL SCHOOL:

Universidad Nacional Autónom de Honduras

Edificio Hernán Corrales Padilla, Calle de La Salud Contiguo al Hospital Escuela, Tegucigalpa. Tel: +504 232 3975. Fax: +504 232 1053. www.unah.hn.

This is the only medical school in Honduras, and you are probably better off applying for electives directly through individual hospitals.

HOSPITALS :

A fantastic site is www.project honduras.com. A subweb of this (www.projecthonduras.com/healthcare providers) lists hospitals, e-mail addresses and even 'wish lists' of equipment needed by many hospitals, some of which are quite remote. Some charities, including the Lions Club of San Pedro, can provide information on hospitals in need.

Main hospitals :
Hospital General San Felipe, Boulevard San Felipe, Avenida Los Prceres, Tegucigalpa, MDC. Tel: +504 336 7698.

Hospital Leonard Martinez, 9–10 Avenida, 7 Calle, SO No 56, San Pedro Sula. Tel: +504 550 8415.

Some small hospitals and clinics:
Centro de Cancer Emma Romero de Callejas, Tegucigalpa DC, Francisco Morazán. Tel: +504 231 0813.
Centro Medico Bayan, Palacios Gracias a Diós. (This is a small hospital in a remote village of 700 people.)
Clinica Esperanza y Vida, Colonia Las Brisas Danli, El Pariaso. Tel: +504 883 2347.
Clinica Materna de Corquín, Corquín, Comayagua.
Clinica de Ojos Fraternidad, San Pedro Sula, Sula Cortés. Tel: +504 553 0631.
Clinica Solidaridad y Vida, Tegucigalpa DC, Francisco Morazán. (This is a small hospital with 10 beds and a clinic.)
Friends Hospital, Rus Rus, Gracias a Diós. (A more remote hospital with 32 beds.)
Hospital Adventista, Valle de Angeles, Francisco Morazán. (With 65 beds.)
Hospital del Area, Puerto Cortés. (With 72 beds.)
Hospital Divina Providencia de Corquín, Corquín, Comayagua.
Hospital Evangelico, Siguatepeque, Comayagua. Tel: +540 773 0170.
Hospital Gabriela Alvarado, Danlí.
Hospital Suizo Hondureño, La Ceiba, Atlántida. Tel: +504 441 2029/0069. (With 30 beds.)
Instituto Nacional Cardiopulmonar, Colonia Lara, Boulevard de los Proceres Tegucigalpa DC, Francisco Morazán. (This is the country's national heart and lung hospital.)

DIVING MEDICINE

If it's diving medicine you're after, there's a recompression chamber at **Anthony's Key Resort** (Hyperbaric Chamber Roatan, Bay Island. Tel +504 45 1049. Fax: +504 45 1049).

Mexico

Population: 94 million
Language: Spanish
Capital: Mexico City
Currency: Mexican new peso
Int Code: +52

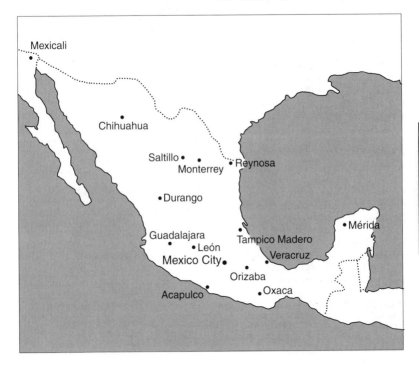

Mexico has been independent from Spain since 1836 but still retains a great deal of Spanish as well as its own culture. It straddles the whole of Central America. There are enormous wealth disparities. The slums of Mexico are some of the poorest in the world; 16% live in extreme poverty. On the other hand, there are a number of billionaires who don't even pay tax. Mexico has some amazing beaches (Acapulco, Yucatán) and a great deal of Aztec history, making it a popular tourist destination. It is not, however, a popular elective destination. This is probably because of the definite need for fluent Spanish. For this reason, only a few hospitals and the major medical schools are outlined below.

✪ Medicine:

There are two main healthcare institutions; the **Mexican Institute of Social Security**, which has recently been privatized, and the **Institute of Social Service and Security for State Employees**, the government-funded public welfare system. The latter provides health services, loans and pensions, and sets health and safety standards. Mexico is renowned for having good surgery and dentistry, but this is really only in the private sector. There is a mixture of 'developed country' diseases among the rich and infectious diseases, including TB, among the poor. What you see depends on where you go.

➲ Visas and work permits:

The embassy states that students need a student entry permit requiring:
- A passport (valid for more than one year)
- A completed application form
- A letter of acceptance from a university in Mexico
- A letter indicating you can fund yourself (a minimum of US$500 a month)
- Photographs (six full-face and five right-side profile).

You have to go personally to the consular office to sign and fingerprint the entry document.

Obtaining a visa for short-term work (less than six months) is extremely difficult. If you have an offer of work from a Mexican institute, they should apply to the immigration authorities in Mexico City to issue a working visa. This can take some time. Contact the Mexican embassy for more details.

USEFUL ADDRESSES:

International Relations Department of the Health Ministry: Secretaría de Salud, Dirección General de Asuntis se Asuntos Internacionales, Dr Rafael Alvarez Cordero, Director General, Francisco P Miranda No 177–4o piso, 06100 México DF. Tel: +52 5 651 0828. Fax: +52 5 583 0833. www.ssa.gob.mx.

Mexican Medical Association: Asociación Nacional de Colegios, Médicos Estatales Rosalio Bustamante No 224, Col. Esfuerzo nacional, CD, Madero, Tams CP 89470. Tel: +52 12 17 0388. Fax: +52 12 13 1969.

Mexican Nurses Association: Colegio nacional de Enfermeras AC, Czda Obrero Mundial 229, Cal del Valle, Apartado Postal 12-986, 03100 México DF. Tel: +52 5 543 6637. Fax: +52 5 669 4031.

Mexican Dental Association: Asociación Dental Mexicana AC, Ezequiel Montes No 92, Col. Revolución, Delegación Cuahternoc, 06030 México DF. Tel: +52 5 5566 6133.

MAIN MEDICAL SCHOOLS:

Mexico City
Escuela Nacional de Medicina y Homeopatia (Instituto Politécnico Nacional), Arroyo de Guadalupe No 239, Fraccionamiento La Escalera, Colonia Ticomán, 07320 México. Tel: +52 5 586 9449. Fax: +52 5 586 5524. www.ipn.mx.

Universidad Autónoma Metropolitana, División de Ciencias Biológicas y de la Saud, Unidad Zochimilco, Calzada del Hueso No 1100, Colonia Villa Quietud, Delegación Coyoacán, 04960 México 21. Tel: +52 5 483 7200. Fax: +52 5 483 7200. cueyatl.uam.mx.

Universidad National Autónoma de México, Facultad de Medicina, Ciudad Universitaria, México 20. Tel: +52 5 616 1162. Fax: +52 5 616 1616. www.facmed.unam.mx. (This is the oldest and probably the largest medical school in Mexico, founded in 1572.)

Universidad La Salle, Escuela Mexicana de Medicina, Fuentes 31, Tlalpan, Apartado Postal 22271, 14000 México. Tel: +52 5 606 2657. Fax: +52 5 606 3157. www.ulsa.mx.

OTHER MEDICAL SCHOOLS:

Universidad Autónoma de Baja California, Escuela de Medicina, Calle los Misioneros, Centro Civico Comercial de Mexicali, 21000 Mexicali, Baja California Norte. Tel: +52 65 571 622. Fax: +52 65 572 658. www.facmed.unam.mx.

Universidad Autónoma Benito Juárez de Oxaca, Escuela de Medicina y Cirugía, Calzada Porfirio Díaz, Oxaca de Juárez, Oxaca. Tel: +52 95 153 058. Fax: +52 95 153 058. www.uabjo.mx.

Universidad Autónoma de Chihuahua, Facultad de Medicina, Avenida Colón y Rosales, Apartado Postal 1090, 31350 Chihuahua. Tel: +52 14 152 059. Fax: +52 14 152 543. www.uach.mx.

Universidad Autónoma de Coahuila, Escuela de Medicina, Francisco Murguia Sur No 205, 25000 Saltillo, Coahuila. Tel: +52 84 128 095. Fax: +52 84 128 095. www.uadec.mx.

Universidad Autónoma de Nuevo León, Facultad de Medicina, Hospital Universitario Dr José E. Gonzales, Avenida Francisco I Madero al Poniente y Gonzalitos, Monterrey, NL 64460. Tel: +52 83 294 153. Fax: +52 83 485 477. www.medicina.uanl.mx.

Universidad Autónoma de Tamaulipas, Facultad de Medicina, Centro Universitario Tampico Madero, Apartado Postal C-33, 89339 Tampico, Veracruz. Tel: +52 12 270 576. Fax: +52 12 270 586. www.uat.mx.

Universidad de Guadalajara, Facultad de Medicina, Centro Médico, Colonia Independencia, Guadalajara, 44340 Jalisco. Tel: +52 3 617 5022. Fax: +52 3 617 5506. www.udg.mx.

Universidad de Guanajuato, Facultad de Medicina de León, 20 de Enero 929, León, CP 37320. Tel: +52 47 148 455. Fax: +52 47 142 522. www.ugto.mx.

Universidad Juáeez del Estado de Durango, Escuela de Medicina Humana, Avenida Universidad y Fanny Anitúa, Apartado Postal 229, 34000 Durango. Tel: +52 18 121 779. Fax: +52 18 130 527. www.ujed.mx.

Universidad Valle del Bravo, Escuela de Medicina, Hospital Universitario, Calle Septima y Rio Mante, Colonia Longoria, Ciudad Reynosa, 88700 Tamaulipas. Tel: +52 89 234 722. Fax: +52 89 239 447.

Universidad Veracruzana, Facultad de Medicina, Sedán e Iturbide, Hidalgo Carrillo Puerto, Ciudad Mendoza, 94740 Veracruz. Tel: +52 272 63 309. Fax: +52 272 71 209. www.uv.mx.

Universidad de Yucatán, Facultad de Medicina, Avenida Itzáez No 498, Apartado Postal 1225, Mérida, 97000 Yucatán. Tel: +52 99 240 554. Fax: +52 99 233 297. www.uady.mx.

RURAL WORK:

Programa de Ampliacion de Cobertura (PAC)

Jurisdiccion, Orizaba, Veracruz.

PAC is an initiative founded in 1996 by the Mexican Secretariat of Health to take basic health services and health education to the most isolated indigenous communities of the country. The initiative started in just one state (Veracruz). From a base in the city of Orizaba, ten 'modules', each consisting of about six individuals – doctors, nurses, dentists and social workers – disperse each Monday morning to their own substation, often many hours' drive up into the mountains. One such settlement is a tiny community called Tehuilango. From here each morning, the team walks for two to three hours to little Indian settlements on the hills to hold a clinic and various education seminars. These rural people are incredibly tough and most of the time is spent educating, vaccinating, pulling teeth and suturing. As secondary referral is virtually impossible, serious but otherwise treatable conditions (such as obstetric complications) are often fatal.

Nicaragua

Population: 4.5 million
Language: Spanish
Capital: Managua
Currency: Córdoba oro
Int Code: +505

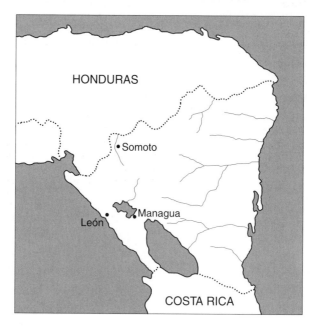

Nicaragua lies in the heart of Central America and has ocean to the east and west. It is the poorest country in Central America (some places won't be able to afford a stamp to write back to you) as a result of 40 years of dictatorship and then an 11-year civil war. Despite that, Nicaragua is a beautiful place and well worth visiting. You must be very confident in your Spanish as no one speaks a word of English. It is not a common elective destination because of this.

The **Nicaragua Health Fund** (83 Margaret Street, London W1N 7NB, UK) can arrange electives with the medical schools in Managua and also work in rural health centres.

✪ Medicine:

Infectious diseases, especially TB, are common. Violence and accidents also provide plenty of work. There are 27 hospitals in total though this is rapidly increasing. Nicaragua has three medical schools: one in León and two in Managua.

◎ Climate:

Nicaragua has a tropical climate, being particularly hot between March and

May. The occasional hurricane and earthquake make it that bit more exciting.

USEFUL ADDRESS:

Ministry of Health, Complejo, Concepcion Palacios, Managua. Tel: +505 2 897 1509. Fax: +505 2 897 483. www.ops.org.ni.

Managua

Universidad Nacional Autónoma de Nicaragua

Facultad de Ciencias Médicas, Managua. Tel: +505 2 277 1850. Fax: +505 2 278 6782. www.unan.edu.ni.
This is the medical school for the capital. (*See* above for electives here.)

Universidad Americana

Facultad de Medicina, Campus Universitario, Camino de Oriente, PO Box A-139, Managua. Tel: +505 278 3800, ext 314. Fax: +505 278 2577. www.uam.edu.ni.

León

Universidad Autónoma de Nicaragua

Facultad de Ciencias Médicas, Apartado Postal 608, Edificio Central UNAN -

León, Costado Norte Iglesia La Merced, León. Tel: +505 311 4475. Fax: +505 311 4970. www.unanleon.edu.ni.
This is an old medical school that uses:

Hospital Escuela Dr Oscar

Danilo Rosales Arguello, León.
The hospital: This is an extremely busy tertiary referral centre in Nicaragua's second-largest city. Conditions are very grim, but it is an incredible experience. Lots of tropical pathology and practical procedures for students but not many investigations. Doctors get paid $30 a month here. León is 20 minutes from the coast.

RURAL WORK:

Centro de Solvo

Jaro Bismark Moncada, Somoto Madriz.
The hospital: A health centre in the mountains on the border with Honduras. It is in Madriz, the poorest area of Nicaragua, and is incredibly poor. The medicines are provided by charity and the doctors do very well with their limited resources. Many patients have to walk for three days to get here. Lots of malaria, TB, dengue fever and other tropical diseases. It's very busy. There are also mobile clinics to surrounding areas. An excellent elective experience – highly recommended if you have good Spanish.

Paraguay

Population: 5 million
Languages: Spanish and Guaraní
Capital: Asunción
Currency: Guaraní
Int Code: +595

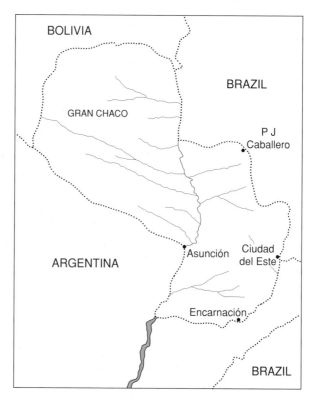

Paraguay has only recently struggled out of a military dictatorship. It is a landlocked country with the River Paraguay dividing it. In the east are hills and fields that are home to 90% of the people. The west (Chaco) is virtually uninhabited. It is not a popular elective destination, presumably because of the need for fluent Spanish.

✪ Medicine:

Basic sanitation is still not available only a third of people being able to access safe drinking water. Resources are really only available in Asunción, where over half of the county's hospital beds are. Infectious diseases (including TB) and obstetric complications are commonly seen.

⮑ Visas and work permits:

No clear information on requirements for electives can be obtained. A tourist visa at least will be needed. The embassy then states that to reside permanently in Paraguay, you would need:

- A passport
- A good conduct certificate from your police
- A birth certificate
- A marriage certificate
- A special certificate from the Department of Informatica if you are over 18
- A good conduct certificate from INTERPOL in Asunción (Cnel Gracia 468 y Tte Rodi)
- A health certificate
- A certificate of life from the local police(!)
- Proof of legal entrance issued by customs
- Two passport photos
- A tourist visa from the Paraguayan consulate.

If you are there temporarily, the embassy claims that you need all the above plus a letter from the employer or a copy of the labour contract with the certificate of studies or degree. You are best to contact the embassy yourself.

USEFUL ADDRESS:

Ministry of Health: Ministerio de Salud Publica y Bienestar Social, Av Pettirossi y Brasil, Asunción. Tel: +595 21 207 328 Fax: +595 21 206 700.

MEDICAL SCHOOL:

Universidad Nacional de Asunción, Facultad de Ciencias Médicas, Casilla de Correo No 1102, Avenida Dr Montero 658, Asunción. Tel: +595 21 481 549. Fax: +595 21 480 130. www.una.py. (Founded in 1898.)

HOSPITALS IN ASUNCIÓN:

Barrio Oberero, Yegros y 11 Pdta, Asunción. Tel: +595 21 72 989.
Cruz Roja, Brasil 216 or José Berges c/Brasil, Asunción. Tel: +595 21 200 004/22 797/208 199.
Hijas de la Caridad, Dr Montero y Lagerenza, Asunción. Tel: +595 21 420 868.
Hospital Bauista, Rca Argentina y Campos Cervera (RA), Asunción. Tel: +595 21 600 171. Fax: +595 21 602 212.
Hospital de Clinicas, Dr Montero y Lagerenza, Asunción. Tel: +595 21 420 982/420 983.
Hospital Nacional de Itagua, Itagua. Tel: +595 21 24 450 Fax: +595 21 24 459.
Hospital Privado Frances, Brasilia e/Insurralde, Asunción. Tel: +595 21 295 250.
Hospital Privado Salem, Colon y Holanda, Asunción. Tel: +595 21 80 199/80 532.
Instituto del Cancer y del Quemado, Asunción. Tel: +595 21 291 227/242.
Lacimet, Avda, Venezuela, Asunción. Tel: +595 21 292 652.
Metropolitano SRL, Tte Ettiene c/Ruta Mcal Estigarribia, Asunción. Tel: +595 21 501 270.
Militar Central, Gral Diaz y Don Bosco, Asunción. Tel: +595 21 494 601.
Pediatrico, Taruma 1038, Asunción. Tel: +595 21 552 459.
Primeros Auxilios, Brasil e/FR Moreno y M Dominguez, Asunción. Tel: +595 21 203 113.
Samaritano, Fdo de la Mora 2248 (RA), Asunción. Tel: +595 21 550 121.
Sanatorio Juan Max Boettner, Avenida Venezuela y Sol, Asunción. Tel: +595 21 290 288.
Sanatorio Migone Battilana, Eligio Ayala 1293, Ciudad de Asunción. Tel: +595 21 498 200. Fax: +595 21 5630.
Universitario NTRA SRA de fa Asunción, Lilio y E Miranda, Asunción. Tel: +595 21 602 236.

HOSPITAL IN OTHER REGIONS:

Hospital Regional de Ciudad del Este, Ciudad del Este. Tel: +595 61 50 0485.
Hospital Regional Coronel Oviedo, Ciudad de Cnel Oviedo. Tel: +595 521 2167.
Hospital Regional Encarnatión, Ciudad de Encarnación. Tel: +595 71 2271.
Hospital Regional Pedro Juan Caballero, Ciudad de Pedro Juan Caballero. Tel: +595 36 2208.

Paraguay

Peru

Population: 24 million
Languages: Spanish, Quechua and Aymará
Capital: Lima
Currency: New sol
Int Code: +51

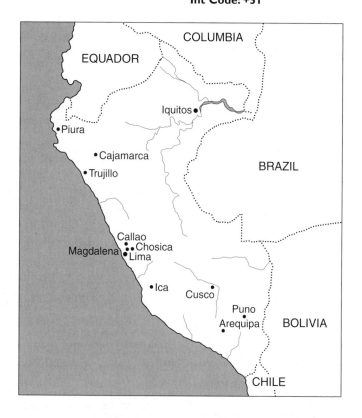

Situated on the west coast of South America, Peru has gained fame from themes as diverse as its great Inca Empire and Paddington Bear. Until relatively recently it has had a turbulent economic and political history, although since the election of Alberto Fujimori in 1990, the situation has greatly improved. Fifty per cent of Peru's 24 million population live in rural areas. Seven million live in Lima. The population structure includes 50% Indian and 33% Mesi. Food is cheap but dangerous. Travel round Peru is best achieved by air and a trip to the Andes is a must. The two official languages are Spanish *and Quechua; however, there are a number of different dialects in the jungles and highlands. You must have a good knowledge of Spanish, especially if going anywhere remote.*

○ Medicine:

Peru's public healthcare system has really gone to pot. There is no free cover and no GP service. On top of that, infectious diseases are becoming more and more prevalent as social deprivation increases. Cases are often very advanced by the time they get to hospital. Malaria and TB are widespread and in recent years cholera has returned to epidemic proportions. Dengue fever, dysentry, trypanosomiasis and leishmaniasis all occur. You really need to go to a private clinic if you want good treatment. The lack of iodine in the mountains has also meant that between 40% and 90% of children get goitres. Beware of altitude sickness if you are flying up to Cusco.

◎ Climate and crime:

There are a number of different climates: an arid desert with cool winters, the chilly Andes and the tropical Amazon Basin. It is warmest around Christmas. Peru is not that safe, and there are several no-go areas in Lima. There is the odd kidnapping.

⊃ Visas and work permits:

Nationals of countries including the UK, Australia, New Zealand, the USA and most of Europe can stay for 90 days without a permit, but they are required to have a return ticket. British volunteer workers should obtain a visa either before they go or once in Peru. Student visas can easily be obtained with a letter from the institution in Peru, a couple of photos, a passport and a copy of your last bank statement. If you are going to work for pay, the institution has to apply to its department of immigration. If you are working for a charity, their sponsors must apply to the **Secretaria Ejecutiva de Coperacion Technica International of the Ministerio de la Presidencia**. The Peruvian Immigration

Service can then authorize a visa. Alternatively, you can go out as a tourist and apply for a visa when there. The embassy can provide a list of clinics and hospitals across Peru.

Work:

Most Westerners work with an international organization. Organizations working in Peru include:

Comite Internacional de la Cruz Roja (Red Cross International Committee), Avenida Juan d Aliaga 620, Magdalena. www.icrc.org/spa
Organizacion Panamericana de la Salud (Pan-American Health Organization), Los Cedros 269, Lima 27.
UNICEF, Parqe Melitón Porras 350, Lima 18.

USEFUL ADDRESSES:

Ministry of Health: Ministry de Salud, 8 Cuadra Avda Salaverry, Jesús Maria, Lima 11, Tel: +51 14 326 242. Fax: +51 14 313 671.
Peru Medical Association: Colegio Médico del Perú, Malecón Armendáriz No 791 Miraflores, Lima. Tel: +51 14 474 930. Fax: +51 12 423 917. www.colmed.org.pe.
Peru Dental Association, Los Proceres 261, Urb Santa Constanza, Surco. Tel: +51 14 351 623. Fax: +51 14 351 623.

MEDICAL SCHOOLS:

Over the past five years, the number of medical schools has increased from nine to 22; the orginal nine are listed here. The others can be found on www.medicstravel.org. The three in Lima are:

Universidad Nacional Federico Villarreal, Programa Académico de Medicina Humana, Jr Río Chepen s/n Cuadra 1, Hospital Hipólito Unánue, Lima 10 (El Agustino)
Tel: +51 1 362 1152. Fax: +51 1 362 5545. http://medicinaunfv.org.
Universidad Nacional Mayor de San Marcos, Programa Académico de Medicina Humana, Casilla 529, Avenida Grau 755, Lima 1. Tel: +51 14 328 1154. Fax: +51 14 328 3231. www.unmsm.edu.pe. (This is the oldest one, founded in 1856.)
Universidad Peruana Cayetano Heredia, Apartado 5045, Programa Académico de Medicina, Avenida Honorio Delgado 932, San Martin Porres, Lima 31. Tel: +51 14 820 828. Fax: +51 14 820 828. www.upch.edu.pe.

Some medical schools outside Lima:

Universidad Nacional de la Amazonía Peruna, Programa Académco de Medicina, Apartado 496, Avenida Colonial s/n, Moronillo, Punchana, Apartado 613, Iquitos. Tel: +51 94 251 780. Fax: +51 94 233 228.
www.uniamazonia.edu.pe.

Universidad Nacional de San Agustin, Programa Académico de Medicina, Casilla 1365, Arequipa. Tel: +51 54 233 793. Fax: +51 54 233 803. www.unsa.edu.pe.

Universidad Nacional San Antonio Abad, Programa Académico de Medicina Humana, Avenida de la Cultura s/n, Apartado 921, Cusco. Tel: +51 84 224 905. Fax: +51 84 226 048. www.unsaac.edu.pe.

Universidad Nacional Técnica de Piura, Programa Académico de Medicina Humana, Prolongación Avenia Grau s/n, Apartado 295, Piura. Tel: +51 74 345 259. Fax: +51 74 342 865. www.unp.edu.pe.

Universidad Nacional de Trujillo, Programa Académico de Medicina Humana, Salaverry 545, Apartado 361, Trujillo. Tel: +51 44 232 131. Fax: +51 44 254 482. www.unitru.edu.pe.

Universidad San Luis Gonzaga, Programa Acaedémico de Medicina Humana, Independencia 431, Apartado 106, Ica. Tel: +51 34 223 615. Fax: +51 34 225 262.

Lima

Lima has suffered with overpopulation since the 1920s. It has become polluted, noisy, dirty and rife with theft. There are many shanty towns (pueblos jovenes) in poorer areas. These have come about as migrants have arrived trying to find jobs. In some of these there is no electricity, water or adequate sanitation. This is a great contributing factor to the spread of disease. In recent years cholera has become endemic.

The most popular elective destination in Peru is the tropical medicine institute (**Instituto de Medicina Tropical Alexander von Humboldt**), which is associated with the Universidad Peruano Cayetano Heredia:

Instituto de Medicina Tropical Alexander von Humboldt (Universidad Peruana Cayetano Heredia)

Apartado 5045, Postal 4314, Lima 100. Tel: +51 14 823 401. Fax: +51 14 823 404.
The hospital: In the outpatients department of this tropical diseases hospital, you'll see leishmaniasis, brucellosis, typhoid, viral hepatitis, bartonellosis and other rarer conditions such as spider bites and free-living amoebiasis. Hep B and HIV are also very common. The ward has 30 beds dedicated to tropical diseases and HIV. Facilities are sparse, but there are opportunities for practical procedures such as lumbar punctures.

O Elective notes: Conditions around the hospital, which includes many slums, are extremely poor, to the extent that interns often have to supply their own syringes and needles. Despite this, the staff are incredibly friendly and encourage you to get involved. They charge a fee of $300 per month for teaching. This is well worth it as you are otherwise unlikely to know much about the diseases. A good understanding of Spanish is essential. They can also arrange for you to spend a week in Iquitos in the Amazon jungle (two hours north-east of Lima; $170 for the return flight). There you will see many cases of leprosy, snake bites and leishmaniasis. The hospital here (**Hospital Regional de Loreto**) is again very ill-equipped, but the staff are welcoming.

Accommodation: Difficult unless you have relatives in Peru.

Instituto de Salud del Niño (Children's Hospital of Lima)

Avenida Brasil 600, Breña, Lima 5, Lima. Tel: +51 330 0066. Fax: +51 425 1840. www.isn.gob.pe.
The hospital: The first paediatric hospital in Peru. It has 600 beds and receives children from all over the country.

Hospital de Emergencia Casumiru Ulloa

Avenida Republica de Panama, Miraflores, Lima. Tel: +51 14 455 096.

Cajamarca

Cajamarca is an Andean town in Peru's northern highlands 2700 m above sea level. It has a population of 70 000 and, although not a tourist spot, is rich in Inca and pre-Inca history.

Hospital Regional de Cajamarca
Avenida Mario Urteaga No 500,
Cajamarca. Tel: +51 44 922 414.
The hospital: Has 170 beds and serves a widely dispersed population of 150 000. There are regional outposts with nurses and junior doctors. There is no GP service so everything has to come to one of these. This may mean a few days' walking. Common conditions are TB (the national TB programme does free tests and treatment for anyone with a persistent cough to try to eliminate this), malnutrition and infectious diseases. There is very poor antenatal healthcare as even that has to be paid for.
Accommodation: One of the hospital secretaries has previously rented a room for around US$50 a month (Jiron San Sebastian 332, Cajamarca. Tel: +51 44 821 660). Meals are free in the hospital.

Moyobamba

Moyobamba is a Spanish-speaking town of 25 000 people in the Peruvian jungle in the region of San Martin. It is on a plateau and therefore has a pleasant climate.

Asociación San Lucas
Apartado #2, Moyobamba, San Martin.
The hospital: Run by the Asociación San Lucas, a medical missionary organization holding a GP-type consultation service in the town with healthcare workers in surrounding villages. It provides a free service to under-fives and their mothers, and gives basic advice on sanitation and nutrition. The medical/nursing team also visits the villages from time to time. There is a great deal of parasitic infection, nutritional

problems and skin, chest, gastrointestinal and urinary infections. There is very much a Christian emphasis in the way things are done.
Accommodation: Can usually be arranged with one of the church in Moyobamba's families.

SOME OTHER REGIONAL HOSPITALS:

Hospital Jose Mendoza Olavarria, Avenida 24 de Julio, Tumbles 401. Tel: +51 74 524 775.
Hospital Regional Centro de Salud, 1022 El Sol, Puno. Fax: +51 54 351 020.
Hospital Regional IPSS, Antiguo Aeropuerto s/n Cusco. Tel: +51 84 234 724. Fax: +51 84 234 724.

OTHER PLACES IN PERU:

Asociacion Cristiana Femenina, B Herrera 157B, Lima 14. (YWCA.)
Clinica San Juan de Dios, Plaza Garibaldi s/n, Lima.
Comp Hijas de la Caridad San Vicente de Paul, S/n Hospital Dos de Mayo, San Martin, Lima.
Ejercito de Salvacion, Colón 138, Callao. (Salvation Army.)
Hermanitas de los Ancianos Desamparados, La Florida 339, Chosica. (For the elderly.)
Hijas de Maria Immaculada, Av El Polo 350, Monterrico, Lima 33.
Hogar Clinica San Juan de Dios, Km 1 Carr Central, Lima.
Hospital de Beneficencia de Maternidad, Clinica Sta Maria S/n AM Quesada, Lima.
Iglesia Anglicana Episcopal del Peru, Chacaltana 114, Lima 18. Tel: +51 14 453 044.
Obras Misioales Pontificias, Mrcal Miller 1524, Lima 14.
Puericultorio de Beneficencia Perez Aranibar, Avenida del Ejército, Lima 17.
Sociedad Francesa de Beneficencia, Centro Hospitalario Maison de Sante, M Aljovin 208, Lima.
Union Nacional de Ciegos del Peru, Plaza Bolognesi 479, Lima. Tel: +51 14 230 941. Fax: +51 14 423 8380. E-mail: pattyrenato@hispavista.com. (For blind people.)

Venezuela

Population: 22 million
Language: Spanish
Capital: Caracas
Currency: Bolívar
Int Code: +50

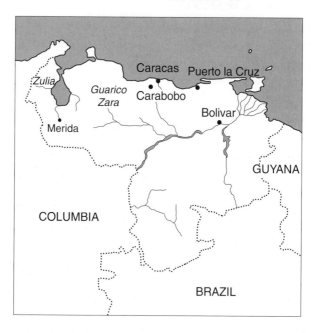

Venezuela is not a common destination. Most of its population lives in very poor conditions in shanty towns. It does, however, have large oil reserves so the economic situation may change over the next few decades. There's a lot to do in Venezuela: trekking and biking in the Andes, Los Llanos (the Plains), the Amazon basin, Gran-Sabana, Angel Falls, diamond mines and the Orinoco delta. Very fluent Spanish is absolutely necessary to work or do an elective here.

✪ Medicine:

Most healthcare is concentrated in the towns, and people from indigenous communities often have to travel long distances to receive treatment. Because of this, many conditions present very late. Venezuela has a reputation for innovative plastic surgery. There are ten medical schools.

USEFUL ADDRESSES:

Ministry of Health, Torre Sur, 5°, Centro Simón Bolivar, Caracas 1010. Tel: +58 2 483 3533.
Venezuela Dental Association, Avenida Guanare, Urb Las Palmas, Edif. COV Piso 3, Apartado de Correos 1341, Caracas. Tel: +58 2 793 6604. Fax: +58 2 793 7494.

MEDICAL SCHOOLS:

Anzoátegui:
Universidad de Oriente (Núcleo Anzoátegui), Escuela de Medicina, Carretera Negra vía el Tigre, Avenida Universidad, Puerto La Cruz, Estado Anzoátegui. Tel: +58 281 262 331. Fax: 281 268 1533. www.anz.udo.edu.ve.

Bolívar:
Universidad de Oriente (Núcleo Bolívar), Escuela de Medicina, Calle Raúl Leoní con Calle Columbo Silva, Ciudad Bolívar, Edo. Bolívar Tel: +58 285 223 738. Fax: +58 285 285 226. www.re.udo.edu.ve.

Carabobo:
Universidad de Carabobo, Facultad de Ciencias de la Salud ñ Escuela de Medicina Bárbula, Valencia, Edo. Carabobo. Tel: +58 41 666 258. Fax: +58 41 666 238. www.uc.edu.ve/fcs/.

Caracas:
Universidad Central de Venezuela, Escuela de Medicina José María Vargas, Ciudad Universitaria, Caracas, Distrito Federal. Tel: +58 2 606 7770. Fax: +58 2 605 3522. www.med.ucv.ve.
Universidad Central de Venezuela, Escuela de Medicina Luis Razetti, Edificio Decanato de Medicina, Urb. Los Chaguaramos, Caracas, Distrito Federal. Tel: +58 2 605 3347. Fax: +58 2 605 3520. www.med.ucv.ve.

Falcón:
Universidad Nacional Experimental Francisco de Miranda, Area Ciencias de la Salud, Edificio Santa Ana, Calle Falcón, Coro, Edo. Falcón. Tel: +58 68 521 668. Fax: +58 68 514 882. www.unefm.edu.ve.

Guárico:
Universidad Nacional Experimental Rómulo Gallegos, Facultad de Medicina, Vía El Castrero San Juan de los Morros, Edo. Guárico. Tel: +58 46 315 726. www.urg.edu.ve.

Lara:
Universidad Centro Occidental Lisandro Alvarado, Facultad de Medicina, Avenida Liberator cruce Calle 22, Zona Hospital Central Antonio María Pineda, Barquisimeto, Edo Lara. Tel: +58 51 519 898. Fax: +58 51 519 589. www.ucla.edu.ve/dmedicin/.

Mérida:
Universidad de los Andes, Facultad de Medicina, Avenida F.F. Cordero, Mérida, Edo Mérida. Tel: +58 74 403 040. Fax: +58 74 403 045. www.ula.ve. (This is a teaching hospital with good teaching, especially in tropical medicine and public health. They can also arrange trips to remote medical centres. Accommodation in Merida guesthouses costs 2670–5340 VEB ($4–8) a night.

Zulia:
Universidad del Zulia, Facultad de Medicina, Avenida 16 Goajira, Edificio Rectorado, Maracaibo, Edo. Zulia. Tel: +58 61 598 540. Fax: +58 61 598 532. www.luz.ve.

A couple of other hospitals previously used are:

Centro Medico Dolente La Trinidad
Avenida Interlomunal El Hatillo, Apdo Postal 80474, Caracas 1080A.
The hospital: This plush private clinic is run as an outpatient department. All specialities up to plastics and ophthalmological surgery are catered for.
O Elective notes: There are no other medical students so you get a great deal of attention. You can run exercise ECGs and pulmonary function tests, do outpatients (very busy) and help in theatre. Staff have previously helped arrange trips down the Amazon to supply medication to rural communities.

Hospital de Los Niños
JM De Los Rios, Caracas.
The hospital: Although many have previously enjoyed time here, reports say that they are not keen on elective students.

USA, BERMUDA and CANADA

Population: 274 million
Language: English
Capital: Washington DC
Currency: US dollar
Tel Code: +1

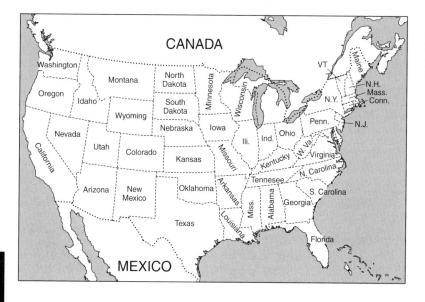

Little needs to be said about the USA. It's big. It offers many sites and activities in a high-tech First World setting. From California to New York, it has something for everyone. You probably already know if American-style medicine is for you. All 126 medical schools and the hospitals commonly visited are listed below. It is a popular elective destination and information is easily available on the Internet. That said, it doesn't make it easy to decide where to go. Each institution claims to be the biggest and best in everything. Every hospital and doctor has been named in a magazine (such as Home and Garden) *as being one of the top ten in America. How will you choose? Look at the speciality you* *want to do and what there is to do in the vicinity. For nurses and other health specialists, virtually every single medical school listed also has a nursing school so just write to the head of nursing at the appropriate address.*

○ Medicine:

The state of medical care in the US is well known and is a constant problem for successive administrations. It has been described as a paradox of excess and deprivation. Although 11% of the GDP is spent on healthcare, 30 million Americans can't afford fees or insurance. There are four sources of funding:

- Patient fees (the very rich)
- Private insurance, with many clauses and limits
- Federally funded Medicare insurance for the elderly and disabled which is not comprehensive
- State-funded Medicare insurance for low-income families, although single people are not eligible (so one-third of children below the poverty line have no insurance).

The **Veterans Affairs Medical Centers** (VAMC) are a group of government-run hospitals (similar to the NHS) established to serve ex-service men, although they now also serve the general community. Despite these, three-quarters of US hospitals are privately owned. US physicians are renowned for using high-tech medicine and many investigations. The use of such tests is high principally because of the high rate of litigation. Patients also tend to be quite knowledgeable and can demand tests and since they (or their insurance company) are paying it's no skin off the doctor's nose. In some cases, the more tests done, the more the doctor gets paid. It really is a huge market. An 'accountant' in the emergency room (ER) counting up the number of cannulae and drugs used in a resuscitation situation is not uncommon but seems strange to those from outside. All this paints a rather bad picture. There are, however, many small hospitals outside the cities. Some are mentioned below, but a good list of hospitals in America is available on http://neuro-www.mgh.harvard.edu/hospitalweb.shtml. Overall, if you want first-class medical experience with cutting-edge technology, the US is probably the place to be.

◎ Climate and crime:

The climate varies considerably across this huge country, from the sunny beaches of Los Angeles to the constant rain of Seattle. The crime rate also varies. Washington, New York and LA are the worst (or the best if you want to do trauma).

⮞ Visas, work permits and exams:

O Electives:

Many students going to America only fill in the visitor's waiver on the plane that lets you stay there as a tourist for three months. Be very careful if you're thinking of doing this. The official line from the US Embassy is that you need a J1 visa (currently costing £30). There are a couple of reasons why it is a good idea to get a visa. Some institutions (especially large research centres such as NASA) need to see the visa to give you a security pass. Not having a visa will therefore ruin any elective plans. Another reason is that if you get caught, you'll jeopardize your chances of ever being allowed to work in the States. For detailed information, contact the **US Embassy** (*see* Section 4). The visa information line in the UK is +44 891 200290 (50p a minute to listen to it being reeled off as slowly as possible) or +44 991 500590 (a criminal £1.50 a minute to speak to someone). They don't make life any easier if you try to visit them. You'll need an appointment (take everything with you: letters from the hospital etc.). For all these reasons, think about getting a visa early.

A few students have been requested to have a medical examination before going to specific hospitals. This is on the whole unusual, but ask the hospital directly whether you need to bring any documents. (A copy of your hep B certificate and immunizations will always stand you in good stead.)

WORKING IN AMERICA AS A DOCTOR:

If you want to work in America, the main problem is not getting in but getting the exams done to obtain licensure. The following are needed before you apply for a work permit:

- You must pass the United States Medical Licensing Examinations (USMLE, www.usmle.org), in three steps (*see* below).

- You must also pass an English language proficiency test
- And a clinical skills assessment
- You need all the appropriate documents from your country stating that you can practise medicine unrestricted
- The Educational Commission for Foreign Medical Graduates (ECFMG) will also need to confirm your medical credentials with your medical school.

The USMLE itself does not give licensure, but the results are given to the appropriate state medical board, which can then grant such licences. Step one concerns basic biomedical science, with an emphasis on the principles and mechanisms of health, disease and modes of therapy. Step two assesses the application of your medical knowledge to clinical science, including health promotion and disease prevention. Step three assesses how you combine your knowledge of biomedical science and clinical medicine to unsupervised patient care. All the steps should be completed within seven years.

A number of medical students are now doing the USMLE exams while doing their undergraduate course (as steps one and two can be done before qualification). This has the obvious advantage that it is all fresh in your mind. If you didn't do them then, don't panic. There are excellent revision courses available specifically for these. A good time to consider doing them is after MRCP/MRCS, but you will also need to revise preclinical medicine and all the specialities, including paeds, psychiatry, etc. You then have to sit an English language proficiency test and a clinical proficiency test (the clinical skills assessment). For detailed information contact the **Educational Commission for Foreign Medical Graduates** (3624 Market Street, Philadelphia, PA 19104. Tel: +1 215 386 5900. Fax: +1 215 386 9196) or visit www.usmle.org or www.ecfmg.org. A good website for information on postgraduate training is www.fulbright.co.uk. Once registered,

you can then apply for specialist training (residency), which takes three to seven years, ending in your becoming a consultant. Full licensure occurs after completing 12 months of residency and passing part III of the USMLE exams. Note: Some specialist training overseas can be counted to reduce the residency programme.

Contact the embassy for information regarding work permits, but by far the biggest hurdle is getting licensed. This licensing makes short-term work opportunities near impossible, although there are plenty of research opportunities since no licence is needed for this. Temporary visas include the J1 (for temporary supervised work sponsored by an educational institution) and the H1 (for those skilled for a job for which a US worker is not available). Once licensed, you then have to register with the appropriate state board.

WORKING AS A NURSE:

Nurses have to have passed the state licensing exam (the National Council of State Boards of Nursing Licensure Examinations, or NCLEX), but before you can do this you will have to sit the Commission on Graduates of Foreign Nursing Schools (CGFNS) exam. This CGFNS exam is required before you can get an H1-A nurses visa.

MALPRACTICE INSURANCE:

For electives, the best and simplest option is to ask the institution accepting you whether they can provide cover as they do for their own students. Some will do this automatically; others may charge you for it. Some may give you an address of a local provider, and a few will say that they don't take foreign medical students at all as they won't accept any cover you can get. With threats of 'Well, we take your students', they may say that they will take you as long as your university takes full liability (which they will not). Another way around this is to ask for a purely observational elective (no touching!); this may be fine in psychiatry but is pretty stupid if doing trauma. The Medical and Dental Defence Union of Scotland (MDDUS) has recently provided cover. Contact your defence union to see whether they can do this and ask your host institution whether they will accept their cover.

For working, the situation is pretty simple: you need to obtain insurance through either the hospital or a recommended broker. The Medical Protection Society (MPS) and MDDUS recommend **Physicians Insurers Association of America** (PIAA; 2275 Research Boulevard, Suite 250, Rockville, MD 20850).

IMPORTANT NOTE ON ELECTIVES:

Some universities in America are incredibly elective-friendly ... no tuition fees and they cover malpractice insurance. Others are completely obstructive and charge exorbitant tuition fees no matter how long or short your elective. For example, Harvard charges over $2000 for a four-week elective. Although some students have said they have found the teaching worth it, many have found it a complete rip-off. If this becomes a problem, DON'T panic; there are ways around it. If you are threatened with extortionate fees, try to find the name of someone in the department you want to visit (either through a hospital contact or from the Internet) and write DIRECTLY to them. If they say that you have to go through the school, try someone else. If you have real problems and a friendly dean, ask him or her to write (your dean may say that your medical school will charge their students silly figures to stop them coming over).

Note: Do try the medical school in the first instance as this makes it official and they can help with accommodation. There is one medical school that actually gives you a grant if you do an elective with them ....

PROFESSIONAL ORGANIZATIONS:

Doctors:
American Medical Association, 515 North State Street, Chicago, IL 60610. Tel: +1 312 464 4677. Fax: +1 312 464 4567. www.ama-assn.org.
Federation of State Medical Boards, Federation Place, 400 Fuller Wiser Road, Suite 300, Euless, TX 76039-3855. Tel: +1 817 868 4000. Fax: +1 817 868 4098. www.fsmb.org.
Educational Commission for Foreign Medical Graduates (ECFMG), 3624 Market Street, Philadelphia, PA 19104-2685. Tel: +1 215 386 5900. Fax: +1 215 387 9963.

Nurses:
American Nurses Association Inc., 600 Maryland Avenue, SW, Suite 100 West, Washington DC 20024. Tel: +1 202 651 7134. Fax: +1 202 651 7001. www.ana.org.
American Association of Colleges of Nursing, One Dupont Circle, NW Suite 530, Washington DC 20036, Tel: +1 202 463 6930. Fax: +1 202 785 8320. www.aacn.nche.edu.
Commision on Graduates of Foreign Nursing Schools (CGFNS), 3600 Market Street, Suite 400, Philadelphia, PA 19104-2651. Tel: +1 215 349 8767. Fax: +1 215 222 8454. www.cgfns.org.
National Council of State Boards of Nursing, 676 N St Clair Street, Suite 550, Chicago, IL 60611-2921. Tel: +1 312 787 6555. www.ncsbn.org.

Dentists:
American Dental Association, 211 East Chicago Avenue, Chicago, IL 60611. Tel: +1 312 440 2500. Fax: +1 312 440 2800. www.ada.org.

Physiotherapists:
American Physical Therapy Association, 111 North Fairfax Street, Alexandria, VA 22314. Tel: +1 703 684 2782. Fax: +1 703 684 7343. www.apta.org.
Federation of State Boards of Physical Therapy, 509 Wythe Street, Alexandria, VA 22314. Tel: +1 703 299 3100. Fax: +1 703 229 3110. www.fsbpt.org.

Occupational therapists:
American Occupational Therapy Association Inc., 4720 Montgomery Lane, PO Box 31220, Bethesda, MD 20824-1220. Tel: +1 301 652 2682. Fax: +1 301 652 7711. www.aota.org.
National Board for Certification in Occupational Therapy, 800 S Frederick Avenue, Suite 200, Gaithersburg, MD 20877-4150. Tel: +1 301 990 7979. Fax: +1 301 869 8492.

Medical specialities:
Family Practitioners: American Academy of Family Physicians, 11400 Tomahawk Creek Parkway, Leawood, KS 66211-2672. Tel: +1 800 274 2237. www.aafp.org.

Obstetrics and gynaecology: American College of Obstetrics and Gynecologists, 409 12th Street SW, PO Box 96920, Washington DC 20090-6920. www.acog.org.

Physicians: American College of Physicians, 190 N Independence Mall West, Philadelphia, PA 19106-1572. Tel: +1 800 523 1546. www.acponline.org.

Radiologists: American College of Radiology, 1891 Preston White Drive, Reston, VA 22091. Tel: +1 703 648 8900. www.acr.org.

Surgeons: American College of Surgeons, 633 North Saint Clair Street, Chicago, IL 60611-3211. Tel: +1 312 202 5000. Fax: +1 312 202 5001. www.facs.org.

ALABAMA

University of Alabama School of Medicine

1530 3rd Avenue South, 306 Medical Education Building, Birmingham, AL 35294-3293. Tel: +1 205 934 1111. Fax: +1 205 934 0333. www.uab.edu/uasom.
Initially founded in Mobile in 1859, the school moved to Birmingham (via Tuscaloosa) in 1945. Birmingham is now the main campus, with medical divisions in Tuscaloosa and Huntsville.

University of South Alabama College of Medicine

Mobile, AL 36688-0002. Tel: +1 334 460 7176. Fax: +1 334 460 6278.
http://southmed.usouthal.edu.
Although the school was not in existence until 1973, the South Alabama Medical Centre has existed since 1831. This is the largest site of the university and has a level 1 trauma centre. Other associated institutions are the **USA Springhill Campus**, Cancer Centre, Health Services building, the **Searcy Hospital**, **Knollwood** and **USA Children's and Women's** hospitals.

ARIZONA

University of Arizona College of Medicine

1501N Campbell Ave, PO Box 245018, Tuscon, AZ 85724-5018. Tel: +1 520 626 7383. Fax: +1 520 626 4884.
www.medicine.arizona.edu.

The college was established in 1967, and the main 30-acre complex (Arizona Health Sciences Center) comprises a number of facilities. Of specialist interest here are centres for cancer, cardiac care (they're big in transplants, especially pioneering artificial ones), arthritis and paediatric research.

POPULAR HOSPITALS IN ARIZONA:

St Joseph's Hospital Trauma Unit

West Thomas Road, Phoenix, AZ.
The hospital: A major trauma centre. It is very busy, with many penetrating injuries.
O Elective notes: Plenty of procedures to do and very friendly staff. ATLS courses are run regularly and there are chances to go out with paramedics/firefighters. Highly recommended.

Mayo Clinic Scottsdale

13400 East Shea Boulevard, Scottsdale, AZ 85259. Tel: +1 602 301 4338.
Fax: +1 602 301 8323.
The hospital: High-tech and advanced. Look under the Mayo Clinic Rochdale for more information.

ARKANSAS

University of Arkansas College of Medicine

4301 West Markham Street, Little Rock, AR 72205-7199. Tel: +1 501 686 5354.
Fax: +1 501 686 5873. www.uams.edu.
This is is the principal biomedical research centre for Arkansas. The college comprises the **University Hospital** (350 beds, with state-of-the-art ITU) and state hospitals, a cancer research centre, the **Harvey and Bernice Jones Eye Institute**, the **Donald Reynolds Centre on Ageing**, the **Arkansas Children's Hospital**, the **VA Medical Centre** and **Arkansas Rehabilitation and Radiation Therapy Institutes**.

CALIFORNIA

University of California School of Medicine

One Shields Avenue, Davis, CA 95616–8661. Tel: +1 530 752 2717. Fax: +1 520 752 2376. www.med.ucdavis.edu.

The school has existed since 1973. It mainly uses the 455-bed **UC Davis Medical Centre** (with a level 1 trauma department) but has connections with the **Shriners Hospital for Children** and the **Ellison Ambulatory Care Centre**.

University of California Irvine College of Medicine

Medical Education Building, Irvine, CA 92697–4089. Tel: +1 949 824 5388 Fax: +1 949 824 2485. www.com.uci.edu.

The medical college of Orange County has existed since 1896 but became part of UCI in 1965. It consists of the UCI medical centre (with level 1 trauma, cancer, burns, transplant and neuropsychiatric centres) on-site and many affiliated hospitals. Research areas include the neurosciences, oncology, imaging, neonatology, cardiovascular, genetics and geriatrics. They have a well-organized elective programme on the web but charge international students $200.

University of California Los Angeles School of Medicine

Box 957035, Los Angeles, CA 90095–7035. Tel: +1 310 825 6373. Fax: +1 310 206 5046. www.medsch.ucla.edu.

Running since the 1950s, UCLA is associated with the **University Medical Centre** (600 beds), the **UCLA Ambulatory Medical Plaza** (with a level 1 trauma centre and specialist intensive care and operating suites), the **Mater Children's Hospital** (120 beds), the **Stein Eye Institute**, the **VA**, **Cedas–Sinai** and **Olive View Medical Centres** and the **Santa Monica Hospital**. UCLA has recently acquired the **Santa Monica UCLA Medical Center** (1250 Sixteenth Street, Santa Monica, CA 90404. Tel: +1 310 319 4000) with 363 beds, an emergency centre, ITU, NICU and a facility for sexually abused children.

University of California San Diego School of Medicine

Medical Teaching Facility, 9500 Gilman Drive, La Jolla, CA 92093–0606. Tel: +1 619 534 3880. Fax: +1 858 822 3067. www.medicine.ucsd.edu.

The medical school is surrounded by a wonderful variety of laboratory teaching and research facilities. Along with the UCSD Medical Centres (**Hillcrest**, 200 West Arbor Drive, San Diego, CA 92103. Tel: +1 619 543 622, and **La Jolla**, 9300 Campus Point Drive, La Jolla, CA 92037. Tel: +1 619 657 7000), it is associated with the **VA**, the **Naval Regional Medical Centre** and eight other hospitals and clinics. Details of their elective programme (costing $250.00 per four-week clerkship) are on their website. Excellent research opportunities exist here.

University of California San Francisco School of Medicine

Third Street and Parnassus Avenue, San Francisco, CA 94143. Tel: +1 415 476 2342. www.som.ucsf.edu.

UCSF Medical Center (505 Parnassus Avenue, San Francisco, CA 94122. Tel: +1 415 476 1000) is a 560-bed hospital near Golden Gate Park that is split between **Moffitt** (built in 1956) and **Long** (built in 1983) hospitals. Cardiac, neurosurgery and many other specialities are provided, and the hospitals have a great history of pioneering medical advances.

UCSF/Mount Zion Medical Center (1600 Divisadero Street, San Francisco, CA 94115. Tel: +1 415 567 6600) is a 365-bed hospital best known for its cancer centre. UCSF is also linked to **San Francisco General Hospital** (724 beds) and **San Francisco VA Medical Center** (500 beds). UCSF has a commitment to increasing the number of doctors from minority groups and has links with Berkeley.

Loma Linda University School of Medicine

Loma Linda, CA 92350. Tel: +1 909 558 4467. Fax: +1 909 422 4558. www.llu.edu. Loma is a very Christian medical school that was founded in 1909. The campus has the **LLU Medical Center** (11234 Anderson Street, Loma Linda, CA 92354. Tel: +1 909 558 4000), including a children's hospital. It has close links with the **LLU Behavioural Medical Center**, the **VA**, the **San Bernardino County General Hospital** and the **Glendale Adventist Medical Center**.

University of Southern California School of Medicine

1975 Zonal Avenue (KAM 100-C) Los Angeles, CA 90033. Tel +1 323 442 2552. www.usc.edu/hsc.
USC is a private, non-religious, co-educational university that established its medical school in 1885. It is opposite the main teaching hospital, the **Los Angeles County and USC Medical Center**. There is also the 284-bed **USC University Hospital**, the **USC Cancer Centre**, the **Doheny Eye Institute**, the **House Ear Institute**, an orthopaedic centre and the **Children's Hospital LA**.

Stanford University School of Medicine

300 Pasteur Drive, Stanford, CA 94305-5302. Tel: +1 650 723 4000. Fax: +1 650 725 7368. www.stanford.edu.
Teaching institutions include **Stanford University Hospital** (663 beds), the **Lucile Packard Children's Hospital** (214 beds; 725 Welch Road, Palo Alto, CA 94304. Tel: +1 650 497 8000), the **Palo Alto VA Hospital** (1000 beds) and the **Santa Clara County Valley Medical Center** (791 beds). The university library has one of the most impressive medical collections anywhere.

POPULAR HOSPITALS IN CALIFORNIA:

San Francisco

With its Golden Gate Bridge and rich culture, San Francisco is often considered to be the most pleasant part of California – a sharp contrast to its nearest neighbour, Los Angeles.

San Francisco General Hospital

1001 Potrero Avenue, San Francisco, CA 94110.
The hospital: SFGH is a county hospital with the only trauma centre in San Francisco, serving a population of 1.5 million. The emergency department treats 70 000 patients a year from a diverse background, many homeless individuals, intravenous drug users and alcoholics. It is world-renowned for having the first ever inpatient ward for HIV/AIDS. This unit receives awards year after year and is leading AIDS research. There is also a large paeds and genetics department.
○ Elective notes: Like everywhere in California, medicine here is very serious … you'll be expected to work long and hard. Four weeks in the ER is well organized with (monitored) eight-hour shifts (four to five days on, one day off), good teaching and a paramedic ride-along. There are plenty of procedures (suturing, central lines and manipulations under supervision) to do. Each day starts at 7 am with breakfast and a tutorial. You are treated as an integral part of the team and are as such expected to conduct 'consults'.

The HIV unit is repeatedly highly recommended. This is a 24-bed ward dedicated to the care of patients with HIV/AIDS. The friendly team on this ward provides an AIDS consult service. The function of this is to assess and make recommendations on any hospitalized patient with HIV/AIDS. There are daily ward rounds and excellent tutorials. Outpatient clinics include dermatology (mainly Kaposi's sarcoma), ophthalmology for cytomegalovirus retinitis and general follow up. To get more involved in the AIDS programme here, you can write to UCSF medical school, but they may say that you can't work here for insurance reasons. In that case, write directly to the department (UCSF AIDS Program, Building 80, Ward 84, San Francisco General Hospital, 995 Potrero Avenue, San Francisco, CA 94110. Tel: +1 415 206 8313. Fax: +1 415 476 6953).

If you just want to do paramedic work, try contacting the **San Francisco Department of Public Health** (Paramedic Division, 2789 25th Street, San Francisco, CA 94110).

Accommodation: Tuition is free but accommodation near impossible (try to make friends). The university can give advice but it's all expensive. You'll also need insurance.

Los Angeles

Famed for 'Baywatch' a huge movie industry and a population of health freaks who jog every morning, you may wonder why LA needs hospitals at all. Fortunately there are also a lot of overweight couch potatoes providing the need for more cardiologists in one city than there are in the entire UK. There is also a huge (often illegal) Hispanic immigrant population who live in poverty and in whom many diseases are far more prevalent. It really is a land of dichotomy, from the incredibly rich to the exceedingly poor.

There are two main teaching hospitals in LA: the **LAC & USC Medical Center** and the **UCLA Medical Center**.

LAC and USC Medical Centre
University of Southern California, GNH 11900, 2025 Zonal Avenue, Los Angeles, CA 90033.
The hospital: The LAC and USC Medical Center is a state-run hospital and one of the largest acute-care hospitals in the USA. It provides a huge range of medical and surgical services, and is a level 1 trauma centre with a busy ER.

Harbour-UCLA Medical Center
1000 West Carson Street, Torrance, California.
The hospital: Harbour UCLA Medical Center is a friendly county hospital just south of central LA. If you can't pay, treatment is free so it is mainly the disadvantaged who are seen. Many patients from Mexico have never seen a doctor before, hence it provides an interesting range of medicine. The hospital has 500 beds and most specialities are catered for.

O Elective notes: You are well looked after in a medical consult team, being given a couple of patients to assess and manage (with supervision). There are two interactive teaching rounds a day with afternoon lectures every day and many seminars, so you're always busy. Don't walk around here at night as it's just outside South-Central. All doorways have metal detectors which tells you something.

Accommodation: Free and in the hospital grounds. There is, however, no heating, no kitchen and nowhere to wash your clothes. Three generous meals a day are provided. It is therefore a relatively cheap elective (until you go touring).

Kaiser Sunset Facility
Sunset Boulevard, Los Angeles, CA.
The hospital: This tertiary referral centre for cardiothoracic surgery and interventional cardiology caters for a population of 2.5 million. It is run as a 'not-for-profit health management organization', which means you still need insurance to go there. It is an excellent place for an elective if you know you want to do cardiology.

COLORADO

Most people who go to Colorado on elective are really looking for a place to go skiing. That said, the following places are recommended. (See also 'Something different' at the end of this chapter.)

University of Colorado School of Medicine

4200 East 9th Avenue, C-297, Denver, CO 80262. Tel: +1 303 315 7565. Fax: +1 303 315 8494. www.uchsc.edu/sm/sm/.
Founded in 1883, the school now uses a number of hospitals throughout the Denver region and clinics throughout Colorado.

POPULAR HOSPITALS IN COLORADO:

University of Colorado Health Sciences Center

4200 East North Avenue, Denver, CO 80262.
The hospital: The hospital complex caters for most specialities and has a busy ER, although the major trauma centre is at Denver General Hospital.
O Elective notes: Organizing electives here has been difficult in the past. In the ER, students do four ten-hour shifts a week and there is plenty to do – lots of procedures. They will let you off to go skiing. Stay in Summit County where there are free buses up to Copper Mountain.

St Anthony Central Hospital

4231 West 16th Avenue, Denver, CO 80204.
The hospital: One of a group of three private hospitals in Denver (there is another in the city and one at Frisco in the Rockies). It has a level 1 trauma centre (which isn't that busy) and a helicopter emergency service.
O Elective notes: The hospital expects you to turn up (try to do four days on, three off), but it is excellent for skiing. You may well need a car though to get to some of the resorts. Allow £200 a week for this.

Boulder

Boulder is a unique enclave of science, research, education, sports and outdoor pursuits. At an altitude of 1630 m and with

350 days of sunshine a year, it attracts a great number of athletes for altitude training. The town has a population of 94 000 served by one large community hospital. The Rockies, with unlimited trails, are on the doorstep. This is definitely the place if you like the outdoors. It is a university town (although there's no medical school).

There are a number of institutes as well as the main hospital. **Boulder Orthopedics** (933 Alpine Avenue, Boulder, CO 80304) sees a great number of sports injuries and is run by four orthopaedic surgeons. **Boulder Heart Institute** (2750 Broadway, Boulder, CO 80304) is a private practice run by two invasive cardiologists. As it's private there are no waiting lists: chest pain on Monday – angiogram on Tuesday – bypass by Friday. **Boulder Valley Oncology LLP** (1155 Alpine Avenue, Suite 360, Boulder, CO 80304, Tel: +1 303 449 9500) is a large private practice right next to the main hospital.
Accommodation: As Boulder is a university town, there is plenty of accommodation available. Expect to spend around $350–400 a month.

CONNECTICUT

University of Connecticut School of Medicine

263 Farmington Avenue, Farmington, CT 06030–1905. Tel: +1 860 679 2385. Fax: +1 860 679 1282. http://medicine.uchc.edu/.
Founded in 1968, the school is part of the University of Connecticut Health Center, consisting of a 204-bed hospital, an ambulatory unit and a large library. It is affiliated with eight hospitals in Hartford and 11 community hospitals.

Yale University School of Medicine

333 Cedar Street, New Haven, CT 06510. Tel: +1 860 785 4672. Fax: +1 203 432 1333. http://info.med.yale.edu.
The school was established in 1810 and, with the nursing school and hospital, forms part of the **Yale–New Haven**

Medical Center. The local **VA**, the **Connecticut Mental Health Center**, the **St Raphael** and **Waterbury Hospitals** and the **Yale Psychiatric** hospitals are associates. It has a huge library.

POPULAR HOSPITALS IN CONNETICUT:

Yale University School of Medicine
333 Cedar Street, New Haven, CT 06510. Tel: +1 860 785 4672. Fax: +1 203 432 1333. http://info.med.yale.edu.
The medical school is particularly well known and hence attracts many students. Skiing in Vermont is easily accessible, and Boston and Washington are short train rides away. To arrange an elective in any of their hospitals, write to the **Office of International Medical Studies** (Yale University School of Medicine, 60 College Street, PO Box 208034, Newhaven, CT 06520–8034 or the address above. Also visit http://info.med. yale.edu). There is a $500 administration fee ($350 if you are only doing four weeks), but this gives use of all the academic and social facilities. Electives here have been highly recommended.
Accommodation: Can be provided in a dormitory adjacent to the school and New Haven Hospital for $110 a week. It has good facilities. Many other students live here too so it is also good socially.

Yale–New Haven Hospital
New Haven, CT.
The hospital: This is a spacious modern (900-bed) teaching hospital with a large children's hospital attached. All specialities are catered for with hi-tech facilities.

WASHINGTON DC

George Washington University School of Medicine
2300 Eye Street, Washington DC 20037. Tel: +1 202 994 3506. Fax: +1 202 994 1753. www.gwumc.edu.

The University Hospital provides a number of research opportunities as well as teaching. The **National Naval Medical Center**, **Washington Hospital Center** and **Children's**, **Fairfax**, **Holy Cross**, **St Elizabeth's** and **VA** hospitals are also linked.

Georgetown University School of Medicine
3900 Reservoir Road, NW Washington DC 20007. Tel: +1 202 687 1154. www.dml.georgetown.edu/schmed.
The medical school (part of the oldest Catholic- and Jesuit-sponsored university in the USA) works with the **University Hospital** (389 beds) and nine federal and community hospitals. The **Medical Center** (the largest in the capital) has a concentrated care centre providing emergency, outpatient, surgery, X-ray and transplant facilities. The **Lombardi Cancer Research Center** is near and there are good sports and dining facilities close by.

Howard University College of Medicine
520 W Street, NW Washington DC 20059. Tel: +1 202 806 9494. Fax: +1 202 806 7934. www.med.howard.edu.
When it was founded in 1868 with seven students, Howard was the only black medical school in the USA. Today, it trains men and women from all backgrounds. Twenty-five per cent of black American doctors are from Howard. The **University Hospital** has 321 beds. Other hospitals used are the **District of Columbia General Hospital**, **St Elizabeth's Hospital**, **US Naval Medical Center**, **Walter Reed Medical Center**, **Washington VA**, **Providence**, **National Rehab**, **Washington** and **Prince George's**.

POPULAR HOSPITALS IN WASHINGTON:

Washington Hospital Center
110 Irving Street, NW, Washington DC 20010–2975. Tel: +1 202 877 5190. Fax: +1 202 877 3173.

The hospital: The Washington Hospital Center is a large general hospital within a campus comprising the **National Children's**, **Washington Heart**, **National Rehabilitation** and **VA** hospitals. Washington has the dubious privilege of being the most violent city in the USA. Much of this trauma is (despite a clean-up campaign) still drugs related and commonly involves the poorer black population. **MedSTAR** (Medical Shock, Trauma and Acute Resuscitation) is the level 1 trauma centre within the hospital and deals purely with major trauma such as gunshot wounds (20%), stabbings, beatings, road traffic accidents (known as MVAs – motor vehicle accidents – 50%), falls and burns. It consists of seven patient bays and two helicopters. There are three surgical trauma teams (one civilian, one US Army, one US Navy) who work a 1:3 rota.

O **Elective notes:** Medical students make an essential part of the team with specific roles and jobs. These jobs are very varied but can be mundane, such as stabilizing cervical spines or writing the history and exam. The reward for this is being allowed to perform procedures ranging from suturing to chest tube insertion, central lines and, for the truly keen, removing bullets. You will be expected to be a house officer to three or four patients. Normal working hours are from 7 am (a ward round with the junior members of the team) until late afternoon, and one night in three you will be expected to assist (and don't expect any sleep … they average 14 trauma responses a day). BEWARE OF THE AMOUNT OF WORK YOU HAVE TO DO (this cannot be overemphasized). You are there every day (including weekends) and average 80 hours a week. Despite this, there is time to see the city. The other students are from the George Washington and Uniformed Services medical schools. This elective comes thoroughly recommended for anyone wishing to pursue a career in ER or surgery. All specialities are catered for in other departments. Malpractice insurance is provided by the hospital.

Accommodation: This includes a swimming pool and satellite TV for $130 a month, although the rooms are shared and not that great. There is an excellent canteen (with Pizza Hut!). The area around the hospital is fairly dodgy and at night a taxi from the hospital to Georgetown or downtown DC is a good idea. During the day, the Metro to downtown is good. Washington is an incredible city with lots of tourist attractions as well as some good bars and clubs in Georgetown and at Du Pont Circle. There are usually a lot of elective students around and the American interns are very sociable, although they apparently insist on wearing white trainers to the pub!

VA Medical Center (George Washington School of Medicine)

50 Irving Street NW, Washington DC 20422.
The hospital: The VA is a large general hospital with most specialities.

O **Elective notes:** Again, there is a great deal of responsibility. The endocrinology unit is friendly but will work you, expecting papers to be reviewed for journal clubs, etc. In return, you will see a great deal of medicine, diabetes, thyroid problems, Klinefelter's syndrome, Paget's disease, osteoporosis …. You will be expected to write a six-page essay (remember this if you're applying for a grant). Expect to work hard, but this is a rewarding experience and comes highly recommended.

Accommodation: This is a major drawback. A retired couple rent out rooms (2045 Park Road NW, Washington DC 20010). This is 20 minutes from the hospital and too dangerous a neighbourhood to walk through so a bus is needed. The accommodation itself is a room in a house. The couple are pleasant, and there are no other students. Go in a pair if you can.

FLORIDA

University of Florida College of Medicine

UF Health Sciences Center, Gainsville, FL 32610–0216. Tel: +1 352 392 4569. Fax: +1 352 846 0622. www.med.ufl.edu.

Founded in 1956, the University Health Center comprises the **Stetson Medical Science Building**, an academic and cancer research building, **Shands Hospital**, the **Brain Institute** and the **VA Jacksonville**.

University of Miami School of Medicine
1600 NW 10th Avenue, PO Box 016159, Miami, FL 33101. Tel: +1 305 213 6545. Fax: +1 305 243 6548. www.miami.edu.
This, the largest and oldest medical school in Florida, is next to the **Jackson Memorial Hospital** (3000 beds) in Miami (50000 admissions a year). With the **VA** it provides most patients. There are also the **Mailman Center for Child Development**, the **Bascom Palmer Eye Institute**, the **Applebaum MRI Center**, the **Ambulatory Care Center**, the **UM Hospital**, **Diabetes Research Institute**, the **Sylvester Comprehensive Cancer Center** (the only one in Florida) and the **Ryder Trauma Center**.

University of South Florida College of Medicine
12901 Bruce B. Downs Boulevard, Tampa, FL 33612 4799. Tel: +1 813 974 2229. Fax: +1 813 974 4990. www.med.usf.edu.
Founded in 1971, the main clinical areas are the USF medical clinics, **Tampa General Hospital**, **Haley Veterans Hospital**, **Shriners Hospital for Children**, **Moffitt Cancer Center**, **Genesis Clinic**, **USY Psychiatry Center** and **Eye Institute**. It also has links with the **All Children's Hospital**, **Bayfont Medical Center**, **Bay Pines Veterans Hospital** (St Petersburg) and **Orlando Regional Medical Center**.

GEORGIA

Emory University School of Medicine
Woodruff Health Sciences Center, Atlanta, GA 30322 4510. Tel: +1 404 727 5640. Fax: +1 404 727 0473. www.emory.edu/WHSC.

Founded in 1915, the medical school has access to over 3000 beds in its teaching hospitals.

Medical College of Georgia School of Medicine
1120 15th Street, Augusta, GA 30912-4760. Tel: +1 706 721 0211. Fax: +1 706 721 0959. www.mcg.edu.
Founded in 1828, this is the 11th-oldest medical school in the US. The main hospital used is the **Medical College of Georgia Hospital**, with 80 speciality clinics and a regional trauma centre. Elective details here and in rural hospitals are on their website.

Mercer University School of Medicine
1550 College St, Macon, GA 31207. Tel: +1 912 301 2542. Fax: + 1 912 301 2547. www.mercer.edu.
MUSM (founded in 1982) uses Mercer Health Systems, consisting of an ambulatory care facility, the **Medical Center of Central Georgia** in Macon, the **Memorial Center** in Savannah and the **Medical Centers** in Rome, Albany and Columbus.

Morehouse School of Medicine
720 Westview Drive, SW Atlanta, GA 30310–1495. Tel: +1 404 752 1500. Fax: +1 404 752 1512. www.msn.edu.
Founded in 1978, Morehouse is historically black. The affiliated hospitals include **Grady Memorial Hospital**, the **Tuskegee VA** (Alabama) and the **Southwest Community Hospital**.

HAWAII

University of Hawaii at Manoa John A. Burns School of Medicine
1960 East-West Road, Honolulu, HI 96822. Tel: +1 808 956 8300. Fax: +1 808 956 9547. http://hawaiimed.hawaii.edu/.
The school is situated in the Manoa campus and **Leahi Hospital**. It uses hospitals and facilities throughout the state. Their

web page has details of elective arrangements.

POPULAR HOSPITALS IN HAWAII:

Since full details of electives on Honolulu are given on the web page, these are not discussed here. If you fancy something a bit smaller, try another hospital or another island:

Kaiser Permanente Medical Center

3288 Moanalua Road, Honolulu, HI 96819. Tel: +1 808 834 5333.

The hospital: A fairly small, friendly, advanced hospital with 260 beds, a 30-bed CCU, six theatres, a cardiac catheterization suite and a very busy ER. It provides care for Kaiser Insurance Members throughout the Hawaiian Islands.

O **Elective notes:** Because of the insurance situation in the USA, you have to sign a contract saying that you won't do anything to patients. This immediately limits practical procedures. There are, however, plenty of patients to clerk and meetings to attend. It is very friendly and many people are keen to teach.

Hilo Medical Center

1190 Waianuenue Avenue, Hilo, HI 96720.

The hospital: Hilo is a small place on a big island. The hospital is pretty small and probably less well run than you might expect from an American hospital. It does, however, provide most basic specialities.

O **Elective notes:** The staff are generally friendly and there's lots of pathology to be seen, but don't expect everyone to be up to date with the latest technologies. Travel around the island, although public transport is incredibly limited. Check out the volcanoes, Waipio Valley, Kona side of the island (stay in Patey's place – cheap and cheerful), do some snorkelling and swim with the dolphins. At night, you can whale watch too! It really is the travelling that makes this elective worth-

while. Hilo is pretty quiet ... if it's nightlife you want, go to Honolulu or Waikiki.
Accommodation: DO NOT let them put you in the hospital accommodation – apparently it's not up to much. Find a student flat with a low rent. If you arrive early, stay at Arnott's Lodge, a really friendly hostel. While you're there you can sort out the accommodation for the rest of your stay.

ILLINOIS

University of Chicago Pritzker School of Medicine

924 E 57th Street, BLSC 104, Chicago, IL 60637 5416. Tel: +1 773 702 1937.
Fax: +1 773 702 2598.
http://pritzker.bsd.uchicago.edu.

The university is in south Chicago (12 minutes from downtown) in the Hyde Park area. The school prides itself on producing academic physicians. The university is a hive of biomedical research. Hospitals used include the **University of Chicago**, the **Weiss** and the **MacNeal**.

Finch University of Health Sciences, Chicago Medical School

3333 Green Bay Road, North Chicago, IL 60064. Tel: +1 847 578 3000.
Fax: +1 847 578 3401. www.finchcns.edu.

Founded in 1912 and based in north Chicago, the school uses **Cook County Hospital**, the **Edward Hines VA Medical Center**, the **North Chicago VA**, the **Illinois Masonic Medical Center**, the **Swedish Covenant Hospital**, **Norwalk Hospital**, the **Lutheran General Hospital**, **Mount Sinai Hospital** and the **Henry Ford Health Sciences Center** (Detroit).

University of Illinois at Chicago College of Medicine

1819 West Polk Street, Chicago, IL 60612-7332. Tel: +1 312 996 3500.
Fax: +1 312 996 9006. www.uic.edu.

Since its foundation in 1881, the

University of Illinois College has run two parallel medical school programmes over four sites. The **College of Medicine at Chicago** is in the Health Sciences Center of the University. The **College of Medicine at Urbana–Champaign** (Medical Sciences Building 190, 506 South Mathews Street, Urbana, IL 61801. Tel: +1 217 333 5469. Fax: +1 217 333 8868. www.med.uiuc.edu) is on a large campus with many academic and multi-faculty contacts. The **College of Medicine at Peoria** (1 Illini Drive, PO Box 1649, Peoria, IL 61605. Tel: +1 309 671 8407. Fax: +1 309 671 8452. www.uicomp. uic.edu) has many community hospitals and a modern campus, and the **College of Medicine at Rockford** (1601 Parkview Avenue, Rockford, IL 61107. Tel: +1 815 395 5600. Fax: +1 815 395 5887. www.rockford.uic.edu) is central and has a number of hospitals attached.

Loyola University of Chicago Stritch School of Medicine

2160 South First Avenue, Maywood, IL 60153. Tel: +1 708 216 3229. www.med-dean.luc.edu.

Founded in 1870, this is private and the largest Catholic university in the USA. The medical school was organized in the 1920s, and in 1969 the **Loyola University Medical Center** was built in Maywood, 19 km west of the Chicago Loop. The centre has the school and the 570-bed **McGaw Hospital**. It also uses the 1022-bed **Hines VA Hospital**.

Northwestern University Medical School

303 East Chicago Avenue, Chicago, IL 60611. Tel: +1 312 503 9443.
Fax: +1 312 908 5502. www.nums.edu.

The medical school (founded 1859) is on the university's lake-front Chicago campus and uses **Glenbrook** (100 beds), **Evanston** (420 beds), **Children's Memorial** (248 beds) and **Northwestern** (659 beds) hospitals as well as the **Rehabilitation Institute of Chicago** and the **Chicago VA**.

Rush Medical College of Rush University

600 South Paulina Street, Chicago, IL 60612. Tel: +1 312 942 6913. Fax: +1 312 942 2333. www.rushu.rush.edu.

Originally founded in 1837, Rush Medical College was closed from 1942 until 1971, when it was made part of the University of Chicago. Today, it uses a number of institutions, including the **Rush–Presbyterian–St Luke's Medical Center** (1653 W Congress Parkway, Chicago, IL 60612. Tel: +1 312 942 5000), which serves 2 million people.

Southern Illinois University School of Medicine

801 North Rutledge Street, PO Box 19620, Springfield, IL 62794-9620. Tel: +1 217 782 3318. Fax: +1 217 524 0786.
www.siumed.edu.

Founded in 1969, the college uses the **Springfield Memorial Medical Center** and **St John's Hospital**.

POPULAR HOSPITALS IN ILLINOIS:

Cook County Hospital

Chicago, IL.

The hospital: The trauma department of this public hospital is famed as the basis for the TV series *ER* and is one of the best in the US. The staff are very friendly. There is a great deal of penetrating trauma (gunshots, stabbings) and road accidents in this very busy department.

Elective notes: There are excellent opportunities for many practical procedures. The teaching is also very good.

Accommodation: A list is provided. Note: The YMCA in downtown is full of drug addicts. Try to arrange to stay with someone from the hospital.

Alexian Brothers Medical Center

800 Biesterfield Road, Elk Grove Village, IL 60007.

The hospital: Alexian Brothers Medical Center is a private hospital situated about 16 km west of Chicago. The hospital has about 500 beds and a staggering 470 physicians/surgeons on the staff. The world of American private medicine is undoubtedly dominated by matters financial, but the Alexian Brothers has succeeded as a non-profit-making organization to become only one of three hospitals in Illinois to be accredited with commendation by the American Medical Association. Medical students are few and far between so people are keen to teach and there are many practical procedures to do, especially in the ER. Facilities are state of the art. This elective is thoroughly recommended.

Accommodation: And meals in the hospital are provided free, but the lack of other students limits your social life to those twice your age.

INDIANA

Indiana University School of Medicine
635 Barnhill Drive, Indianapolis, IN 46254. Tel: +1 317 274 7175. Fax: +1 317 274 4309. www.medicine.iu.edu.

This is the medical school for Indiana (founded in 1903) and has centres in Bloomington, Fort Wayne, Gary, Evansville, Muncie, Lafayette, Terre Haute and South Bend. The university is also a major research centre and has the University Hospital.

IOWA

University of Iowa College of Medicine
Medicine Administration Building, Iowa City, IA 52242–1101. Tel +1 319 335 8052. Fax: +1 319 335 8049.
www.medicine.uiowa.edu.

Since its foundation in 1868, the college has become a major part of the state's health. The health sciences campus comprises the University of Iowa Hospitals and Clinics, the **VA** and the **Hardin Health Sciences Library**.

KANSAS

University of Kansas School of Medicine
3901 Rainbow Boulevard, Kansas City, KS 66160 7301. Tel: +1 913 588 5245. Fax: +1 913 588 5259. www.kumc.edu.

Founded in 1899, the Medical Center campus includes the **Leid Biomedical Research Building**, the Dykes Library and the University Hospital (with 485 beds). A separate campus is allied to four Wichita hospitals.

KENTUCKY

University of Kentucky College of Medicine
301 East Main Street, Suite 400, Lexington, KY 40507-1507. Tel: +1 859 257 5320. Fax: +1 859 3232437.
www.mc.ky.edu.

The college (founded in 1956) is part of the University of Kentucky Chandler Medical Center on the university campus in Lexington. Hospitals used include the **University of Kentucky Hospital** (473 beds), the **VA** (662 beds) and hospitals throughout Lexington and Kentucky. The campus also has critical care, cancer, ageing and MRI centres.

University of Louisville School of Medicine
Abell Administration Center, 323 East Chestnut, Louisville, KY 40202–3866. Tel: +1 502 852 5193. www.louisville.edu.

Founded in 1833, the school is part of the **Health Sciences Center** in downtown Louisville. Hospitals used include the 404-bed acute and trauma **University Hospital**, the **Kosair-Children's Hospital**, the **Jewish Hospital**, the **Norton Hospital** and the **VA**. Also affiliated are the **Kentucky Lions Eye Research Institute**, **James Brown Cancer Center**, **Child Evaluation Center** and **Fazier Rehabilitation Center**.

LOUISIANA

Louisiana State University School of Medicine in New Orleans
1901 Perdido Street, New Orleans, LA 70112–1393. Tel: +1 504 568 4006. Fax: +1 504 568 4008.
www.medschool.lsumc.edu.
Since its establishment in 1931, the school has grown and now uses a number of buildings and hospitals, principally the **Medical Center of Louisiana** and the **University Hospital**. Outside, the **Medical Center** in Lafayette and the **Long Hospital** in Baton Rouge are used.

Louisiana State University School of Medicine in Shreveport
PO Box 33932, Shereveport, LA 71130–3932. Tel: +1 318 675 5190. Fax: +1 318 675 5244. www.sh.lsumc.edu/.
Founded in 1969, the school uses two main hospitals: the **Louisiana State University Hospital** (650 beds) and the affiliated **Shreveport VA Hospital** (450 beds).

Tulane University School of Medicine
1430 Tulane Avenue, SL67, New Orleans, LA 70112–2699. Tel: +1 504 588 5187. Fax: +1 504 988 6735.
www.mcl.tulane.edu.
Established in 1834, this private non-sectarian school is in downtown New Orleans near the Superdrome and Vieux Carre (French Quarter). It uses the

Charity Hospital of New Orleans, the **VA** and the **Tulane University Hospital**. There are also public health, tropical medicine, bioenvironmental health, children's, neurological, cardiovascular, geriatric, cancer, transplant, women's and sports centres.

MARYLAND

Johns Hopkins University School of Medicine
720 Rutland Avenue, Baltimore, MD 21205–2196. Tel: +1 410 955 8401., Fax: +1 410 955 2522.
www.hopkinsmedicine.org.
The school is a private, non-denominational institution founded in 1893 that uses the **Johns Hopkins Hospital** (600 N Wolfe Street, Baltimore, MD 21287–4606). There is a school of hygiene and public health, and a number of affiliated centres, such as the **Krieger Institute** for children with brain disorders. The **Sinai Hospital** (2401 West Belvedere Avenue, Baltimore, MD 21215–5271) is a 500-bed community hospital with strong links to Johns Hopkins School of Medicine. To do an elective at the Johns Hopkins Hospital, the elective fee is currently £156 and insurance with them costs around £102. Teaching is of a high quality, and it's recommended for electives.

University of Maryland School of Medicine
655 West Baltimore Street, Baltimore, MD 21201. Tel: +1 410 706 7478.
www.umm.edu.
Having been founded in 1808, this school is the fifth oldest in the US. It is on the Baltimore City Campus of the university (with law, science and other faculties) and next to the downtown Charles Center, Inner Harbour and Oriole Park. It has access to 2300 beds through various hospitals.

USA

Uniformed Services University of the Health Sciences F. Edward Herbert School of Medicine

4301 Jones Bridge Road, Bethesda, MD 20814 4799. Tel: +1 800 772 1743. Fax: +1 301 295 1960. www.usuhs.mil.

The USUHS was founded in 1976 to prepare health workers for the services. The school is in the Naval Hospital in Bethesda. It collaborates with federal health resources in Washington DC and serves to select medical officers. The school of nursing has the same address. A few people who have done electives here have done intensive courses in ATLS, ALS and military medicine.

MASSACHUSETTS

Boston University School of Medicine

715 Albany Street, Boston, MA 02118. Tel: +1 617 638 4630/5300. Fax: +1 617 638 5258. www.bumc.bu.edu.

Originally the New England Female Medical College (founded in 1848), the school became part of the university in 1873. The school, with the **University Hospital** and other departments, makes up the **Boston Medical Center** (1 Boston Medical Center Place, Boston, MA 02118. Tel: +1 800 841 4325. Fax: +1 617 638 8000), a 547-bed private hospital and level 1 trauma centre in Boston's South End. It also uses the **Boston VA Hospital**.

Harvard Medical School

25 Shattuck Street, Boston, MA 02115–6092. Tel: +1 617 432 0442. Fax: +1 617 432 0446. www.med.harvard.edu.

A catalogue of their electives can be found at: http://medcatalog.harvard.edu. Note: The current cost is $2650 a month, and the maximum allowed (if you can afford it!) is three four-week electives.

The school (which has produced 12 Nobel Laureates) has been based in the Longwood Avenue Quadrangle since 1906, although it was actually established in 1782. A number of hospitals are used. These include the **Massachusetts General** (MGH), **Children's**, **Brigham and Women's**, **Beth Israel Deaconess Medical Center**, **Mount Auburn**, **Dana-Farber Cancer Institute**, **Massachusetts Eye and Ear** and **Cambridge** hospitals. The **Massachusetts Mental Health Center** and the **McLean** hospitals provide psychiatric services. **Harvard Vanguard Medical Associates** and others provide community facilities. Other institutions include the **Shriners Burns Institute**, the **West Roxbury** and **Brockton VA Medical Centers** and the **Spaulding Rehab Hospital**. There are close links with the Massachusetts Institute of Technology.

University of Massachusetts Medical School

55 Lake Avenue, North Worcester, MA 01655. Tel: +1 508 856 8989. Fax: +1 508 856 5536. www.umassmed.edu.

Established in 1962, the UMass medical school uses the **UMass Memorial Medical Center**, comprising 761 beds over two acute hospitals and a number of community hospitals, for its clinical teaching. **UMass Worcester** is next to the Biotechnology Research Park and has a molecular medicine and cancer center.

Tufts University School of Medicine

136 Harrison Avenue, Boston, MA 02111. Tel: +1 617 636 7000. Fax: +1 617 636 0375. http://tufts.edu/med.

The university was established in 1852, although the medical school was founded in Boston in 1893. Thirty hospitals are associated, and a number of departments, including the **New England Medical Center** (750 Washington Street, Boston MA 02111), a specialized diagnostic and referral hospital with a paediatric trauma institute, the **Baystate Medical Center**

(759 Chestnut Street, Springfield, MA 01199), a 700-bed centre providing comprehensive care to the million people in west Massachusetts, and **Faulkner Hospital**, in Jamaica Plain, are used.

POPULAR HOSPITALS IN MASSACHUSETTS:

Boston

Boston is a great city, with good shops, public transport and night-life. Most people go here because of the reputation of Harvard and the many world-renowned institutions.

To arrange an elective in any Harvard-associated hospital you are supposed to write to Harvard Medical School at the above address. The application form is available on the Internet at www.harvard.edu. Alternatively, e-mail exclerks@warren.med.harvard.edu. The application form gives you five or six choices. The big three hospitals are the MGH, the Beth Israel and the Brigham and Women's. To apply, you need to send $100 with a medical and a report of a clear chest X-ray from the previous six months.

The current fee to do a four-week elective here is a mind-blowing $2650, and this goes up year on year. This gives full Harvard student privileges (such as e-mail ... woopy doo!). You also get a certificate to state that you've been to Harvard. The package has previously also included malpractice insurance. If you happen to have this spare cash lying around or rich relatives, great. A number of people have said that the teaching is so good that it's worth every dollar. Realistically, this is way out of most people's reach. There are, however, ways around it, although this is becoming increasingly difficult. A few scholarships exist; ask Harvard or your own medical school for information on these. The most common tactic is to use a contact that someone in your hospital has. You need to apply directly to a consultant there. Many will turn round and say that

you must apply through the school so try someone else. There are lists of consultants in every department on the web. Don't give up.

This is, of course, unofficial advice as the university expects students to apply directly though them. However, with charges as high as they are and while their students can visit other hospitals for free, they should expect people to try to get round it. In general, an elective in any hospital here is hard work, but you don't pay that kind of money just to swan about Boston.

Note: MGH, the Brigham and Women's, the Children's, the Beth Israel and the New England Deaconess Hospitals as well as Harvard Medical School are in the Longwood area of Boston (*see* the map on the website). It is a great area for academics but there's not much else close by.

Accommodation: Usually provided in Vanderbilt Hall. Add another $700 to your bill for rent here. (It's a room with a desk but no sink or bedding.) The hall is a good 15 minutes from the city centre but is next to Harvard Medical School and close to the Brigham and Women's, Beth Israel and Children's Hospital. If you want a sink and a heated room for the same $700, you can stay at Mrs Weinstein's Guesthouse (48 Temple Street, Boston, MA 02214. Tel: +1 617 227 4062). Also try the YMCA in Charlestown (with a free shuttle bus to the General Hospital).

Full details of all the hospitals are given on the EXCELLENT website www.hmcnet.harvard.edu and hence only addresses (and occasional notes) are given below.

Massachusetts General Hospital
55 Fruit Street, Boston, MA 02114–2696.
The hospital: Founded in 1811, it now provides 820 beds and is renowned for being at the forefront of technology, with nearly all medical and surgical subspecialities. Its emergency centres are on the main campus and in Chelsea.
O Elective notes: The ER has extremely good teaching and is well

timetabled. Once the attending physician has seen you with a few patients, you are allowed to see patients on your own and then just get them to review things. The trauma team is extremely well trained and impressive to watch. In anaesthetics, the surgical ITU has good teaching and is very enjoyable. If interested in intensive care, this is worthwhile.

Beth Israel Deaconess Medical Center
330 Brookline Avenue, Boston, MA 02215. Tel: +1 617 667 7000.
The hospital: This is another large Harvard teaching hospital. It has excellent reports for cardiothoracic and plastic surgery, although both are very busy.

Children's Hospital
300 Longwood Avenue, Boston, MA 02115
The hospital: This is the major paeds referral centre.

Brigham and Women's Hospital
221 Longwood Avenue, Boston, MA 02115.

Shriners Hospital for Crippled Children Burns Institute
St Blossom Street, Boston, MA 02114-2699.
The hospital: Some people have found that they won't provide indemnity cover, and there are few patients and so not much teaching.

Mount Auburn Hospital
330 Mount Auburn Street, Cambridge, MA 02238. Tel: +1 617 492 3500.
The hospital: A smaller, highly specialized community hospital in Cambridge but still under Harvard Medical School.

Whitehead Institute
Nine Cambridge Center, Cambridge, MA 02142.
The institute: The Whitehead Institute has seven different research groups, including oncological. It is linked to MGH where clinics can be attended.
Accommodation: Book early as Boston is expensive.

Joslin Diabetes Center
The centre: This centre offers good opportunities for those who want to do research.

Lahey Hitchcock Medical Center
30 Mall Road, Burlington, MA 01803.
The hospital: This is very high-tech, with a good cardiology department.
O Elective notes: There is the opportunity to see advanced procedures but very little hands-on (e.g. ECHO rather than auscultation).
Accommodation: This can usually be arranged in a private house.

Veterans Administrative Hospital
1100 VW Parkway, West Roxbury, Boston, MA.
The hospital: A very busy hospital about 13 km from the centre of Boston.
O Elective notes: It's associated with Harvard, hence there are many medical students around. It's hard work, seeing your own patients in clinic, who you then discuss with a senior.
Accommodation: Has not been provided in the past.

Schepen's Eye Research Institute
20 Staniford Street, Boston, MA 02114.
Tel: +1 617 912 0100.
Schepen's is a major eye research centre, now pioneering retinal transplantation research.

Massachusetts Eye and Ear Infirmary
243 Charles Street, Boston, MA 02114.
Tel: +1 617 573 5520. Fax: +1 617 573 344.

MICHIGAN

Michigan State University College of Human Medicine
East Lansing, Michigan 48824–1317, USA
Tel: (517) 353 9620 Fax: 432 0021.
www.chm.msu.edu.
The CHM was originally designed in 1964 to create more primary care physi-

cians. The first two years of training are on the East Lansing campus, students are then sent to one of six community hospitals (Flint, Grand Rapids, Lansing, Saginaw, Kalamazoo or the Upper Peninsula).

University of Michigan Medical School
Ann Arbor, MI 48109–0611. Tel: +1 734 764 6317. Fax: +1 734 763 0453. www.med.umich.edu/medschool/.
Covering 84 acres with 30 buildings, the medical centre claims to be the world's largest one-site complex devoted to health education, research and clinical care. The university hospitals have 888 beds in total and treat over half a million patients a year. In addition to the university hospitals, **St Joseph Mercy Hospital**, the **VA**, **Oakwood Hospital** and the **William Beaumont Hospital** are used.

Wayne State University School of Medicine
540 East Canfield, Detroit, MI 48201. Tel: +1 313 577 1466. Fax: +1 313 577 1330. www.med.wayne.edu.
The **Detroit Medical Center** houses the medical school, the Lande Medical and Elliman Clinical Research Buildings, the Harper-Grace, Hutzel and Children's Hospitals, the University Health Center (ambulatory care), the Detroit Receiving Hospital, the Rehabilitation Institute and the VA hospitals. Outside, the **Sinai**, **Saint John**, **Oakwood**, **William Beaumont**, **Providence** and **Saint Joseph Mercy** hospitals are used.

POPULAR HOSPITALS IN MICHIGAN:

Providence Hospital
16001 West Nine Mile Road, 3rd Floor Fischer Centre, Southfield, MI 48075.
The hospital: This is a world-leading institute for craniofacial and reconstructive surgery.

○ Elective notes: It is very hard work but very rewarding. They show a great deal of interest in students. This is highly recommended to anyone interested in plastics, ENT or max-fax.

MINNESOTA

Mayo Medical School
200 First Street, SW Rochester, MN 55905. Tel: +1 507 284 3671. Fax: +1 507 284 2634.
www.mayo.edu/education/mms/intro.htm.
The Mayo Foundation and Mayo Clinic is the world's largest group practice, and the medical school is an important part of it. The clinics (run as outpatients) are in three locations: Rochester (Minnesota), Jacksonville (Florida) and Scottsdale (Arizona). Four hospitals (**St Mary's Rochester**, **Rochester Methodist**, **St Luke's, Jacksonville** and **Mayo Clinic Hospital, Scottsdale**) are linked for tuition and the referral of patients (*see* below). All offer very high-tech subspecialities. There are also rural health centres. There are great research opportunities with Mayo, and because of the small class size, one-to-one teaching is common.

University of Minnesota Duluth School of Medicine
10 University Drive, Duluth, MN 55812. Tel: +1 218 726 7571. Fax: +1 218 726 6235. http://penguin.d.umn.edu.
UMD provides two years' preclinical training before students are transferred to the University of Minnesota Medical School for the clinical component. Links are with the **St Mary's/Duluth Clinic**, **Miller–Dwan Medical Centers** and **St Luke's Hospital**.

University of Minnesota Medical School Minneapolis
420 Delaware Street, SE, Minneapolis, MN 55455–0310. Tel: +1 612 626 4949. Fax: +1 612 626 6491 1. www.med.umn.edu.
The school is on the Minneapolis campus of the University of Minnesota and

part of the University of Minnesota Academic Health Center with which all the major hospitals in the Minneapolis–St Paul area are associated (*see* University of Minnesota Hospital below).

POPULAR HOSPITALS IN MINNESOTA:

Mayo Medical School and its hospitals
200 First Street SW, Rochester, MN 55902. Tel: +1 507 284 3671 Fax: +1 507 284 2634.
The hospital: The medical school has only 40 places a year but 4000 applicants. This tells you what type of institution it is. The Mayo clinics are renowned for their excellence all over the world. The Rochester was the first, but two others (Jacksonville, Florida, and Scottsdale, Arizona) have followed. It has a multidisciplinary approach and is an international front-runner for thoracic surgery. One-third of patients seen are under Medicare. The Rochester site encompasses the clinic (outpatients), **St Mary's Hospital** (1216 Second Street, SW Rochester, MN 55905) and **Rochester Methodist Hospital** (201 Center St W, Rochester, MN 55905).

St Mary's Hospital was founded in 1883 by Mother Mary Alfred Moes on the condition that the Mayo family provide the medical care; it then had 27 beds. The current 1157-bed hospital is now leading the way in many fields and many specialities: neurosurgery, cardiac and lung transplants and rehabilitation to name but a few. It has a trauma unit with Mayo One, Minnesota's air ambulance. There are eight ITUs! Rochester Methodist Hospital, with 794 beds and 34 operating rooms, provides liver, kidney, pancreas and bone marrow transplant services, O&G and dermatology departments among other specialities.
O Elective notes: The facilities and doctors are outstanding, though surprisingly not intimidating. No one tries to

impress you ... they don't need to. There are opportunities to do research if you wish. You are a total team member and that includes beers after work, ice-skating, skiing, etc. This is an excellent package although the hours can be very long. Thoracics has excellent staff and teaching although you start at around 6 am. The patients get superb care. The major setback is that Rochester doesn't have much entertainment. Try to meet up with friends. There is an application fee of $50 but no elective fees, and malpractice insurance is covered by the Mayo.
Accommodation: The Mayo compiles a list of private homes that elective students can stay at for very reasonable rates. Alternatively, you can stay at the Kahler hotel for a very reduced rate.

University of Minnesota Hospital
Minneapolis, MN.
The hospital: This is the major teaching hospital for the university and accordingly has all specialities.
O Elective notes: To come here write to the Office of Curriculum Affairs at the medical school address. As in many American hospitals, electives here tend to consist of long days and hard work, although it is very friendly and they understand you want to go sightseeing. Indemnity cover is provided for around £70.
Accommodation: The university is very helpful in organizing this.

MISSISSIPPI

University of Mississippi School of Medicine
2500 North State Street, Jackson, MS 39216–4505. Tel: +1 601 984 5010. Fax: +1 601 984 1013. http://medicine.umc.edu/.
Since 1955, the school has used the University of Mississippi Medical Center in Jackson, which comprises the 593-bed **University Hospital**. The

Guyton Research Building and Batson Children's Hospital are also on campus. The VA and McBryde Rehab Center for the Blind are also linked.

MISSOURI

University of Missouri Columbia School of Medicine

One Hospital Drive, Columbia, MO 65212. Tel: +1 573 882 2923. Fax: +1 573 884 4808. www.hsc.missouri.edu.
Established in 1872, the school is on the Columbia Campus with the Health Sciences Center, comprising the University Hospital, Truman VA, Mid-Missouri Mental Health Center, Rusk Rehab Center, Mason Institute of Ophthalmology, Cosmopolitan International Diabetes Center and Ellis–Fischel Cancer Center. In total there are 1000 beds. Affiliations with clinics and hospitals outside are also maintained.

University of Missouri Kansas City School of Medicine

2411 Holmes, Kansas City, Missouri 64108. Tel: +1 816 235 1870. Fax: +1 816 235 5277. http://research.med.umkc.edu.
The medical school (established in 1969) is on the Hospital Hill campus and is near other colleges in the university and community hospitals.

Saint Louis University School of Medicine

1402 South Grand Boulevard, St Louis, MO 63104. Tel: +1 314 577 8622. Fax: +1 314 771 9316. www.slu.edu/colleges/med/.
The school was initially privately endowed by the Jesuits in 1818. The University Hospital, Wohl Memorial Mental Health Institute, Busch Eye Institute and Cardinal Glennon Hospital for Children are on-site. Affiliations are with the Deaconess, DePaul, St John's Mercy and St Mary's medical centers and the St Louis VA.

Washington University School of Medicine

660 South Euclid Avenue, #8107, St Louis, MO 63110. Tel: +1 314 362 6857. Fax: +1 314 362 4658. http://medschool.wustl.edu.
Since its establishment in 1891, the Washington University Medical Center has grown to 230 acres, housing the Barnes-Jewish Hospital (1737 beds), the St Louis Children's Hospital (a leading hospital) and the Central Institute for the Deaf.

NEBRASKA

Creighton University School of Medicine

2500 California Plaza, Omaha, NE 68178. Tel: +1 402 280 2900., Fax: +1 402 280 2599. www.creighton.edu.
The school, founded by Jesuits in 1892, uses St Joseph's Hospital (403 beds) as its main teaching hospital. The Children's Memorial, VA and Alegent Health System hospitals are also used.

University of Nebraska College of Medicine

600 South 42nd Street, Omaha, NE 68198-6585. Tel: +1 402 559 4204. Fax: +1 402 559 4148. www.unmc.edu/UNCOM.
Founded in 1880, the college uses the Nebraska Health System (University Hospital and Clarkson Hospital), University Geriatric Center, Eppley Cancer Research Institute and Meyer Children's Rehab Institute as well as the VA and eight private hospitals. In total it has access to 2800 beds.

NEVADA

University of Nevada School of Medicine

Mail Stop 357, Reno, NV 89557. Tel: +1 775 784 6063. Fax: +1 775 784 6194. www.unr.edu.

USA

This is a state-supported, community-based, university-integrated school that uses community medicine and primary care physicians as its teachers.

NEW HAMPSHIRE

Dartmouth Medical School

1 Rope Ferry Road, Hanover, NH 03755. Tel: +1 603 650 1200. Fax: +1 603 650 1614. www.dartmouth.edu/dms/.

The school (the fourth-oldest in the USA – 1797) is part of the **Dartmouth–Hitchcock Medical Center** (housing the Mary Hitchcock Memorial Hospital, Cotton Cancer Center and White River Junction VA). The **Dartmouth–Hitchcock Clinic** is very large, serving 1.5 million people and containing 372 beds. **Brattleboro Retreat** (VT), the **Family Medical Institute of Augusta** (ME), **Hartford Hospital** (CT) and **Tuba City Indian Health Service Hospital** (AZ) offer further instruction.

POPULAR HOSPITALS IN NEW HAMPSHIRE:

Littleton Regional Hospital

262 Cottage Street, Littleton, NH 03561.

The hospital: Littleton is a town in the north-east consisting of 12 000 people. The hospital serves this and the nearby small towns. Although it is small, it is amazingly well equipped in terms of both machines and people (25 consultants). For example, it has a mobile lithotripsy unit, an MRI and a CT scanner. The consultant staff cover many specialities (family practice, internal medicine, cardiology, radiology, oncology, gastroenterology, neurology, anaesthetics, ER, general surgery, orthopaedics, O&G, paeds, pathology, ophthalmology, urology and psychiatry).

O Elective notes: There are no other medical students here so the staff are keen to teach. You can organize what you want to do on a day-to-day basis and do as much (or as little) as you want. Teaching is mainly in an outpatient setting, although some consultants (e.g. in neurology) may well take you further afield to places such as the Dartmouth–Hitchcock Medical Centre for lectures and grand rounds.

Everyone is very friendly ... if you're outgoing, people will always be asking you round for dinner. In the summer there are many outdoor sports and in the winter this is one of the great skiing resorts on the east coast. Public transport isn't very good, but there is a regular bus to and from Boston (airport) and other nearby major cities. It's four hours south to Boston and two hours north to the Canadian border. There's lots to do if you like outdoor pursuits. This elective has been highly recommended if you want to see a not-so-famous part of America that is nothing like the cliché of superficiality and commercialism often associated with the country.

Accommodation: And meals have been free; however, don't expect much as they have no proper accommodation for staff. There is usually an empty room on the medical floor. It's not too bad though, with your own bathroom and cable TV.

NEW JERSEY

UMDNJ – New Jersey Medical School

185 South Orange Avenue, Newark, NJ 07103. Tel: +1 973 972 4631. Fax: +1 973 972 7986. www.umdnj.edu/njmsweb.

The University of Medicine and Dentistry medical school moved to Newark in 1977 to be part of a huge centre containing preclinical buildings, the **University Hospital**, an ambulatory care centre and a community health centre. **East Orange VA**, **Hackensack University Medical Center**, **Morristown Memorial Hospital**, the **Children's Hospital of NJ**, the **Kessler**

Institute and **Bergen Pines Hospital** are also used.

UMDNJ – Robert Wood Johnson Medical School

675 Hoes Lane, Piscataway, NJ 08854–5635. Tel: +1 732 235 4576. Fax: +1 732 235 5078. www.rwjms.umdnj.edu.

The **Robert Wood Johnson University Hospital** (named after the president of the Johnson and Johnson company) is the major teaching facility. The **Cooper Hospital** and the **University Medical Center** in Camden also provide training. There are also the Institutes of Mental Health, Environmental and Occupational Health Science.

A POPULAR HOSPITAL IN NEW JERSEY:

St Barnabas Medical Center

Old Short Hills Road, Livingston, NJ 07039.
The hospital: A medium-sized private hospital with most specialities and an ER. Although not a level 1 trauma centre, it is busy. It is well known for its burns and renal transplant unit. The O&G and neonatal units also have a good reputation. This is a very safe area and Livingston is a nice suburb of New Jersey, about an hour's drive from Manhattan.
O Elective notes: There are plenty of opportunities to see whatever interests you. It is what you make it. From the ER, you can go out with the paramedics and see the inner city hospitals.
Accommodation: Not available within the hospital itself.

NEW MEXICO

University of New Mexico School of Medicine

Albuquerque, NM 87131–5166. Tel: +1 505 272 4766. Fax: +1 505 272 8239.
http://hsc.unm.edu.

Founded in 1964, the medical school facilities are on the North Campus, housing biomedical research buildings, the **UNM Mental Health Center**, a cancer center, the **UNM Children's Psychiatric Hospital** and the **Center for Non-invasive Diagnosis**. The **University of New Mexico Hospital** has 421 beds and the **Regional Federal Medical Center** in Albuquerque (257 beds) is also used.

NEW YORK

Albany Medical College

47 New Scotland Avenue, Albany, NY 12208. Tel: +1 518 262 5548. Fax: +1 518 262 5029. www.amc.edu.

Albany was founded in 1839 and is therefore one of the oldest medical schools in the US. It is non-denominational and privately supported. The **Albany Medical Center** (43 New Scotland Avenue, Albany, NY 12208) contains a 631-bed hospital that serves the local community and acts as a tertiary referral centre for two million residents in east New York and west New England. Other hospitals are also linked.

Albert Einstein College of Medicine of Yeshiva University

Jack and Pearl Resnick Campus, 1300 Morris Park Avenue, Bronx, NY 10461.
Tel: +1 718 430 2106. Fax: +1 718 430 8825.
www.aecom.yu.edu.

This is a privately endowed, non-denominational college in the residential area of north-east Bronx. It serves populations from the Bronx, Queens and Manhattan using the **Jacobi Medical Center** (a municipal hospital) and four private voluntary hospitals: the **Bronx Lebanon**, **Montefiore**, **Beth Israel** and **Long Island Jewish** medical centres. There are also biomedical research institutions and accommodation near and on campus.

University of Buffalo School of Medicine and Biomedical Sciences

132 Biomedical Education Building, Buffalo, NY 14214-3013. Tel: +1 716 829 3467. Fax: +1 716 829 2798. www.smbs.buffalo.edu.

Initially founded in 1846, it joined the State University of New York (SUNY) system in 1962. Its campus is in northeast Buffalo, and it uses nine hospitals in the area, including **Buffalo General Hospital** (742 beds with high-tech cardiac surgery facilities).

Columbia University College of Physicians and Surgeons

630 West 168th Street, New York, NY 10032. Tel: +1 212 305 3595. Fax: +1 212 305 3545. www.columbia.edu/dept/ps/.
Founded in 1767, the college was the first in the US to give official doctor of medicine degrees. It is part of the **Columbia–Presbyterian Medical Center**. This provides clinical teaching, as do the **Roosevelt–St Luke's Hospital** and **Harlem Hospital** centres in Manhattan, the **Bassett Hospital** in Cooperstown, New York, and **Overlook Hospital** in New Jersey.

Mount Sinai School of Medicine of the City University of New York

Annenberg Building, One Gustave L. Levy Place, Box 1002, New York, NY 10029–6574. Tel: +1 212 241 6696. Fax: +1 212 828 4135. www.mssm.edu.
Privately endowed and non-denominational, the school was founded in 1968. The Medical Center has the **Mount Sinai Hospital** (1300 beds) and research laboratories. Additional clinical sites are located throughout New York City, New Jersey, Westchester County and Long Island. Many institutions, including centres for gene therapy, Jewish genetic diseases, the neurobiology of ageing, transplantation and cardiovascular disease, are associated.

New York Medical College

Sunshine Cottage, Valhalla, NY 10595. Tel: +1 914 594 4507. Fax: +1 914 594 4976. www.nymc.edu.
Founded in 1860 (originally as the New York Homeopathic Medical College), the college has a strong Catholic background. The campus is in Westchester, 40 km from New York City. It uses hospitals throughout urban and suburban New York, as well as regional hi-tech tertiary referral centres.

New York University School of Medicine

PO Box 1924, 550 First Avenue, New York, NY 10016. Tel: +1 212 263 5290. www.med.nyu.edu.
Founded in 1841, NYU now has many associated hospitals. The NYU Hospitals Center comprises the **Tisch Hospital** and the **Rusk Institute of Rehabilitation** (*see* below). **Bellevue Hospital** (First Avenue at 27th Street, NY 10016. Tel: +1 212 562 4141) is the original school hospital with many specialities. The **Hospital for Joint Diseases** (301 East 17th Street, NY 10003. Tel: +1 212 598 6000), **NYU Downtown Hospital** (170 William Street, NY 10038. Tel: +1 212 312 5000) and many others are also associated.

University of Rochester School of Medicine and Dentistry

Rochester, NY 14642. Tel: +1 716 275 7711. Fax: +1 716 273 1016.
www.urmc.rochester.edu/smd.
The school was founded in 1920 and the on-site facilities include the **Strong Memorial Hospital**, an **Ambulatory Care Center**, research centres and clinics. Five affiliated hospitals are also used.

State University of New York Health Science Center at Brooklyn College of Medicine (Downstate College)

450 Clarkson Avenue, Brooklyn, NY 11203. Tel: +1 718 270 3776. Fax: +1 718 270 4074. www.hscbklyn.edu.
The college is a descendant of the Long Island College Hospital founded in 1860. It became part of the university in 1950. It uses a number of major hospitals, including its own 406-bed **University Hospital of Brooklyn** (445 Lenox Rd, Brooklyn, NY 11203-2098).

State University of New York at Stony Brook School of Medicine Health Sciences Center

Stony Brook, NY 11794–8434. Tel: +1 631 444 2081. Fax: +1 631 444 2202. www.hsc.stonybrook.edu.

Founded in 1971, the Health Sciences Center uses the 540-bed **University Hospital**.

State University of New York Health Science Center at Syracuse College (Upstate Medical University)

College of Medicine, 750 East Adams Street, Syracuse, NY 13210-2375. Tel: +1 315 464 5540. Fax: +1 315 464 5565. www.hscsyr.edu.

The College was founded as the Geneva Medical College in 1834 and joined Syracuse University in 1872. It then joined SUNY (State University of New York) in 1950.

Weill Medical College of Cornell University

1300 York Avenue, Box 144, New York, NY 10021. Tel: +1 212 746 5454. Fax: +1 212 746 8745. www.med.cornell.edu.

The college, founded in 1898, is in New York, whereas the university is in Ithaca. Many hospitals are used, including the **New York Presbyterian Hospital**, **New York Hospital Medical Center of Queens**, **Hospital for Special Surgery**, **St Barnabas Hospital**, **New York Community Hospital of Brooklyn**, **Memorial Sloan–Kettering Cancer Center**, **Flushing Hospital** in Queens, **Lincoln Medical and Mental Health Center**, **United Hospital** in Port Chester and **Cayuga Medical Center** in Ithaca.

POPULAR HOSPITALS IN NEW YORK:

To do an elective in New York, apply directly to either the hospital or the medical school (Columbia and New York University are popular choices and well organized).

The New York Presbyterian Group comprises the **Columbia Presbyterian Center** and the **New York Weill Cornell Center**, with the nation's busiest burns unit. Electives in this group of hospitals require quite a bit of paperwork, but their electives catalogue can be found on http://cpmcnet.columbia.edu/dept/ps. Elective fees are currently around $500.

Columbia Presbyterian Medical Center

710 West 168th Street, New York, NY 10032.

The centre: Well known for its transplant programme (especially heart transplants) and its neurology department. There is a busy ER. It is a level 2 trauma centre (which can upgrade to level 1 if necessary) but tends to concentrate on acute medical emergencies. (St Luke's–Roosevelt and Harlem hospitals are the level 1 trauma centres.)

Note: Many people in the area speak only Spanish so a knowledge of this language is a great help.

O **Elective notes:** At the time of writing, Columbia University didn't cover for malpractice insurance, hence 'hands on' experience has been limited for some. However, the teaching (in neurology) is excellent, with the opportunity to do research. The ER has long (12-hour) shifts and students get to clerk their own patients. They are pretty flexible though about when you work. The centre also has an Urban Medicine and Immigrant Health Care Programme. They run medical clinics for the homeless and provide palliative care. Write to the Dean (Office for Student Affairs, College of Physicians and Surgeons, 630 West 168th Street, New York, NY 10032) if you are interested.

Accommodation: Contact the Accommodation Office (Health Sciences Block, 50 Haven Avenue, New York, NY). The Bard Hall (160 Street, Manhattan) is a hall for science students and is pretty basic (bring your own sheets). It costs between $270 and $500 a month. There's a gym on-site and a phone in your room. It's not the nicest area of town, but you'll be close to the subway.

Babies and Children's Hospital
(Part of the Columbia–Presbyterian
Medical Center)
3959 Broadway, New York, NY 10032.
The hospital: A major paediatric centre.
It has friendly staff and sees a wide range
of pathologies.
O **Elective notes:** You are treated like a
US student and it comes recommended.
Accommodation: Provided free for one
month.

Harlem Hospital
Harlem, Manhattan, New York.
The hospital: As one of the major
level 1 trauma centres in New York it
receives all major trauma for the area. It
also has many other specialities.
O **Elective notes:** It is a popular destination for trauma. Apply through
Columbia or directly.

St Luke's–Roosevelt Hospital
New York City, NY.
The hospital: This is a new hospital
with a level 1 trauma centre and is associated with Columbia University.

NY Hospital Cornell Medical Centre
1300 York Avenue, New York, NY 10021.
Tel: +1 212 746 0780.
The hospital: Large but best known for
its ER and burns unit.
O **Elective notes:** In ER students are
recognized as part of the team. There is a
fair bit of responsibility but good supervision.
Accommodation: Good.

NYU Hospitals Center
500 First Avenue, NY 10016.
Tel: +1 212 263 7300.
The group: This is part of the NYU medical school and comprises the **Tisch
Hospital** (same address), which has 726
beds with cardiovascular, neurosurgery,
AIDS, cancer, transplant and reconstructive surgery services, and the **Rusk
Institute of Rehabilitation** (400 East
34th Street, NY 10016. Tel: +1 212 263
7300. Fax: +1 212 263 6675), with 174
beds.

O **Elective notes:** The university has a
very well-structured elective programme, ranging from forensic medicine to neurosurgery. There is a $25 reg-
istration fee, and you need malpractice
insurance. Visit the website for information on other hospitals associated with
NYU and for comprehensive elective
details.

Mount Sinai Hospital
One Gustave L. Levy Place, Box 1002,
New York, NY 10029-6574.
The hospital: A 1171-bed premier tertiary referral facility. Its particular specialities include spinal cord and brain
injury rehabilitation, Jewish genetic diseases, AIDS, geriatrics, neonatal and
paediatric respiratory diseases. It is affiliated to the Mount Sinai School and
NYU. Apply through either of these to
do an elective here.

Maimonides Medical Center
4802 10th Avenue, Brooklyn, NY 11219.
The hospital: This is a very large, well-
equipped DGH. It is very busy and has
all major specialities.
O **Elective notes:** This is a good place
to go if you don't want to work directly
in one of the central big teaching hospitals. There's plenty to see and do. Other
students are from New York and
Grenada. Apply directly to the department you want to work in.

RESEARCH OUTSIDE NEW YORK:

Cold Spring Harbor Laboratories
1 Bungtown Road, Cold Harbor, New
York, NY 11724.
The labs: This is a very large, world-
renowned research centre with world
leaders such as David Beach, Scott Lowe
and Bruce Stillman. The director is Dr
James Watson (as in Watson and Crick,
the discoverers of the DNA double
helix). It is very busy in the summer with
visiting scientists. This also makes it
very sociable. The institute has two 30 ft
yachts, *The Double Helix* and *The*

Transposon, on its beach, where they often hold summer parties. The labs are very isolated, being 3–5 km from the nearest town (Huntington) and an hour from Manhattan.

O Elective notes: This is an excellent place to visit if you're interested in molecular research. It is very friendly but also very hard work.

NORTH CAROLINA

Duke University School of Medicine

Box 3250 – Medical Center, Durham, NC 27710. Tel: +1 919 684 0381. Fax: +1 919 684 0208. www2.mc.duke.edu/som.
The college, founded in 1930, uses **Duke Hospital**, a private teaching hospital with 1000 beds (same address) as well as the **Durham VA** (508 Fulton Street, Durham, NC 27705), which has 489 beds. The money for the university came from tobacco and many of the patients in the hospital still work for tobacco companies. DUMC is a very high-tech hospital and the university has quite an Oxbridge feel. The night-life is fairly low key.

East Carolina University School of Medicine

Greenville, NC 27858–4354. Tel: +1 252 816 2984. Fax: +1 252 816 3312.
www.ecu.edu/med.
Founded in the 1970s, the 100-acre Health Sciences Center campus houses the preclinical building and the 731-bed **Pitt County Memorial Hospital**. Other services used include the **Jenkins Cancer Center**, **Child Development Evaluation Clinic**, **Mental Health Center**, **Rehab Centers** and **Neonatal ICU**.

University of North Carolina at Chapel Hill School of Medicine

121 MacNider Hall, Chapel Hill, NC 27599–7000. Tel: +1 919 962 6108.
www.med.unc.edu/.

Founded in 1879, this uses the **University of North Carolina Hospitals**, **Cancer Research Center** and **Biological Sciences Center**, all of which are on-site. A number of hospitals outside are also used.

Wake Forest University School of Medicine

Medical Center Boulevard, Winston-Salem, NC 27157–1090. Tel: +1 336 716 4264. Fax: +1 336 716 5807.
www.wfubmc.edu.
The medical school was founded in 1902 and is part of the Wake Forest University Baptist Medical Center. It uses the 806-bed **North Carolina Baptist Hospitals** and the 896-bed **Forsyth Memorial Hospital**.

NORTH DAKOTA

University of North Dakota School of Medicine and Health Sciences

501 North Columbia Road, Grand Forks, ND 58202–9037. Tel: +1 701 777 4221. Fax: +1 701 777 4942.
www.med.und.nodak.edu/.
When founded in 1905, the college offered a two-year course in basic sciences; the clinical years had to be done elsewhere. In 1981, the school started its own clinical course in North Dakota, using community clinics, hospitals and physicians.

OHIO

Case Western University Reserve School of Medicine

10900 Euclid Avenue, Cleveland, OH 44106–4920. Tel: +1 216 368 2825. Fax: +1 216 368 3013. www.mediswww.cwru.edu.
Case Western is a private, independent university with a very green 600-acre campus 8 km east of downtown Cleveland. Teaching hospitals used include the **University Hospitals of**

Cleveland, St Luke's, MetroHealth Medical Center, Mount Sinai Medical Center, VA Cleveland Medical Center and Henry Ford Health System in Detroit.

University of Cincinnati College of Medicine

PO Box 670552, Cincinnati, OH 45267–0552. Tel: +1 513 558 5575. Fax: +1 513 558 1165. www.med.uc.edu/.
The college offers extensive clinical and research facilities. It uses the huge University of Cincinnati Medical Center, where all specialities are catered for. Full elective details are available on-line, and you actually submit your request directly.

Medical College of Ohio

3000 Arlington Avenue, PO Box 10008, Toledo, OH 43614. Tel: +1 419 381 4000. Fax: +1 419 383 4005. www.mco.edu.
Founded in the early 1970s, this very academic institution offers good teaching and plenty of research. It is located on a 475-acre campus in south Toledo. Hospitals on campus include the Medical College of Ohio Hospital (258 acute beds with a level 1 trauma centre and transplant specialities), the MCO/Mercy Rehab Hospital (36 beds) and the Kobaker Center for emotionally disturbed children.

Northeastern Ohio Universities College of Medicine

PO Box 95, Rootstown, OH 44272–0095. Tel: +1 330 325 2511/800 686 2511. Fax: +1 330 325 8372. www.neoucom.edu.
NEOUCOM is publicly supported and has its preclinical campus in Rootstown, three major public universities and 16 community hospitals in Akron, Youngstown and Canton areas. In total, there are 6500 beds.

Ohio State University College of Medicine and Public Health

370 West Ninth Avenue, Columbus, OH 43210–1238. Tel: +1 614 292 2220. Fax: +1 614 292 1544. http://medicine.osu.edu/.

The university is one of the largest in the country and the medical college was founded in 1914. The main campus in Columbus uses the University Hospitals and the OSU Cancer Center, as well as rural hospitals.

Wright State University School of Medicine

PO Box 1751, Dayton, OH 45401–1751. Tel: +1 937 775 2934. Fax: +1 937 775 3322. www.med.wright.edu/.
The school, on the university campus in Fairborn, was established in 1973. It uses seven teaching hospitals totalling 3823 beds.

POPULAR HOSPITALS IN OHIO:

Cleveland Clinic Foundation

9500 Euclid Avenue, Cleveland, OH 44195.
The hospital: The hospital is very proud of the fact that it is the sixth-best hospital in America. There are 985 beds, of which over 100 are devoted to critical care. It is privately run by a board of trustees and does not have official links with any medical school. Students are therefore a bit of a novelty and get treated pretty well. The critical care unit boasts, with some justification, that it provides some of the best acute medical and surgical care anywhere, and the hospital has an 'international' feel that is unusual and distinctive for a hospital in the Midwest.

O **Elective notes:** There are many serious and interesting cases. As a student in critical care, you can get to insert CVP lines and Swan–Ganz catheters. It's a work hard, play hard environment. In neurology, you're expected to get involved and do consults. You'll also do admissions. These consults and admissions become *your* patients, and you're responsible for information gathering and presenting them on ward rounds. A few reports show that some teams are not all that friendly.

Accommodation: Free and pretty good (single rooms with a shower and toilet between two). In the past, they have even contributed towards your plane ticket (a $200 voucher with $70 deducted for rent)!

OKLAHOMA

University of Oklahoma College of Medicine
PO Box 26901, Oklahoma City, OK 73190. Tel: +1 405 271 2331. Fax: +1 405 271 3032. www.ouhsc.edu.
This very modern college offers teaching centres in Oklahoma City and Tulsa. In Oklahoma City, the college has a 200-acre complex, with 17 public and private institutions making up the Oklahoma Health Center.

OREGON

Oregon Health Sciences School of Medicine
3181 SW Sam Jackson Park Road, Portland, OR 97201-3098. Tel: +1 503 494 4329. Fax: +1 503 494 3400. www.ohsu.edu.
The school was founded in 1887 and is situated on a 100-acre campus in Sam Jackson Park overlooking the city and only 2.5 km from the business centre. The two hospitals on-site provide 509 beds. The **Child Development and Rehab Center** and **Crippled Children's Division** are also on-site. The **VA** (563 beds) is also affiliated. As in much of America, an elective here can be hard work.
Accommodation: In the university halls of residence (708 SW Sam Jackson Rak Road) and cheap and convenient. You really need a car to explore outside Portland.

PENNSYLVANIA

Jefferson Medical College of Thomas Jefferson University
1025 Walnut Street, Philadelphia, PA 19107. Tel: +1 215 955 6983. Fax: +1 215 923 6939. www.tju.edu.
Founded in 1824, teaching is at the Thomas Jefferson University Hospital (111 South 11th Street, Philadelphia, PA 19107. Tel: +1 215 955 6000), a regional trauma and spinal injuries centre with specialities such as liver transplantation and AIDS, and 15 associated hospitals. The college is developing research opportunities.

MCP Hahnemann University School of Medicine
2900 Queen Lane, Philadelphia, PA 19129. Tel: +1 215 991 8100. Fax: +1 215 843 0214. www.mcphu.edu.
When it was founded in 1850, MCP was the first medical school for women, but it became co-educational in 1969. It still seeks diverse students. The Hahnemann University is a private institution.
The college uses a large network of hospitals, including **Hahnemann University Hospital** (Broad and Vine Streets, Philadelphia, PA 19102. Tel: +1 215 762 7000), with 618 beds. It has high-tech specialities such as cardiac transplantation, as well as a level 1 trauma centre and aeromedical transport programme.

Pennsylvania State University College of Medicine
PO Box 850, Hershey, PA 17033. Tel: +1 717 531 8755. Fax: +1 717 531 6225. www.hmc.psu.edu.
The medical college was founded after a generous grant from the Hershey Foundation in 1963. It utilizes the **Pennsylvania State University Hospital**. The 550-acre campus is in hills 13 km from the capital, Harrisburg, and has the 504-bed **Milton Hershey Medical Center**, with a children's

hospital, emergency department (level 1 adult and paeds trauma centre) and rehabilitation hospital. There is a helipad for the LIFE LION aeromedical service.

University of Pennsylvania School of Medicine

3450 Hamilton Walk, Suite 100, Philadelphia, PA 19104-6087.

Tel: +1 215 898 8034. Fax: +1 215 898 0833. www.med.upenn.edu/.

Founded in 1765 by Benjamin Franklin, the school claims to have been the first medical school in the US. It is well known as one of the Ivy League universities. Affiliated hospitals include the **University of Pennsylvania Hospital**, the **VA**, the **Children's Hospital of Philadelphia**, **Phoenixville** and **Pennsylvania Hospitals** and the **Presbyterian Medical Center**.

University of Pittsburgh School of Medicine

Scaife Hall, Pittsburgh, PA 15261.

Tel: +1 412 648 8975. Fax: +1 412 648 1236. www.dean-med.pitt.edu.

The school (founded in 1886) is in the Oakland district of Pittsburgh and uses the huge University of Pittsburgh Medical Center, which has the **UPMC Presbyterian** and **Shadyside** hospitals and a number of speciality hospitals. Nine community hospitals are associated. It also uses the **Children's Hospital of Pittsburgh** and the **VA Medical Center**.

Temple University School of Medicine

3400 N Broad Street, Philadelphia, PA 19140. Tel: +1 215 707 7000. Fax: +1 215 707 6932.

www.temple.edu/medschool/.

The school, situated within the Temple Hospital, was founded in 1901. Clinical teaching is at the **New Temple University Hospital**, the **New Temple University Children's Medical Center**, the **Albert Einstein Medical Center** and 23 other centres.

POPULAR HOSPITALS IN PENNSYLVANIA:

Hospital of the University of Pennsylvania

Spruce Street, Philadelphia, PA 19104–6021.

The hospital: Being the main hospital for the University of Pennsylvania, it is busy and has all specialities.

O Elective notes: Whatever department you work in, be prepared to work very hard. Cardiothoracic surgery is busy, with ward rounds at 5.30 am and theatre starting at 8 am. This is excellent if you like cardiothoracic surgery, not good if you want a holiday. Other departments are a bit more relaxed than this. Write to the **Office of International Relations** (1007 Blockley Hall, 423 Guardian Drive, Philadelphia, PA 19104-6021).

Accommodation: This may be arranged for $500+ (£375) a month. Stay in International House – it's friendly.

Veterans Administration Medical Centre

University Avenue, Philadelphia, PA.

The hospital: This is also associated with the University of Pennsylvania and has most general specialities.

O Elective notes: Again, be prepared to work incredibly hard (5.45 am ward rounds in general surgery). There is a fantastic amount of responsibility, but students have occasionally felt that they were treated poorly and have not enjoyed the long days.

Pittsburgh Medical School

(See address above)

Full details of this incredibly expensive elective can be found on the web (where there is an application form for the truly rich). Quoting from their website: 'there is a non-refundable application fee $50. Tuition expense (flat rate for four to eight weeks) is $2100'. They then estimate monthly expenses (including rent at $595) to total another $1074. You have therefore spent $3224 and haven't even bought your airline ticket yet. This can really only be described as criminal since their students can visit hospitals in Europe and Australia for free (including free rent). Ask your dean to write and say that your hospital will charge their students silly figures too. Surf the net ... find the department you want to do an elective in and apply directly. *See* Harvard for more tips on how to get around stupid fees. You have to ask yourself whether you really want to go there if they are making it that awkward!

RHODE ISLAND

Brown University School of Medicine
97 Waterman St, Providence, RI 02912–9706. Tel: +1 401 863 2149. Fax: +1 401 863 2660. www.brown.edu. The school (which, unusually, has an eight-year college and medical course) is affiliated with **Rhode Island Hospital** (with 719 beds the largest hospital in the state). The **Bradley** (child psychiatric centre), **Butler** (psychiatric), **Miriam** (247-bed general hospital with research), **Memorial** (294-bed general/rehabilitation hospital), **Women** (obstetrics), **Infants** and the local **VA** hospitals are also associated. For electives there are no tuition fees and malpractice insurance is around $70.

SOUTH CAROLINA

Medical University of South Carolina College of Medicine
171 Ashley Avenue, Charleston, SC 29425. Tel: +1 803 792 2300. Fax: +1 803 792 3764. www.musc.edu. The oldest medical school in the South was founded in 1824. Hospitals utilized including the **Medical University Hospital**, **Children's Hospital**, **Storm Eye Institute**, **Psychiatric Institute** and

Hollings Cancer Center, which make up the MUSC Medical Center. The **Charleston Memorial** and **VA Hospitals** and local hospitals are also linked.

University of South Carolina School of Medicine
Columbia, SC 29208. Tel: +1 803 733 3325. Fax: +1 803 733 3328. www.med.sc.edu. The school is relatively new (1974) and situated on a newly renovated, 93-acre campus. The **Palmetto Richland Memorial Hospital** (649 beds), **William Hall Psychiatric Hospital** (270 beds), **Dorn Veterans Hospital** (530 beds), **Moncrief Army Hospital** and others are the main teaching sites.

SOUTH DAKOTA

University of South Dakota School of Medicine
2501 West 22nd Street, Sioux Falls, SD 57105. Tel: +1 605 357 1300. Fax: +1 605 357 1311. www.usd.edu/med. Initially (in 1907), the school had only a basic sciences course, but there are now three clinical sites (Yankton, Sioux Falls and Rapid City). Its prime objective is to create primary care doctors for South Dakota.

TENNESSEE

East Tennessee State University James H. Quillen College of Medicine
PO Box 70580, Johnson City, TN 37614 0580. Tel: +1 423 929 6327. Fax: +1 423 975 8340. http://qcom.etsu.edu. Situated in a large metropolitan area of Tennessee, Quillen (founded in 1978) uses a number of hospitals (many rural) to specialize in training primary care physicians. Hospitals in Johnson City

(the medical centre), Kingsport, Bristol and Elizabethton provide the school with 3000 beds.

Meharry Medical College School of Medicine

1005 DB Todd Boulevard, Nashville, TN 37208. Tel: +1 615 327 6204. Fax: +1 615 327 6568. www.mmc.edu.

Meharry when founded in 1876, was designed to educate freed slaves and the poor. Today the school provides excellent training for African Americans and other minorities. The **Metropolitan Nashville General Hospital**, **Blanchfield Community**, **York VA** and **Murfreesboro VA** hospitals are affiliated.

University of Tennessee Memphis College of Medicine

62 South Dunlap, 420 Hyman Boulevard, Memphis, TN 38163-2101. Tel: +1 901 448 5506. Fax: +1 901 448 7683. www.utmem.edu.

Founded in 1851, the **University of Tennessee Bowld Hospital**, **St Jude Children's Hospital**, **Baptist Memorial Hospital**, **VA** and **LePasses Rehabilitation Center** make up the 6000 beds on the 41-acre campus.

Vanderbilt University School of Medicine

209 Light Hall, Nasville, TN 37232–0685. Tel: +1 615 322 2145. Fax: +1 615 343 8397. www.mc.vanderbilt.edu/medschool/.

The school is on the Vanderbilt campus and uses 5000 beds in a number of hospitals.

TEXAS

Baylor College of Medicine

1 Baylor Plaza, Houston, TX 77030. Tel: +1 713 798 4451. Fax: +1 713 798 5563. www.bcm.tmc.edu.

Founded in 1900, Baylor moved to Houston in 1943. It is one of the medical schools in the huge 356-acre Texas

Medical Center in Houston containing 13 hospitals and four nursing schools and providing 4200 beds in the pleasant south-west area of Houston.

Texas A&M University System Health Science Center College of Medicine

159 Joe Reynolds Medical Building, College Station, TX 77843-1114. Tel: +1 409 845 7743. Fax: +1 409 845 5533. www.medicine.tamushsc.edu/.

This large university (founded in 1971) has one of the top five research budgets in the US. The Central Texas Medical Center on campus consists of a number of hospitals and clinics. It also uses the **Teague Veteran's Center** in Temple, TX, the **Driscoll Children's Hospital** in Corpus Christi, TX, and others. In total there are 1976 beds with a two million outpatient turnover.

Texas Tech University Health Sciences Center School of Medicine

3601 4th Street, Lubbock, TX 79430. Tel: +1 806 743 3000. Fax: +1 806 743 3021. www.ttuhsc.edu.

The school, established in 1969, uses hospitals in Lubbock (the main campus), Amarillo and El Paso. These, along with other community hospitals, provide 2900 beds.

University of Texas Southwestern Medical Center at Dallas Southwestern Medical School

5323 Harry Hines Boulevard, Dallas, TX 75235–9096. Tel: +1 214 648 6776/5617. Fax: +1 214 648 3289. www.swmed.edu.

Founded in 1943, the 100-acre campus just north of Dallas offers good facilities. The **Parkland Memorial**, **Lipshy University** and **Presbyterian Hospitals**, along with the **Children's Medical Center**, **Baylor University Medical Center**, **St Paul Medical Center**, **Texas Scottish Rite Hospital for Children** and **Southwestern Institute of Forensic Sciences** are all affiliated.

University of Texas Medical School at Galveston

Ashbel Smith Building, Galveston, TX 77555–1317. Tel: +1 409 772 1011. Fax: +1 409 772 6216. www.utmb.edu.

Established in 1891, the medical branch uses eight hospitals (providing 923 beds), the **Marine Biomedical Institute**, the **Institute for the Medical Humanities** and the **Shriners Burns Institute**.

University of Texas Houston Medical School

PO Box 20708, Houston, TX 77225. Tel: +1 713 500 5116. Fax: +1 713 500 0604. www.med.uth.tmc.edu.

The **Hermann Hospital** (650 beds) is the main hospital for the Texas Medical Center in Houston. The school (founded in 1969) makes use of this and many other institutions in the centre. Other hospitals include the **University of Texas**, **Anderson Cancer Center**, **Southwest Memorial Hospital**, **St Joseph** and **Lyndon Baines Johnson Hospitals**.

University of Texas Medical School at San Antonio

Health Sciences Center at San Antonio, 7703 Floyd Curl Drive, San Antonio, TX 78284–7702. Tel: +1 210 567 2665. Fax: +1 210 567 2685. www.uthscsa.edu.

Founded in 1959, the school's main hospitals include the **University Hospital and Health Centre** and **Murphy VA**. Affiliated hospitals include **Wilford Hall USAF Hospital**, the **Aerospace Medical Division of USAF**, **Brooke Army Hospital**, **Baptist Memorial Hospital** and **Santa Rosa Medical Center**.

POPULAR HOSPITALS IN TEXAS:

Texas Medical Center

Houston, TX.

The centre: The world's largest medical centre. With 42 institutions, it is said to have 100 000 visitors a day. It has many world-leading pioneers and even the smallest speciality is catered for. There is a free bus service around the centre although a car is really needed to get around Houston. Note: The **Ben Taub** is the county hospital providing free care to those without insurance.

The **Hermann Hospital** (6411 Fannin, Houston, TX 77030) has a busy ER (but with not as much trauma as, for example, Washington or New York). The **Methodist Hospital** is a private hospital with advanced neurosurgery. There is also the **Texas Children's Hospital**. The **Texas Heart Institute** (at St Luke's Episcopal Hospital, PO Box 20345, Houston, TX 77225–0345) has good elective reports. It is a (non-profit) private institution founded in 1962 and claims to be the largest cardiovascular centre in the world. The first heart transplant in the USA and the first artificial heart were implanted here. No fee is charged and malpractice insurance is not required. Contact the **Surgical Associates of Texas PA**, Texas Heart Institute. The affiliates for each medical school are listed above.

Accommodation: The various medical schools or institutions normally help out, but if you have major problems contact University Housing (7900 Cambridge, Houston, TX 77054. Tel: +1 713 792 8112) or the Texas Women's University Director of Housing (1130 M.D. Anderson Boulevard, Houston, TX 77030. Tel: +1 713 794 2157). Linda Vista Apartments (1303 Eaton Street, Houston, TX) comes recommended and costs $500 a month.

VA Medical Center

2002 Holcombe Boulevard, Houston, TX 77030.

The hospital: A busy general hospital also in Houston.

O Elective notes: Prepare to work hard. General and vascular surgery, for example, have ward rounds at 6 am, and the day finishes at 7 pm. There's also a 6 am ward round on Saturdays. Elective students are integrated into the local student programme. The theatre time is excellent

... students are allowed to scrub up and close the abdomen. Minor procedures can also be performed under supervision. The staff and students are extremely friendly. If you can take long days, this is a good experience. Note: To organize this you have to apply to the Baylor College of Medicine ... early.

Accommodation: Arranged through Baylor and is very good.

UTAH

University of Utah School of Medicine

50 North Medical Drive, Salt Lake City, UT 84132. Tel: +1 801 581 7498. Fax: +1 801 585 3300.

http://medstat.med.utah.edu/som.

Established in 1904, the school is part of a multifaculty university using its own **University Hospitals**, **Howard Hughes Medical Institute**, **Utah Genome Center**, **Utah Cancer Center**, **Moran Eye Center** and other specialized institutions.

VERMONT

University of Vermont College of Medicine

Burlington, VT 05405. Tel: +1 802 656 2154. www.med.uvm.edu.

Burlington, on the eastern shores of Lake Champion, is the home to Vermont (established in 1822). It uses the **Fletcher Allen Health Care's Medical Center Hospital** (500 beds) on campus.

VIRGINIA

Eastern Virginia Medical School of the Medical College of Hampton

721 Fairfax Avenue, Norfolk, VI 23507–2000. Tel: +1 757 446 5812. Fax: +1 757 446 5896. www.evms.edu.

This is a community-based teaching institution founded in 1973. It aims to produce top-notch primary care doctors. Using 33 community-based institutions, it provides healthcare for a third of Virginia. On campus is **Sentara Norfolk General Hospital**, the tertiary referral centre.

Virginia Commonwealth University School of Medicine

1101 East Marshall Street, PO Box 980565, Richmond, VA 23298. Tel: +1 804 828 9790. Fax: +1 804 828 5115.

www.vcu.edu.

The school (founded in 1838) is very near the governmental area of downtown Richmond and therefore centrally located. It has an excellent clinical research center and a 1000-bed hospital on the main campus, with the largest neonatal ITU and ER in Virginia. It also uses 800 beds at a new **VA Hospital**.

University of Virginia School of Medicine

Box 395, Charlottesville, VA 22908. Tel: +1 804 924 8418. Fax: +1 804 982 0874.

www.med.virginia.edu.

The school (founded in 1825) is situated with the **University Hospital** in the grounds of the university. The medical centre has 552 beds with seven separate ITUs. In total there are 27 000 inpatients a year. It is also associated with the **Veteran Affairs Medical Center** (Roanoke–Salem Program, VAMC, Medical Service (111), 1970 Roanoke Boulevard, Salem, VA 24153). This has some good elective reports especially for ITU.

WASHINGTON

University of Washington School of Medicine

Health Sciences Center, Seattle, WA 98195–6340. Tel: +1 206 543 7212. Fax: +1 206 543 3639.

www.washington.edu/medical/som/.

The school was established in 1945 and uses a number of hospitals. Note: The children's hospital refuses to take elective students.

POPULAR HOSPITALS IN SEATTLE:

Harborview Medical Center
325 Ninth Avenue, Seattle, WA 98104-2499. Tel: +1 206 731 3263. Fax: +1 206 731 3563.
The hospital: This has the only level 1 trauma centre in a large area of northwest USA. There is plenty of trauma (road traffic accidents, stabbings). Other specialities are also provided.
O Elective notes: ER shifts are 12 hours long. Lots of experience and procedures. The paramedics are some of the best in the world.

WEST VIRGINIA

Marshall University School of Medicine
1600 Medical Center Drive, Huntingdon, WV 25701-3655. Tel: +1 304 691 1700. Fax: +1 304 691 1744.
www.musom.marshall.edu.
Marshall has been committed since its foundation in the early 1980s to encouraging primary healthcare physicians, and a community-based course is used. An ambulatory care centre, the VA and rural clinics are utilized. The **Marshall University Medical Center** has medicine (including cardiovascular), O&G, paeds and surgery departments. There is also a large forensic science programme.

West Virginia University School of Medicine
Health Sciences Center, PO Box 9815. Morgantown, WV 26506. Tel: +1 304 293 3521. Fax: +1 304 293 7968.
www.hsc.wvu.edu/som/.
Although basic sciences have been taught since the turn of the 20th century,

the school has been clinical only since the second half. The **Ruby Memorial** (400 beds), **Chestnut Ridge Psychiatric** (80 beds) and **Mountainview Rehabilitation** (80 beds) hospitals are affiliated.

WISCONSIN

Medical College of Wisconsin
8701 Watertown Plank Road, Milwaukee, WI 53226. Tel: +1 414 456 8246.
www.mcw.edu.
The school (originating at the turn of the 20th century) is in the **Milwaukee Regional Medical Center**. Affiliated hospitals include the **Froedtert Memorial Lutheran Hospital** (469 beds with cancer, transplant, trauma and neurology/surgery centres), the **Children's Hospital of Wisconsin** (222 beds, with 24 in paediatric intensive care) and the **Zablocki VA**, providing over 7000 beds in total.

University of Wisconsin Medical School
Medical Sciences Center, 1300 University Avenue, Madison, WI 53706. Tel: +1 608 263 4925. Fax: +1 608 262 2327.
www.medsch.wisc.edu.
The **University of Wisconsin Center for Health Sciences** houses the medical school (founded 1907), University Hospital and clinics on its campus in Madison.

SOMETHING DIFFERENT:

Forensic medicine
America is a pretty good place to do forensic medicine. It's not all murders as you might expect, but there are a great deal more than in Europe, Australia or New Zealand. Africa does have high rates of violence and murder, but there isn't the system to investigate it. For these reasons, America is ideal. In a land where medical care costs a small fortune,

USA

you'll be pleased to know that everyone has the right to a free autopsy if the family wishes. There are a number of places to look for information. A good place to start is to visit www.criminalistics.com. This lists all institutions with a forensic science programme, for example the **Marshall University Forensic Science Programme** (1542 Spring Valley Drive, Huntington, WV 25755-9310. Tel: +1 304 696 7394. http://meb.marshall.edu/forensic). The most popular elective destination for forensic medicine is New York.

Office of the Chief Medical Examiner
520 First Avenue, New York, NY 10016.
The office: The OCME investigates sudden, unexpected, suspicious and violent deaths, as well as fatalities in special legally defined circumstances, such as those in public institutions, resulting from occupational diseases, or from communicable diseases that are a threat to public health, and those resulting from diagnostic or therapeutic procedures. Of the 10 million people living in New York, 70 000 deaths occur each year, half of which get referred to the OCME.

○ **Elective notes:** If you've a strong stomach and are genuinely interested, this is an excellent place to do an elective. There are opportunities to go out to the scene of death and to court. Note: After getting the OK from the OCME, you have to go through the NYU.

Accommodation: NYU can offer accommodation in New York for a hefty $500 a week, but there are plenty of hostels.

Skiing, diving and NASA
For skiing, diving medicine and NASA, *see* Section 3.

Bermuda

Population: 60 000
Language: English
Capital: Hamilton
Currency: Dollar
Int Code: +1

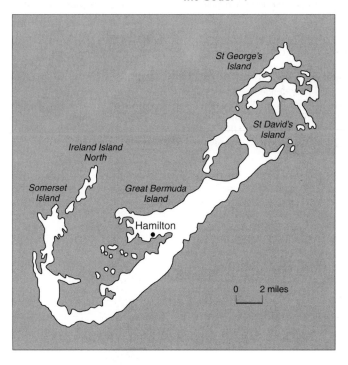

The 138 islands that comprise Bermuda lie in the North Atlantic, 909 km due east of the nearest land at Cape Hatteras in North Carolina. Together they form an area of just over 20 square miles. Of the 60 000 inhabitants, 60% are black, the remainder being of mixed race or white (of British or Portuguese descent). The numbers swell by half a million when the tourists arrive. It has been a British Crown colony since 1612 and is now a tourist and tax haven. Bermuda has one of the highest per capita incomes in the world and a recent campaign by the former leader to gain independence from the UK was firmly rejected.

Bermuda has two hospitals: the King Edward VII Memorial Hospital, a general hospital, and St Brendan's, a psychiatric unit.

◎ Climate:

Normally mild and humid as a result of the Gulf Stream, but hurricanes can cause havoc between June and November.

USEFUL ADDRESS:

Ministry of Health, Old Hospital Building, 7 Pint Finger Road, Paget DV 04. Tel: +1 236 0224. Fax: +1 236 3971.

King Edward VII Memorial Hospital

PO Box HM 1023, Hamilton, Bermuda HM DX.

The hospital: Officially opened in the 1960s and having had extensions, the hospital now has 323 beds. There are six wards (two general surgical, two general medical, one maternity and one children's) plus an extended care and intensive care unit. It is well equipped, with a CT scanner. There's one junior doctor (often an SHO from the UK) looking after each ward, but it is the GPs who are actually responsible for their patients while in hospital and therefore visit at least once every day. The healthcare system is insurance-based like that in the US. There are many conditions to see here, but HIV is extremely common.

Accommodation: Has previously been provided free. Apply early as the hospital can only accept three students simultaneously and gives priority to Bermudans. Write to the **Bermuda Hospitals Board** at the above address.

St Brendan's Hospital

PO Box 501 DV, Devonshire.

The hospital: St Brendan's is the only psychiatric hospital in Bermuda. The population is generally affluent with very low unemployment. There are two organized sessions a week, but the doctors give informal teaching.

Canada

Population: 29.5 million
Languages: English and French
Capital: Ottawa
Currency: Canadian dollar
Int Code: +1

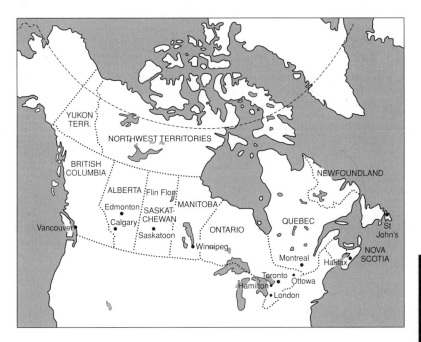

Canada, the world's second-largest country, stretches across five time zones and is made up of ten provinces and two territories. Forty per cent of the population is British in origin, 27% French, 20% from other European countries and only 4% indigenous. Because of its size, Canada has had to develop a good transportation system. The rail and road systems reach far into the north.

✪ Medicine:

A national insurance scheme provides state health service for the entire popula-tion. However, approximately 25% choose to use private healthcare. As with many developed nations, the costs of newer treatments and an ageing popula-tion is putting a strain on the system. The doctor:patient ratio is 1:455. The typical big Western killers – heart, respiratory diseases and cancers – bump most people off.

All medical students have a degree before starting medical school. Many also have a PhD. Because of this, their first pre-clinical years are very clinically orientated and they then do only two clinical years. The students have patients to look after hence elective students will too. This is why malpractice insurance is vital.

Patients do not pay for consultations and can access specialists without the need for GP referral.

◎ Climate and crime:

Canada is cold. In the south (Vancouver), it is cold but can occasionally get warm. In the north (Ellesmere Island), it is polar and consistently freezing. Canada has a much better crime record than neighbouring USA. This is mostly attributable to strict gun laws and safer cities.

➲ Visas and work permits:

British citizens do not need a visa to stay in Canada for up to six months as a tourist; however, you may be asked to prove sufficient funds and a return ticket on arrival. Those studying (including medical students) need to get authorization from the Canadian High Commission. To work, you need employment authorization from the High Commission before you leave your country. An agreement exists whereby if you are in full-time education and aged between 18 and 30, you may be allowed to work temporarily if returning to full-time education.

For both electives and work, you will be required to have a medical. The medical has to be done by an approved GP (costing around £60, but plead poverty of course). You'll also need a chest X-ray and syphilis screen (£15). To try to save some cash, see whether your hospital can do the X-ray and visit your local STD clinic (paper bag on head) to get a free VDRL blood test. The reports of these then need to be sent to the Canadian High Commission who then write a letter of facilitation saying you are fit to work in Canada. This must be presented to the Canadian immigration officer upon arrival. Also ask your host hospital what they need. They may want a doctor's certificate saying what vaccinations you have had, in which case get it done while having your medical.

Note: Quebec has similar but separate immigration procedures (*see* Section 4). Check out www.hc-sc.gc.ca/english for their Department of Health's advice on working in Canada.

If you're wanting to work in Canada, you can write directly to hospitals, hence addresses have been included. Community hospitals are often desperate for staff. You will need to contact the appropriate area medical board for registration. This can be a problem in some areas because of complete American-style rules that cannot be bent. You may, for example, just want to do ER, or you may be a specialist in a specific field. If you've not done four weeks of paeds or O&G, however, your application may be refused. This is because they have to do these subjects in their residency year. You can argue till you are blue in the face, but some of the boards will stick to their guns. Try asking the hospital offering work to help you out.

EXAMS:

To work permanently in Canada, you'll need to get the Medical Council of Canada Evaluating Examination (MCCEE), which is taken in March and September, to register as a doctor. You will then need to sit the Licensure Qualifying Examination Part I between one and two years later, after postgraduate training in a Canadian hospital. Twelve months after that, you can sit the Part II, which gives you a full licence to practise. To work temporarily in an undersubscribed speciality or unpopular area (e.g. Newfoundland), the above procedure can, however, be waived. Check out the **Society of Rural Physicians of Canada** website for adverts for such jobs (www.srpc.ca).

MALPRACTICE INSURANCE:

For an elective, first find out whether the host institution covers you as it would its own students. They may charge you for this or recommend a broker. Ask your defence union/protection society whether they will cover you. They may for electives (e.g. the MDDUS does) but probably not for working. If they can, ask your host institution whether it will accept this cover. If not, contact the Canadian Medical Protection Association (PO Box 8225, Stn T, Ottawa. Tel: +1 613 725 2000. Fax: +1 613 725 1300).

PROFESSIONAL ORGANIZATIONS:

Doctors:
Canadian Medical Association, 1867 Alta Vista Drive, Ottawa, Ontario K1G 5W8. Tel: +1 613 731 9331. Fax: +1 613 731 1779. www.cma.ca.
Federation of Medical Licensing Associations of Canada, PO Box 8234, Ottawa, Ontario K1G 3H7. Tel: +1 613 738 0372. Fax: +1 613 738 8977.
Medical Council of Canada, PO Box 8234, Station T, Ottawa, Ontario K1G 3H7. Tel: +1 613 521 6012. Fax: +1 613 521 9417. www.mcc.ca.

Nurses:
Canadian Nurses Association, 50 The Driveway, Ottawa, Ontario K2P 1E2. Tel: +1 613 237 2133. Fax: +1 613 237 3520. www.can-nurses.ca.

Dentists:
Canadian Dental Association, 1815 Alta Vista Drive, Ottawa, Ontario K1G 3Y6. Tel: +1 613 523 1770. Fax: +1 613 523 7736. www.cda-adc.ca.
Royal College of Dentists, 365 Bloor Street East, Suite 1706, Toronto, Ontario. Tel: +1 416 929 2722. Fax: +1 416 929 5924. www.rcdc.ca.
National Dental Examining Board, 100 Bronson Avenue, Suite 203, Ottawa, Ontario K1R 6G8. Tel: +1 613 236 5912. Fax: +1 613 236 8386.

Physiotherapists:
Canadian Physiotherapy Association, 2345 Yonge Street, Suite 410, Toronto, Ontario M4P 2E5. Tel: +1 416 932 1888. fax: +1 416 932 9708. www.physiotherapy.ca.

Occupational therapists:
Canadian Association of Occupational Therapists, Carleton Technology and Training Centre, Suite 3400, 1125 Colonel Bay Drive, Ottawa, Ontario K1S 5R1. Tel: +1 613 523 2268. Fax: +1 613 523 2552. www.caot.ca.

Pharmacists:
Canadian Pharmacists Association, 1785 Alta Vista Drive, Ottawa, Ontario K1G 3Y6. Tel: +1 613 523 7877. Fax: +1 613 523 0445. www.cdnpharm.ca.

Medical specialities:
College of Family Physicians of Canada: 2630 Skymark Avenue, Mississauga, Ontario L4W 5A4. www.cfpc.ca.
Royal College of Physicians and Surgeons, 774 Promenade Echo Drive, Ottawa, Ontario K1S 5N8. Tel: +1 613 730 8177. Fax: +1 613 730 8830. www.rcpsc.medical.org.

USEFUL ADDRESSES

For French speakers:
Association des médicins de langue française du Canada, 8355 boul Saint-Laurent, Montréal, PQ H2P 2Z6. Tel: +1 514 388 2228. www.amlfc.com.
Collège des Médecins. www.cmq.org.

There are 16 medical schools in Canada, listed here by region.

BRITISH COLUMBIA

Vancouver

With a population of 1.8 million Vancouver is a great city with loads to see and do. Stanley Park, Chinatown and Downtown must all be visited (but steer clear of East Hastings, which is a bit dodgy). The other great boon for skiers is Whistler, only two hours away.

University of British Columbia
Point Grey Campus: Faculty of Medicine, 317–2194 Health Sciences Mall, Vancouver, British Columbia V6T 1Z3.
Tel: +1 604 822 2421. Fax: +1 604 822 6061. www.med.ubc.ca.
Vancouver Hospital: Faculty of Medicine, Deans Office, Vancouver Hospital and Health Sciences Centre 3250–910 West 10th Avenue, Vancouver, British Columbia V5Z 4E3. Tel: +1 604 875 4500. Fax: +1 604 875 5611.

Founded in 1950, the faculty uses the on-site **Vancouver Hospital** and **Health Sciences Centre** (with 240 acute, 300 extended care and 60 psychiatric beds), **St Paul's Hospital** and the **Children's**

and Women's Health Centre of British Columbia.

The university can arrange electives in any of the hospitals in British Columbia (write to the clinical clerkship elective programme at the Vancouver Hospital address); however, note that they recently placed restrictions on elective students visiting their main teaching hospitals (**Vancouver Hospital** – UBC and Oak sites, **St Paul's**, **BC's Children's Hospital**, **BC Women's** and **Sunnyhill**). You can still apply, but they may not accept you to these teaching centres (some people have phoned directly to find a couple of spaces available so it's worth a try). They will try to put you in a community hospital: **Burnaby**, **Chilliwack General**, **Dawson Creek and District**, **Delta**, **Fort St John General**, **GR Baker Memorial**, **Greater Victoria**, **Kelowna General**, **Kimberley and District**, **Kitimat General**, **Kootenau Lake District**, **Maple Ridge**, **Matsqui-Suma-Abbotsford General**, **Mills Memorial**, **Nanaino Regional General**, **Peace Arch District**, **Penticton Regional**, **Powell River General**, **Prince George Regional**, **Prince Rupert Regional**, **Queen Charlotte Islands General**, **Queen Victoria**, **Richmond**, **Royal Inland**, **St Joseph's General**, **St Mary's**, **St Vincent's**, **Surrey Memorial**, **Trail Regional**, **Vernon Jubilee**, **Victoria General**, **West Coast General**, **WCB Rehab Centre**, **United Church of Canada**: **Bella Coola General**, **RW Large Memorial** and **Wrinck Memorial Hospitals**.

UBC charges an elective fee of around $250 (£110), but that includes malpractice insurance. They have previously helped with accommodation for those in Vancouver, but it's not great value. Most students stay either in youth hostels (HI Downtown has been recommended) or in the YMCA/YWCA, costing about £400 for seven weeks. Shaughnessy Village (1125 West 12th Avenue, Vancouver, British Columbia. Tel: +1 604 736 5511) is also recommended. Community hospitals all provide lodgings.

Vancouver General Hospital and Health Sciences Centre

899 West 12th Avenue, Vancouver V5Z 1M9. Tel: +1 604 875 4111.
www.vanhosp.bc.ca.
The hospital: When it first opened in 1886, Vancouver hospital was a nine-bed tent used to treat injured railway workers. Now it is split over four sites: **Vancouver General Hospital**, **UBC Hospital**, the **GF Strong Rehab Centre** and the **George Pearson Centre**. Today this totals 1900 beds. Vancouver General Hospital is a large, modern, friendly hospital providing virtually every speciality bar paeds and maternity. Trauma, burns, multiple sclerosis, sports medicine, transplantation, epilepsy surgery and brain/spinal cord injury are just a few of its specialized services.

O **Elective notes:** Students are responsible for the patients they clerk in, organizing CTs, taking bloods, etc. It's a busy place. Teaching, however, often ends up cancelled. In neurology, the twice-daily rounds mean that you may be there until 7 or 8 pm. Cadiothoracics has had good reports. For forensics, *see* the end of this section.

St Paul's Hospital

1081 Burrard Street, Vancouver, British Columbia V6Z 1Y6.
The hospital: As one of the main hospitals affiliated to UBC, this is a busy hospital situated in downtown Vancouver. It is particularly known for its cardiology and pathology. It also receives all the major trauma.

O **Elective notes:** The ER is a great place for an elective. It is very near the YMCA.

BC Children's Hospital

Vancouver, British Columbia. Tel: +1 604 875 2345.
www.childhosp.bc.cs/Childrens/bcch.HTM.
The hospital: This is a very friendly 242-bed hospital catering for children up to 16 years of age throughout British Columbia. It has all paeds specialities. It is also a teaching and research centre.

The cardiology department has had good elective reports.

St Vincent's Hospital

744 West 33rd Avenue, Vancouver, British Columbia U52 2K4.

The hospital: A friendly community hospital. It is a peripheral hospital with mainly geriatric and psychiatric specialities. There is a small ER open from 8 am to 8 pm.

O **Elective notes:** Although some have found being the only student in the operating theatre good for teaching, others have found it incredibly dull and had wished they had chosen somewhere more central. For specialities such as orthopaedics, urology, ophthalmology and cardiothoracic surgery you need to visit St Paul's Hospital. To do an elective here, you still need to apply through UBC.

BC Women's Hospital and Health Centre

4500 Oak Street, Vancouver, British Columbia V6H 3N1.

www.childhosp.bc.ca/womens/.

The hospital: Vancouver's specialist maternity hospital.

Sunnyhill Health Centre for Children

3644 Slozan Street, Vancouver, British Columbia V5M 3E8. Tel: +1 604 434 1331.

The hospital: A centre for children with developmental disabilities.

COMMUNITY HOSPITALS IN BRITISH COLUMBIA:

To do electives in these, you should apply through UBC.

Note: If it's skiing you're after, the snow usually settles between November and March.

Kootenay Lake District Hospital

3 View Street, Nelson, British Columbia V1L 2V1.

The hospital: Small and very friendly, and seeing a lot of skiing accidents. It's also very busy as the next nearest hospital is over 160 km away. Nelson is a small town of 10 000–15 000 people that lies approximately 600 km east of Vancouver. It is situated on the shore of Kootenay Lake amidst the Kootenay Mountains (at 3000 ft) and was a common destination for the hippies and draft dodgers of the 1970s. Many of these people are still here, along with the more recent influx of New Age people, altogether making Nelson a very colourful and active community. It is also a beautiful place to visit. The skiing (£12 a day) is some of the best. From May, water sports on the lake take over.

O **Elective notes:** It is a popular destination for Canadian as well as foreign elective students. Many specialities are catered for, but you are free to do as you please. There is no schedule, but the informal teaching is good. The ER and internal medicine are recommended. The staff are very friendly, giving you an ample social life and opportunities to explore the beautiful scenery.

Accommodation: Basic but with beautiful mountain views. Both the accommodation and the food are currently free, although this may soon change. Don't panic though – there is a good youth hostel in town.

Dawsons Creek and District Hospital

816–103rd Avenue, Dawsons Creek, British Columbia V1G 2G1.

The hospital: A small, friendly district general hospital (18 hours by coach or two hours by plane from Vancouver), serving the population of Dawson (11 000) and the surrounding areas. It has surgery, medicine, O&G, and psychiatric wards as well as an ER. Some of the cases in the ER are the results of the social antagonism within the community (especially towards native Indians). There is a large GP input into the hospital.

O **Elective notes:** You can do as much or as little as you want.

Kimberley and District Hospital

260 Fourth Avenue, Kimberley, British Columbia VIA 2R6.

The hospital: This small, GP-run hospital has 35 beds. It is 56 km from the nearest speciality hospital. Six GPs run the clinics from 10 am to 5 pm and also run the hospital. They do their own deliveries, including Caesarean sections. In the ski season (February and March), there are plenty of orthopaedic injuries from the ski slope five minutes away. A few specialists visit to do clinics.

O Elective notes: This is a good place to learn a lot, and there's plenty of experience. It is frowned on if you don't turn up, but days off for skiing are encouraged. The nearest airport is Cranbrook.

Trail Regional Hospital

1200 Hospital Bench Trail, British Columbia VIR 4MI.

The hospital: Pretty small but medicine, surgery, paeds, ER and anaesthetics are all catered for.

O Elective notes: You can do whatever you want; the doctors are pleased to have a student about. It's in the middle of nowhere and can get a bit lonely, but it's pretty easy to get to the ski hills.

Accommodation: And food are free.

Vernon Jubille Hospital

31st Street, Vernon, British Columbia. Tel: +1 250 549 5225.

The hospital: A medium-sized DGH, with an ER, major specialities and family practice.

O Elective notes: There is good practical teaching. No other students are around and there's a flexible timetable (for the good skiing nearby).

Royal Inland Hospital

Kamloops, British Columbia.

The hospital: A nice clean hospital in the centre of Kamloops.

O Elective notes: Unfortunately, Kamloops is a fairly small city, but there are excellent ski resorts nearby and friendly doctors who let you do what you want. You are advised to go with friend.

Accommodation: A good room with phone. The food in the canteen is reasonable.

Chilliwack General Hospital

45600 Menholm Road, Chilliwack, British Columbia V2P 5J4.

The hospital: A medium-sized, mainly GP-run hospital. There are some permanently employed specialists who work mostly in ER. Chilliwack is a nice town about an hour from the nearest ski slopes.

Surrey Memorial Hospital

13750 96th Avenue, Surrey, British Columbia V3V 1Z2.

The hospital: This community hospital rarely has students. It's a friendly place with good teaching.

FORENSIC MEDICINE:

Department of Forensic Pathology

1st Floor Laurel Pavillion, Vancouver Hospital Health Services CTR, 855 West 12th Avenue, Vancouver, British Columbia V5Z 1M9.

Forensic medicine at the hospital comes thoroughly recommended. The chap in charge is very friendly. Most of the work is finished by 2–3 pm, giving you the evenings free. Hob-nob with the police and try to get a day with them. Students can help in about three or four autopsies a day.

ALBERTA

Calgary

Calgary is a fairly large city ... most of which seems to have been built for the 1988 winter Olympics. Banff National Park in the heart of the Rockies is only one-and-a-half hours away. The pubs and clubs shut at 2 am so there's a good night-life.

University of Calgary
Faculty of Medicine, 3330 Hospital Drive, NW Calgary, Alberta T2N 4N1. Tel: +1 403 220 4262. www.ucalgary.ca.
The medical faculty was founded in 1970 and is situated in the Calgary Health Sciences Centre. They can arrange electives in Calgary's hospitals. There's a charge of around $200. The only Calgary hospital to provide accommodation is the Foothills. Students have previously stayed in university digs (around $300 a month), handy for downtown.

Alberta Children's Hospital
1820 Richmond Road SW, Calgary, Alberta T2T 5C7.
The hospital: This fairly large, modern hospital is the paediatric tertiary referral hospital for Alberta and hence has all specialities. It is a 10–15-minute bus ride from downtown Calgary.
O **Elective notes:** The staff and other medical students are very welcoming. They organize the programme for you ... a typical rotation being one week emergency, one week neonatology and four weeks general. They do expect you to work, but as a student you are given quite a lot of responsibility.
Accommodation: None is available in the hospital. You can stay at the Foothills Hospital, a 10–15-minute bus ride away.

Calgary General Hospital
841 Centre Avenue East, Calgary, Alberta T2E 0A1.
The hospital: This is one of Calgary's main hospitals and was located on two sites, Bar Valley and Peter Longheed, although the Bar Valley site has recently been closed. The ER is a busy department seeing many acute surgical and medical emergencies; however, most trauma goes to Calgary's other main hospital, the Foothills.
O **Elective notes:** As a student in ER, you are given a rota with different supervisors. You are never expected to work overnight.
Accommodation: Cannot be provided

in the hospital, but if you apply to the Foothills Hospital, you can stay there.

Foothills Hospital
1403–29 St NW, Calgary, Alberta T2N 2T9.
The hospital: A large, well-equipped friendly hospital. It has many specialities including Calgary's trauma department.
O **Elective notes:** You can do as much or as little as you want. Trauma comes highly recommended.
Accommodation: Basic ... no cooking facilities and no sheets or pillows are provided, but it is cheap. It's in the Foothills grounds – great as you can lie in before work, but you are a fair way out from the night-life. The public transport is good, but you'll need to get a taxi back from the night clubs.

FORENSIC MEDICINE:

Office of the Chief Medical Examiner
6070 Bowness Road NW, Calgary, Alberta T3B 3R7.
There are plenty of autopsies and court visits. The office is very friendly, work is usually finished by early afternoon and the staff positively encourage you to go out and see Calgary and the Rockies.

University of Alberta
Faculty of Medicine, 2J2.00 Walter C. Mackenzie Health Sciences Centre Edmonton, Alberta T6G 2R7.
Tel: +1 403 492 6350. Fax: +1 403 492 9531. www.med.ualberta.ca.
Founded in 1913, the University campus has the **Walter Mackenzie Health Sciences Centre** on-site. The university also uses the **Royal Alexandra**, **Alberta**, **Glenrose**, **Edmonton General**, **Misericordia**, **Grey Nuns** and **Charles Camsell** hospitals as well as the **Cross Cancer Institute**. It's not a common elective destination for students from the UK. Write to the school for elective opportunities in any of their hospitals.

SASKATCHEWAN

University of Saskatchewan
College of Medicine, Health Sciences Building, 107 Wiggins Road, Saskatoon, Saskatchewan S7N 5E5. Tel: +1 306 966 8554. Fax: +1 306 966 6164.
www.usask.ca/medicine.
Established in 1926, clinical teaching is now carried out at the **Royal University Hospital**, **St Paul's** and **Saskatoon City Hospitals** in Saskatoon, and the **Plains Health Centre** and **General Hospital** in Regina.

MANITOBA

University of Manitoba
Faculty of Medicine, 753 McDermot Avenue, Winnipeg, Manitoba R3E 0W3. Tel: +1 204 789 3569. Fax: +1 204 789 3929. www.umanitoba.ca.
The college was founded in 1883 and today is situated opposite the **Winnipeg Health Sciences Centre** (which is separate from the rest of the university). Within the Health Sciences Centre, there are children's, adult's, women's, respiratory and rehabilitation hospitals totalling over 1000 beds. Other hospitals used include the **Boniface General** (900 beds), **Misericordia** (409 beds), **Seven Oaks** (336 beds), **Deer Lodge Veterans** (500 beds), **Grace** (306 beds) and **Victoria** (254 beds) hospitals.

Flin Flon General Hospital
Flin Flon, Manitoba R8A 1N2.
The hospital: Flin Flon is a mining town that lies between the provinces of Manitoba and Saskatchewan. It is a small northern Canadian town with a total population of 15 000 (including the neighbouring native Canadian reserves). The hospital has 100 beds and is staffed by ten doctors. It is well equipped with two theatres, an X-ray and ultrasound department, an ITU and an ER. Each of the doctors is employed by the regional health authority and works both as a spe-

cialist and as a GP in the town. Two or three times a week they fly out to native Canadian reserves in northern Saskatchewan. The clinics here can be a real eye-opener as there are terrible political problems. The native population live in very poor conditions on designated reserve land. Alcohol and drug abuse are huge problems and the clinics are very busy.

O **Elective notes:** A typical day starts with a ward round reviewing any patients admitted in the night and then going to theatre. There could be specialist or minor surgical procedures to get involved in. The afternoon is usually spent in a clinic in the town or flying to clinics further north. Your help is greatly appreciated here. When you are on call, there are many opportunities to perform procedures such as chest drains.

The coldest time is from January through to March, when the temperature ranges from 0 to -37°C. Winter activities include ice fishing, ice hockey, ski-dooing, curling, etc. There's plenty to do in the days, but at night ... the nearest cinema is one-and-a-half hours away and the nearest city (Winnipeg or Saskatoon) about eight.

ONTARIO

Toronto

Toronto is a pleasant lively modern city with skyscrapers, a beautiful harbour, museums, ice rinks and good restaurants. CN Tower and a Blue Jays game must be seen.

University of Toronto
Faculty of Medicine, Toronto, Ontario M5S 1A8. Tel: +1 416 978 2717. Fax: +1 416 971 2163.
www.library.utoronto.ca/medicine.
This large faculty is associated with eight teaching hospital units. Those on University Avenue include the **University Health Network** (Toronto General, which has merged with Toronto

Western, and Princes Margaret), the **Hospital for Sick Children** and **Mount Sinai Hospital**. Others are **St Michael's**, the **Toronto Rehab Institute**, the **Sunnybrook and Women's College Health Sciences Centre**, the **Clarke Institute of Psychiatry** and the **Baycrest Centre for Geriatric Care**.

To do an elective anywhere in Toronto you should first write to the **Visiting Electives Coordinator** (Room 2124, Medical Sciences Building, Faculty of Medicine, University of Toronto, 1 King's College Circle, Toronto, Ontario M5S 1A8. Tel: +1 416 978 2691. Fax: +1 416 971 2163). Elective information is on the university website.

They charge from C$216 for one to two weeks up to C$432 for an eight-week long elective. You MUST apply at least four months before the proposed elective date or they will fine you another C$50. Then add on a bit for malpractice insurance (around C$100 per four weeks; this can be arranged through the university). Don't pay for insurance until they have confirmed your elective. APPLY EARLY … especially if you want to do something popular (e.g. trauma).

Accommodation: Try Student Housing (Koffler Student Centre, University of Toronto, 214 College Street, Toronto, Ontario M5T 1R2. Tel: +1 416 978 8045). Many stay at Tartu College (310 Bloor Street West, Toronto, Ontario M5S 1W4. Tel: +1 416 925 9405. Fax: +1 416 925 2295). Another place to try is the Toronto General Hospital Residence (90 Gerrard Street West, Toronto, Ontario M5G 1J6. Fax: +1 416 340 3923). This costs about $200 a week. Some have saved money by getting right out of town (a 50-minute train ride from centre) to Hospitality York (York University, 4200 Keele St, North York, Ontario; only £6 a night). If you're really stuck, try Toronto Tourist Information (Toronto Eaton Centre, 1 Dundas Street West, Toronto, Ontario M5G 1Z3).

Warning: You may be expected to work quite hard in Toronto. Here, electives can make up to 50% of Canadian students' study and are therefore considered an integral part of the course. They may not understand that it's supposed to be a cleverly disguised holiday.

The University Health Network comprises the **Toronto General, Toronto Western** and **Princess Margaret Hospitals**. All are in downtown and on www.uhealthnet.on.ca.

Toronto General Hospital

200 Elizabeth Street, University Avenue, Toronto. Tel: +1 416 340 3131.
The hospital: A huge teaching hospital with numerous specialities, including heart disease, transplantation, tropical disease, eating disorders and a busy emergency department treating 30 000 cases a year. The hospital has had some pretty amazing firsts including the development of insulin, the invention of the pacemaker and world's first single and double lung transplants. It has Canada's largest HIV clinic and first eating disorders clinic.
O Elective notes: The day starts early, at 7.30 am, so try to get accommodation nearby.

Toronto Western Hospital

399 Bathurst Street, Toronto.
Tel: +1 416 603 5801.
The hospital: Here they are doing a great deal of research into brain, spinal cord, lung and vision diseases. It has a busy ER seeing 40 000 a year.

Princess Margaret Hospital

610 University Avenue, Toronto, Ontario M5G 2M9. Tel: +1 416 946 2000.
The hospital: With its research arm, the Ontario Cancer Institute, this is regarded as one of the top cancer centres in the world. It is a beautiful, well-equipped hospital with very friendly and good teaching staff.

Hospital for Sick Children

555 University Avenue, Toronto M5G 1X8.
The hospital: The Hospital for Sick Children ('Sick Kids') is one of the

largest paeds academic health science centres in the world. It is a very modern (opened in 1993) and well-equipped tertiary referral institution for the whole of the Toronto–Ontario area. As such, it sees a wide variety of rare diseases. The entrance hall has fluffy toys and a Disney store and patients have their own rooms.

O **Elective notes:** This is highly recommended if you are interested in paeds. Apply over a year in advance. There are some excellent teachers (especially in cardiology). Bear in mind that subjects such as infectious diseases are mainly ward work, whereas cardiology has many more outpatient clinics. Students tend to be taught rather than given house officer jobs. When applying, you have to select a subspeciality from adolescent medicine, cardiology, genetics, emergency, endocrinology, gastrointestinal medicine and nutrition, haematology, hepatology, infectious diseases, neonatology, neurology, perinatology, respiratory medicine and rheumatology.

Accommodation: This is in a building just across the road from the hospital. It costs C$150 a week. The hospital can provide you with details.

St Michael's Hospital

30 Bond Street, Toronto, Ontario M5B 1W8. Tel: +1 416 360 4000. Fax: +1 416 864 5870.

The hospital: Is part of the University of Toronto and has the busiest of the three emergency departments in the city.

O **Elective notes:** In the ER, hours are fairly flexible and offer excellent experience: clerking patients, doing the preliminary investigations and suturing. Teaching is good, but the staff are often too busy.

Queens Street Mental Health Centre

1001 Queen St West, Toronto, Ontario.

The hospital: This is Toronto's main psychiatric facility. An elective here is very supervisor-dependent. As with most psychiatry, admissions can take a great deal of time, and unless you get good teaching, you may get bored.

Sunnybrook and Women's College Health Sciences Centre

Toronto, Ontario. www.sunnybrook.utoronto.ca.

The hospital: Has 1300 beds and was originally for veterans but is now an acute care civilian hospital.

St Joseph's Health Centre

30 The Queensway, Toronto, Ontario M6R 1B5.

The hospital: This lies 2 km from downtown, with a good transport system (buses, street cars and a subway). Although not the largest hospital in Toronto, it has the main specialities and offers good opportunities to see and assist in general surgery and a busy ER.

Accommodation: The residences are sparse and basic (C$25 a week), but it's easy to get into the city centre.

Hamilton

Hamilton is a large town between Toronto and Niagara Falls. It has a large industrial base and is therefore not the prettiest town in Canada.

McMaster University

Health Sciences Centre, 1200 Main Street West, Hamilton, Ontario L8N 3Z5. Tel: +1 905 525 9140. Fax: +1 905 527 2707. www.fhs.mcmaster.ca.

The university offers an undergraduate medical programme and postgraduate medical education. The clinical components of the undergraduate course occur in the McMaster Division of the Hamilton Health Sciences Corporation and other hospitals in Hamilton.

St Peter's Hospital

Mapel Wood Road, Hamilton, Ontario.

The hospital: One of Hamilton's teaching hospitals.

O **Elective notes:** It is good for care of the elderly and you can use McMaster's facilities. However, you really need a car to get around from here.

St Joseph's Hospital

50 Charlton Avenue, Hamilton, Ontario L8N 4A6.

The hospital: Most specialities are available.

O Elective notes: Some have found it a bit isolated and lonely.

Hamilton Psychiatric Hospital

100 West 5th Street, Hamilton, Ontario L8N 3K7.

The hospital: The psychiatry is practised with a great deal of compassion and innovation. As a quaternary referral centre (affiliated to McMaster University), there is a great deal of pathology to be seen.

Accommodation: Cheap, comfortable, convenient and organized by McMaster University.

University of Ottawa

Faculty of Medicine, 451 Smyth Road, Ottawa, Ontario K1H 8M5. Tel: +1 613 562 5800. Fax: +1 613 562 5457. www.uottawa.ca.

Within the university are the faculty of medicine and schools of nursing and human kinetics. Due to a change in policy, since December 1997 the University of Ottawa no longer accepts foreign elective students.

The University of Ottawa serves three hospitals in Ottawa, one being **Ottawa Civic Hospital** (1053 Carling Avenue, Ottawa, Ontario K1Y 4E9). This is both English- and French-speaking.

Queen's University

Faculty of Health Sciences School of Medicine, Kingston, Ontario K7L 3N6. Tel +1 613 533 2542. Fax: +1 613 533 6884. http://meds.queensu.ca/medicine.

Founded in 1854, the university campus is in Kingston on Lake Ontario. The three major hospitals (currently in process of reforms) are the **Kingston General Hospital** (for acute inpatient care), the **Hotel Dieu Hospital** (for ambulatory care) and the **St Mary's of the Lake Hospital** (for elderly, rehabilitation and palliative care).

Kingston General Hospital

76 Stuart Street, Kingston, Ontario K7L 2V7.

The hospital: A large teaching hospital on the North Shore of Lake Ontario about three hours by train from Toronto and Montreal. The senior staff are friendly and encourage evidence-based medicine.

O Elective notes: Sign-in rounds occur daily, and you will be given patients to assess. It can be very hard work, and the finalists will spend most of the time in the library rather than coming out to play. This is a great elective and you will learn a lot (especially cardiology). However, it's not so great if you really just want to travel and see Canada.

University of Western Ontario

Faculty of Medicine and Dentistry, Medical Sciences Building, London, Ontario N6A 5C1. Tel: +1 519 661 3744. Fax: +1 519 661 3797. www.med.uwo.ca.

The medical faculty has been around since 1882. It's a private University based in London, Ontario, and uses a number of local hospitals.

QUEBEC

Montreal

Montreal is a great city with much to do in June, July and August. In the winter, the temperature goes down to −20°C, so don't go then if you don't like the cold. This is arguably the most beautiful time of the year though. There is also a jazz festival as an added incentive. It helps to be able to speak some French as about half the population is French-speaking.

The two universities in Montreal are the **McGill** (English-speaking) and the **Université de Montréal** (French-speaking). Beware of going to a French-speaking hospital as the French is slightly different from European French and you may have problems.

McGill University

Faculty of Medicine, 3655 Drummond Street, Montreal, Quebec H3G 1Y6. Tel: +1 514 398 3517. Fax: +1 514 398 4631. www.mcgill.ca.

McGill came about in 1811 when James McGill bequeathed his estate. With the Montreal General Hospital, the medical school was set up and became the first medical faculty in Canada in 1821. Today, it has grown considerably and uses the **Montreal Children's**, **Montreal General**, **Montreal Neurological**, **Sir Mortimer B Davis–Jewish General**, **Shriner's Crippled Children's**, **Douglas** and **Royal Victoria** hospitals. Many hospitals outside Quebec are also associated. Instruction in McGill institutions is in English.

Apply to McGill for electives at any of their institutions. They can also help out with accommodation. Try to stay at the McGill-affiliated halls of residence … you'll get to meet more people. The order of preference is:

- Royal Victoria College ($50 (£25) a week)
- Montreal Diocesan College
- Presbyterian College.

These are all near University Street. Neither of the last two are religious!

Royal Victoria Hospital

Avenue Des Pins Ouest (or 687 Pine Avenue), Montreal, Quebec H3A 1A1.

The hospital: Is huge and the main hospital for McGill University medical school. The renal department is world-renowned and the teaching is excellent. Both staff and students are very friendly. There is a very team-based approach to medicine. Nearly all specialities are catered for. English is used most commonly.

O Elective notes: There are good reports from the cardiology and general medicine departments. If doing O&G, medical students take it in turn to be on call at nights and catch deliveries. Apply early – it's popular.

Montreal General Hospital/Hôpital General de Montreal

1650 Cedar Avenue, Montreal, Quebec H3G 1A4. Tel: +1 514 937 6011.

The hospital: Hosts many specialities and has a busy ER.

O Elective notes: There are many opportunities for practical procedures and the teaching is very good. Medical intensive care comes recommended.

Montreal Neurological Institute and Hospital

3801 University Street, Montreal, Quebec H3A 2B4. www.mcgill.ca/mni/.

The hospital: This is *the* place to do neurology in Canada and has a world-wide reputation. Its long history includes the development of the EEG. It is a very friendly place. The hospital is central so clubs and bars are near by.

O Elective notes: At 8 am there is a signing-in session at which interesting cases are presented. Then there is a teaching ward round. The rest of the day you're admitting patients and following them around the hospital. It can be very hard work but comes thoroughly recommended by all who have been there.

Sir Mortimer B. Davis–Jewish General Hospital

3755 Cote St Catherine Road, Montreal, Quebec H3T 1EZ. Tel: +1 514 30 8222. Fax: +1 514 340 7510.

The hospital: Has 675 beds.

Université de Montréal

School of Medicine, PO Box 6128, Station Centre-Ville, Montreal, Quebec H3C 3J7. Tel: +1 514 33 6265. Fax: +1 514 343 6629. www.umontreal.ca.

The medical school was founded in 1843 and today uses 14 teaching hospitals and research centres. Note: All instruction is in French.

QUEBEC MEDICAL SCHOOLS OUTSIDE MONTREAL:

Université Laval

Faculty of Medicine, Ste-Foy, Quebec G1K 7P4. Tel: +1 418 656 2131. Fax: +1 418 656 2733. www.ulaval.ca.

Established in 1852 by Royal Charter, the university uses its health sciences centre and an affiliated hospital for its teaching.

University of Sherbrooke

Faculty of Medicine, Sherbrooke, Quebec J1H 5N4. Tel: +1 819 564 5208. Fax: +1 819 564 5378. www.usherb.ca.

This relatively new faculty (admitting since 1966) is entirely French-speaking. It is multidisciplinary, with a faculty of nursing. Its Health Sciences Centre includes a 700-bed teaching hospital. Twelve other hospitals are also used.

NOVA SCOTIA

Halifax has a population of 700 000 but has four universities. This is therefore very much a student city.

Dalhousie University

Faculty of Medicine, 5849 University Avenue, Halifax, Nova Scotia B3H 4H7. Tel: +1 902 494 6592. Fax: +1 902 494 7119 www.mcms.dal.ca.

The faculty, founded in 1868, covers the three Maritime Provinces of Canada (Nova Scotia, New Brunswick and Prince Edward Island), with a population of 1.7 million. The teaching hospitals total 2300 beds. The major teaching hospitals used include **Queen Elizabeth II Health Sciences Centre** (www.qe2-hsc.ns.ca) in the heart of Halifax (including Camp Hill, Victoria General, Nova Scotia Rehab and New Halifax Infirmary). This is the major referral centre for Maritime Canada, **IWK Grace Health Centre**, **Nova Scotia Hospital** (psychiatric), **St John Regional Hospital**, a large modern hospital in New Brunswick.

To do electives in these write to the university. They have previously been awkward about malpractice insurance, though their position may have changed.

Victoria General Hospital

Halifax, Nova Scotia.
The hospital: Is the largest teaching

hospital in Nova Scotia with a full range of medical specialities and research facilities. It is in downtown Halifax next to the children and maternity hospitals, a stone's throw from the medical campus.

NEWFOUNDLAND

Newfoundland, right in the far east of Canada, has a population of 500 000, most of whom live in St John's. St John's itself is built around a pleasant harbour.

Memorial University of Newfoundland

Faculty of Medicine, St John's, Newfoundland A1B 3V6. Tel: +1 709 737 6615. Fax: +1 709 737 5186. www.med.mun.ca/med/.

Founded in 1925, Memorial is the only university in Newfoundland. The Health Sciences Centre includes the general hospital with 530 beds. A number of other hospitals in St John's are also used. To do an elective in these hospitals, you'll need to apply to the university. They have a fee of around C$100 and can provide malpractice cover for around C$137.

Memorial University Hospital

St John's, Newfoundland A1B 3V6.
The hospital: This provides nearly all specialities, but the **Grace Hospital** provides obstetric care and the **Charles Janeway Children's Hospital** (Pleasantville, St John's) paediatric care. These hospitals provide tertiary referral care for a massive area up to Labrador, hence rescue flights are common. The Janeway and Grace are soon to close so everything will be at the Memorial.

Charles S. Curtis Memorial Hospital

Grenfell Regional Health Services, St Anthony, Newfoundland A0K 4S0. Tel: +1 709 454 3333. Fax: +1 709 454 2052.
The hospital: In St Anthony (population 3200), the healthcare here is very much

GP- ('family medicine') orientated. The GPs run clinics in the hospital and admit directly. Once patients have been admitted, the GPs can then direct their care. The hospital has 60 beds and six ITU beds. Family practice also covers obstetrics, gynaecology and emergency medicine. The CCMH covers a large area ... the northern Newfoundland peninsula, coastal Quebec and southern Labrador. Because of the great distances, flying is an integral part of medical practice, bringing in patients from far-out nursing stations or taking more serious ones to St Johns. The obstetrics department receives on average 250 deliveries a year and, with the gynaecology unit, has two antenatal and two general outpatient clinics a week.

O **Elective notes:** This is an incredibly popular destination for students – hence the length of this section. As a student, you go out to the local communities for clinics and are involved with the hospital care. You therefore get a great deal of experience in a number of specialities and in the hospital you are given a great deal of responsibility. In surgery you effectively work as a JHO. Here they actually NEED you and you become a valued member of the team. There is a rota (no more then 1:3) for on call where the medical students cover the entire hospital and admit in ER. If doing surgery, you are the assistant. Don't go here if you don't like being isolated.

Note: In O&G, there have apparently been some problems between staff (nursing and medical) and students as sometimes a bit too much is expected of students and there is not much teaching. Other branches are great though.

St Anthony is a town where cod fishing and moose hunting are the topics of the day and the locals really do wear red and black lumberjack shirts. The population is rapidly diminishing as people move to the cities. There is high unemployment (20%) since cod fishing (the main industry) was made illegal in 1992 to preserve fish stocks. In the winter, there are whales, icebergs and moose to see and the opportunity to try 'ski-dooing'. You can also visit the only Viking settlement in North America (L'Anse aux Meadows). In July and August, it can be warm (20°C), but fog is still common. During January to March, it is very cold with snow storms. Many festivals occur in the summer. Corner Brook is the nearest town (six hours in the car), and Gros Morne National Park is great for hiking. The local ice rink does not hire skates and there are no commercial ski-hire businesses. Transport is also a major problem.

Accommodation: If you stay for eight weeks, accommodation, food and money towards your airfare (C$1000) are currently provided by CCMH, but this is in the process of changing. The accommodation was with other elective students (there are no resident students) and very friendly.

Section 3
Adventure
Medicine

Medicine is your passport to travel! And if you fancy an adventure you have a world of possibilities. This new section gives you information on a few organizations that may provide a bit more adrenaline. It is by no means exhaustive – but it should help to set the ball rolling! Remember, you don't have to work through an organization to do something a bit different. There are many remote hospitals listed in this book that will in their own way provide an adventure. Take a look at www.medicstravel.org as this has databases of people wanting to work overseas and organizations/remote hospitals requiring medics.

Expedition medicine

Expedition medicine is becoming big business and there is plenty for doctors and nurses to get involved in. As 'adventure tourism' increases, so does the need for medics who are happy to work in remote environments. The deal is usually that the medic gets to go at a slightly reduced rate, rarely is it free and virtually never is it paid. There are a few things to think about:

- What type of expedition are you interested in – mountain, polar, rainforest, rafting, etc.? Some previous experience usually helps you get selected
- What is your liability if you cock up? Contact your defence union for advice – it is not a 'good samaritan' act if you have received any kind of inducement to be there
- Will you be OK not earning for a while?
- Also note that being the 'medic' may involve a bit more than you thought – you will have to get a kit, and you may be required to organize vaccinations and pre-trip medicals.

There are many organizations and private companies you may want to approach; *see* the 'Mountain medicine' section for some contacts.

Royal Geographical Society

Expedition Advisory Centre, 1 Kensington Gore, London SW7 2AR, UK. Tel: +44 20 7591 3030. Fax: +44 20 7591 3031. www.rgs.org.
The RGS holds a database of expeditions that are planned. This *Bulletin of Expedition Vacancies* is available for purchase and says which ones require medics. They also have a *Register of Personnel* of those wanting to go on expeditions (doctors, nurses, etc.) to which you can add your name for free. Just fill in the form on the website and send it back. The RGS also runs *Medical Cell*, a discussion forum for those in remote areas. They have produced a book, *Expedition Medicine* (edited by Warrell and Anderson), which is essential reading before joining an expedition.

The section on NGOs in Section 4 contains more addresses, but a couple of organizations that regularly require medics are:

Raleigh International, 27 Parsons Green Lane, London SW6 4HZ, UK. www.raleigh.org.uk.
Trekforce, 34 Buckingham Palace Road, London SW1 0RE, UK. www.trekforce.org.uk.

There are a number of chairites arranging 'sponsor my holiday'-style trips (you know – bike-ride Vietnam sort of thing). If that's what you want to help out on take a look at www.acrossthedivide.co.uk. Incidentally, the overall donations from such trips came to £12 million in 2001, whereas the costs of the trips came to £10.5 million, not that there's any suggestion that some middle-men might be doing quite well out of it.

See the end of this chapter for training organizations.

When thinking about applying to a particular diving institution consider which components of diving medicine interest you. Do you want diving research (mainly physiology), training (medic diver qualifications), performing 'fitness to dive' medical examinations or do you want to treat diving-related injuries? Bear in mind, however, that the provision of care is only necessary if there is a problem so basing yourself at a site that has only a decompression chamber may provide weeks of inactivity (but plenty of time for diving!). Ideally, you should be somewhere that provides many aspects of diving medicine or somewhere with an affiliated hospital enabling you to see other patients as well. Being in the Navy opens other avenues.

GENERAL DIVING MEDICAL WEBSITES:

Diving Medicine Online
This excellent site has information on everything from diving with asthma to diving with a coronary stent. It also lists all the decompression chambers and dive medicine centres country by country. www.scuba-doc.com.

Divers' Alert Network
This gives safety advice to civilian divers and information on training and research. www.diversalertnetwork.org.

Undersea and Hyperbaric Medicine Society
The members of this international, non-profit-making organization are mostly doctors and hyperbaric scientists. www.uhms.org.

European Underwater and Baromedical Society
This publishes the *European Journal of Underwater and Hyperbaric Medicine*. www.eubs.org.

UK:

Diving Disease Research Centre
Hyperbaric Medical Centre, Tamar Science Park, Rsearch Way, Plymouth PL6 8DU. Tel: +44 1752 209999. Fax: +44 1752 209115. www.ddrc.org.
This centre is affiliated with Derriford Hospital and has become a leader in diving physiology research since the 1980s (in areas such as diving with diabetes, disabilities and asthma). The research centre runs extensive training programmes and treats decompression illness, carbon monoxide and cyanide poisoning, smoke inhalation and soft tissue infections such as necrotizing fasciitis.

National Hyperbaric Centre
This centre, located in Aberdeen, is a leading hyperbaric testing, training and research centre. It provides medical cover for a large part of north-eastern Scotland, including the commercial divers of the oil and gas industry. www.demon.co.uk/hyperbar.

Scottish Diving Medicine
This is the homepage of the recompression chambers in Scotland that provide care for NHS patients with diving-related illness. www.sams.ac.uk/sdm.

RED SEA:

Sharm El Sheikh Hyperbaric Medical Centre
Based in the busiest dive area of the Red Sea, this centre is happy to take elective students and foreign doctors (for more information see the elective report by Kevin Bailey at www.studentbmj.com/back issues/1001/life/385.html). www.sharm-chamber.org.

SAUDI ARABIA:

This site lists dozens of dive centres in Saudi Arabia. www.saudidiving.com/dive-centers.htm.

USA:

There are many academic centres with an interest in diving medicine in the US. The Divers' Alert Network (based at Duke University) is a good place to start. Also look at Diving Medicine Online (*see* above).

AUSTRALIA AND THE SOUTH PACIFIC:

The South Pacific Underwater Medicine Society

This is the main site for Oceania, with information on dive centres in the region and courses that tend to be run in Australia. It also has a journal section where you might be able to find who is doing the type of research you are interested in. www.spums.org.au.

PACIFIC ISLANDS:

Luganville Hospital, Luganville, Espirito Santo Island, Vanuatu.

This hospital has the hyperbaric chamber for the Pacific islands and can provide a fantastic elective.

OTHER USEFUL WEBSITES:

British Sub Aqua Club: www.bsac.com.
PADI Diving: www.padi.com.

Spending some time as part of an elective or working on an overseas trip with a mountain rescue association can be quite easy to organize. There are many to be found, from the Himalayas to the Alps, the Rookies to the Blue Mountains of Australia. Lots more information can be found by doing a Google search, but here are some top sites.

SKI PATROLS AND SEARCH AND RESCUE TEAMS:

For a useful set of links, try www.patrol.org and www.ski-injury.com.

Australian Ski Patrol Association:
www.skipatrol.org.au.
New South Wales Ski Patrol:
www.nsw-ski-patrol.org.au.
Austrian ski patrols: www.bergrettung.at.
British Association of Ski Patrollers:
Tel: +44 1855 811443. www.basp.org.uk.
Canadian ski patrols: www.cspc.ca.
French ski patrols: www.anps.asso.fr.
Italian ski patrols: www.fisps.it.
New Zealand Search and Rescue:
www.nzlsar.org.nz.
Swiss ski patrols: www.skipatrol.ch.
Rega Swiss Air Rescue: www.rega.ch.
US National Ski Patrol: www.nsp.org.
Venezuelan Rescue Association:
www.rescate.org.
Also try www.emergencyrescue.com.

A couple of places previously visited by medical students:

Eldora Ski Patrol
Eldora Mountain Resort, Eldora, Colorado, USA. (Write to the Ski Patrol Director.)
Eldora is a small resort at 3076 m (10 000 ft) one hour away from Denver. Day trippers come from Denver and Boulder to ski here. Approximately eight patrollers ensure that the slopes are safe in the morning and then attend to the injured during the day. Trauma resulting

from falls and collisions is common, as is acute mountain sickness.

Vail Valley Medical Center
Vail, Colorado, USA. www.vvmc.com.
Vail is one of the largest ski areas in America with 8000 skiers on the slope a day and 30 patrollers. Because of its size, Vail has its own hospital (with CT and MRI) in the village. There are opportunities here to both go on the slopes and work in a fully equipped hospital.

MOUNTAIN MEDICINE WEBSITES:

General information:
International Society for Mountain Medicine:
www.ismmed.org.
British Mountaineering Council:
www.bmc.co.uk.

UK:
Patterdale Mountain Rescue Team:
www.mountainsrescue.org.uk.

USA:
Mountain Rescue Association: www.mra.org.
Portland Mountain Rescue: www.pmru.org.

Europe:
Alps/Pyrennes: Mountain Medicine and Traumatology Department of Chamonix Hospital (DMTM): www.perso.wanadoo.fr/dmtmcham/rescue.
Iceland: Mountain Rescue Team – Iceland: www.eh.est.ic/fbsa/.

Nepal:

Himalayan Rescue Association
Head Office, Dhobichaur, Lazimpat, PO Box 4944, Thamel, Kathmandu. Tel: +977 1 440 292. E-mail: hra@mail.com.np.
www.himalayanrescue.com.
They have two posts in the Himalayas. One is in Periche (near the Everest Base Camp). This sees mainly Western trekkers with minor injuries and acute mountain sickness. Qualified volunteers

are required to work for periods of three months. The other post is in Manang (Himalayan Rescue Association Post, Manang, Manang District; write early as a porter has to carry this letter 140 km from the nearest road up 3800 m). This is on the Annapurna circuit and sees locals as well as trekkers. Neither is allowed to take elective students for a full elective, but you are usually welcome to pop by and spend a couple of days there. Occasionally, students (usually with projects) have been allowed to stay at the Manang site. Check the website for more details.

Also check out www.medex.org.uk, which organizes high-altitude research in the region.

ROYAL FLYING DOCTOR SERVICE OF AUSTRALIA:

Think of Australia and think of medicine and this is what you get. Because of this, an elective with one of the 14 stations operating a Flying Doctor service is extremely hard to come by. Over the past few years they have really restricted it to Australian students (for insurance reasons), but don't let that put you off. If you apply early (very early … two or more years in advance) and to as many places as possible, you are in with a chance. It is certainly worth it.

The Royal Flying Doctor Service (RFDS) is legendary around the world and is still providing for the needs of thousands. Eighty per cent of Australia is RFDS territory. Reverend John Flynn started it all. In 1912 he wanted to be able to provide a medical service to those terribly isolated in Australia's interior. Many people had died horrible, lonesome deaths in these very isolated parts. But there were two major problems: first, how could the patient alert the doctor, and second, how could the doctor get there? Two very new inventions solved these: the radio and the aeroplane. Most people laughed off the idea, but Flynn persisted, and in 1933 the Australian Aerial Medical Service was born. Today, the RFDS flies 6.5 million km a year, makes 169 000 patient contacts a year (3000 a week), carries out 17 000 emergency evacuations and conducts 5000 clinics (95 a week) in places that would otherwise be entirely isolated. All this is done with just 350 staff. They also conduct radio clinics, send 2500 medical packs to isolated areas and have provided the communication network for the School of the Air.

The administration of the 14 bases is divided between seven sections, each of which is completely autonomous, meeting the particular needs of its area. Generally speaking, the sections follow a state pattern. There are, however, exceptions: the Victorian section's field of operations is in the Kimberley region in the north-west of Western Australia, with radio bases at Derby and Wyndham. Two other sections operate in Western Australia. These are the Western Australian Section (Port Hedland, Jandakot, Carnarvon and Meekatharra) and the Eastern Goldfields Section (Kalgoorlie). The South Australia Section is responsible for both South Australia (Port Augusta) and the Northern Territory (Alice Springs). The other three sections are New South Wales (Broken Hill), Queensland (Charleville, Mount Isa and Cairns) and Tasmania.

Addresses:

The website is at www.rfds.org.au.

Superintendent, Alice Springs RFDS, Alice Springs, NT 0870.
Director of the New South Wales RFDS Section and Base, PO Box 463, Broken Hill Airport, Broken Hill, NSW 2880.
Superintendent, Cairns RFDS, 1 Junction Street, Cairns, QLD 4870.
General Manager, Royal Flying Doctor Service, 29 Douglas Street, Carnarvon, WA 6071.
General Manager, Central Section of the RFDS, 2 Beulah Road, Kent Town, SA 5067.
Superintendent, Charleville RFDS, Old Cauuamulla Road, Charleville, QLD 4470.
General Manager, Eastern Goldfields RFDS Section and Base, 56 Piccadilly Street, Kalgoorlie, WA 6430.
General Manager, Royal Flying Doctor Service, The Main Street, Meekatharra, WA 6642.
Superintendent, Mount Isa RFDS, Barkly Highway, Mount Isa, QLD 4825.
General Manager, Port Augusta RFDS, 4 Vincent Terrace, Port Augusta, SA 5700.
General Manager, Royal Flying Doctor Service, The Esplanade, Port Hedland, WA 6721.
General Manager, RFDS Queensland Section GPO Box 550, QLD 4001.
General Manager, Royal Flying Doctor Service, Tasmanian Section, PO Box 199, Launceston, TAS 7250.
General Manager, Victoria RFDS Base, Clarendon Street, Derby, WA 6728.
General Manager, Victoria RFDS, 2a River Street, South Yarra, VIC 3141.
General Manager, Western Australia RFDS Section, 3 Eagle Drive, Jandakot Airport, WA 6164.

Flying Obstetrics and Gynaecology Service

124 McDowall Street, PO Box 264, Roma, QLD 4455 Tel: +61 7622 2966. Fax: +61 7622 3520.

This is based in Roma, about eight hours west of Brisbane. Every day, the eight-seater plane flies out with a consultant and registrar in O&G, and an anaesthetist. In the remote hospitals in the outback, one of the seniors runs a clinic while the other runs the surgery. Surgery includes D&Cs, laparoscopies, hysterectomies and the odd Caesarean section. The group running the service is very friendly.

O **Elective notes:** This is an excellent elective (if you don't get air-sick). You are often really needed in theatre and are made to feel part of the team. With supervision they let you do a number of procedures. You must apply at least a year in advance as this is very popular.

Accommodation: Provided in the nurses' quarters of the hospital in Roma.

AFRICAN FLYING DOCTORS:

There are a couple of services in addition to individual hospital services that run in various regions of Africa:

East Africa Flying Doctors Society (AMREF)

11 Old Queen Street, London SW1H 9IA, UK. Tel: +44 20 7233 0066. Fax: +44 20 7233 0099. www.amref.org.

AMREF is an not-for-profit organization to which tourists can pay a kind of insurance. In return, they are provided with an air evacuation service across East Africa. With the money this service generates AMREF, then runs clinics and emergency services for local people.

Flying Doctors Society of Africa

PO Box 30125, Nairobi, Kenya. Tel: +254 2 501300/501301/501302/501303/500508. Tel/fax: +254 2 601594. E-mail: flyingdocs@net2000ke.com. www.flyingdoctorsocietyafrica.com. One branch of this is:

Arusha Flying Doctor Services

PO Box 944, Arusha, Tanzania. Tel: +255 27 250 1593.

There are literally hundreds of private companies throughout the world that provide a retrieval service for insurance companies. They can be found very easily by doing a Google search.

If you're interested in basic physiology you'll love aviation and space medicine. There are probably more organizations you can apply to than you think. NASA is obviously the famous one, but look at some of the links listed below.

NASA

www.nasa.gov.

Doing some research for NASA has become increasingly popular over the last ten years. This, and the state of heightened terrorism alert in the US, has made things much more difficult for the visiting medic. When I originally worked for NASA in 1994 I just faxed some NASA laboratories and got a very positive response. Today the process has been very much formalized. Information and application forms are available from NASA's website. With the recent threats of terrorism, NASA has massively clamped down on security. If you're applying from the US, you may get in; if from outside, chances are you will not. At the time of writing, things are about to change. Check www.medicstravel.org for the latest details.

The main NASA bases doing medical research are **NASA Johnson** (www.jsc.nasa.gov – where the shuttle is controlled from in Houston), **NASA Kennedy** (www.ksc.nasa.gov – where the shuttle takes off in Florida) and **NASA–Ames Space and Research Centres** (www.arc.nasa.gov – a medical and jet propulsion centre just up the San Francisco Bay). There has, however, been a shift from research being done at NASA (a bureaucratic, currently underfunded organization) to getting it done at more fluid, dynamic universities. And this is where a golden opportunity arises. Get to do the same work through the back door – with a NASA-affiliated group. The easiest way to find out about such groups is to use Medline and search for 'NASA', 'gravity' and any other key words that you're interested in (e.g. 'sleep disturbance' or 'space adaptation syndrome'). Look at where the research in these areas is being done and write to them directly. You have a much greater chance of getting a positive response and, since things tend to be less bureaucratic, a greater chance of getting some research done in a limited time.

RUSSIAN SPACE ORGANIZATIONS:

Russian Aviation and Space Agency: www.rosaviakosmos.ru.
Russian Space Research Institute: www.iki.rssi.ru.

The School of Russian and Asian Studies has set also up space medicine programmes: www.sras.org.

OTHER SPACE AGENCIES AND ORGANIZATIONS:

Brazilian Space Agency: www.inpe.br.
British National Space Centre: www.bnsc.gov.uk.
European Space Agency: www.esrin.esa.it.
International Academy of Aviation and Space Medicine: www.iaasm.org.
Italian Space Agency: www.asi.it.
Japanese Space Agency: www.nasda.go.jp.

AMERICAN AVIATION ORGANIZATIONS:

Aerospace Medical Association: www.asma.org.
Civil Aviation Medical Association: www.civilavmed.com.
FAA Civil Aeromedical Institute: www.cami.jccbi.gov.
Flight Safety Foundation Human Factors and Aviation Medicine home page: www.flightsafety.org.

International Civil Aviation Organization: www.icao.org.
USAF School of Aerospace Medicine: www.brooks.af.mil.

UK AVIATION ORGANIZATIONS:

Civil Aviation Authority of the United Kingdom: www.caa.co.uk.

For academic aviation medicine, try the Aviation Medicine Department, RAF Farnborough, Hertfordshire, UK.

AUSTRALIAN AND NEW ZEALAND MEDICAL ORGANIZATIONS:

Aviation Medical Society Australia and New Zealand: www.amsanz.org; New Zealand: www.avmed.org.nz.

OTHER AVIATION ORGANIZATIONS:

Austrian Society for Aerospace Medicine: www.asm.at.
French Aviation and Medicine Society (SOFRAMAS): www.soframas.asso.fr.
German Society of Aviation and Space Medicine: www.dglrm.de.
Israel Aerospace Medicine Institute: www.iami.org.il.

EXPEDITION TRAINING ORGANIZATIONS:

Frontline Medical Services Ltd: Tel: +44 1389 87781. www.frontlinemedics.com.
Plas Y Brenin: National Mountain Centre. www.pyb.co.uk.
Wilderness Medical Society: www.wms.org.
Wilderness Medical Training: The Coach House, Thorny Bank, Skelsmergh, Kendal LA8 9AW, UK. Tel: +44 1539 823183. www.wildernessmedicaltraining.co.uk.

Section 4
The Appendix

Non-governmental and missionary organizations

There are hundreds of non-governmental (NGO) and missionary organizations, many specializing in a particular medical field or geographical area. Remember to check out www.medicstravel.org for up-to-date listings of work available (both voluntary and paid). The World Service Enquiry (WSE) maintains a list of organizations offering placements for volunteers and paid employment. WSE's Guide to Working for Development at Home and Overseas is available online at www.wse.org.uk. British Overseas NGOs for Development (BOND; www.bond.org.uk) holds contact details for over 200 UK-based organizations involved in development. The volunteer recruitment website www.do-it.org.uk has launched a one-stop guide to help people who are interested in volunteering overseas. The site lists organizations offering volunteering opportunities throughout the world for new and experienced volunteers, in addition to case studies and online diaries. For missionary work, there is a fantastic website called www.mfinder.org, which has dozens of opportunities overseas. www.idealist.org has a database of volunteer opportunities.

The UK Department of Health has produced a 'toolkit' giving advice on planning overseas work into your career. It can be found at:
www.doh.gov.uk/internationalhumanitarianand healthwork.

Key:
† = missionary organization
* = only takes those with considerable experience.

*Acord – www.acord.org.uk
Dean Geadley House, 52 Horseferry Road, London SW1P 2AF, UK. Tel: +44 20 7227 8600. Fax: +44 20 7799 1868.

Acord has offices in and sends volunteers to Angola, Botswana, Burkina Faso, Burundi, Chad, the Congo, Eritrea, Ethiopia, Guinea, Liberia, Mali, Mauritania, Mozambique, Namibia, Rwanda, Somalia, Sudan Tanzania and Uganda.

Action against Disability
Regional Rehab Centre, Hunters Road, Newcastle-upon-Tyne NE2 4NR, UK.

Action against Hunger – www.aahuk.org
Unit 7B Larnaca Works, Grange Walk, London SE1 3EW, UK. Tel: +44 20 7394 6300. Fax: +44 20 7237 9960.
Action against hunger provides relief and development to over 40 countries (including parts of Africa, South America and Russia). They offer one-year contracts that incorporate food, travel and accommodation expenses as well as an allowance. Nutritionalists, doctors and nurses are often required.

Action Aid – www.actionaid.org
Hamlyn House, MacDonald Road, London N19 5PG, UK. Tel: +44 20 7561 7561. Fax: +44 20 7272 0899. (They also have offices in Guatemala, Thailand, Zimbabwe and the USA – see their website.)
Action Aid provides help to some of the poorest countries in Africa, South America and Asia.

Action on Disability and Development – www.add.org.uk
Vallis House, 57 Vallis Road, Frome, Somerset BA11 3EG, UK.
Tel: +44 1373 473064. Fax: +44 1373 452075. E-mail: info@add.org.uk.

ADD is a UK-based agency that works with disabled people in 12 of the poorest countries in Africa and Asia.

Action Health
This has now been incorporated into Skillshare (see below).
Action Partners Ministries –
www.actionpartners.org.uk
Bawtry Hall, Bawtry, Doncaster DN10 6JH, UK. Tel: +44 1302 710750.
Fax: +44 1302 719399.
This is a small Christian organization that has links with many hospitals in Africa (Cameroon, Chad, Egypt, Kenya, Ghana, Congo, Sudan and Nigeria). Most of their work concerns rural development, however, there are often places available for doctors and nurses.

†Africa Evangelical Fellowship
6 Station Court, Station Approach, Borough Green, Sevenoaks, Kent TN15 8AD, UK.
The Africa Evangelical Fellowship provides missions to Angola, Botswana, Malawi, Mozambique, Namibia, South Africa, Swaziland, Tanzania, Zambia, Zimbabwe and the Islands of Madagascar, Mauritius and Réunion.

†Africa Inland Mission –
www.aim-us.org or www.aim-eur.org
2 Vorley Road, Archway, London N19 5HE, UK. Tel: +44 20 7281 1184.
Fax: +44 20 7281 4479.
AIM is a missionary organization that runs a number of missionary hospitals in 13 countries in Africa, including Angola, Central African Republic, Comores, Chad, Congo, Kenya, Lesotho, Madagascar, Mayotte, Mozambique, Namibia, Seychelles, Sudan, Tanzania and Uganda. They have previously been very good at aranging short-term placements and electives.

African Medical and Research Foundation (AMREF) –
www.amref.org
11 Old Queen Street, London SW1H 9LA, UK.
AMREF is based in Nairobi and has country offices in Kenya, Uganda, Tanzania and South Africa. There are field offices in Mozambique and Ethiopia, and major programmes in South Sudan, Somalia and Rwanda. AMREF's priority intervention areas are HIV/AIDS, TB, STDs, malaria, water and basic sanitation, disaster management and response, family health, clinical outreach services to remote areas, the development of health learning materials, training and undertaking consultancies. See Section 3 for AMREF's Flying Doctor Service.

Agency for Personal Service (APSO) – www.apso.ie
APSO Head Office, Bishops Square, Redmonds Hill, Dublin 2, Ireland. Tel: +353 1 478 9400. Fax: +353 1 475 1006.
This is the central organization for all of Ireland's NGOs. They can provide information on work throughout Africa and Central America.

American Refugee Committee – www.archq.org
2244 Nicolette Avenue, Suite 250, Minneapolis, MN 55404, USA Tel: +1 612 872 7060. Fax: +1 612 872 4309.

Australian Volunteers International – www.ozvol.org.au
71 Argyle Strett, PO Box 350, Fitzroy, VIC 3065, Australia. Tel: +61 3 9279 1788.
Fax: +61 3 9419 4280.
Australian Volunteers International sends (as its name implies) Australian volunteers to over developing 50 countries. It also sends volunteers to remote Aboriginal settlements throughout Australia. Volunteers have to be Australian, be at least 20 and have at least two years' previous work experience. Posts are usually for a minimum of two years and are salaried at a level comparable to local wages at your destination, hence food and lodging should be covered.

†Baptist Missionary Society – www.bms.org.uk
PO Box 49, Baptist House, 129 Broadway, Didcot, Oxon OX11 8XA, UK. Tel: +44 1235 512 077. Fax: +44 1235 511 265.

The Baptist Missionary Society has a variety of posts, but most useful to readers will be the short-term medical posts. You are usually required to pay towards working with them, but costs are reasonable. Check their website for current availablility.

British Council – www.britishcouncil.org

Bridgewater House, 58 Whitworth Street, Manchester M1 6BB, UK. Tel: +44 161 957 7755. Fax +44 161 957 7762.

The British Council serves to form connections with people worldwide. Their website provides many links.

British Executive Service Overseas (BESO) – www.beso.org

164 Vauxhall Bridge Road, London SW1V 2RB, UK. E-mail: team@beso.org.

BESO works in 146 countries providing professional expertise to other organizations. Medics of all descriptions are often required. There is no upper or lower age limit.

British Nepal Medical Trust – www.bnmt.org.np

130 Vale Road, Tonbridge, Kent TN9 1SP, UK. Tel: +44 1732 360284. Fax: +44 1732 363876.

Working in the eastern region of Nepal, BNMT implements, in close collaboration with the government, three major programmes: TB and leprosy control and management; essential drugs supply and rational use; and community health and development.

†CAFOD – www.cafod.org.uk

2 Romero Close, Stockwell Road, London SW9 9TY, UK.

CAFOD works with partners overseas but does not send people directly – contact Christians Abroad (*see* below).

Calcutta Rescue Fund – www.calcuttarescue.nl

PO Box 16163, Clapham, London SW4 7ZT, UK. Tel: +44 1483 44094.1 Fax: +44 1483 573184.

This organization was set up by Dr Jack Preger, a British National who has made working in Calcutta his life's work.

Nurses, pharmacists, physiotherapists and podiatrists are required with a minimum of 12 months' commitment.

*CARE International UK – www.careinternational.org.uk

Tower House, 8–14 Southampton Street, London WC2E 7HA, UK. Tel: +44 20 7379 5247. Fax: +44 20 7379 0543.

CARE is a very large relief organization concentrating on Africa, South America, Asia and Eastern Europe. It takes only professionals with extensive experience in the areas that are relevant to CARE's current projects. Three years of professional expereince in a developing country and a masters in public health or a diploma in tropical medicine and hygiene are also often required. CARE keep a register of suitable applicants so applying directly is worthwhile. Adverts for specific projects can be found in the *Guardian* newspaper on Thursdays or on the CARE website.

Catholic Institute for International Relations – www.ciir.org

Unit 3, Canonbury Yard, 190a New North Road, London N1 7BJ, UK. Tel: +44 20 7354 0883. Fax +44 20 7359 0017.

The CIIR has a subsection entitled International Cooperation for Development. This is a Skillshare programme that provides healthcare and other workers to around 11 developing countries in Africa, South America, the Caribbean and the Middle East. This includes doctors, nurses, physiotherapists, occupational therapists, pharmacists and midwives. You must be two years post-qualification and contracts are usually for two years.

†Catholic Medical Mission Board – www.cmmb.org

10 West 17th Street, New York, NY, USA. Tel: +1 212 242 7757. Fax: +1 212 807 9161.

CMMB is an American organization that places US and Canadian doctors and nurses in Catholic mission hospitals in Africa, South America, Eastern Europe, the Caribbean and Papua New Guinea. Posts can last from one month to two years and the amount of assistance is proportional to the length of the contract.

†Catholic Network of Volunteer Services – www.cnvs.org

This organization runs an excellent website that connects volunteers to many vacancies in a number of Catholic organizations. Jobs in Africa and South America for doctors, surgeons and nurses are often listed.

Children's Aid Direct

6–8 Crown Street, Reading, Berkshire RG1 2SE, UK. Tel: +44 1189 584000. Fax: +44 1189 581230.

†Christian Aid – www.christian-aid.org.uk

PO Box 100, London SE1 7RT, UK.
While Christian Aid works with many partners overseas, it does not place volunteers there directly. Contact Christians Abroad for overseas work (*see* below).

†Christian Medical Fellowship – www.cmf.org

157 Waterloo Road, London SE1 8XN, UK. Tel: +44 20 7928 4694.

†Christian Outreach Relief and Development – www.cord.org.uk

1 New Street, Leamington Spa, Warwickshire CV31 1HP, UK. Tel: +44 1926 315301. Fax: +44 1926 885786.
CORD currently works in Afghanistan, Cambodia, Mozambique, Rwanda, Tanzania, Vietnam and Zambia. They require committed Chrisians for (initially) one year. All types of health professional are required. Accommodation, expenses and a small salary are usually provided.

†Christians Abroad – www.cabroad.org.uk

1 Stockwell Green, London SW9 9HP, UK. Tel: +44 20 7346 5951.
Fax: +44 20 7346 5955.
Christians Abroad have a number of vacancies. Accomodation, transport and a small local salary are usually provided.

The site is also home to the World Service Enquiry, a database of overseas workers. A monthly listing of overseas jobs (*Opportunities Abroad*) is also published.

†Christoffel Blindenmission – www.cbmi.de

Orwell House, Cowley Road, Cambridge CB4 4WY, UK. Nibelungenstrasse 124, D-6140 Bensheim 4, Germany. Tel: +49 48 6251 1310. Fax: +49 62 5113 1165.
CBM is a Christian organization that prevents and treats blindness and rehabilitates the disabled in around 100 developing countries. Because of this mission, they tend to recruit ophthalmologists, orthopaedic surgeons and physiotherapists for a minimum of two years.

†Church Missionary Society – www.cms-uk.org

Partnership House, 157 Waterloo Road, London SE1 8UU, UK. Tel: +44 20 7928 8681. Fax: +44 20 7401 3215.
CMS has many opportunities for Christians over 18 years of age. Missions can last from three weeks to six years, and all kinds of volunteers (doctors, nurses, teachers, accountants …) are required.

†Church of Scotland World Mission – www.churchofscotland.org.uk

121 George Street, Edinburgh EH2 4YN, UK.

Commonwealth Society for the Disabled

Dilke House, Malet Street, London WC1E 7JA, UK.

Concern Universal – www.concern-universal.org

21 King Street, Hereford HR4 9BX, UK. Tel: +44 1432 355111. Fax: +44 1432 355086.
Concern Universal works in a number of countries in South America and Africa.

Concern Worldwide UK – www.concern.ie

47 Frederick Street, Belfast BT1 2LW, UK.
52–55 Camden Street, Dublin 2, Ireland.

248–250 Lavender Hill, London SW11 1LJ, UK. Tel: +44 20 7738 1033.
Fax: +44 20 7738 1032.

Concern Worldwide provides both emergency relief and long-term development projects to over 20 countries including Angola, Afghanistan, Burundi, Bangladesh, Cambodia, the Congo, East Timor, Ethiopia, Haiti, Honduras, India, Kosovo, Laos, Liberia, Mozambique, North Korea, Rwanda, Sierra Leone, Somalia, Tanzania and Uganda. Applicants must be at least 21 years old, with 18 months of post-qualification work experience. Contracts can last three to six months for emergency relief situations or up to two years for longer-term projects.

CUSO – www.cuso.org

400-2255 Carling Avenue, Ottawa, Ontario K2B 1A6, Canada. Tel: +1 613 829 7445. Fax: +1 613 829 7996.

CUSO supplies Canadian volunteers to Africa, Asia, South America and the Caribbean, and to local projects in Canada itself. They provide a salary to cover living expenditure in your destination, as well as flights, insurance and a lump resettlement cost. Usually only Canadians can volunteer.

Department for International Development – www.dfid.gov.uk

Abercombie House, Eaglesham Road, East Kilbride G75 8EA, UK. 94 Victoria Street, London SW1E 5JL, UK. Tel: +44 20 7917 0107. Fax: +44 20 7917 0174.

DFID does not actually place volunteers overseas although their website has a number of useful links.

Edinburgh Medical Missionary Society – www.emms.org

7 Washington Lane, Edinburgh EH11 2HA, UK. Tel: +44 131 313 3828. Fax: +44 131 313 4662.

The EMMS has links with hospitals in Africa, Asia and South America. They have previously been very good at helping with electives.

Emmanuel Hospital Association – www.eha.org.uk

European Fellowship, PO Box 43, Sutton, Surrey SM2 5WL, UK. Head Office: 808/92 Deepali Building, Nehru Place, North Delhi 19, India. Tel/Fax: +91 11 643 2055.

EHA provides healthcare via 19 hospitals and 27 community projects across Northern India. Basic healthcare needs such as hygiene and literacy are an intergral part of their projects. They recruit most medical and surgical specialities as well as dentists, nurses, other healthcare workers and non-medical people such as architects, teachers, accountants and builders. Contracts are for between six months and two years and an allowance to cover living costs in India is provided. The volunteer has to provide the travel costs.

Friends of Ludhiana – www.friendsofludhiana.org.uk

157 Waterloo Road, London SE1 8UU, UK. Tel: +44 20 7928 1173.

This is the UK support centre for the Christian Medical College, Ludhiana, Punjab, India.

Goal UK – www.goal.ie

c/o Mean Road, London W3 8AN, UK or PO Box 19, Dun Loaghaire, County Dublin, Ireland. Tel: +252 1 280 9779. Fax: +353 1 280 9215.

Halo Trust – www.halotrust.org

PO Box 7905, Thornhill, DG3 5WA, UK Fax: +44 1848 331122.

The Halo Trust specializes in mine clearance. Specialist personnel only are required.

Handicap International – www.handicap-international.org

14 Avenue Bethelot, 69361 Lyon, France. Tel: +334 7869 7979. Fax: +334 7869 7994.

Hands around the World – www.handsaroundtheworld.org.uk

PO Box 25, Coleford, Gloucestershire GL16 7YL, UK. Tel: +44 1594 560223.

HATW specializes in sending individuals to provide help in developing countries.

Healthnet International – www.healthnetinternational.org

Singel 540, 1017 Amsterdam, The Netherlands. Tel: +31 20 512 0640. Fax: +31 20 420 1503.

Healthnet is a Dutch organization that sends volunteers to areas of chronic crisis and post-conflict situations.

Health Unlimited – www.healthunlimited.org

Prince Consort House, 27–29 Albert Embankment, London SE1 7TS, UK. Tel: +44 20 7582 5999. Fax: +44 20 7582 5900.

Health Unlimited provides help to indigenous people in Brazil, Burma, Cambodia, China, El Salvador, Guatemala, Laos, Namibia, Nicaragua, Peru and Somalia. Most of their work is of a public health nature, promoting disease prevention by working with local people and promotions such as radio campaigns. For these reasons, public health rather than clinical specialists are usually recruited. Contracts are usually for around two years and salary and flights are paid. Vacancies can be found on their website, in the *Guardian* newpaper and in the International Health Exchange's magazine.

Health Volunteers Overseas – www.hvousa.org

PO Box 65157, Washington DC 20035-5157, USA. Tel: +1 202 296 0928. Fax: +1 202 296 8018.

HVO provides volunteers to teach healthcare in Africa, Asia, the Caribbean and South America. Anaesthetists, surgeons (especially maxillary-facial and orthopaedic), paediatricians, dentists and nurses are usually required. Note: The prinicple of HVO is to teach rather than actually provide healthcare. Most posts last for two to four weeks. Any nationality can apply, but expenses (usually around $3000 for a month) have to be covered by the volunteers themselves.

*HelpAge International – www.helpage.org

67–74 Saffron Hill, London EC1N 8QX, UK. Tel: +44 20 7404 7201.

HelpAge supports disadvantaged older people in over 49 countries throughout Africa, Asia and South America. They run emergency programmes following disasters and conflicts.

HMD Response International – www.hmdresponse.org

3 Pembridge Square, London W2 4DR, UK. Tel: +44 20 7229 7447. Fax: +44 20 7229 3434.

Response International has both paid and volunteer work in areas of recent conflict (Bosnia, Kosovo, Lebanon and Pakistan). Doctors (GPs), nurses and physiotherapists as well as those with public health skills are required.

Institute for Health Sector Development – www.Ihsd.org

27 Old Street, London EC1V 9HL, UK.

IHSD sends its own in-house consultants to advise on major projects overseas.

Institute for International Cooperation and Development – www.Iicd-volunteer.org

PO Box 520, Williamstown, MA 01267, USA. Tel: +1 413 458 9828. Fax: +1 413 258 3323.

The IICD organizes voluntary work in India, Africa and South America for periods of 6–18 months. Volunteers have to pay a fee (usually US$3000–6000).

Interaction – www.Interaction.org

1717 Massachusetts Avenue NW, Suite 701 Washington DC 20036, USA. Tel: +1 202 667 8227.

Interaction is an alliance of 160 US NGOs that cover every developing country. Check out their website for details.

International Care and Relief – www.icrcharity.com

27 Church Road, Tunbridge Wells, Kent TN1 1HT, UK. Tel: +44 1892 519619. Fax: +44 1892 529029.

ICR works in some of the world's poorest areas to provide sanitation, basic needs and primary healthcare while teaching self-sustainability.

International Child Care Trust
Unit 3L, Leroy House, 436 Essex Road, London N1 3QP, UK.

International Health Exchange –
www.ihe.org.uk
134 Lower Marsh Road, London SE1 7AE, UK. Tel: +44 20 7620 3333. Fax: +44 20 7620 2277. E-mail: info@ihe.org.uk.
The IHE is a central organization that helps to recruit health professionals to many international organizations. It lists available jobs in its two magazines – *The Health Exchange* and *Job Supplement* – and also on the web. It runs a number of courses for those planning to work overseas.

International Medical Corps –
www.imcworldwide.org
US address: 11500 West Olympic Boulevard, Suite 506, Los Angeles, CA 90064-1524, USA. Tel: +1 310 826 7800. Fax: +1 310 442 662. UK address: 3 Anselm Road, Hatch End, Pinner, Harrow, Middlesex HA5 4LH, UK.
Tel: +44 208 428 4025.
IMC is an American-based, non-profit-making organization that provides medical and other staff to areas of war, disaster or longstanding poverty. They offer a good salary and cover costs.

†International Nepal Fellowship –
www.inf.org.np
Nepal head office: PO Box 5, Pokhara, Nepal. Tel: +977 6 120 111. Fax: +977 6 120 430. UK office: 69 Wentworth Road, Harborne, Birmingham B17 9SS, UK.
Tel: +44 121 427 8833.
Fax: +44 121 428 3110.
The INF has many projects across Nepal, but areas of particular speciality include TB, leprosy, HIV and community health. They require a broad range of health professionals for both hospital and community-based work. Volunteers have to pay expenses. Check their website for placement availability. Note: You should be a practising Christian to work with INF.

International Rescue Committee –
www.theirc.org
122 East 42nd Street, 12th Floor, New York, NY 10168–1289, USA.
Tel: +1 212 551 3000. Fax: +1 212 551 3180.
The IRC is a non-profit-making, non-sectarian organization providing aid for refugees around the world. Founded by Albert Einstein to aid those being oppressed by war and violence, their current emphasis is on helping those in Afghanistan although they have projects in 30 countries. They provide emergency medical and public health support.

International Rescue Corps –
www.intrescue.org
8 Kings Road, Grangemouth, Stirlingshire FK3 8HW, UK.
The IRC is a frontline search and rescue organization that has participated in work after a number of disasters in the UK and overseas.

International Service –
www.Internationalservice.org.uk
Suite 3a, Hunter House, 57 Goodramgate, York YO1 7FX, UK. Tel: +44 1904 647799. Fax: +44 1904 652353.
International Service takes doctors, nurses and other health professionals to a number of countries in South America, the Middle East and Africa to collaborate with local organizations. Missions are for two years minimum, but flights, accomodation and an allowance are provided.

International Voluntary Service Inc
1424 16th Street NW, Suite 504, Washington DC 20036, USA.

†Interserve – www.interserve.org
325 Kennington Park Road, London SE11 4QH, UK. Tel: +44 20 7735 8227. Fax: +44 20 7587 5362.
Interserve is a Christian organization that sends all kinds of professionals (doctors, nurses, dentists, accountants, teachers, engineers, etc.) on both short- and long-term missions to many countries in the developing world. Their website lists current vacancies.

Jerusalem Princes Basma Centre for Disabled Children

PO Box 19764, Jerusalem 91197, Israel.
Tel: +972 2 626 4536. Fax: +972 627 4449.
The Princes Basma provides rehabilitation, hydrotherapy and physiotherapy for disabled children. The minimum stay is three months. A small sum of 'pocket money' is provided.

Latin Link – www.latinlink.org

175 Tower Bridge Road, London SE1 2AB, UK. Tel: +44 20 7939 9000.
Fax: +44 20 7939 9015.
Latin Link works in Argentina, Bolivia, Brazil, Costa Rica, Ecuador, Nicaragua and Peru. It performs both medical and community development work and takes doctors, nurses and medical students (on electives). All must be committed Christians and ideally speak Spanish or Portuguese (depending on the destination). Most work is for a minimum of three years, although there are some short contracts of one to two years.

LEPRA – www.lepra.org.uk

Fairfax House, Causton House, Colchester CO1 1PU, UK.
LEPRA works in a number of countries including India, Nepal, China, Brazil and Madagascar to try to eliminate leprosy. They are interested to hear from any medical volunteers.

†Leprosy Mission – www.leprosymission.org

International office: 80 Windmill Road, Middlesex TW8 0QH, UK. Tel: +44 20 8569 7292. Fax: +44 20 8569 7808. UK office: Goldhay Way, Orton Goldhay, Peterborough PE2 5GZ, UK. Tel: +441733 370505. Fax: +44 1733 370960.
The Leprosy Mission is a Christian organization that works in over 30 countries throughout Africa and Asia. Doctors, surgeons, occupational therapists and physiotherapists are required. All must be at least two years post-qualification and be committed, practising Christians (of a Protestant or Reformed denomination).

*Marie Stopes International – www.mariestopes.org.uk

153–157 Cleveland Street, London W1P 5PG, UK. Bruce Mackay, 62 Grafton Way, London W1P 5LD, UK.
Tel: +44 20 7574 7423.
It is principally concerned with providing reproductive and sexual health information in 38 countries. It also runs clinics in countries such as Kenya.

Marlborough Brandt Group – www.mgb.org

1a London Road, Malborough, Wiltshire SN8 1PH, UK. Tel: +444 1672 514078.
Fax: +44 1672 514922.
This UK-based charity has links with the village of Gunjur in the Gambia, West Africa.

MEDAIR – www.medair.org

13 Highfield Oval, Ambrose Lane, Harpenden AL5 4BX, UK.
MEDAIR provides relief and rehabilitation in favour of the most vulnerable, mostly women, children and the sick, in countries affected by war or natural disaster. They go to areas of greatest need, often very inaccesible areas. At the time of writing, such areas include Afghanistan, Angola, Uganda, Sudan and Madagascar. They require doctors and nurses who are committed Christians to work for a minimum of (usually) one year. They provide flights and training and pay $100 a month for the first year, increasing to $1000 a month thereafter. Unlike many agencies, you only need to have one year post-qualification experience (you don't need a PhD in public health, etc.). Vacancies are listed on their website.

Médecins du Monde UK – www.medecinsdumonde.org

11 Sovereign Close, Sovereign Court, London E1 9HW, UK. Tel: +44 20 7488 4888.
Médecins du Monde needs medical workers for nearly 300 projects in 57 countries. They will take volunteers for as little as three months.

**Médecins sans Frontières –
www.msf.org**
International office: Rue de la Tourelle 39,
B-1040 Brussels, Belgium. Tel: +32 2 280
1881. Fax: +32 2 280 0173. UK office:
124–132 Clerkenwell Road, London EC1R
5DL, UK. Tel: +44 20 7713 5600. Fax: +44
20 7713 5004. US office: 6 East 39th
Street, 8th Floor, New York, NY 10016,
USA. Tel: +1 212 679 6800. Fax: +1 212
679 7016. Canadian office: 720 Spadina
Avenue, Suite 402, Toronto, Ontario M5S
2T9, Canada. Tel: +1 416 964 0619. Fax: +1
416 963 8707. Australian office: PO Box
847, Broadway, NSW 2007, Australia. Tel:
+61 2 9552 4933. Fax: +61 2 9552 6539.
MSF is the world's largest independent
organization for emergncy medical relief,
operating in over 80 countries where
there have been either natural or man-
made disasters. They want skilled medical and technical people aged over 25 for
a minimum of nine months, although surgeons (who need to have three years of
higher surgical training) and anaethetists
can get shorter posts of between six
weeks and three months post-conflict.
Doctors need to be two years post-
registration, and nurses two years' post-
qualification. Experience in general
practice, O&G, paeds and tropical
disesases (ideally the diploma) are very
desirable. The cost to the volunteer is nil.

Medical Aid for Iraq
Unit 16, Foundation House, 38 Kingsland
Road, London E2 EDQ, UK.

Medical Aid for Palestinians
33a Islington Park Street, London
N1 1QB, UK. Tel: +44 20 7226 4114.
Fax: +44 20 7226 0880.
Placements, for six months (and longer),
mainly in the West Bank, Gaza Strip and
Lebanon, are given to experienced doctors
and nurses to provide emergency relief and
long-term training. Flights, accommodation and a living allowance are provided.

**Medical Emergency Relief
International – www.merlin.org.uk**
14 David Mews, London W1M 1HW, UK.
Tel: +44 20 7487 2505.
Fax: +44 20 7487 4042.

MERLIN provides emergency relief following natural disasters, conflicts or epidemics regardless of religion or politics.
They particularly target areas where the
local health infrastructure has collapsed.
Ideally, they stabilize the area over six to
twelve months and then withdraw. You
can register with them to be considered
for work as a doctor/surgeon or nurse. A
background in public health or tropical
medicine is especially desirable.
Contracts are for six to twelve months
and an allowance is provided.

**†Medical Missionaries for Mary –
www.medical-missionaries.com**
66 Newland Street, Silvertown, London
E16 2HN, UK.

**Mercy Corps –
www.mercycorps.org**
UK office: 11 Grovelands Avenue,
Swindon, Wiltshire SN1 4ET, UK.
Tel: +44 1793 486 036.
Fax: +44 1793 643 383. US office: 3015
SW First Avenue, Portland, OR 97201,
USA. Tel: +1 800 292 3355.
The website lists (mainly non-health-
related) jobs around the world.

**†Methodist Church Overseas
Division**
Reverend Winston Graham, Overseas
Division, 25 Marylebone Road, London
NW1 5JR, UK. Tel: +44 20 7486 5502.
Fax: +44 20 7487 4042.

**†Mid Africa Ministry –
www.midafricaministry.org**
Partnership House, 157 Waterloo Road,
London SE1 8UY, UK. Tel: +44 20 7928
8681. Fax: +44 20 7401 2910.

**Mines Advisory Group –
www.mag.org.uk**
47 Newton Street, Manchester M1 1FT,
UK. Tel: +44 161 236 4311.
Fax: +44 161 236 6244.

**†Nepal Leprosy Trust –
www.rec.org.uk/nlt**
Nepal office: PO Box 96, Kathmandu,
Nepal. UK office: 15 Duncan Road,

Richmond, Surrey TW9 2JD, UK. Tel: +44 181 332 9023. Fax: +44 181 948 2703.

The NLT helps to rehabilitate those with leprosy and TB in Western Terai, Nepal.

Ockenden Venture –
www.ockenden.org.uk

Constitution Hill, Woking, Surrey GU22 7UU, UK. Tel: +44 1483 772012. Fax: +44 1483 750774.

The Ockenden Venture works to promote self-reliance for refugees, displaced people, returnees and their host communities throughout the world.

One World Action –
www.oneworldaction.org

Bradley's Close, White Lion Street, London NW1 9PF, UK. Tel: + 44 20 7833 4075. Fax: +44 20 7833 4102.

This group works in Angola, Bangladesh, Cape Verde, El Salvador, Guatemala, Honduras, Namibia, Nicaragua, the Philippines, South Africa and the Western Sahara.

Operation Crossroads Africa –
www.igc.org/oca

475 Riverside Drive, Suite 1366, New York, NY 10115, USA Tel: +1 212 870 2106. Fax: +1 212 870 2644.

Operation Crossroads Africa is geared to sending pre-medical/nursing as well as medical and nursing students on community and medical projects in Brazil and 12 African countries. They also take qualified volunteers to help training. There are usually around ten volunteers per group and projects last six weeks. The projects are based in rural communities and run from mid-June to mid-August. Applicants should be between 17 and 35 years old. The fee is $3500 but help with fundraising can be provided. There is a (compulsory) three-day orientation course in New York.

*Oxfam – www.oxfam.org

274 Banbury Road, Oxford OX2 7DZ, UK. Tel: +44 1865 311311. Fax: +44 1865 312380.

They tend only to organize work in the country in which they are based but may offer advice on work overseas.

Plan International –
www.plan-international.org

5–6 Underhill Street, London NW1 7HS, UK. Tel: +44 20 7482 9777. Fax: +44 20 7482 9778.

Population Concern –
www.populationconcern.org.uk

Studio 325, Highgate Studios, 53–79 Highgate Road, London NW5 1TL, UK. Tel: +44 870 770 2476. Fax: +44 20 7267 6788.

Project Hope –
www.projecthope.org

Wilson Building, Stockley Park West, Uxbridge UB1 1BT, UK. Tel: +44 208 990 2864. Fax: +44 208 990 4383.

Health Opportunities for People Everywhere works in 30 countries.

Quaker Peace and Service Friends House

173 Euston Road, London NW1 2BJ, UK.

Raleigh International –
www.raleigh.org.uk

27 Parsons Green Lane, London SW6 4HZ, UK.

Raleigh is a youth development charity organizing community and environmental expeditions around the world. Applicants are usually aged between 17 and 25 (over 25s are staff). Expeditions usually take three months and you have to raise some funds. Medical staff (doctors and nurses, mimimum age 25) are also required.

*Red Cross Society –
www.redcross.org.uk
(www.redcross.org in USA)

9 Grosvenor Crescent, London SW1X 7EJ, UK. Tel: +44 20 7235 5454. Fax: +44 207 245 6315. Australian Red Cross: PO Box 100, East Melbourne, VIC 3002. Tel: +61 3 9418 5200. Fax: +61 3 9419 0404. New Zealand Red Cross: Red Cross House, 14 Hill Street, Wellington 1, PO Box 12-140, New Zealand. Tel: +64 4 472 3750. Fax: +64 4 473 0315. American Red Cross: Office of the President, 17th and D

Streets, Washington DC 20006, USA.
Tel: +1 202 728 6600. Fax: +1 202 775
0733. Canadian Red Cross: 1800 Alta Vista
Drive, Ottawa, Ontario K1G 4JG, Canada.
Tel: +1 613 739 3000.
Fax: +1 613 731 1411.
The Red Cross, together with the Red
Cresent, provides professional volunteers following natural disasters and
conflicts. The headquarters is in
Geneva (International Committee of the
Red Cross, 19 Avenue de la Paix, CH
1202, Geneva, Switzerland. Tel: +41 22
734 6001. Fax: +41 22 733 2057.
www.icrc.org), but your first point of
contact should be the society in your
own country. The Red Cross provides
professional aid to a number of
countries. This can be short term after a
disaster or conflict, or more long term.
Doctors and nurses with an acute
surgical or anaesthetic skill are therefore
required, especially in conflict or disaster situations. Primary healthcare skills
are also important. They keep a register
of potential volunteers. You must be
between 25 and 50 years of age for your
first secondment and registered with the
General Medical Council if you are a
doctor or with the United Kingdom
Central Council for Nursing, Midwifery
and Health Visiting if a nurse from the
UK. Doctors need to be registrar or consultant level, and nurses should be at
least three years post-qualification. For
community projects, a degree in public
health or tropical medicine is often
required. Flights, a local allowance and a
salary are provided.

Rescue and Preparedness in Disasters – www.rapidsar.org.uk
Beech Lodge, Jacobstowe, Okehampton,
Devon EX20 3RG, UK.
RAPID is an emergency response organization that sends trained volunteers out
to areas following conflicts and natural
disasters.

Rotary Doctor Bank of GB and Ireland
Alan Thomas, Morawelon, St Hilary,
Cowbridge CF71 7DP, UK.

Ryder–Cheshire Foundation – www.rydercheshire.org.uk
82 Queen's Road, Brighton BN1 3XE, UK.
Tel: +44 1273 821056.
Fax: +44 1273 821059.
The foundation can place physiothera-
pists.

†Salvation Army – www.salvationarmy.org
Health Services, 101 Queen Victoria
Street, PO Box 249, London EC4 4EP, UK.
Tel: +44 20 7332 0101.
Fax: +44 20 7236 4981.
The Salvation Army has links with many
mission hospitals around the world.

Sandy Gall's Afghanistan Appeal – www.sandygallsafghanistanappeal.org
PO Box 145, Tonbridge, Kent TN11 8SA, UK.
This organization helps with prosthetics,
orthotics and physiotherapy in
Afghanistan.

†SAO Cambodia (formerly Southeast Asian Outreach) – www.sao-cambodia.org
Bawtry Hall, Bawtry, Doncaster
DN10 6JH. Tel: +44 1302 714004.
Fax: +44 1302 710027.
SAO has a number of development pro-
jects in Cambodia. Qualified healthcare
workers can apply for both short- and
long-term missions.

*Save The Children Fund – www.savethechildren.org.uk
Leonie Lonton, 17 Grove Lane,
Camberwell, London SE5 8RD, UK.
Tel: +44 20 7703 5400.
Fax: +44 20 7703 2278.
Save the Children encourages locals to
work and rarely sends out volunteers.
Only highly qualified people are required.

†Scottish Churches World Exchange – www.worldexchange.org.uk
7 Randolf Crescent, Edinburgh EH3 7TH,
UK.
The World Exchange offers both short
visits and longer-term (one year)
exchanges all over the world.

Scottish European Aid
5 Lemington Terrace, Edinburgh,
EH10 4JW, UK.

Skillshare International – www.skillshare.org
126 New Walk, Leicester LE1 7JA, UK.
Tel: +44 116 254 1862.
Fax: +44 116 254 2614.
Action Health has now merged with Skillshare. They sends professional volunteers to Botswana, India, Lesotho, Mozambique, Namibia, South Africa, Swaziland and Tanzania, and to train local people in inexpensive, effective healthcare skills. They provide costs but you must be between 21 and 63 years of age, have skills and work for a minimum of six months. You have to have at least two years of post-qualification experience, although not necessarily have previous overseas work experience. Applications from all healthcare professionals (including those as couples or with families) are welcome. Note: You will be required to do some fundraising before you go. Accommodation, food and transport costs as well as a small monthly allowance are provided.

†Tear Fund – www.tearfund.org
Anthea Fisher, 100 Church Road, Teddington, Middlesex TW11 8QR, UK. Tel: +44 20 8977 9144. Fax: +44 20 8943 3594.
Tearfund works with Christian groups in over 90 countries on relief and development projects. Community-based health professionals are required and a salary, as well as travel costs, is provided.

Terre des Hommes – www.terredeshommes.org
PO Box 388, 1000 Lausanne, Switzerland.

†Trocaire – www.trocaire.org
169 Booterstown Avenue, Blackrock, Co Dublin, Ireland. Tel: +353 1 288 5385.
This is the Irish Catholic Agency for World development. Trocaire provides support both to development and disaster relief projects.

Tropical Health and Education Trust – www.thet.org
Professor Eldryd Parry, 24 Eversholt Street, London NW1 1AD, UK.
Tel: +44 20 7679 8127/8128/8129.
Fax: +44 20 7679 8190.
THET aims to relieve the disadvantages in training for healthcare in poorer tropical countries and to promote health through collaboration in teaching and research. It has many links between UK and African hospitals. Medical staff from all disciplines (including, for example, laboratory technicians) are required to train local people.

Ugandan Society for Disabled Children
68 Adrian Road, Abbots Langley, Hertfordshire WD5 0AQ, UK. Tel. +44 1923 263102. Fax: +44 1923 267838. E-mail: ugandasoc@aol.com.

*UNICEF UK – www.unicef.org
UK offices: Africa House, 64–78 Kingsway, London WC2B 6NB, UK. 55 Lincolns Inn Fields, London WC2, UK. Tel: +44 20 7405 5592. Fax: +44 20 7405 2332. Geneva office: Palais des Nations, 1211 Genève 10, Switzerland. US office: UNICEF House, 3 United Nations Plaza, New York, NY 10017, USA.
Although UNICEF does not send volunteers overseas directly, it does run the United Nations Volunteer programme (www.unv.org). Applications can be made online.

United Nations Association International Service
Stella Hobbs, Suite 3a, Hunter House, 57 Goodramgate, York YO1 2LS, UK. Tel: +44 1904 647799. Fax: +44 1904 652 353.
UNAIS works with locally managed initiatives in Bolivia, Brazil, Burkina Faso, Mali and the West Bank and Gaza Strip. Primary healthcare is a particular priority. You must be over 18 and two years' commitment is usually required, but costs are covered.

United Nations Volunteers –
www.unv.org
Postfach 260 111, D-53153 Bonn, Germany. Tel: +49 228 815 2000. Fax: +49 228 815 2001. But send CVs to: United Nations Volunteers Offshore Processing Centre, PO Box 25711, 1311 Nicosia, Cyprus.

UNVs are currently working in 150 countries; many volunteers are doctors, nurses and midwives acting to help develop health services within communities. Seventy per cent of UNVs are themselves from developing countries. The average length of an assignment is two years.

United Society for the Propagation of the Gospel –
www.uspg.org.uk
Partnership House, 157 Waterloo Road, London SE1 8XA, UK. Tel: +44 020 7928 8681. Fax: +44 20 7928 2371.

URBANAID
79 Amsterdam Road, London Yard, London E14 3UU, UK. Tel: +44 20 7515 7366.

Voluntary Services Overseas –
www.vso.org.uk
317 Putney Bridge Road, London SW15 2PN, UK. Tel: +44 20 8780 7500. Fax: +44 20 8780 7207.

VSO is the largest overseas volunteer recruiting agency in the world and sends professionals to Africa, Asia, the Pacific Islands and Eastern Europe. Their website has a database of work available for pharmacists, doctors, dentists, midwives, nurses, health educators/administrators, radiographers, dieticians, occupational therapists, physiotherapists and speech therapists. You have to be two years post-qualification. Most posts are of two years' duration (though some as short as three months are occasionally available). Flights, accommodation and a living allowance are provided.

Volunteer Missionary Movement –
www.vmmusa.org or www.iol.ie
1 Stockwell Green, London SW9 9JF, UK. Tel: +44 20 7737 3678. Fax: +44 20 7346 5955.

This ecumenical organization recruits and prepares volunteers for a number of skills in Africa (Uganda, Kenya, Tanzania, Zambia) and Central America (Guatemala). You must be over 24 years old and a commitment of two years is normally required.

Wateraid – www.wateraid.org.uk
Prince Consort House, 27–29 Albert Embankment, London SE1 7UB, UK. Tel: +44 20 7793 4500. Fax: +44 20 7793 4545.

Although primarily involved with the supply of water to areas in Asia and Africa, Wateraid also has a hygiene programme that requires healthcare workers. Placements are usually advertised in the *Guardian* newspaper and on their website.

World Church and Mission
8 Tavistock Place, London WC1H 9RT, UK.

World Exchange –
www.worldexchange.org.uk
St Colm's International House, Inverleith Terrace, Edinburgh EH3 5NS, UK. Tel: +44 131 315 4444.

World Exchange has information on exchanges (usually lasting a year) all over the world.

*World Health Organization –
www.who.org
Personnel Officer, Avenue Apia 20, 1211 Geneva 27, Switzerland.

†World Service Enquiry –
www.wse.org.uk
233 Bon Marché Centre, 241–251 Ferndale Road, London SW9 8BJ, UK. Tel: +44 870 770 3274. Fax: +44 870 770 7991.

This organization provides vocational information to both Christians and non-Christians. They have information on voluntary and paid opportunities for short- (from two weeks) or long-term work in aid, development and mission agencies. They cater for the skilled and unskilled over 18 years of age.

†Worldvision –
www.worldvision.org.uk
World Vision House, 599 Avebury Boulevard, Milton Keynes MK9 3PG, UK. Tel: +44 1908 841000. Fax: +44 1908 841001. Worldvision is a large Christian organization providing development and relief projects to over 100 countries.

†Worldwide Evangelisation for Christ International –
www.wec-int.org
Bulstrode, Oxford Road, Gerrards Cross, Buckinghamshire SL9 8SZ, UK. Tel: +44 1753 884631. Fax: +44 1753 882470.

WEC is an interdenominational organization working in over 60 countries. Medical posts for doctors, nurses, midwives and physiotherapists are available in the Middle East, Ghana, Chad, the Congo and Guinea Bissau.

Youth Vision with a Mission
Highfield Oval, Ambrose Lane, Harpenden AL5 4BX, UK.

The number of grants available is phenomenal. The best place to start is www.rdinfo.org.uk. Another site with many useful links is www.man.ac.uk/rcn/ukwide/ukrfund.html. Below are a few of the more commonly used ones.

AH Bygott Undergraduate Scholarships

Secretary to the Academic Trust Funds Committee, University of London, Senate House (Room 234), Malet Street, London WC1E 7HU, UK. Tel: +44 20 7862 8041. Fax: +44 20 7862 8042. E-mail: L.West@acadmic.lon.ac.uk.

This is only for London medical/dental students doing electives in public health. Awards of up to £750 are made. Note: They also give a £1500 award to a postgraduate for research work, including travel in public health and related subjects.

Alchemy Foundation

Trevereux Manor, Limpsfield Chart, Oxted, Surrey RH8 0TL, UK.

Anglo French Medical Society – www.anglofrenchmedical.org

They give £250 for an elective in a French-speaking country.

Anglo-Israel Association

9 Bentinck Street, London W1M 5RP, UK. Tel: +44 20 7486 2300. Fax: +44 20 7935 4690.

The Wyndham Deedes Memorial Travel Scholarship is open to graduates or senior students who travel to Israel to study an aspect of Israeli life (economical, cultural, scientific, etc.). Each scholarship is valued up to £2000. You must stay at least six weeks and write a 5000 word essay.

Association for the Study of Medical Education – www.asme.org.uk

12 Queen Street, Edinburgh EH2 1JE, UK. Tel: +44 131 225 9111. Fax: +44 131 225 9444. E-mail: info@asme.org.uk.

They offer a £300 prize for a piece of work/survey or research in a field of medical education.

Association of Anaesthetists of Great Britain and Ireland

Honorary Secretary, 9 Bedford Square, London WC1B 3RA, UK.

The association offers prizes for essays written.

British Association of Dermatologists

19 Fitzroy Square, London W1T 6EH, UK. Tel: +44 20 7383 0266. Fax: +44 207 388 5263. E-mail: admin@bad.org.uk.

They offer ten grants of £500 for undergraduate projects on dermatology or skin biology – 'The effect of too much sun during my elective'!

British Association of Forensic Medicine

Department of Forensic Pathology, Medico-Legal Centre, Watery Street, Sheffield S3 7ES, UK. Tel: +44 114 2738721.

They offer a prize (awarded retrospectively) of around £200 for the best elective report on a project undertaken in forensic medicine. It needs to be a scientific-type presentation of around 2000 words.

British Association of Plastic Surgeons – www.baps.co.uk

Royal College of Surgeons, 35–43 Lincoln's Inn Fields, London WC2A 3PN, UK.

They have 10 annual elective grants of around £500 each. Applications in the form of a letter giving an itinerary and costs, together with a brief CV, should be submitted to the Chairman of the Education and Research Sub-Committee. A report is required three months after your return. The closing date for application is the end of January each year.

British Federation of Women Graduates

28 Great James Street, London WC1N 3ES, UK. Tel: +44 20 7404 6447. Fax: +44 20 7404 6505.

They have previously helped with living expenses.

British Geriatrics Society for the Health of the Aged

1 St Andrew's Place, Regents Park, London NW1 4LB, UK.

The society offers awards of up to £500 to UK medical students doing electives concerned with health/healthcare in old age.

British Medical and Dental Student's Trust

Secretary, Mackintosh House, 120 Blythswood Street, Glasgow G2 4EA, UK. Tel: +44 141 221 5858. Fax: +44 141 228 1208.

They give a number of awards, often around the £150–600 mark.

British Nutrition Foundation – www.nutrition.org.uk

High Holborn House, 52–54 High Holborn, London WC1V 6RQ, UK. Tel: +44 20 7404 6504. Fax: +44 20 7404 6747.

The foundation runs the following two schemes. **The Nestlé Bursary Scheme**: Since 1978, the *BNF* and Nestlé Charitable Trust have aimed to 'help medical students to undertake an elective concerned with nutritional problems encountered in the Third World, associated with adults in apparent health and disease states, including the special areas of maternal health and infant nutrition'. Twelve bursaries of up to £500 are available. A report is required five months after your return. The **Dennis Burkitt Study Awards**: This is also run by the *BNF* (in conjunction with Kellogg's).

The ten awards (a tribute to Burkitt, as in lymphoma and research into diet and worldwide disease) are for students of medicine, nutrition science and related subjects who undertake studies into food and nutrition, especially in developing countries. Awards of up to £750 are made.

British Society for Haematology

Scientific Secretary, 2 Carlton House Terrace, London SW1Y 5AF, UK.

Eight scholarships, each a maximum of £600, are awarded to medical students wishing to do an elective project involving haematology. Send a letter outlining the project and costs, and letters from your dean and the host institution.

Cancer UK

10 Cambridge Terrace, London NW1 4JL, UK.

Cancer UK gives ten bursaries of £1000 each to UK medical students doing an elective involving the prevention, detection, treatment or management of cancer. There is a maximum of one per school and a six-page report is required within three months of your return.

Child Health Research Appeal Trust

Institute of Child Health, University of London, 30 Guildford Street, London WC1N 1EH, UK.

Five awards of £125 a week are offered nationally for those undertaking epidemiological, psychiatric or community-based clinical work in the UK only. Apply to the Registrar.

Clegg Scholarship

BMJ, BMA House, Tavistock Square, London WC1H 9TR, UK.

This is for an elective with the *BMJ* to learn about medical journalism.

Commonwealth Foundation Medical Elective Bursaries

The foundation offers awards for senior medical students doing electives in developing Commonwealth countries.

They are not available for Australia, the UK, Canada or New Zealand. Countries covered include the following. *Africa*: Botswanna, Cameroon, the Gambia, Ghana, Kenya, Lesotho, Malawi, Mauritius, Mozambique, Namibia, South Africa, Swaziland, Tanzania, Uganda, Zambia and Zimbabwe. *Caribbean*: Belize, Dominica, Grenada, Guyana, Jamaica, St Lucia, St Vincent, Trinidad and Tobago. *Asia*: Bangladesh, India, Malaysia, Pakistan, Singapore and Sri Lanka. *Pacific*: Fiji, Kiribati, Nauru, Papua New Guinea, Solomon Islands, Tonga, Tuvalu, Vanuatu and Western Samoa. Approximately 50 awards of up to £1000 are offered for tenure in May each year; you should apply via your dean before January. A report is required on your return. The award is given on (1) the feasibility and scientific merit of the attachment proposed and its usefulness to the student and receiving institution, and (2) the educational record and motivation of the student.

Eating Disorders Association
Sackville Place, 44 Magdalen Street, Norwich, Norfolk NR3 1JU, UK.
This offers prizes for essay writing.

Edinburgh Medical Missionary Society – www.emms.org
The society offers £200 travel bursaries to committed Christian students arranging electives.

Edward Boyle Memorial Trust
Six elective bursaries of up to £500 each are offered. A separate application is not required if you are applying to the Commonwealth Foundation.

Faculty of Public Health Medicine of the Royal Colleges of Physicians of the UK
4 St Andrew's Place, London NW1 4LB, UK.
The faculty offers the Cochrane Prize for UK medical students doing an educational activity in public health.

Israel Medical Association
22 Macheson Road, London NW3 2LU, UK. Tel: +44 20 7267 6784. Dr Lionel Balfour-Lynn, 120 Harley St, London W1N 1AG, UK.
There are eight £300 awards for medical students doing their elective in a hospital in Israel. Include your CV, a proposal of what you will be doing and a letter from your host.

Jacki Deakin Dystonia Prize – www.dystonia.org.uk
Prizes of £1000, £500 and £250 are awarded.

Kabi Pharmacia Elective Grant
Kabi Pharmacia Ltd, Knowhill, Milton Keynes MK5 8PH, UK.
They make six awards of £250 for those doing electives in developing countries. Awards are made on the basis of a written application of no more that 400 words. Write to Dr Richard Wild, Haderburg Medical Director at the above address.

LEPRA (British Leprosy Relief Association)
Fairfax House, Causton Road, Colchester, Essex CO1 1PU, UK. Tel: +44 1206 5662286. Fax: +44 1206 762151.
LEPRA offers awards for essays.

Leukaemia Research Fund
43 Great Ormond Street, London WC1N 3JJ, UK. Tel: +44 20 7405 0101. Fax: +44 20 7242 2488.
They make five awards of up to £600 for electives allied to the study of haematological malignancy.

Lord Mayor's 800th Anniversary Awards Trust
401 Salisbury House, London Wall, London EC2M 5RR, UK. Tel: +44 20 7638 8358. Fax: +44 20 7638 9681.
They have previously given awards to medical students going on elective. Preference is given to those who have a connection with the City of London. Applicants need to be aged between 17 and 25, and grants are normally around £500.

Medical Research Council
20 Park Crescent, London W1N 4AL, UK.
Tel: +44 20 7636 5422. Fax: +444 20 7636 3427.
The MRC runs the Rogers Fund for an elective period in the tropics.

Medical Society for the Study of Veneral Diseases
1 Wimpole Street, London W1M 8AE, UK.
The society offers a £200 prize for a report (maximum 2000 words) on STD or genitourinary or HIV medicine.

Medical Women's Federation Student Elective Bursaries
62 Denbigh Street, London SW1V 2EX, UK.
One award of £300 is made to a London student studying maternal or child health in a developing country. Submit a CV and a project outline.

Medicine Group and The Glaxo Wellcome Medical Fellowship
Medicine Group (Journals) Ltd, Freespost, Elective Grant Co-ordinator, Publishing House, 62 Stret Street, Abingdon, Oxon OX14 3BR, UK. Tel: +44 1235 555770.
Fax: +44 1235 554691.
Annually (on 31st March) the group awards one £400 prize to an applicant from each UK medical school for an elective in the following 12 months. One top award of £1000 is given. Send a CV and comprehensive description of your proposed elective and your reasons for doing it, confirmation from your host (if available) and the names of two referees (your dean and a consultant).

Mental Health Foundation – www.mentalhealth.org.uk
20/21 Cornwall Terrace, London NW1 4QL, UK. Tel: +44 20 7535 7400.
Fax: +44 20 7535 7474.
This is for electives in psychiatry and may require an essay. Eight awards of up to £400 are made.

Milupa Student Elective Grant Fund
Milupa Ltd, Milupa House, 1390 Uxbridge Road, Hillingdon, Middlesex UB10 0NE, UK. Tel: +44 20 8573 9966.
Fax: +44 20 8569 2175.
Ten awards of up to £500 are given nationally for an elective with research into paediatric nutrition. Write to the Managing Director.

National Birthday Trust Fund
27 Sussex Place, Regent's Park, London NW1 4SP, UK.
The fund provides two awards of £250 for those doing electives in obstetrics or neonatology.

Newby Trust Limited
Hill Farm, Froxfield, Petersfield, Hampshire GU32 1BQ, UK.

Pathological Society of Great Britain and Ireland
Education Secretary, Royal College of Pathologists, 2 Carlton House Terrace, London SW1Y 5AF, UK.
Awards are made of up to £50 a week for a maximum of 12 weeks. You will need to submit a report within three months of your return; £150 is given to the best.

Renal Association
Triangle House, Broomhill Road, London SW18 4HX, UK. Tel: +44 20 8875 2413.
Fax: +44 20 8877 9308.
There are four bursaries of £250 for medical students doing an elective of which renal medicine is a significant component.

Royal College of General Practitioners
The RCGP offers elective prizes for primary care/GP electives.

Royal College of Obstetricians and Gynaecologists
27 Sussex Place, Regent's Park, London NW1 4RG, UK. Tel: +44 20 7262 5425.
Fax: +44 20 7723 0575.
Prizes are offered for students showing the greatest understanding of a clinical

problem in O&G. Provide a case history with a maximum of 3000 words.

Royal College of Surgeons of England – research@rcseng.ac.uk

Preiskel Elective Prize in Surgery, Research and Audit Board, 35/43 Lincoln's Inn Fields, London WC2A 3PN, UK
Tel: +44 20 7312 6672.
Fax: +44 20 7831 5741.
The college gives awards of between £500 and £1000 for students wishing to pursue a career in surgery who do a surgical elective in the developing world. Send six copies of: your CV, details of the proposed project, a letter from your dean and a letter from the surgeon at the host institution.

Royal Society of Medicine – anaesthesia@rsm.ac.uk

Section of Anaesthesia, 1 Wimpole Street, London W1G 0AE, UK. Tel: +44 20 7290 2986. Fax: +44 20 7290 2989.

Royal Society of Medicine

Section of the History of Medicine, 1 Wimpole Street, London W1M 8AE, UK.
Tel: +44 20 7290 2985.
Fax: +44 20 7290 2989.
They offer the Norah Schuster Prize to preclinical, clinical and dental students.

Royal Society of Tropical Medicine and Hygiene

Manson House, 26 Portland Place, London W1N 4EY, UK. Tel: +44 20 7580 2127.
Fax: +44 20 7436 1389.
There is an award of £500 for an account of any work carried out by a medical student of any nationality during an elective in a tropical/developing county. It is awarded on originality and contribution to the knowledge/understanding of tropical diseases.

St Francis Leprosy Guild

21 The Boltons, London SW10 9SU, UK.
The guild has previously given elective awards of up to £600 for those doing electives involving leprosy.

Scottish Eastern Association of the Medical Women's Federation

Royal Hospital for Sick Children, 2 Rillbank Crescent, Edinburgh EH9 1LF, UK.
This is open to female medical students in Aberdeen, Dundee and Edinburgh, with awards of £200 twice a year.

Sir John Cass's Foundation

PO Box 853, 31 Jewry Street, London EC3N 2HA, UK. Tel: +44 20 7480 5884.
They can offer awards to students who have been residents in inner London for the previous three years and who are under 25 years of age.

Society of Occupational Medicine

6 St Andrew's Place, Regent's Park, London NW1 4LB, UK. Tel: +44 20 7486 2641. Fax: +44 20 7486 0028.
The Thackrah Award for Undergraduate Study of Occupational Medicine is offered at up to £1000 for research or an elective in occupational medicine. It is funded by Nestlé UK.

Vandervell Foundation

Bridge House, 181 Queens Street, London EC4 4DD, UK. Tel: +44 20 7248 9045.

Wellbeing (The Health Research Charity for Women and Babies)

27 Sussex Place, Regent's Park, London NW1 4SP, UK. Tel: +44 20 722 5337.
Fax: +44 17 724 7725.
They run the National Birthday Trust Fund that each year gives two bursaries of £250 to elective students studying obstetrics or neonatal paediatrics.

Winston Churchill Memorial Trust – www.wcmt.org.uk

15 Queen's Gate Terrace, London SW7 5PR, UK. Tel: +44 20 7584 9315.
Fax: +44 20 7581 0410.
Set up to commemorate Winston Churchill, the trust offers around 100 awards a year (totalling around £500 000). Each year, they produce a leaflet suggesting categories to apply for. They can be very broad e.g. 'Health

Promotion for Young People' or 'Leadership in the Community'. Any medical staff could therefore apply if they are doing anything that is either personally or community-enhancing.

Other bursaries that are available only through your clinical school registry are:

Churchill Livingstone Student Bursary: one award of £1000 for an essay.

Clinical Endocrinology Trust Elective Bursaries: 10 awards of £500 are made nationally.

Cow and Gate Prize: medical schools (departments of paediatrics) often have information on a number of their prizes.

Dr Robert Malcolm Trust Awards: a £300 award is available for every medical school.

Royal College of Physicians: Oscar Reginald Lewis Wilson Scholarship: a £250 award is awarded to an applicant from each medical school that is British or a member of the Commonwealth. Applications are viewed in terms of a proposed project and the student's financial situation.

University of London Convocation: two awards of variable amounts are made per school.

Wellcome Trust student elective prizes: this is open to UK medical students who must do a research project under supervision in any discipline bar cancer. One-third of awards are for tropical medicine. Up to £1000 can be given for personal support and up to £600 for the costs of the project. Nominations are only accepted from the dean of your medical school (or the director of an overseas Wellcome Trust); do not contact the Wellcome Trust directly. Each school has a quota of awards, and a 1500-word essay is required on your return. Contact addresses for two Wellcome Trust Overseas units are as follows. *Kenya*: Dr W. Watkins, Wellcome Trust Laboratories, PO Box 43640, Nairobi, Kenya. Tel: +254 2 711673. *Thailand and Vietnam*: Grants Administrator, Nuffield Department of Clinical Medicine Room 5803, John Radcliffe Hospital, Headington, Oxford OX3 9DU, UK.

GRANTS FOR NURSES AND OTHER HEALTHCARE PROFESSIONALS:

The fantastic website www.rdinfo.org.uk lists virtually all funding for travel and research. Try searching on this site for your speciality and 'travel'. Other good places to start are the finacial support section of the RCN's website – www.rcn.org.uk/support/support_financial_rcn.html – and www.man.ac.uk/rcn/ukwide/ukrfund.html.

USEFUL READING

Career Development for Nurses – Opportunities and Options by J Sanderson (1993. Scutari Press, 17–19 Peterborough Road, Harrow-on-the-Hill, Middlesex HA1 2AX, UK.) This has a section on funding and finance.

Sponsorship for Students by R. Theodorou (1999. Hobsons. Contact the Careers and Occupations Information Centre (COIC), Room E455, Moorfoot, Sheffield S1 4PQ, UK).

Students Grants and Loans – a Brief Guide (Department for Education and Employment, Student Support Division, Mowden Hall, Staindrop Road, Darlington DL3 9BG, UK. Tel: +44 1325 392822. Also obtainable from any local education authority).

Charities Digest by C. Rios (2002. Family Welfare Association, 501–505 Kingsland Road, London E8 4AA, UK).

The Directory of Grant Making Trusts by D. Casson et al (2003–2004. Charities Aid Foundation. Available from main nursing reference libraries and large reference libraries).

The Grants Register (2003. Palgrave Macmillan, 4 Little Essex Street, London WC2R 3LD, UK).

The Pocket Guide to Grant Applications by I.K. Crombie and C. du V. Florey

(1998. BMJ Books, London). This provides advice on how to approach organizations and contains guidelines on drawing up grant applications.
The Springboard Sponsorship and Funding Directory (2000. Careers Research and Advisory Centre).

A few popular grants include those from the:

British Association of Critical Care Nurses, Administration, Crown House, 28 Winchester Road, Romsey, Hampshire SO51 8AA, UK. Tel: +44 1794 521767. www.baccn.org.uk. (They offer grants of up to £2000.)

Nuffield Trust RCN Travel Fellowship, www.rcn.org.uk. (The trust offers up to £5000 for overseas work.)

Scottish Hospital Endowments Research Trust, Princes Exchange, 1 Earl Grey Street, Edinburgh EH3 9EE, UK. Tel: +44 131 659 8800. Fax: +44 131 228 8118. www.shert.com. (They offer travel grants of up to £1500.)

Chartered Society of Physiotherapy Research and Clinical Effectiveness Unit, 14 Bedford Row, London WC1R 4ED, UK. Tel: +44 20 7306 6666/6617. www.csp.org.uk. (Awards of up to £15 000 are offered.)

The following section contains pretty comprehensive lists of embassies in the UK, Australia and America. Embassies occasionally move or change phone number. If you have any problems, either look in the phone book, do a search on the Internet or visit www.embassyworld.com, which lists all the major embassies.

Embassies in the UK

Afghanistan: Embassy of the Islamic State of Afghanistan, 31 Princes Gate, London SW7 1QQ. Tel: +44 20 7589 8891/8892. Fax: +44 20 7589 3452.

Albania: Embassy of the Republic of Albania, 4th Floor, 38 Grosvenor Gardens, London SW1W OEB. Tel: +44 20 7730 5709. Fax: +44 20 7730 5747.

Algeria: Algerian Embassy, 54 Holland Park, London W11 3RS. Tel: +44 20 7221 7800. Fax: +44 20 7221 0448. E-mail: mail@admi.freeserve.co.uk. www.personal.u-net.com/~consalglond/.

Angola: Angolan Embassy, 98 Park Lane, London W1Y 3TA. Tel: +44 20 7495 1752. Fax: +44 20 7495 1635.

Argentina: Embassy of Argentina, 65 Brook Street, London W1Y 1YE. Tel: +44 20 7318 1300. Fax: +44 20 7318 1301. E-mail: blj@atina.ar. www.argentine-embassy-uk.org/.

Armenia: Embassy of the Republic of Armenia, 25a Cheniston Gardens, London W8. Tel: +44 20 7938 5435.

Australia: Australian High Commission, Australia House, The Strand, London WC2B 4LA. Tel: +44 20 7379 4334. Fax: +44 20 7240 5333. www.australia.org.uk/. Consulate (Immigration Managed Post): Chatsworth House, Lever Street, Manchester M1 2DL. Tel: +44 161 228 1344. Fax: +44 161 236 4074.

Austria: Austrian Embassy and Consular Section, 18 Belgrave Mews West, London SW1X. Tel: +44 20 7235 3731.

Azerbaijan: Republic Embassy of Azerbaijan, 4 Kensington Court, London W8. Tel: +44 20 7938 3412.

Bahamas: Bahamas High Commission, 10 Chesterfield Street, London W1X. Tel: +44 20 7408 4488.

Bahrain: Embassy of the State of Bahrain, 98 Gloucester Road, London SW7. Tel: +44 20 7370 5132.

Bangladesh: Bangladesh High Commission, 28 Queens Gate, London SW7. Tel: +44 20 7584 0081.

Barbados: Barbados High Commission, 1 Great Russell Street, London WC1. Tel: +44 20 7631 4975.

Belarus: Embassy of the Republic of Belarus, 6, Kensington Court, London W8 5DL. Tel: +44 20 7937 3288. Fax: +44 20 7361 0005.

Belgium: Belgian Embassy, 103 Eaton Square, London SW1W 9AB. Tel: +44 20 7470 3700. Fax: +44 20 7259 6213. www.belgium-embassy.co.uk/.

Belize: Belize High Commission, 22 Harcourt House, 19 Cavendish Square, London W1M. Tel: +44 20 7499 9728.

Benin: Benin Consulate, Dolphin House, 16 The Broadway, Stanmore, Middlesex HA7 4DW. Tel: +44 20 8954 8800. Fax: +44 20 8954 8844.

Bermuda: Bermuda Society and Secretariat, Five Trees Wood Lane, Stanmore, Middlesex HA7. Tel: +44 20 8954 0652.

Bolivia: Bolivian Embassy, 106 Eaton Square, London SW1W 9AD. Tel: +44 20 7235 4248 or +44 20 7235 4255 (consulate). Fax: +44 20 7235 1286.

Bosnia and Herzegovina: Embassy of Bosnia and Herzegovina, 320 Regent Street, 4th Floor, London W1R 5AB. Tel: +44 20 7255 3758. Fax: +44 20 7255 3760.

Botswana: Botswana High Commission, 6 Stratford Place, London W1N 9AE. Tel: +44 20 7499 0031.

Brazil: Brazilian Embassy, 32 Green Street, London W1Y 4AT. Tel: +44 20 7499 0877. Fax: +44 20 7493 5105. www.brazil.org.uk/.

Brunei: Brunei Darussalam High Commission, 19–20 Belgrave Square, London SW1X. Tel: +44 20 7581 0521.

Bulgaria: Embassy of the Republic of Bulgaria, 186–188 Queens Gate, London. Tel: +44 20 7584 9400.

Cameroon: Cameroon Embassy, 84 Holland Park, London W11. Tel: +44 20 7727 0771.

Canada: Canadian High Commission, 1 Grosvenor Square, London W1X 0AB. Tel: +44 20 7258 6601. Fax: +44 20 7258 6506. www.canada.org.uk.

Caribbean: Eastern Caribbean Commission, 10 Kensington Court, London W8. Tel: +44 20 7937 9522.

Cayman Islands: Cayman Islands Government Office in the UK, 6 Arlington Street, London SW1A 1RE. Tel: +44 20 7491 7772. Fax: +44 20 7491 7944.

Chile: Chilean Embassy, 12 Devonshire Street, London W1N. Tel: +44 20 7580 6392.

China: Embassy of the People's Republic of China, 31 Portland Place, London W1N 3AG. Tel: 0891 990909 or +44 20 7631 1430. Manchester: Denison House, 49 Denison Road, Manchester M14 5RX. Tel: +44 161 224 8672. Edinburgh: 43 Station Road,

Edinburgh EH12 7AF. Tel: +44 131 316 4789.
www.chinese-embassy.org.uk.
Colombia: Colombian Embassy, 3 Hans Crescent,
London SW1X. Tel: +44 20 7589 9177.
Congo, Democratic Republic of: Congolese
Embassy, 26 Chesham Place, London SW1X 8HH.
Tel: +44 20 7235 6137. Fax: +44 20 7235 9048.
Also 12 Caxton Street, London SW1H.
Tel: +44 20 7222 7575.
Costa Rica: Costa Rican Embassy, Flat 1, 14
Lancaster Gate, London W1 3LH. Tel: +44 20 7706
8844. Consulate: Flat 2, 38 Redcliffe Square,
London SW10 9JY. Tel: +44 20 7373 7973.
Cote d'Ivoire: Embassy of the Republic Cote
d'Ivoire, 2 Upper Belgrave Street, London SW1.
Tel: +44 20 7235 6991.
Croatia: Embassy of the Republic of Croatia,
21 Conway Street, London W1P.
Tel: +44 20 7387 1144.
Cuba: Commercial Office of the Cuban Embassy,
167 High Holborn, London WC1V.
Tel: +44 20 7240 2488.
Cyprus: Cyprus High Commission, 93 Park Street,
London W1Y. Tel: +44 20 7499 8272.
Czech Republic: Czech Embassy, 26 Kensington
Palace Gardens, London W8 4QY. Tel: +44 20 7243
1115/7900. Fax: +44 20 7727 9654.
Denmark: Royal Danish Embassy, 55 Sloane
Street, London SW1X 9SR. Tel: +44 20 7333 0200.
Fax: +44 20 7333 0270. www.denmark.org.uk/.
Consulate in Edinburgh: 4 Royal Terrace, Edinburgh,
UK. Tel: +44 131 556 4263.
Dominica: Dominican High Commission,
1 Collingham Gardens, London W8.
Tel: +44 20 7370 5194.
Ecuador: Embassy of Ecuador, Flat 3b,
3 Hans Crescent, London SW1X.
Tel: +44 20 7584 1367.
Egypt: Embassy of the Arab Republic of Egypt,
2 Lowndes Street, London SW1X.
Tel: +44 20 7235 9719.
El Salvador: Embassy of El Salvador, Tennyson
House, 159 Great Portland Street, London W1N.
Tel: +44 20 7436 8282.
Eritrea: Consulate of the State of Eritrea,
96 White Lion Street, London N1.
Tel: +44 20 7713 0096.
Estonia: Estonian Embassy, 16 Hyde Park Gate,
London SW7 5DG. Tel: +44 20 7589 3428.
Fax: +44 20 7589 3430. E-mail: loa@estonia.gov.uk.
www.estonia.gov.uk/.
Ethiopia: Ethiopian Embassy, 17 Princes Gate,
London SW7. Tel: +44 20 7589 7212.
Europe: Commission of the European
Communities, 8 Storeys Gate, London SW1P.
Tel: +44 20 7973 1992.
Fiji: Embassy of Fiji, 34 Hyde Park Gate, London
SW7. Tel: +44 20 7584 3661.
Finland: Finnish Embassy, 38 Chesham Place,
London SW1X 7JT. Tel: +44 20 7838 6200. Fax: +44
20 7235 3680. E-mail: sanomat.lon@formin.fi.
www.finemb.org.uk.
France: French Embassy, 58 Knightsbridge, London
SW1X 7JT. Tel: +44 20 7201 1000/7838 2055.
Fax: +44 20 7201 1004. www.ambafrance.org.uk/.
Gabon: Gabonese Embassy, 27 Elvaston Place,
London SW7. Tel: +44 20 7823 9986.

Gambia: Gambia High Commission,
57 Kensington Court, London W8.
Tel: +44 20 7937 6316.
Georgia: Georgian Embassy, 3 Hornton Place,
Kensington, London W8. Tel: +44 20 7937 8233.
Germany: German Embassy, 23 Belgrave Square,
London SW1X. Tel: +44 20 7824 1300. Fax: +44 20
7824 1435. E-mail: mail@german-embassy.org.uk.
www.german-embassy.org.uk/.
Ghana: High Commission for Ghana, 104 Highgate
Hill, London N6. Tel: +44 20 8342 8686.
Greece: Consulate General of Greece, 1a Holland
Park, London W11. Tel: +44 20 7221 6467.
Guatemala: Embassy of Guatemala, 13 Fawcett
Street, London SW10. Tel: +44 20 7351 3042.
Fax: +44 20 7376 5708.
Guyana: Guyana High Commission, 3 Palace
Court, Bayswater Road, London W2 4LP.
Tel: +44 20 7229 7684/7688.
Fax: +44 20 7727 9809.
Honduras: Embassy of Honduras, 115 Gloucester
Place, London W1H 3PJ. Tel: +44 20 7486 4880.
Fax: +44 20 7486 4550.
Hungary: Embassy of Hungary, 35B Eaton Place,
London SW1X 8BY. Tel: +44 20 7235 2664.
Visa line: 0891 171204. Fax: +44 20 7235 8630.
Iceland: Icelandic Embassy, 1 Eaton Terrace,
London SW1W. Tel: +44 20 7590 1100.
Fax: +44 20 7730 1683.
India: High Commission of India, India House,
Aldwych, London WC2B. Tel: +44 20 7836 8484.
www.hcilondon.org/. *Consulate in Glasgow:* Fleming
House, 6th Floor, 134 Renfrew Street, Glasgow G3
7ST. Tel: +44 141 331 0777. Fax: +44 141 331 0666.
E-mail: cgiglasgow@btinternet.com.
Indonesia: Indonesian Embassy, 38 Grosvenor
Square, London W1X. Tel: +44 20 7499 7661.
Iran: Embassy of Iran, 16 Princes Gate, London
SW7. Tel: +44 20 7225 3000.
Iraq: Iraqi Embassy, 21 Queens Gate, London
SW7. Tel: +44 20 7584 7141.
Ireland: Embassy of Ireland, 17 Grosvenor Place,
London SW1X 7HR. Tel: +44 20 7235 2171.
Fax: +44 20 7245 6961.
Israel: Israeli Embassy, 2 Palace Green,
London W8 4QB. Tel: +44 20 7957 9500. Fax: +44
20 7957 9555. E-mail: isr-info@dircon.co.uk.
www.israel-embassy.org.uk/london/.
Italy: Italian Embassy, 14 Three Kings Yard, London
W1Y 2EH. Tel: +44 20 7312 2200. 24 hour
information line: 0891 600340 (50p a minute).
Fax: +44 20 7312 2283. E-mail:
emblondon@embitaly.org.uk.
www.embitaly.org.uk/. *Edinburgh consulate general*:
32 Melville Street, Edinburgh EH3 7HA. Tel: +44
131 226 3631/220 3695. Fax: +44 131 226 6260.
London consulate general: 38 Eaton Place,
London SW1X 8AN. Tel: +44 20 7235 9371.
Fax: +44 20 7823 1609.
Jamaica: Jamaican High Commission, 1–2 Prince
Consort Road, London SW7 2BZ. Tel: +44 20 7823
9911. Fax: +44 020 7589 5154. E-mail:
jamhigh@jhcuk.com. www.jhcuk.com/.
Japan: Embassy of Japan, 101–104 Piccadilly,
London W1V 9FN. Tel: +44 20 7465 6500. Fax: +44
20 7491 9347. E-mail: info@embjapan.org.uk.
www.embjapan.org.uk/.

Embassies

Jordan: Embassy of the Hashemite Kingdom of Jordan, 6 Upper Phillimore Gardens, London W8 7HB. Tel: +44 20 7937 3685. Fax: +44 20 7937 8795. www.jordanembassyuk.gov.jo/.

Kazakstan: Embassy for the Republic of Kazakstan, 33 Thurloe Square, London SW7. Tel: +44 20 7581 4646.

Kenya: Kenya High Commission, 45 Portland Place, London WIN. Tel: +44 20 7636 2371.

Korea: Embassy of the Republic of Korea, 4 Palace Gate, London W8 5NF. Tel: +44 20 7581 0247/3330 (visa section). Fax: +44 20 7581 8076.
Also 60 Buckingham Gate, London SW1.
Tel: +44 20 7227 5500.

Kuwait: Embassy of the State of Kuwait, 2 Alberts Gate, London SW1X. Tel: +44 20 7590 3400.

Kyrgz Republic: Kyrgz Republic Embassy, 119 Crawford Street, London W1H 1AF.
Tel: +44 20 7935 1462. Fax: +44 20 7935 7449.
E-mail: embassy@kyrgyz-embassy.org.uk.
www.kyrgyz-embassy.org.uk/.

Latvia: Latvian Embassy, 45 Nottingham Place, London W1M 3FE. Tel: +44 20 7312 0040 Fax: +44 20 7312 0042. E-mail: latemb@dircon.co.uk.

Lebanon: Lebanese Embassy, 21 Kensington Palace Gardens, London W8. Tel: +44 20 7229 7265.

Lesotho: High Commission of the Kingdom of Lesotho, 7 Chesham Place, Belgravia, London SW1 8HN. Tel: +44 20 7235 5686.

Liberia: Liberian Embassy, 2 Pembridge Place, London W2. Tel: +44 20 7221 1036.

Libya: Libyan Interests Section, 119 Harley Street, London. Tel: +44 20 7486 8250.

Lithuania: Embassy of the Republic of Lithuania, 84 Gloucester Place, London W1H.
Tel: +44 20 7486 6401.

Luxembourg: Luxembourg Embassy, 27 Wilton Crescent, London SW1X. Tel: +44 20 7235 6961.

Macedonia: Embassy of the Republic of Macedonia, 10 Harcourt House, 19a Cavendish Square, London W1M 9AD. Tel: +44 20 7499 5152. Fax: +44 20 7499 2864.

Madagascar: Consulate of the Republic of Madagascar, 16 Lanark Mansions, Pennard Road, London W12. Tel: +44 20 8746 0133.

Malawi: Malawian Embassy, 33 Grosvenor Street, London W1X 0DE. Tel: +44 20 7491 4172.
Fax: +44 20 7491 9916.

Malaysia: Malaysian Embassy, 45 Belgrave Square, London SW1 8QT. Tel: +44 20 7235 8033.

Malta: Malta High Commission, Malta House, 36–38 Piccadilly, London W1V. Tel: +44 20 7292 4800.

Mauritius: Mauritius High Commission, 32 Elvaston Place, London SW7. Tel: +44 20 7581 0284.

Mexico: Mexican Embassy, 42 Hertford Street, London W1Y 7TF. Tel: +44 20 7499 8586. Fax: +44 20 7495 4035. E-mail: mexuk@easynet.co.uk. www.demon.co.uk/mexuk/. *Consular section:* 8 Halkin Street, London SW1X 7DW. Tel: +44 20 7235 6393. Fax: +44 20 7235 5480. E-mail: consullondon@easynet.co.uk.

Monaco: Consulat Général de Monaco, 4 Cromwell Place, London SW7 2JE. Tel: +44 20 7225 2679. Fax: +44 20 7581 8161.

Mongolia: Mongolian Embassy, 7 Kensington Court, London W8. Tel: +44 20 7937 5238.

Morocco: Moroccan Embassy, 49 Queens Gate Gardens, London SW7. Tel: +44 20 7581 5001.

Mozambique: Mozambique High Commission, 21 Fitzroy Square, London W1. Tel: +44 20 7383 3800.

Myanmar: Embassy of the Union of Myanmar, 19a Charles Street, London W1X. Tel: +44 20 7499 8841.

Namibia: Namibian High Commission, Centre Link, 34 South Molton Street, London W1Y 2BP. Tel: +44 20 7344 9706. Fax: +44 20 7409 7306. Also 6 Chandos Street, London W1M 0LQ. Tel: +44 20 7636 6244. Fax: +44 20 7637 5694.

Nepal: Royal Nepalese Embassy, Visa Section, 12A Kensington Palace Gardens, London W8 4QU. Tel: +44 20 7229 1594. Fax: +44 20 7792 9861.

Netherlands: Royal Netherlands Embassy, 38 Hyde Park Gate, London SW7. Tel: +44 20 7590 3200.

New Zealand: New Zealand High Commission, New Zealand House, Haymarket, London SW1Y 4TQ. Tel: +44 20 7930 8422 (chancery), +44 20 7973 0366, +44 20 7973 0370 (immigration/visas), +44 20 7930 8422/020 7839 4580 (consular/ passports), +44 20 7973 0363/7839 8929 (tourism). www.nzembassy.com.

Nicaragua: Nicaraguan Consulate, 58 Kensington Church Street, London W8. Tel: +44 20 7938 2373.

Nigeria: Nigeria High Commission, 56–57 Fleet Street, London EC4Y 1BT. Tel: +44 20 7353 3776. Visas: +44 20 7353 3776, ext. 227–229. Fax: +44 20 7353 4352. Also Nigeria House, 9 Northumberland Avenue, London WC2N. Tel: +44 20 7839 1244.

Norway: Royal Norwegian Embassy, 25 Belgrave Square, London SW1X 8QD. Tel: +44 20 7591 5500. Fax: +44 20 7245 6993. E-mail: morten@embassy.norway.org.uk.
www.norway.org.uk.

Oman: Embassy of the Sultanate of Oman, 167 Queens Gate, London SW7. Tel: +44 20 7225 0001.

Pakistan: High Commission for Pakistan (Medical Division), 36 Lowndes Square, London SW1X 9JN. Tel: +44 20 7664 9200. Fax: +44 20 7664 9224.

Panama: Embassy of Panama, 48 Park Street, London W1Y. Tel: +44 20 7493 4646. *Consulate:* 40 Hertford Street, London. Tel: +44 20 7409 2255.

Papua New Guinea: Visa Section, PNG High Commission, 14 Waterloo Place, London SW1Y 4AR. Tel: +44 20 7930 0922/0926.

Paraguay: Embassy of Paraguay, Braemar Lodge, Cornwall Gardens, London SW7 4AQ. Tel: +44 20 7937 1253/6629. Fax: +44 20 7937 5687.

Peru: Peruvian Consulate General, 52 Sloane Street, London SW1X 9SP. Tel: +44 20 7235 6867 Fax: +44 20 7823 2789.

Philippines: Philippines Embassy, 9a Palace Green, London W8 4QE Tel: +44 20 7937 1600. Fax: +44 20 7937 2125.

Poland: Embassy of Poland, Chancery, 47 Portland Place, London W1N 4JH. Tel: +44 20 7580 4324. Fax: +44 20 7323 4018. www.poland-embassy.org.uk/. *Edinburgh consulate general:* 2 Kinner Road, Edinburgh EH3 5PE.
Tel: +44 131 552 0301. Fax: +44 131 552 1086.

Portugal: Portuguese Embassy, 11 Belgrave Square, London SW1X. Tel: +44 20 7235 5331.

Qatar: Qatar Embassy, 30 Collingham Gardens, London SW5. Tel: +44 20 7370 6871.

Romania: Embassy of Romania, 4 Palace Green, London W8. Tel: +44 20 7937 9666.
Russian Federation: Russian Federation Embassy, 13 Kensington Palace Gardens, London W8 4QX. Tel: +44 20 7229 3628/3629. Fax: +44 20 7727 8624/7727 8625/7299 5804. *Consulate:* 5 Kensington Palace Gardens, London W8 4QS. Tel: +44 20 7229 8027. Recorded visa message: 0891 171271. Fax: +44 20 7229 3215. *Consulate in Edinburgh:* Tel: +44 131 225 7098. Fax: +44 131 225 9587.
Rwanda: Embassy of the Republic of Rwanda, 58–59 Trafalgar Square, London WC2N. Tel: +44 20 7930 2570.
Saudi Arabia: Royal Embassy of Saudi Arabia, 119 Harley Street, London W1N. Tel: +44 20 7935 9931.
Senegal: Senegalese Embassy, 11 Phillimore Gardens, London W8 7QG. Tel: +44 20 7937 0925/0926. Fax: +44 20 7937 8130. Also 39 Marioes Road, London W8. Tel: +44 20 7938 4048.
Seychelles: Seychelles Embassy, PO Box 4PE, 2nd Floor, Eros House, 11 Baker Street, London W1M 1FE. Tel: +44 20 7224 1660. Fax: +44 20 7487 5756. www.seychelles.uk.com/.
Sierra Leone: Sierra Leone High Commission, 33 Portland Place, London W1N. Tel: +44 20 7636 6483.
Singapore: Singapore High Commission, 9 Wilton Crescent, London SW1X 8RW. Fax: +44 20 7245 6583/7235 8315.
Slovakia: Embassy of the Slovak Republic, 25 Kensington Palace Gardens, London W8 4QY. Tel: +44 20 7243 0803. Fax: +44 20 7727 5824.
Slovenia: Embassy of Slovenia; Cavendish Court, 11–15 Wigmore Street, London W1H 9LA. Tel: +44 20 7495 7775. Fax: +44 20 7495 7776. E-mail: slovene-embassy.london@virgin.net. www.embassy-slovenia.org.uk/.
South Africa: South African High Commision, South Africa House, Trafalgar Square, London WC2N 5DP. Tel: +44 20 7451 7299. Fax: +44 20 7451 7284. www.southafricahouse.com.
Spain: 39 Chesham Place, London SW1X 8SB. Tel: +44 20 7235 5555. Fax: +44 20 7235 9905. *Consulate general:* 20 Draycott Place, London SW3 2RZ. Tel: +44 20 7589 8989.
Sri Lanka: High Commission of the Democratic Socialist Republic of Sri Lanka, 13 Hyde Park Gardens, London W2 2LU. Tel: +44 20 7262 1841/1842/1843/1844/1845/1846. Fax: +44 20 7262 7970. E-mail: lancom@easynet.co.uk. http://ourworld.compuserve.com/homepages/lanka/.
Swaziland: Kingdom of Swaziland High Commission, 20 Buckingham Gate, London SW1E. Tel: +44 20 7630 6611.
Sweden: Embassy of Sweden, Consular Section, 11 Montagu Place, London W1H 2AL. Tel: +44 20 7724 2101/7917 6400. Fax: +44 20 7917 6475/6476. E-mail: embassy@swednet.org.uk. www.swedish-embassy.org.uk/ embassy/index.html.
Switzerland: Swiss Embassy, 16–18 Montagu Place, London W1H 2BQ. Tel: +44 20 7616 6000. Fax: +44 20 7724 7001. E-mail: vertretung@lon.rep.admin.ch. www.swissembassy.org.uk/.
Syria: Syrian Embassy, 8 Belgrave Square, London SW1X. Tel: +44 20 7245 9012.

Tanzania: Tanzania High Commission, 43 Hertford Street, London W1Y 8DB. Tel: +44 20 7499 8951. Fax: +44 20 7491 9321. E-mail: Balozi@tanzania-online.gov.uk. www.tanzania-online.gov.uk.
Thailand: Royal Thai Embassy, 29–30 Queen's Gate, London SW7 5JB. Tel: +44 20 7589 2944. Fax: +44 20 7823 9695. E-mail: dx42@cityscape.co.uk. http://thaidip.mfa.go.th/london/.
Tonga: Tonga High Commission, 36 Molyneux Street, London W1H 6AB. Tel: +44 20 7724 5828. Fax +44 20 7723 9074.
Trinidad and Tobago: Trinidad and Tobago High Commission, 42 Belgrave Square, London SW1X. Tel: +44 20 7245 9351.
Tunisia: Tunisian Embassy, 29 Princes Gate, London SW7 1QG. Tel: +44 20 7584 8117. Fax: +44 20 7225 2884.
Turkey: Turkish Embassy, 43 Belgrave Square, London SW1X 8PA. Tel: +44 20 7393 0202 Fax: +44 20 7393 0066. E-mail: info@turkishembassy-london.com. www.turkishembassy-london.com/. *Consulate:* www.turkconsulate-london.com/.
Turkmenistan: Embassy of Turkmenistan, 2nd Floor, 14 Wells Street, London W1. Tel: +44 20 7255 1071.
Uganda: Ugandan High Commission, Uganda House, 58–59 Trafalgar Square, London WC2N 5DX. Tel: +44 20 7839 5783. Fax: +44 20 7839 8925.
Ukraine: Embassy of Ukraine, 78 Kensington Park Road, London W11. Tel: +44 20 7727 6312.
United Arab Emirates: Embassy of the United Arab Emirates, 30 Princes Gate, London SW7. Tel: +44 20 7589 3434.
Uruguay: Uruguayan Consulate, 140 Brompton Road, London SW3. Tel: +44 20 7589 8735.
USA: American Embassy, 24 Grosvenor Square, London W1A 1AE. Tel: +44 20 7499 9000. Fax: +44 20 7894 0699. www.usembassy.org.uk/. *Consulate in Belfast:* Tel: +44 28 328 239. Fax: +44 28 224 8482. *Consulate in Edinburgh:* 3 Regent Terrace, Edinburgh, EH7 5BW. Tel: +44 131 556 8315. Fax: +44 131 557 6023.
Uzbekistan: 41 Holland Park, London W11. Tel: +44 20 7229 7679.
Venezuela: Consular Section, 56 Grafton Way, London W1P 5LB. Tel: +44 20 7387 6727. Fax: +44 20 7383 3253. E-mail: venezlon@venezlon.demon.co.uk. www.venezlon.demon.co.uk/.
Vietnam: Vietnam Embassy, 12 Victoria Road, London W8. Tel: +44 20 7937 3174.
Yemen: Embassy of the Republic of Yemen, 57 Cromwell Road, London SW7. Tel: +44 20 7584 6607.
Zaire: Diplomatic Mission of the Republic of Zaire, 26 Chesham Place, London SW1X. Tel: +44 20 7235 6137.
Zambia: Zambian High Commission, 2 Palace Gate, London W8 5NG. Tel: +44 20 7589 6655. Fax: +44 20 7581 1353.
Zimbabwe: High Commission of the Republic of Zimbabwe, Zimbabwe House, 429 Strand, London WC2R 05A. Tel: +44 20 7836 7755. Fax: +44 20 7379 1167.

Embassies

Embassies in Australia

Afghanistan: Consulate of the Islamic State of Afghanistan, PO Box 88, Canberra, ACT 2601. Tel: +61 2 629 8024.

Argentina: Argentina Embassy, 1 Alfred Street, Piso 13, Suite 1302, Gold Fields House, Circular Quay, Sydney, NSW 2000. Tel: +61 2 9251 3402. Fax: +61 2 9251 3405. E-mail: mail@consarsydney.org.au. www.consarsydney.org.au/. Embassy of Argentina, MLC Tower Philip, Canberra. Tel: +61 2 6282 4555.

Austria: Austrian Embassy, 12 Talbot Street, Forest, Canberra, ACT 2603. Tel: +61 2 6295 1533. Fax: +61 2 6239 6751. www.austriaemb.org.au.

Bangladesh: Bangladesh High Commission, PO Box 5, Red Hill, ACT 2603. Tel: +61 2 6290 0511. Fax: +61 2 6290 0544. http:\\users.cyberone.com.au/bdeshact/.

Belgium: Belgian Embassy, Arkana Street Yarralumla, Canberra, ACT 2600. Tel: +61 2 6273 2501. Fax: +61 6 273 33 92. *Consulate general:* 12a Trelawney Street, Woollahra, Sydney, NSW 2025. Tel: +61 2 9327 8377. Fax: +61 2 9328 7924.

Bosnia and Herzegovina: Embassy of the Republic of Bosnia and Herzegovina, 15 State Circle Forest, Canberra, ACT. Tel: +61 2 6239 5955.

Brazil: Brazilian Embassy, 19 Forster Crescent, Yarralumla, Canberra, ACT 2600. Tel: +61 2 6273 2372. Fax: +61 2 6273 2375. http://people.interconnect.com.au/~aasbrem/emb.htm. *Consular section:* 19 Forster Crescent, Yarralumla, Canberra, ACT 2600. Tel: +61 2 6273 4837. Fax: +61 2 6273 4837.

Burma: National Coalition Government of the Union of Burma, PO Box 2024, Queanbeyan, NSW 2620. Tel: +61 2 6297 7734.

Cambodia: Royal Embassy of Cambodia, 5 Canterbury Crescent, Deakin, Canberra, ACT. Tel: +61 2 6273 1259/1154. Fax: +61 2 6273 1053.

Cameroon: Consulate of the Republic of Cameroon, 65 Bingara Road, Beecroft, NSW 2119. Tel: +61 2 9876 4544. Fax: +61 2 9869 2470. E-mail: consular@tig.com.au. www.cameroonconsul.com/.

Canada: Canadian Embassy, Level 5, Quay West, 111 Harrington Street, Sydney, NSW 2000. Tel: +61 2 364 3050. Fax: +61 2 364 4099. *High Commission of Canada:* Yarralumla, Commonwealth Avenue Canberra, ACT 2600. Tel: +61 2 6270 4000. Fax: +61 2 6273 3285. Visas: Tel: +61 2 9364 3050. Fax: +61 2 9364 3099. www.dfait-maeci.gc.ca/australia/menu-en.asp.

Chile: Chilean Embassy, 10 Culgoa Circuit, O'Malley, ACT 2606. Postal address: PO Box 69, Monaro Crescent, Canberra, ACT 2603. Tel: +61 2 6286 2430. E-mail: echileau@dynamite.com.au. www.netinfo.com.au/chile/. *Consulate in Sydney:* 8th Floor, National Mutual Centre, 44 Market Street, Sydney, NSW 2000. Tel: +61 2 9299 2533. Fax: +61 2 9299 2868. *Consulate in Melbourne:* Level 43, Nauru House, 80 Collins Street, Melbourne, VIC 3000. Tel: +61 3 9654 4479. Fax: 03 9650 8290. E-mail: cgmelbau@magna.com.au.

China: Embassy of the Peoples Republic of China, 15 Coronation Drive, Yarralumla, Canberra, ACT. Tel: +61 2 6273 4780.

Colombia: Embassy of Colombia, 101 Northbourne Avenue, Turner, Canberra, ACT 2612. Tel: +61 2 6257 2027.

Croatia: Embassy of the Republic of Croatia, 14 Jindalee Crescent, O'Maly, Canberra, ACT. Tel: +61 2 6286 6988.

Cyprus: Cyprus High Commission, 30 Beale Crescent, Deakin, Canberra, ACT. Tel: +61 2 6281 0834.

Czech Republic: Czech Embassy, 38 Culgoa Circuit, O'Maly, Canberra, ACT 2606. Tel: +61 2 6290 1386. Fax: +61 2 6290 0006.

Denmark: Danish Embassy, 15 Hunter, Yarralumla, Canberra, ACT. Tel: +61 2 6273 2195. Fax: +61 2 6273 3864. *Consulate general:* Gold Fields House, 1 Alfred Street, Circular Quay, Sydney, NSW 2000. Tel: +61 2 9247 2224. Fax: +61 2 9251 7504. E-mail: dkconsul@dkconsul-sydney.org.au. www.dkconsul-sydney.org.au/.

Egypt: Embassy of the Arab Republic of Egypt, 1 Darwin Avenue, Yarralumla, Canberra, ACT. Tel: +61 2 6273 4437.

European Union: Delegation of the European Commission, 18 Arkana, Yarralumla, Canberra, ACT. Tel: +61 2 6271 2777. Fax: +61 2 6273 4445. E-mail: australia@ecdel.org.au. www.ecdel.org.au/.

Fiji: Embassy of the Republic of Fiji, 19 Beale, Deakin, Canberra, ACT. Tel: +61 2 6239 6872. Also 97 Mugga Way, Red Hill, Canberra, ACT. Tel: +61 2 6260 5115.

Finland: Finnish Embassy, 10 Darwin Avenue, Yarralumla, Canberra, ACT 2600. Tel: +61 2 6273 3800. Fax: +61 2 6273 3603. E-mail: sanomat.can@formin.fi. www.finland.org.au/. *Consulate in Sydney:* 537 New South Head Road, Double Bay, NSW 2028. Tel: +61 2 9327 7904. Fax: +61 2 9327 7528. E-mail: finconsul@hartingdale.com.au.

France: French Embassy, 6 Perth Avenue, Yarralumla, Canberra, ACT 2600. Tel: +61 2 6216 0100. Fax: +61 2 6216 0156. E-mail: embassy@france.net.au. www.france.net.au/frames_eng.html.

Germany: Embassy of the Federal Republic of Germany, 119 Empire Circuit, Yarralumla, Canberra, ACT 2600. Tel: +61 2 6270 1911. Fax: +61 2 6270 1951. E-mail: embgerma@bigpond.net.au. www.germanembassy-canberra.com.

Greece: Greek Consulate General, Stanhill House 34 Queens Road, Melbourne, VIC 3004. Tel: +61 3 9866 4524/4525. Fax: +61 3 9866 4933. Also Embassy of Greece, Corner Turrana and Empire Circuit, Yarralumla, Canberra, ACT. Tel: +61 2 6273 3011.

Hungary: Hungarian Embassy, 17 Beale Crescent, Deakin, Canberra, ACT. Tel: +61 2 6282 3226.

India: High Commission of India, 3 Moonal Place, Yarralumla, Canberra, ACT. Tel: +61 2 6273 3999.

Indonesia: Indonesian Embassy, 8 Darwin Ave, Yarralumla, Canberra, ACT. Tel: +61 2 6273 3222/6250 8600. *Consulates: Adelaide:* Tel: +61 8 8223 6535. *Darwin:* Tel: +61 89 8981 9352. *Melbourne:* Tel: +61 3 9690 7811. *Perth:* Tel: +61 9 9219 8212. *Sydney:* Tel: +61 2 93449933.

Iran: Embassy of the Islamic Republic of Iran, 25 Culgoa Circuit, O'Maly, Camberra, ACT. Tel: +61 2 6290 2421. Fax: +61 2 6290 2431.

Iraq: Embassy of Republic of Iraq, 48 Culgoa Circuit, O'Maly, Canberra, ACT. Tel: +61 2 6286 1333.

Ireland: Embassy of Ireland, 20 Arkana Street, Yarralumla, Canberra, ACT 2600. Tel: +61 6 273 3022/3201. Fax: +61 6 273 3741.

Israel: Israeli Embassy, 6 Turrana Street, Yarralumla, Canberra, ACT 2600. Tel: +61 2 6273 1309/1300. Fax: +61 2 2734273. E-mail: Isremb.Canberra@U030.Aone.Net.Au. *Consulate:* 37 York Street, Sydney, NSW 2000. Tel: +61 2 264 7933. Fax: +61 2 290 2259.

Italy: Italian Embassy, 12 Grey Street Deakin, Canberra, ACT 2600. Tel: +61 6 273 3333. Fax: +61 2 6273 4223. www/ambitalia.org.au.

Japan: Embassy of Japan, 112 Empire Circuit, Yarralumla, Canberra, ACT. Tel: +61 2 6273 3244.

Jordan: Embassy of the Hasemite Kingdom of Jordan, 20 Roebuck, Red Hill, Canberra, ACT. Tel: +61 2 6295 9951.

Kenya: Kenya High Commission, 33 Ainslie Avenue, Canberra City, Canberra, ACT. Tel: +61 2 6247 4788.

Korea: Embassy of the Republic of Korea, 113 Empire Circuit, Yarralumla, Canberra, ACT. Tel: +61 2 6273 3044.

Kuwait: Kuwait Military Liasion Office, 37 Culgoa Circuit, O'Maly, Canberra, ACT. Tel: +61 2 6286 2516.

Laos: Embassy of Laos Peoples Democratic Republic, 1 Dalman Crescent, O'Maly, Canberra, ACT. Tel: +61 2 6286 6933.

Lebanon: Embassy of Lebanon, 27 Endeavour Red Hill, Canberra, ACT. Tel: +61 2 6295 7378.

Malaysia: Malaysian High Commision, 7 Perth Avenue, Yarralumla, Canberra, ACT. Tel: +61 2 6273 1543.

Malta: Malta High Commission, 261 La Perouse, Red Hill, Canberra, ACT. Tel: +61 2 6295 1586. *Consulate general:* Level 5, 343 Little Collins Street, Melbourne, VIC 3000. Tel: +61 3 9670 8427. Fax: +61 3 9670 9451. E-mail: maltacg@alphalink.com.au. www.vu.edu.au/malta/.

Mauritius: Mauritius High Commission, 2 Beale Crescent, Deakin, Canberra, ACT. Tel: +61 2 6281 1203.

Mexico: Embassy of Mexico, 14 Perth Ave, Yarralumla, Canberra, ACT. Tel: +61 2 6273 3963.

Myanmar: Embassy of the Union of Myanmar, 22 Arkana, Yarralumla, Canberra, ACT. Tel: +61 2 6273 3811.

Netherlands: Embassy of the Netherlands, 120 Empire Circuit, Yarralumla, Canberra Tel: +61 2 6273 3111. Fax: +61 2 6273 3206.

New Zealand: New Zealand High Commission, Commonwealth Avenue, Canberra, ACT 2600. Tel: +61 2 6270 4211. Fax: +61 2 6273 3194. *Consulates:* Watkins Place Building, 288 Edward Street (GPO Box 62), Brisbane, QLD 4001. Tel: +61 7 221 9933. Fax: +61 7 229 7495. *Melbourne:* 60 Albert Road, South Melbourne, VIC 3205. Tel: +61 3 9696 0501. Fax: +61 3 9696 0391. *Sydney:* Level 14, Gold Fields Building, 1 Alfred Street, Circular Quay (GPO Box 365), Sydney, NSW 2000. Tel: +61 2 247 1999. Fax: +61 2 247 1754.

Nigeria: Nigeria High Commission, 7 Terrigal Circuit, O'Maly, Canberra, ACT. Tel: +61 2 6286 1322. Fax: +61 2 6286 5332.

E-mail: nigeria_act@netinfo.com.au.

Norway: Embassy of Norway, 17 Hunter, Yarralumla, Canberra, ACT. Tel: +61 2 6273 3444. Also 80 Mugga Way, Red Hill, Canberra, ACT. Tel: +61 2 6295 1048.

Pakistan: High Commission for Pakistan, 4 Timbarra Crescent, O'Maly, Canberra, ACT. Tel: +61 2 6290 1676.

Palestine: Palestinian Delegation, 19 Carnegie Crescent, Narbndh, Canberra, ACT. Tel: +61 2 6925 0222.

Papua New Guinea: High Commission of Papua New Guinea, 39–41 Forster Crescent, Yarralumla, Canberra, ACT. Tel: +61 2 6273 3322. Fax: +61 2 6273 3732.

Peru: Embassy of Peru, 43 Culgoa Circuit, O'Maly, Canberra, ACT. Tel: +61 2 6290 0922.

Philippines: Embassy of the Philippines, 1 Moonah Place, Yarralumla, Canberra, ACT. Tel: +61 2 6273 2535. Fax: +61 2 6273 3984.

Poland: Embassy of the Republic of Poland, 6 Turrana, Yarralumla, Canberra, ACT. Tel: +61 2 6273 1208.

Portugal: Embassy of Portugal, 23 Culgoa Circuit, O'Maly, Canberra, ACT Tel: +61 2 6290 1733.

Romania: Embassy of Romania, 4 Dalman Crescent, O'Maly, Canberra, ACT. Tel: +61 2 6286 2343.

Russian Federation: Russian Federation Embassy, 78 Canberra Avenue, Griffith, Canberra, ACT 2603. Tel: +61 6 295 9033/9474.

Saudi Arabia: Embassy of Saudi Arabia, 8 Culgoa Circuit, O'Maly, Canberra, ACT. Tel: +61 2 6286 2099.

Singapore: High Commission of Singapore, 17 Forster Crescent, Yarralumla, Canberra, ACT. Tel: +61 2 6273 3944. Fax: +61 2 6273 3260. E-mail: singaporehc@u030.aone.net.au.

Slovakia: Embassy of the Slovak Federal, 47 Culgoa Circuit, O'Maly, Canberra, ACT. Tel: +61 2 6290 1516.

Slovenia: Embassy of Slovenia, Level 6, 60 Marcus Clarke Street. Postal address: PO Box 284, Civic Square, Canberra, ACT 2601. Tel: +61 2 6243 4830. Fax: +61 2 6243 4827. E-mail: embassyofslovenia@webone.com.au. http://slovenia.webone.com.au/.

Solomon Islands: Solomon Islands High Commission, 19 Napier Close, Deakin, Canberra, ACT. Tel: +61 2 6282 7030.

South Africa: High Commission of South Africa, State Circle, Yarralumla, Canberra, ACT. Tel: +61 2 6273 2424.

Spain: Embassy of Spain, 15 Arkana, Yarralumla, Canberra, ACT. Tel: +61 2 6273 3555.

Sri Lanka: Sri Lankan High Commission, 35 Empire Circuit, Forrest, Canberra, ACT 2603. Tel: +61 6 239 7041/7042. Fax: +61 6 239 6166. E-mail: slhc@atrax.net.au. http://slhccanberra.webjump.com/.

Sweden: Embassy of Sweden, Turrana Street, Yarralumla, Canberra, ACT. Tel: +61 2 6270 2700.

Switzerland: Embassy of Switzerland, 7 Melbourne Avenue Forest, Canberra, ACT. Tel: +61 2 6273 3977.

Thailand: Royal Thai Embassy, 111 Empire Circuit, Yarralumla, Canberra, ACT 2600. Tel: +61 6 273 1149. Fax: +61 6 273 1518. E-mail: Thai@csccs.com.au. www.geocities.com/CapitolHill/7789/.

Embassies

Turkey: Turkish Embassy, 60 Mugga Way, Red Hill, Canberra, ACT 2603. Tel: +61 2 6295 0227/0228. Fax: +61 2 6239 6592. E-mail: turkembs@ozemail.com.au. www.ozemail.com.au/~turkembs/. *Consulate in Sydney*: 66 Ocean Street, Woollahra, Sydney, NSW 2025. Tel: +61 29 327 6629. Fax: +61 29 362 4730. E-mail: dtsid@adcom.com.au. www.adcom.com.au/dtsid/.
UK: British High Commission, Commonwealth Avenue, Yarralumla, Canberra, ACT 2600. Tel: +61 2 6270 6666. Fax: +61 2 6270 6653 (chancery), +61 2 6270 6606 (information). www.uk.emb.gov.au/. *Canberra: Passport/visa/consular section*: Level 10, CBS Tower, Canberra City, ACT 2601. Tel: +61 2 6257 2434 (passports), +61 2 6257 1982 (entry clearances). Fax: +61 2 6257 5857. *British consulates: Adelaide*: 22nd Floor, 25 Grenfell Street, Adelaide, SA. Tel: +61 8 212 7280/7281. Fax: +61 8 212 7283. *Brisbane*: Level 26, Waterfront Place, 1 Eagle Street, Brisbane, QLD 4000. Tel: +61 7 3236 2575/2577/2581. Fax: +61 7 3236 2576. *Melbourne*: 17th Floor, 90 Collins Street, Melbourne, VIC 3000. Tel: +61 3 9650 2990. Fax: +61 3 9650 2990. *Perth*: Level 26, Allendale Square, 77 St George's Terrace, Perth, WA 6000. Tel: +61 9 221 5400. Fax: +61 9 221 2344. *Sydney*: Level 16, The Gateway, 1 Macquarie Place, Sydney Cove, Sydney, NSW 2000. Tel: +61 2 247 7521. Fax: +61 2 251 6201.
Uruguay: Embassy of the Uruguay Chancery, 24 Brisbane Avenue, Brtn, Canberra. Tel: +61 2 6282 4800.
USA: Embassy of the United States of America, 21 Moonah Place, Yarralumla, Canberra, ACT 2600. Tel: +61 2 6270 5000. Fax: +61 2 6270 5970/5940. E-mail: usiscanb@ozemail.com.au. www.usis-australia.gov/embassy.html. *Consulate generals: Melbourne*: Level 6, 553 St Kilda Road, Melbourne, VIC. Tel: +61 3 9526 5900. www.ozemail.com.au/~usaemb/melbourne/. *Sydney*: Level 59, MLC Centre, 19–29 Martin Place, Sydney, NSW 2000. Tel: +61 2 9373 9200 (reception). Fax: +61 2 9373 9107. www.ozemail.com.au/~usaemb/sydney/. *Perth*: 16 St Georges Terrace, Perth, WA 6000. Tel: +61 8 9231 9400. Fax: +61 8 9231 9444. www.ozemail.com.au/~usaemb/perth/.
Venezuela: Embassy of Venezuela, 5 Culgoa Circuit, O'Maly, Canberra, ACT. Tel: +61 2 6290 2900. E-mail: venezuela@linkpro.com.au. www.linkpro.com.au/venezuela/.
Vietnam: Embassy of the Socialist Republic of Vietnam, 6 Timbara Crescent, O'Maly, Canberra, ACT. Tel: +61 2 6286 6059.
Yugoslavia: Embassy of Federal Republic of Yugoslavia, 11 Nuyts Red Hill, Canberra, ACT. Tel: +61 2 6295 1458.

Embassies in the USA

Afghanistan: Embassy of the Republic of Afghanistan, 2341 Wyoming Ave, NW, Washington DC 20008. Tel: +1 202 234 3770. Fax: +1 202 328 3516.

Albania: Embassy of the Republic of Albania, 2100 S Street, NW, Washington DC 20008. Tel: +1 202 223 4942. Fax: +1 202 628 7342.
Algeria: Embassy of the Democratic and Popular Republic of Algeria, 2118 Kalorama Road NW, Washington DC 20008. Tel: +1 202 265 2800. Fax: +1 202 667 2174. E-mail: embalgus@cais.com. www.algeria-us.org/.
Angola: Embassy of Angola, 1615 M Street, NW Suite 900, Washington DC 20036. Tel: +1 202 785 1156. Fax: +1 202 785 1258. E-mail: angola@angola.org. www.angola.org/.
Antigua and Barbuda: Embassy of Antigua and Barbuda, 3216 New Mexico Avenue, NW, Washington DC 20016. Tel: +1 202 362 5122. Fax: +1 202 362 5225.
Argentina: Embassy of the Argentine Republic, 1600 New Hampshire Avenue, NW, Washington DC 20009. Tel: +1 202 238 6400. Fax: +1 202 332 3171. E-mail: embajadaargentina@worldnet.att.net. www.embassyofargentina-usa.org/.
Armenia: Embassy of the Republic of Armenia, 2225 R Street, Washington DC 20008. Tel: +1 202 319 1976. Fax: +1 202 319 2982. www.armeniaemb.org/.
Australia: Embassy of Australia, 1601 Massachusetts Avenue, NW, Washington DC 20036. Tel: +1 202 797 3000. Fax: +1 202 797 3168. www.austemb.org/.
Austria: Embassy of Austria, 3524 International Court, NW, Washington DC 20008. Tel: +1 202 895 6700. Fax: +1 202 895 6750.
Azerbaijan: Embassy of the Republic of Azerbaijan, 927 15th Street, NW, Suite 700, Washington DC 20035. Tel: +1 202 842 0001. Fax: +1 202 842 0004. E-mail: azerbaijan@tidalwave.net. www.azembassy.com/.
Bahamas: Embassy of the Commonwealth of the Bahamas, 2220 Massachusetts Avenue, NW, Washington DC 20008. Tel: +1 202 319 2660. Fax: +1 202 319 2668.
Bahrain: Embassy of the State of Bahrain, 3502 International Drive, NW, Washington DC 20008. Tel: +1 202 342 0741. Fax: +1 202 362 2192. E-mail: info@bahrainembassy.org. www.bahrainembassy.org/.
Bangladesh: Embassy of the People's Republic of Bangladesh, 2201 Wisconsin Avenue, NW, Suite 300, Washington DC 20007. Tel: +1 202 342 8372. Fax: +1 202 333 4971. E-mail: BanglaEmb@aol.com. http://members.aol.com/banglaemb/index.html.
Barbados: Embassy of Barbados, 2144 Wyoming Avenue, NW, Washington DC 20008. Tel: +1 202 939 9200. Fax: +1 202 332 7467.
Belarus: Embassy of the Republic of Belarus, 1619 New Hampshire Avenue, NW, Washington DC 20009. Tel: +1 202 986 1604. Fax: +1 202 986 1805.
Belgium: Embassy of Belgium, 3330 Garfield Street, NW, Washington DC 20008. Tel: +1 202 333 6900. Fax: +1 202 333 3079. E-mail: washington@diplobel.org. www.diplobel.org/usa/ default.htm.
Belize: Embassy of Belize, 2535 Massachusetts Avenue, NW, Washington DC 20008. Tel: +1 202 332 9636. Fax: +1 202 332 6888.

Benin: Embassy of the Republic of Benin, 2737 Cathedral Avenue, NW, Washington DC 20008. Tel: +1 202 232 6656. Fax: +1 202 265 1996.
Bhutan: Embassy of Bhutan (Consulate-General). 2 UN Plaza, 27th Floor, New York, NY 10017. Tel: +1 212 826 1919. Fax: +1 212 826 2998.
Bolivia: Embassy of Bolivia, 3014 Massachusetts Avenue, NW, Washington DC 20008. Tel: +1 202 483 4410. Fax: +1 202 328 3712.
Bosnia and Herzegovina: Embassy of Bosnia and Herzegovina, 2109 East Street NW, Washington DC 20037. Tel: +1 202 337 1500. Fax: +1 202 337 1502. E-mail: Embofbih@aol.com.
www.bosnianembassy.org/.
Botswana: Embassy of Botswana, 1531–1533 New Hampshire Avenue, NW, Washington DC 20036. Tel: +1 202 244 4990. Fax: +1 202 244 4164.
Brazil: Embassy of Brazil, 3006 Massachusetts Avenue, NW, Washington DC 20008. Tel: +1 202 238 2700. Fax: +1 202 238 2827. E-mail: scitech@brasil.emb.nw.dc.us.
www.brasil.emb.nw.dc.us/.
Brunei: Embassy of Brunei, Watergate, Suite 300, 2600 Virginia Avenue, NW, Washington DC 20037. Tel: +1 202 342 0159. Fax: +1 202 342 0158.
Bulgaria: Embassy of the Republic of Bulgaria, 1621 22nd Street, NW, Washington DC 20008. Tel: +1 202 387 7969. Fax: +1 202 234 7973. E-mail: bulgaria@access.digex.net.
www.bulgaria-embassy.org.
Burkina Faso: Embassy of Burkina Faso, 2340 Massachusetts Avenue, NW, Washington DC 20008. Tel: +1 202 332 5577. Fax: +1 202 265 6972.
Burundi: Embassy of the Republic of Burundi, 2233 Wisconsin Avenue, NW, Suite 212, Washington DC 20007. Tel: +1 202 342 2574. Fax: +1 202 342 2578.
Cameroon: Embassy of the Republic of Cameroon, 2349 Massachusetts Avenue, NW, Washington DC 20008. Tel: +1 202 265 8790. Fax: +1 202 387 3826.
Canada: Embassy of Canada, 501 Pennsylvania Avenue, NW, Washington DC 20001. Tel: +1 202 682 1740. Fax: +1 202 682 7726. www.cdnemb-washdc.org/.
Cape Verde: Embassy of the Republic of Cape Verde, 3415 Massachusetts Avenue, NW, Washington DC 20007. Tel: +1 202 965 6820. Fax: +1 202 965 1207. E-mail: cvefont@sysnet.net.
www.capeverdeusembassy.org/.
Central African Republic: Embassy of the Central African Republic, 1618 22nd Street, NW, Washington DC 20008. Tel: +1 202 483 7800. Fax: +1 202 332 9893.
Chad: Embassy of the Republic of Chad, 2002 R Street, NW, Washington DC 20009. Tel: +1 202 462 4009. Fax: +1 202 265 1937. E-mail: info@chadembassy.org.
www.chadembassy.org.
Chile: Embassy of Chile, 1732 Massachusetts Avenue, NW, Washington DC 20036. Tel: +1 202 785 1746. Fax: +1 202 887 5579.
China: Embassy of the People's Republic of China, 2300 Connecticut Ave, NW, Washington DC 20008. Tel: +1 202 328 2500. Fax: +1 202 588 0032. E-mail: webmaster@china-embassy.org.
www.china-embassy.org/.

Colombia: Embassy of Colombia, 2118 Leroy Place, NW, Washington DC 20008. Tel: +1 202 387 8338. Fax: +1 202 232 8643. E-mail: webmaster@colombiaemb.org.
www.colombiaemb.org/.
Comoros: Embassy of the Federal and Islamic Republic of the Comoros, 336 East 454th, 2nd Floor, New York, NY 10017. Tel: +1 212 972 8010.
Congo: Embassy of the Republic of Congo, 4891 Colorado Avenue, NW, Washington DC 20011. Tel: +1 202 726 5500. Fax: +1 202 726 1860. Also Embassy of the Democratic Republic of Congo, 1800 New Hampshire Avenue, NW, Washington DC 20009. Tel: +1 202 234 7690. Fax: +1 202 237 0748.
Costa Rica: Embassy of Costa Rica, 2114 S Street, NW, Washington DC 20008. Tel: +1 202 234 2945. Fax: +1 202 265 4795.
www.costarica.com/embassy/.
Cote d'Ivoire: Embassy of the Republic of Cote d'Ivoire (Ivory Coast), 2424 Massachusetts Avenue, NW, Washington DC 20008. Tel: +1 202 797 0300.
Croatia: Embassy of the Republic of Croatia, 2343 Massachusetts Avenue, NW, Washington DC 20008. Tel: +1 202 588 5899. Fax: +1 202 588 8936. E-mail: croatia@mail.idt.net. http://idt.net/~croatia/.
Cuba: Cuba Interests Section, 2630 and 2639 16th Street, NW, Washington DC 20009. Tel: +1 202 797 8518.
Cyprus: Embassy of the Republic of Cyprus, 2211 R Street, NW, Washington DC 20008. Tel: +1 202 462 5772. Fax: +1 202 483 6710.
Czech Republic: Embassy of the Czech Republic, 3900 Spring of Freedom Street, NW, Washington DC 20008. Tel: +1 202 274 9100. Fax: +1 202 966 8540. E-mail: washington@embassy.mzv.cz.
www.czech.cz/washington/.
Denmark: Royal Danish Embassy, 3200 Whitehaven Street, NW, Washington DC 20008. Tel: +1 202 234 4300. Fax: +1 202 328 1470. E-mail: ambadane@erols.com.
www.denmarkemb.org/.
Djibouti: Embassy of the Republic of Djibouti, 1156 15th Street, NW, Suite 515, Washington DC 20005. Tel: +1 202 331 0270.
Dominica: Embassy of the Dominican Republic, 1715 22nd Street, NW, Washington DC 20008. Tel: +1 202 332 6280. Fax: +1 202 265 8057. E-mail: embdomrepusa@msn.com. www.domrep.org/.
Ecuador: Embassy of Ecuador, 2535 15th Street, NW, Washington DC 20009. Tel: +1 202 234 7200.
www.ecuador.org.
Egypt: Embassy of the Arab Republic of Egypt, 3521 International Court, NW, Washington DC 20008. Tel: +1 202 966 6342.
El Salvador: Embassy of El Salvador, 2308 California Street, NW, Washington DC 20008. Tel: +1 202 265 9671. E-mail: cbartoli@elsalvador.org.
www.elsalvador.org.
Equatorial Guinea: Embassy of Equatorial Guinea, 1721 I Street NW, Suite 400, Washington DC 20006. Tel: +1 914 738 9584.
Eritrea: Embassy of Eritrea, 1708 New Hampshire Avenue, NW, Washington DC 20009. Tel: +1 202 319 1991. Fax: +1 202 319 1304. E-mail: veronica@embassyeritrea.org.

Estonia: Embassy of Estonia, 2131 Massachussets Avenue, NW, Washington DC 20008. Tel: +1 202 588 0101. Fax: +1 202 588 0108. www.estemb.org/.
Ethiopia: Embassy of Ethiopia, 2134 Kalorama Road NW, Suite 1000, Washington DC 20008. Tel: +1 202 234 2281. Fax: +1 202 483 8407. E-mail: ethiopia@tidalwave.net. www.ethiopianembassy.org/.
Fiji: Embassy of Fiji, 2233 Wisconsin Avenue, NW, Suite 240, Washington DC 20007. Tel: +1 202 337 8320. Fax: +1 202 337 1996. E-mail: fijiemb@earthlink.net.
Finland: Embassy of Finland, 3301 Massachusetts Avenue, NW, Washington DC 20008. Tel: +1 202 298 5800. Fax: +1 202 298 6030. E-mail: info@finland.org. www.finland.org/.
France: Embassy of France, 4101 Reservoir Road, NW, Washington DC 20007. Tel: +1 202 944 6000 Fax: +1 202 944 6072. www.info-france-usa.org/.
Gabon: Embassy of the Gabonese Republic, 2034 20th Street, NW, Suite 200, Washington DC 20009. Tel: +1 202 797 1000. Fax: +1 202 332 0668.
Gambia: Embassy of the Gambia, 1155 15th Street, NW, Suite 1000, Washington DC 20005. Tel: +1 202 785 1399. E-mail: gamembdc@gambia.com. www.gambia.com/index.html.
Georgia: Embassy of the Republic of Georgia, 1511 K Street, NW, Suite 400, Washington DC 20005. Tel: +1 202 393 5959. Fax: +1 202 393 4537. E-mail: 73324.1007@compuserve.com. www.steele.com/embgeorgia/.
Germany: Embassy of Germany, 4645 Reservoir Road, NW, Washington DC 20007 1998. Tel: +1 202 298 4000. Fax: +1 202 298 4249/333 2653. www.germany-info.org/.
Ghana: Embassy of Ghana, 3512 International Drive NW, Washington DC 20008. Tel: +1 202 686 4520. E-mail: hagan@cais.com. www.ghana-embassy.org/.
Greece: Embassy of Greece, 2221 Massachusetts Avenue, NW, Washington DC 20008. Tel: +1 202 939 5800. www.greekembassy.org/.
Grenada: Embassy of Grenada, 1701 New Hampshire Ave, NW, Washington DC 20009. Tel: +1 202 265 2561.
Guatemala: Embassy of Guatemala, 2220 R Street, NW, Washington DC 20008. Tel: +1 202 745 4952. Fax: +1 202 745 1908. E-mail: Embaguat@sysnet.net. www.mdngt.org/agremilusa/ embassy.html.
Guinea: Embassy of the Republic of Guinea, 2112 Leroy Place, NW, Washington DC 20008. Tel: +1 202 483 9420.
Guinea-Bissau: Embassy of the Republic of Guinea-Bissau, 918 16th Street, NW (Mezzanine Suite), Washington DC 20006.
Guyana: Embassy of Guyana, 2490 Tracy Place, NW, Washington DC 20008. Tel: +1 202 265 6900. E-mail: guyanaem@erols.com. www.wam.umd.edu/~swi/ embassy.htm.
Haiti: Embassy of the Republic of Haiti, 2311 Massachusetts Avenue, NW, Washington DC 20008. Tel: +1 202 332 4090. Fax: +1 202 745 7215. www.haiti.org/embassy.
Honduras: Embassy of Honduras, 3007 Tilden Street, NW, Washington DC 20008. Tel: +1 202 966 7702.

Hungary: Embassy of the Republic of Hungary, 3910 Shoemaker Street, NW, Washington DC 20008. Tel: +1 202 362 6730. Fax: +1 202 686 6412. www.hungaryemb.org/.
Iceland: Embassy of Iceland, 1156 15th Street, NW, Suite 1200, Washington DC 20005 1704. Tel: +1 202 265 6653. Fax: +1 202 265 6656. E-mail: icemb.wash@utn.stjr.is. www.iceland.org/.
India: Embassy of India, 2107 Massachusetts Avenue, NW, Washington DC 20008. Tel: +1 202 939 7000. www.indianembassy.org/.
Indonesia: Embassy of the Republic of Indonesia, 2020 Massachusetts Avenue, NW, Washington DC 20036. Tel: +1 202 775 5200. http://kbri.org/.
Iran: Iranian Interests Section, 2209 Wisconsin Avenue NW, Washington DC 20007. Tel: +1 202 965 4990. www.daftar.org/default_eng.htm.
Iraq: Iraqi Interests Section, 1801 P Street, NW, Washington DC 20036. Tel: +1 202 483 7500. Fax: +1 202 462 5066.
Ireland: Embassy of Ireland, 2234 Massachusetts Avenue, NW, Washington DC 20008. Tel: +1 202 462 3939. www.irelandemb.org/.
Israel: Embassy of Israel, 3514 International Drive, NW, Washington DC 20008. Tel: +1 202 364 5500. Fax: +1 202 364 5423. E-mail: ask@israelemb.org. www.israelemb.org/.
Italy: Embassy of Italy, 1601 Fuller Street, NW, Washington DC 20009. Tel: +1 202 328 5500. Fax: +1 202 462 3605. www.italyemb.nw.dc.us/italy/index.html.
Jamaica: Embassy of Jamaica, 1520 New Hampshire Avenue, NW, Washington DC 20036. Tel: +1 202 452 0660. Fax: +1 202 452 0081. E-mail: emjam@sysnet.net. www.caribbean-online.com jamaica/embassy/washdc/.
Japan: Embassy of Japan, 2520 Massachusetts Avenue NW, Washington DC 20008. Tel: +1 202 238 6700. Fax: +1 202 328 2187. www.embjapan.org/.
Jordan: Embassy of the Hashemite Kingdom of Jordan, 3504 International Drive, NW, Washington DC 20008. Tel: +1 202 966 2664. Fax: +1 202 966 3110. www.jordanembassyus.org/.
Kazakhstan: Embassy of the Republic of Kazakhstan, 1401 16th Street, NW, Washington DC 20036. Tel: +1 202 232 5488.
Kenya: Embassy of Kenya, 2249 R Street, NW, Washington DC 20008. Tel: +1 202 387 6101. Fax: +1 202 462 3829. E-mail: info@kenyaembassy.com. www.kenyaembassy.com/.
Korea: Embassy of the Republic of Korea, 2450 Massachusetts Avenue, NW, Washington DC 20008. Tel: +1 202 939 5600. www.koreaemb.org/.
Kuwait: Embassy of the State of Kuwait, 2940 Tilden Street, NW, Washington DC 20008. Tel: +1 202 966 0702.
Kyrgyz: Embassy of the Kyrgyz Republic, 1732 Wisconsin Avenue, NW, Washington DC 20007. Tel: +1 202 338 5141. Fax: +1 202 338 5139. E-mail: Embassy@kyrgyzstan.org. www.kyrgyzstan.org/.
Laos: Embassy of the Lao People's Democratic Republic, 2222 S Street, NW, Washington DC 20008. Tel: +1 202 332 6416. Fax: +1 202 332 4923. www.laoembassy.com/.
Latvia: Embassy of Latvia, 4325 17th Street, NW, Washington DC 20011. Tel: +1 202 726 8213. Fax:

+1 202 726 6785. E-mail:
latvia@ambergateway.com. www.latvia-usa.org/.
Lebanon: Embassy of Lebanon, 2560 28th Street,
NW, Washington DC 20008. Tel: +1 202 939 6300.
Fax: +1 202 939 6324. E-mail:
EmbLebanon@aol.com. www.erols.com/lebanon/.
Lesotho: Embassy of the Kingdom of Lesotho,
2511 Massachusetts Avenue, NW, Washington DC
20008. Tel: +1 202 797 5533.
Liberia: Embassy of the Republic of Liberia, 5201
16th Street, NW, Washington DC 20011.
Tel: +1 202 723 0437.
Lithuania: Embassy of Lithuania, 2622 Sixteenth
Street, NW, Washington DC 20009 4202. Tel: +1
202 234 5860. Fax: +1 202 328 0466. E-mail:
admin@ltembassyus.org. www.ltembassyus.org/.
Luxembourg: Embassy of Luxembourg, 2200
Massachusetts Avenue, NW, Washington DC
20008. Tel: +1 202 265 4171.
Macedonia: Embassy of the Republic of
Macedonia, 3050 K Street, NW, Suite 210,
Washington DC 20007. Tel: +1 202 337 3063. Fax:
+1 202 337 3093. E-mail: rmacedonia@aol.com.
Malawi: Embassy of Malawi, 2408 Massachusetts
Avenue, NW, Washington DC 20008. Tel: +1 202
797 1007.
Malaysia: Embassy of Malaysia, 2401 Massachusetts
Avenue, NW, Washington DC 20008. Tel: +1 202
328 2700.
Mali: Embassy of the Republic of Mali, 2130 R Street,
NW, Washington DC 20008. Tel: +1 202 332 2249. Fax:
+1 202 332 6603. E-mail: info@maliembassy-usa.org.
www.maliembassy-usa.org.
Malta: Embassy of Malta, 2017 Connecticut
Avenue NW, Washington DC 20008. Tel: +1 202
462 3611.
Marshall Islands: Embassy of the Republic of the
Marshall Islands, 2433 Massachusetts Avenue, NW,
Washington DC 20008. Tel: +1 202 234 5414. Fax:
+1 202 232 3236. E-mail: info@rmiembassyus.org.
www.rmiembassyus.org/ usemb.html.
Mauritania: Embassy of the Islamic Republic of
Mauritania, 2129 Leroy Place, NW, Washington DC
20008. Tel: +1 202 232 5700. Fax: +1 202 232 5701.
Mauritius: Embassy of Mauritius, 4301
Connecticut Avenue, NW, Suite 441, Washington
DC 20008. Tel: +1 202 244 1491. Fax: +1 202 966
0983. www.idsonline.com/usa/ embassydc.html.
Mexico: Embassy of Mexico, 1911 Pennsylvania
Avenue, NW, Washington DC 20006. Tel: +1 202
728 1600. www.embassyofmexico.org/.
Micronesia: Embassy of the Federated States of
Micronesia, 1725 N Street, NW, Washington DC
20036. Tel: +1 202 223 4383.
Moldova: Embassy of the Republic of Moldova,
2101 S Street, NW, Washington DC 20008. Tel: +1
202 667 1130/1131/1137. Fax: +1 202 667 1204.
E-mail: embassy@moldova.org. www.moldova.org/.
Mongolia: Embassy of Mongolia, 2833 M Street
NW, Washington DC 20007. Tel: +1 202 333 7117.
http://members.aol.com/monemb/.
Morocco: Embassy of the Kingdom of Morocco,
1601 21st Street, NW, Washington DC 20009.
Tel: +1 202 462 7979.
Mozambique: Embassy of the Republic of
Mozambique, 1990 M Street, NW, Suite 570,
Washington DC 20036. Tel: +1 202 293 7146.

Myanmar: Embassy of the Union of Myanmar,
2300 S Street, NW, Washington DC 20008.
Tel: +1 202 332 9044.
Namibia: Embassy of the Republic of Namibia,
1605 New Hampshire Avenue, NW, Washington
DC 20009. Tel: +1 202 986 0540.
Nepal: Embassy of Nepal, 2131 Leroy Place, NW,
Washington DC 20008. Tel: +1 202 667 4550.
Netherlands: Embassy of the Netherlands, 4200
Linnean Avenue, NW, Washington DC 20008.
Tel: +1 202 244 5300. Fax: +1 202 362 3430.
www.netherlands-embassy.org/.
New Zealand: Embassy of New Zealand, 37
Observatory Circle, Washington DC 20008. Tel: +1
202 328 4800. Fax: +1 202 667 5227. E-mail:
nzemb@dc.infi.net. www.emb.com/nzemb/.
Nicaragua: Embassy of Nicaragua, 1627 New
Hampshire Avenue, NW, Washington DC 20009.
Tel: +1 202 939 6570. Fax: +1 202 939 6542.
E-mail: embanic_usa@amdyne.net.
http://members.aol.com/embanic1/.
Niger: Embassy of the Republic of Niger, 2204 R
Street, NW, Washington DC 20008.
Tel: +1 202 483 4224.
Nigeria: Embassy of the Federal Republic of
Nigeria, 1333 16th Street, NW, Washington DC
20036. Tel: +1 202 986 8400. Fax: +1 202 775 1385.
http://tribeca.ios.com/~n123/.
Norway: Royal Embassy of Norway, 20 34th
Street, NW, Washington DC 20008. Tel: +1 202 333
6000. www.norway.org/.
Oman: Embassy of the Sultanate of Oman, 35
Belmont Road, NW, Washington DC 20008.
Tel: +1 202 387 1980.
Pakistan: Embassy of the Islamic Republic of
Pakistan, 15 Massachusetts Avenue, NW,
Washington DC 20008. Tel: +1 202 939 6200.
E-mail: info@pakistan-embassy.com.
www.pakistan-embassy.com/.
Panama: Embassy of the Republic of Panama,
2862 McGill Terrace, NW, Washington DC 20008.
Tel: +1 202 483 1407.
Papua New Guinea: Embassy of Papua New
Guinea, 1779 Massachusetts Avenue, NW, Suite
805, Washington DC 20036. Tel: +1 202 745 3680.
Fax: +1 202 745 3679. E-mail:
Kunduwash@aol.com. www.pngembassy.org.
Paraguay: Embassy of Paraguay, 2400
Massachusetts Avenue, NW, Washington DC
20008. Tel: +1 202 483 6960.
Peru: Embassy of Peru, 1700 Massachusetts
Avenue, NW, Washington DC 20036. Tel: +1 202
833 9860. Fax: +1 202 659 8124. E-mail:
peru@peruemb.org. www.peruemb.org.
Philippines: Embassy of the Philippines, 1600
Massachusetts Avenue, NW, Washington DC
20036. Tel: +1 202 467 9300. Fax: +1 202 467 9417.
http://us.sequel.net/RpinUS.
Poland: Embassy of Poland, 2640 16th Street, NW,
Washington DC 20009. Tel: +1 202 234 3800. Fax:
+1 202 328 6271. E-mail: embpol@dgs.dgsys.com.
www.polishworld.com/polemb/.
Portugal: Embassy of Portugal, 2125 Kalorama
Road, NW, Washington DC 20008. Tel: +1 202 328
8610. Fax: +1 202 462 3726. E-mail:
portugal@portugalemb.org.
www.portugalemb.org/.

Embassies

Qatar: Embassy of the State of Qatar, 4200 Wisconsin Avenue, NW, Suite 200, Washington DC 20016. Tel: +1 202 274 1600. Fax: +1 202 237 0061.
Russia: Embassy of the Russian Federation, 2650 Wisconsin Avenue, NW, Washington DC 20007. Tel: +1 202 298 5700. Fax: +1 202 298 5749.
www.russianembassy.org.
Rwanda: Embassy of the Republic of Rwanda, 1714 New Hampshire Avenue, NW, Washington DC 20009. Tel: +1 202 232 2882. Fax: +1 202 232 4544. www.rwandemb.org/.
St Kitts and Nevis: Embassy of St Kitts and Nevis, 3216 New Mexico Avenue, NW, Washington DC 20016. Tel: +1 202 833 3550.
www.stkittsnevis.org/.
St Lucia: Embassy of St Lucia, 3216 New Mexico Avenue, NW, Washington DC 20016. Tel: +1 202 364 6792/6793/6794/6795. Fax: +1 202 364 6723.
St Vincent and the Grenadines: Embassy of St Vincent and the Grenadines, 3216 New Mexico Avenue, NW, Washington DC 20016.
Tel: +1 202 364 6730. Fax: +1 202 364 6736.
Saudi Arabia: Royal Embassy of Saudi Arabia, 601 New Hampshire Avenue, NW, Washington DC 20037. Tel: +1 202 337 4076. E-mail:
info@saudiembassy.net. www.saudiembassy.net/.
Senegal: Embassy of the Republic of Senegal, 2112 Wyoming Avenue, NW, Washington DC 20008.
Tel: +1 202 234 0540.
Seychelles: Chancery, Embassy of the Republic of Seychelles, 800 Second Avenue, Suite 400C, New York, NY 10017. Tel: +1 212 972 1785.
Fax: +1 212 972 1786.
Sierra Leone: Embassy of Sierra Leone, 1701 19th Street, NW, Washington DC 20009.
Tel: +1 202 939 9261.
http://amenhotep4.virtualafrica.com/slmbassy/.
Singapore: Embassy of the Republic of Singapore, 3501 International Place, NW, Washington DC 20008. Tel: +1 202 537 3100. Fax: +1 202 537 0876. E-mail: singemb@bellatlantic.net.
www.gov.sg/mfa/washington/.
Slovakia: Embassy of the Slovak Republic, 2201 Wisconsin Avenue, NW, Suite 250, Washington DC 20007. Tel: +1 202 965 160. Fax: +1 202 965 5166. E-mail: svkemb@concentric.net.
www.slovakemb.com/.
Slovenia: Embassy of the Republic of Slovenia, 1525 New Hampshire Avenue, NW, Washington DC 20036. Tel: +1 202 667 5363. Fax: +1 202 667 4563. www.embassy.org/slovenia/.
South Africa: Embassy of South Africa, 3051 Massachusetts Avenue, NW, Washington DC 20008. Tel: +1 202 232 4400. Fax: +1 202 265 1607. E-mail: safrica@southafrica.net.
www.southafrica.net/.
Spain: Embassy of Spain, 2375 Pennsylvania Avenue, NW, Washington DC 20037. Tel: +1 202 452 0100. Fax: +1 202 833 5670.
www.spainemb.org/ information/.
Sri Lanka: Embassy of Sri Lanka, 2148 Wyoming Avenue, NW, Washington DC 20008. Tel: +1 202 483 4025/4026/4027/4028. Fax: +1 202 232 7181/483 8017. E-mail: slembassy@clark.net.
www.slembassy.org.
Sudan: Embassy of the Republic of the Sudan, 2210 Massachusetts Avenue, NW, Washington DC

20008. Tel: +1 202 338 8565. Fax: +1 202 667 2406. E-mail: info@sudanembassyus.org.
www.sudanembassyus.org/.
Surinam: Embassy of the Republic of Surinam, 4301 Connecticut Avenue, NW, Suite 460, Washington DC 20008. Tel: +1 202 244 7488. Fax: +1 202 244 5878.
Swaziland: Embassy of the Kingdom of Swaziland, 3400 International Drive, NW, Washington DC 20008. Tel: +1 202 362 6683. Fax: +1 202 244 8059.
Sweden: Embassy of Sweden, 1501 M Street, NW, Washington DC 20005. Tel: +1 202 467 2600. Fax: +1 202 467 2656. www.swedenemb.org/.
Switzerland: Embassy of Switzerland, 2900 Cathedral Avenue, NW, Washington DC 20008. Tel: +1 202 745 7900. Fax: +1 202 387 2564.
www.swissemb.org/.
Syria: Embassy of the Syrian Arab Republic, 2215 Wyoming Avenue, NW, Washington DC 20008. Tel: +1 202 232 6313. Fax: +1 202 234 9548.
Taiwan: Republic of China on Taiwan, 4201 Wisconsin Avenue, NW, Washington DC 20016. Tel: +1 202 895 1800. Fax: +1 202 966 0825.
Tanzania: Embassy of the United Republic of Tanzania, 2139 R Street, NW, Washington DC 20008. Tel: +1 202 939 6125. Fax: +1 202 797 7408.
Thailand: Royal Thai Embassy, 1024 Wisconsin Avenue, NW, Suite 401, Washington DC 20007. Tel: +1 202 944 3600. Fax: +1 202 944 3611. E-mail: thai.wsn@thaiembdc.org. www.thaiembdc.org/.
Togo: Embassy of the Republic of Togo, 2208 Massachusetts Avenue, NW, Washington DC 20008. Tel: +1 202 234 4212. Fax: +1 202 232 3190.
Tonga: Embassy of the Kingdom of Tonga (based in London), c/o Tonga High Commission, 36 Molyneux Street, London W1H 6AB, UK. Tel: +44 20 7724 5828. Fax: +44 20 7723 9074.
Trinidad and Tobago: Embassy of the Republic of Trinidad and Tobago, 1708 Massachusetts Avenue, NW, Washington DC 20036. Tel: +1 202 467 6490. Fax: +1 202 785 3130.
Tunisia: Embassy of Tunisia, 1515 Massachusetts Avenue, NW, Washington DC 20005. Tel: +1 202 862 1850.
Turkey: Embassy of the Republic of Turkey, 1714 Massachusetts Avenue, NW, Washington DC 20036. Tel: +1 202 659 8200. Fax: +1 202 659 0744.
www.turkey.org/turkey/.
Turkmenistan: Embassy of Turkmenistan, 2207 Massachusetts Avenue, NW, Washington DC 20008. Tel: +1 202 588 1500. Fax: +1 202 588 0697. E-mail: turkmen@earthlink.net.
www.embassyofturkmenistan.org.
Uganda: Embassy of the Republic of Uganda, 5911 16th Street, NW, Washington DC 20011. Tel: +1 202 726 7100. Fax: +1 202 726 1727. E-mail: ugaembassy@rocketmail.com.
www.ugandaweb.com/ugaembassy/.
UK: Embassy of the United Kingdom of Great Britain and Northern Ireland, 3100 Massachusetts Avenue, NW, Washington DC 20008. Tel: +1 202 588 6500. Fax: +1 202 588 7870.
www.britainusa.com/bis/ embassy/embassy.stm.
Ukraine: Embassy of Ukraine, 3350 M Street, NW, Washington DC 20007. Tel: +1 202 333 7507. Fax: +1 202 333 7510. E-mail: infolook@aol.com.
www.ukremb.com/.

United Arab Emirates: Embassy of the United Arab Emirates, 1255 22nd Street, NW, Suite 700, Washington DC 20037. Tel: +1 202 955 7999.

Uruguay: Embassy of Uruguay, 2715 M Street, NW, 3rd Floor, Washington DC 20007. Tel: +1 202 331 1313. Fax: +1 202 331 8142. E-mail: uruguay@embassy.org. www.embassy.org/uruguay/.

Uzbekistan: Embassy of the Republic of Uzbekistan, 1746 Massachusetts Avenue, NW, Washington DC 20036. Tel: +1 202 887 5300. Fax: +1 202 293 6804. www.uzbekistan.org/.

Venezuela: Embassy of the Republic of Venezuela, 1099 30th Street NW, Washington DC 20007. Tel: +1 202 342 2214. Fax: +1 202 342 6820. E-mail: embavene@dgsys.com. www.embavenez-us.org/.

Vietnam: Embassy of the Socialist Republic of Vietnam, 1233 20th Street NW, Suite 400, Washington DC 20037. Tel: +1 202 861 0737. Fax: +1 202 861 0917. E-mail: vietnamembassy@msn.com. www.vietnamembassy-usa.org/.

Western Samoa: Embassy of Western Samoa, 800 Second Avenue, Suite 400D, New York NY 10017. Tel: +1 212 599 6196.

Yemen: Embassy of the Republic of Yemen, 2600 Virginia Avenue, NW, Suite 705, Washington DC 20037. Tel: +1 202 965 4760. Fax: +1 202 337 2017. E-mail: info@yemenembassy.org. www.yemenembassy.org.

Yugoslavia: Embassy of the Former S F Republic of Yugoslavia, 2410 California Street, NW, Washington DC 20008. Tel: +1 202 462 6566. E-mail: yuembassy@compuserve.com. http://ourworld. compuserve.com/homepages/yuembassy/.

Zambia: Embassy of the Republic of Zambia, 2419 Massachusetts Avenue, NW, Washington DC 20008. Tel: +1 202 265 9717.

Zimbabwe: Embassy of the Republic of Zimbabwe, 1608 New Hampshire Avenue, NW, Washington DC 20009. Tel: +1 202 332 7100. www.zimweb.com/ Embassy/ Zimbabwe/.

Embassies

Travel vaccinations

Polio and tetanus boosters are recommended for all countries listed, but see item marked†

Destination	Typhoid	Hepatitis A	Diphtheria	Tuberculosis	Hepatitis B	Rabies	Men. meningitis	Yellow fever	Jap B enceph	Tick-borne encephalitis	Malaria risk	HIV Prevalence (est. 1999)
Afghanistan	R	R	S			S	S				✓	less than 0.01% (1999 est.)
Albania	S	S	S			S	S			S		less than 0.01% (1999 est.)
Algeria	S	S	S			S	S					0.07% (1999 est.)
American Samoa	R	R	S		S							NA
Andorra												NA
Angola	R	R	S			S	S	R			✓	2.78% (1999 est.)
Anguilla	S	S	S		S							NA
Antigua & Barbuda	S	S	S	S	S							NA
Argentina	S	R	S	S	S	S					✓	0.69% (1999 est.)
Armenia	S	S	S	S	S	S				S		0.01% (1999 est.)
Aruba	S	S	S		S							NA
Australia												0.15% (1999 est.)
Austria										S		0.23% (1999 est.)
Azerbaijan	S	S	R	S	S	S				S	✓	less than 0.01% (1999 est.)
Azores												
Bahamas, The	S	S	S	S	S							4.13% (1999 est.)
Bahrain	S	S	S			S	S					0.15% (1999 est.)
Bangladesh	R	R	S	S	S	S			S		✓	0.02% (1999 est.)
Barbados	S	S	S	S	S							1.17% (1999 est.)
Belarus	S	S	S	S	S	S				S		0.28% (1999 est.)

†The Americas are now polio-free and boosters may be omitted for short-term travellers

Key to immunization recommendations

M = immunization mandatory
R = immunization recommended as risk of infection is substantial
S = immunization sometimes recommended

Vaccines recommended in some circumstances S are for more than three visits in a year, or a stay of more than three months in a rural area, or if the traveller is in a high-risk occupation. Seek specialist advice for complex itineraries.

NB Receiving country outside a yellow fever zone may require a valid yellow fever certificate from travellers going through yellow fever countries.

No vaccines recommended

There are no particular health or vaccine recommendations for the following countries, but travellers to these and all other countries should have their tetanus and polio immunizations up to date.

- Australia
- Austria✣
- Azores
- Belgium
- Canada
- Canary Islands*
- Corfu*
- Corsica
- Crete*
- Cyprus
- Denmark
- Falkland Islands
- Finland✣
- France
- Germany
- Gibraltar
- Greece*
- Hawaii
- Hungary✣
- Ibiza*
- Iceland
- Ireland
- Italy
- Luxembourg
- Madeira*
- Majorca*
- Malta*
- Minorca*
- Monaco
- Netherlands
- New Zealand
- Norway✣
- Portugal*
- Sardinia
- Spain*
- Sweden✣
- Switzerland✣
- USA

*Longer-term travellers should also consider hepatitis A immunization.
✣Longer-term travellers should also consider tick-borne encephalitis immunization.

Polio and tetanus boosters are recommended for all countries listed, but see item marked†

Destination	Typhoid	Hepatitis A	Diphtheria	Tuberculosis	Hepatitis B	Rabies	Men. meningitis	Yellow fever	Jap B enceph	Tick-borne encephalitis	Malaria risk	HIV Prevalence (est. 1999)
Belgium												0.15% (1999 est.)
Belize	R	R	S	S	S	S					✓	2.01% (1999 est.)
Benin	R	R	S		S	S	S	M			✓	2.45% (1999 est.)
Bermuda					S							NA
Bhutan	R	R	S		S	S			S		✓	less than 0.01% (1999 est.)
Bolivia	R	R	S	S		S		R			✓	0.1% (1999 est.)
Bosnia and Herzegovina		S	S	S	S	S				S		0.04% (1999 est.)
Botswana		R	S	S	S	S					✓	35.8% (1999 est.)
Brazil	R	R	S	S	S	S		R			✓	0.57% (1999 est.)
British Virgin Islands	S	S	S		S							NA
Brunei	S	S	S	S	S	S			S			0.2% (1999 est.)
Bulgaria		S	S		S	S				S		0.01% (1999 est.)
Burkina Faso	R	R	S		S	S	S	M			✓	6.44% (1999 est.)
Burma	S	S	S		S	S			S		✓	1.99% (1999 est.)
Burundi	R	R	S		S	S	S	R			✓	11.32% (1999 est.)
Cambodia	S	S	S		S	S			S		✓	4.04% (1999 est.)
Cameroon	R	R	S		S	S	S	M			✓	7.73% (1999 est.)
Canada												0.3% (1999 est.)
Canary Islands												
Cape Verde	R	R	S		S	S		R				NA
Cayman Islands	S	S	S	S	S							NA

†The Americas are now polio-free and boosters may be omitted for short-term travellers

No vaccines recommended

There are no particular health or vaccine recommendations for the following countries, but travellers to these and all other countries should have their tetanus and polio immunizations up to date.

Australia	Austria✣	Azores	Belgium	Canada	Canary Islands*
Corfu*	Corsica	Crete*	Cyprus	Denmark	Falkland Islands
Finland✣	France	Germany	Gibraltar	Greece*	Hawaii
Hungary✣	Ibiza*	Iceland	Ireland	Italy	Luxembourg
Madeira*	Majorca*	Malta*	Minorca*	Monaco	Netherlands
New Zealand	Norway✣	Portugal*	Sardinia	Spain*	Sweden✣
Switzerland✣	USA				

*Longer-term travellers should also consider hepatitis A immunization.
✣Longer-term travellers should also consider tick-borne encephalitis immunization.

Destination	Typhoid	Hepatitis A	Diphtheria	Tuberculosis	Hepatitis B	Rabies	Men. meningitis	Yellow fever	Jap B encephalitis	Tick-borne encephalitis	Malaria risk	HIV Prevalence (est. 1999)
Central African Republic	R	R	S		S	S	S	M			✓	13.84% (1999 est.)
Chad	R	R	S		S	S	S	R			✓	2.69% (1999 est.)
Chile	S	R	S	S	S	S						0.19% (1999 est.)
China	S	R	S	S	S	S			S		✓	0.07% (1999 est.)
Christmas Island												NA
Cocos (Keeling) Islands												NA
Colombia	R	R	S	S	S	S		R			✓	0.31% (1999 est.)
Comoros	R	R	S		S	S					✓	0.12% (1999 est.)
Congo, Democratic Republic of the	R	R	S		S	S	S	M			✓	5.07% (1999 est.)
Congo, Republic of the	R	R	S		S	S		M			✓	6.43% (1999 est.)
Cook Islands	R	R	S	S	S							NA
Corsica												
Costa Rica	R	R	S		S	S					✓	0.54% (1999 est.)
Cote d'Ivoire	R	R	S		S	S	S	M			✓	10.76% (1999 est.)
Crete												
Croatia		S	S	S	S	S				S		0.02% (1999 est.)
Cuba	S	S	S	S	S	S						0.03% (1999 est.)
Cyprus												0.1% (1999 est.)
Czech Republic		S	S		S					S		0.04% (1999 est.)

†The Americas are now polio-free and boosters may be omitted for short-term travellers

Key to immunization recommendations

M = immunization mandatory

R = immunization recommended as risk of infection is substantial

S = immunization sometimes recommended

Vaccines recommended in some circumstances S are for more than three visits in a year, or a stay of more than three months in a rural area, or if the traveller is in a high-risk occupation. Seek specialist advice for complex itineraries.

NB Receiving country outside a yellow fever zone may require a valid yellow fever certificate from travellers going through yellow fever countries.

No vaccines recommended

There are no particular health or vaccine recommendations for the following countries, but travellers to these and all other countries should have their tetanus and polio immunizations up to date.

Australia	Austria✤	Azores	Belgium	Canada	Canary Islands*
Corfu*	Corsica	Crete*	Cyprus	Denmark	Falkland Islands
Finland✤	France	Germany	Gibraltar	Greece*	Hawaii
Hungary✤	Ibiza*	Iceland	Ireland	Italy	Luxembourg
Madeira*	Majorca*	Malta*	Minorca*	Monaco	Netherlands
New Zealand	Norway✤	Portugal*	Sardinia	Spain*	Sweden✤
Switzerland✤	USA				

*Longer-term travellers should also consider hepatitis A immunization.

✤Longer-term travellers should also consider tick-borne encephalitis immunization.

Polio and tetanus boosters are recommended for all countries listed, but see item marked†

Destination	Typhoid	Hepatitis A	Diphtheria	Tuberculosis	Hepatitis B	Rabies	Men. meningitis	Yellow fever	Jap B enceph	Tick-borne encephalitis	Malaria risk	HIV Prevalence (est. 1999)
Denmark												0.17% (1999 est.)
Djibouti	R	R	S		S	S		R			✓	11.75% (1999 est.)
Dominica	S	S	S		S							NA
Dominican Republic	S	S	S	S	S	S					✓	2.8% (1999 est.)
Ecuador	R	R	S	S	S	S		R			✓	0.29% (1999 est.)
Egypt	S	S	S		S	S					✓	0.02% (1999 est.)
El Salvador	R	R	S		S	S					✓	0.6% (1999 est.)
Equatorial Guinea	R	R	S		S	S		R			✓	0.51% (1999 est.)
Eritrea	R	R	S		S	S	S				✓	2.87% (1999 est.)
Estonia			S		S	S				S		0.04% (1999 est.)
Ethiopia	R	R	S		S	S	S	R			✓	10.63% (1999 est.)
Falkland Islands (Islas Malvinas)												NA
Faroe Islands												NA
Fiji	R	R	S	S	S							0.07% (1999 est.)
Finland										S		0.05% (1999 est.)
France												0.44% (1999 est.)
French Guiana	R	R	S		S			M			✓	NA
French Polynesia	R	R	S		S			S				NA
Gabon	R	R	S		S	S		M			✓	4.16% (1999 est.)
Gambia, The	R	R	S	S	S	S	S	R			✓	1.95% (1999 est.)
Gaza Strip												NA

†The Americas are now polio-free and boosters may be omitted for short-term travellers

Key to immunization recommendations

M = immunization mandatory
R = immunization recommended as risk of infection is substantial
S = immunization sometimes recommended

Vaccines recommended in some circumstances S are for more than three visits in a year, or a stay of more than three months in a rural area, or if the traveller is in a high-risk occupation. Seek specialist advice for complex itineraries.

NB Receiving country outside a yellow fever zone may require a valid yellow fever certificate from travellers going through yellow fever countries.

No vaccines recommended

There are no particular health or vaccine recommendations for the following countries, but travellers to these and all other countries should have their tetanus and polio immunizations up to date.

Australia	Austria✣	Azores	Belgium	Canada	Canary Islands*
Corfu*	Corsica	Crete*	Cyprus	Denmark	Falkland Islands
Finland✣	France	Germany	Gibraltar	Greece*	Hawaii
Hungary✣	Ibiza*	Iceland	Ireland	Italy	Luxembourg
Madeira*	Majorca*	Malta*	Minorca*	Monaco	Netherlands
New Zealand	Norway✣	Portugal*	Sardinia	Spain*	Sweden✣
Switzerland✣	USA				

*Longer-term travellers should also consider hepatitis A immunization.
✣Longer-term travellers should also consider tick-borne encephalitis immunization.

Destination	Typhoid	Hepatitis A	Diphtheria	Tuberculosis	Hepatitis B	Rabies	Men. meningitis	Yellow fever	Jap B enceph	Tick-borne encephalitis	Malaria risk	HIV Prevalence (est. 1999)
Georgia		S	S			S	S			S		less than 0.01% (1999 est.)
Germany												0.1% (1999 est.)
Ghana	R	R	S	S	S	S	S	M			✓	3.6% (1999 est.)
Gibraltar												3.6% (1999 est.)
Greece		S										0.16% (1999 est.)
Greenland						S						NA
Grenada	S	S	S	S		S	S					NA
Guadeloupe	S	S	S				S					NA
Guam	R	R	S				S					NA
Guatamala	R	R	S	S	S	S					✓	1.38% (1999 est.)
Guernsey												NA
Guinea	R	R	S		S	S	S	R			✓	1.54% (1999 est.)
Guinea-Bissau	R	R	S		S	S	S	R			✓	2.5% (1999 est.)
Guyana	R	R	S	S	S	S		R			✓	3.01% (1999 est.)
Haiti	S	S	S	S	S	S					✓	5.17% (1999 est.)
Hawaii												
Honduras	R	R	S	S	S	S					✓	1.92% (1999 est.)
Hong Kong	S	S	S	S	S	S					✓	0.06% (1999 est.)
Hungary										S		0.05% (1999 est.)
Ibiza												
Iceland												0.14% (1999 est.)
India	R	R	S	S	S	S			S		✓	0.7% (1999 est.)

†The Americas are now polio-free and boosters may be omitted for short-term travellers

Key to immunization recommendations

M = immunization mandatory

R = immunization recommended as risk of infection is substantial

S = immunization sometimes recommended

Vaccines recommended in some circumstances S are for more than three visits in a year, or a stay of more than three months in a rural area, or if the traveller is in a high-risk occupation. Seek specialist advice for complex itineraries.

NB Receiving country outside a yellow fever zone may require a valid yellow fever certificate from travellers going through yellow fever countries.

No vaccines recommended

There are no particular health or vaccine recommendations for the following countries, but travellers to these and all other countries should have their tetanus and polio immunizations up to date.

Australia	Austria✜	Azores	Belgium	Canada	Canary Islands*
Corfu*	Corsica	Crete*	Cyprus	Denmark	Falkland Islands
Finland✜	France	Germany	Gibraltar	Greece*	Hawaii
Hungary✜	Ibiza*	Iceland	Ireland	Italy	Luxembourg
Madeira*	Majorca*	Malta*	Minorca*	Monaco	Netherlands
New Zealand	Norway✜	Portugal*	Sardinia	Spain*	Sweden✜
Switzerland✜	USA				

*Longer-term travellers should also consider hepatitis A immunization.

✜Longer-term travellers should also consider tick-borne encephalitis immunization.

Polio and tetanus boosters are recommended for all countries listed, but see item marked†

Destination	Typhoid	Hepatitis A	Diphtheria	Tuberculosis	Hepatitis B	Rabies	Men. meningitis	Yellow fever	Jap B enceph	Tick-borne encephalitis	Malaria risk	HIV Prevalence (est. 1999)
Indonesia	S	S	S		S	S			S		✓	0.05% (1999 est.)
Iran	S	S	S		S	S					✓	less than 0.01% (1999 est.)
Iraq	R	R	S		S	S					✓	less than 0.01% (1999 est.)
Ireland												0.1% (1999 est.)
Israel	S	S	S	S	S	S						0.08% (1999 est.)
Italy												0.35% (1999 est.)
Jamaica	S	S	S	S	S							0.71% (1999 est.)
Japan	S	S	S						S			0.02% (1999 est.)
Jersey												NA
Jordan	S	S	S	S	S	S						0.02% (1999 est.)
Kazakhstan	S	S	S		S	S				S		0.04% (1999 est.)
Kenya	R	R	S	S	S	S	S	R			✓	13.95% (1999 est.)
Kiribati	R	R	S		S							NA
Korea, North	S	S	S		S	S			S			NA
Korea, South	S	S	S		S	S			S			0.01% (1999 est.)
Kuwait	S	S	S		S	S						0.12% (1999 est.)
Kyrgyzstan	S	S	S		S	S						less than 0.01% (1999 est.)
Laos	S	S	S		S	S			S		✓	0.05% (1999 est.)
Latvia			S		S	S				S		0.11% (1999 est.)
Lebanon	S	S	S		S	S						0.09% (1999 est.)
Lesotho	S	S	S	S	S	S						23.57% (1999 est.)
Liberia	R	R	S		S	S		M			✓	2.8% (1999 est.)

†The Americas are now polio-free and boosters may be omitted for short-term travellers

Key to immunization recommendations

M = immunization mandatory
R = immunization recommended as risk of infection is substantial
S = immunization sometimes recommended

Vaccines recommended in some circumstances S are for more than three visits in a year, or a stay of more than three months in a rural area, or if the traveller is in a high-risk occupation. Seek specialist advice for complex itineraries.

NB Receiving country outside a yellow fever zone may require a valid yellow fever certificate from travellers going through yellow fever countries.

No vaccines recommended

There are no particular health or vaccine recommendations for the following countries, but travellers to these and all other countries should have their tetanus and polio immunizations up to date.

Australia	Austria✤	Azores	Belgium	Canada	Canary Islands*
Corfu*	Corsica	Crete*	Cyprus	Denmark	Falkland Islands
Finland✤	France	Germany	Gibraltar	Greece*	Hawaii
Hungary✤	Ibiza*	Iceland	Ireland	Italy	Luxembourg
Madeira*	Majorca*	Malta*	Minorca*	Monaco	Netherlands
New Zealand	Norway✤	Portugal*	Sardinia	Spain*	Sweden✤
Switzerland✤	USA				

*Longer-term travellers should also consider hepatitis A immunization.
✤Longer-term travellers should also consider tick-borne encephalitis immunization.

Polio and tetanus boosters are recommended for all countries listed, but see item marked†

Destination	Typhoid	Hepatitis A	Diphtheria	Tuberculosis	Hepatitis B	Rabies	Men. meningitis	Yellow fever	Jap B enceph	Tick-borne encephalitis	Malaria risk	HIV Prevalence (est. 1999)
Libya	S	S	S			S	S					0.05% (1999 est.)
Liechtenstein												NA
Lithuania			S			S	S			S		0.02% (1999 est.)
Luxembourg												0.16% (1999 est.)
Macau	S	S	S			S	S					NA
Macedonia, The Former Yugoslav Republic of	S	S	S			S						less than 0.01% (1999 est.)
Madagascar	R	R	S	S	S	S					✓	0.15% (1999 est.)
Madeira												
Majorca												
Malawi	R	R	S	S	S	S					✓	15.96% (1999 est.)
Malaysia	S	S	S	S	S	S			S		✓	0.42% (1999 est.)
Maldives	R	R	S	S	S	S						0.05% (1999 est.)
Mali	R	R	S			S	S	M			✓	2.03% (1999 est.)
Malta												0.52% (1999 est.)
Man, Isle of												NA
Marshall Islands	R	R	S			S						NA
Martinique	S	S	S			S						NA
Mauritania	R	R	S			S	S	M			✓	1.8% (2000 est.)
Mauritius	R	R	S	S	S	S					✓	0.08% (1999 est.)
Mayotte	R	R	S			S	S				✓	NA

†The Americas are now polio-free and boosters may be omitted for short-term travellers

Key to immunization recommendations

M = immunization mandatory
R = immunization recommended as risk of infection is substantial
S = immunization sometimes recommended

Vaccines recommended in some circumstances S are for more than three visits in a year, or a stay of more than three months in a rural area, or if the traveller is in a high-risk occupation. Seek specialist advice for complex itineraries.

NB Receiving country outside a yellow fever zone may require a valid yellow fever certificate from travellers going through yellow fever countries.

No vaccines recommended

There are no particular health or vaccine recommendations for the following countries, but travellers to these and all other countries should have their tetanus and polio immunizations up to date.

Australia	Austria✤	Azores	Belgium	Canada	Canary Islands*
Corfu*	Corsica	Crete*	Cyprus	Denmark	Falkland Islands
Finland✤	France	Germany	Gibraltar	Greece*	Hawaii
Hungary✤	Ibiza*	Iceland	Ireland	Italy	Luxembourg
Madeira*	Majorca*	Malta*	Minorca*	Monaco	Netherlands
New Zealand	Norway✤	Portugal*	Sardinia	Spain*	Sweden✤
Switzerland✤	USA				

*Longer-term travellers should also consider hepatitis A immunization.
✤Longer-term travellers should also consider tick-borne encephalitis immunization.

Destination	Typhoid	Hepatitis A	Diphtheria	Tuberculosis	Hepatitis B	Rabies	Men. meningitis	Yellow fever	Jap B enceph	Tick-borne encephalitis	Malaria risk	HIV Prevalence (est. 1999)
Mexico	R	R		S	S	S	S				✓	0.29% (1999 est.)
Micronesia, Federated States of	R	R		S			S					NA
Minorca												
Moldova			S	S	S	S				S		0.2% (1999 est.)
Monaco												NA
Mongolia	S	S		S		S	S					less than 0.01% (1999 est.)
Montserrat	S	S		S			S					NA
Morocco	S	S				S	S					0.03% (1999 est.)
Mozambique	R	R		S	S	S	S	S			✓	13.22% (1999 est.)
Namibia	R	R		S	S	S	S	S			✓	19.54% (1999 est.)
Nauru	R	R		S			S					NA
Nepal	R	R		S	S	S	S		S		✓	0.29% (1999 est.)
Netherlands												0.19% (1999 est.)
Netherlands Antilles	S	S		S			S					NA
New Caledonia	R	R		S			S					NA
New Zealand												0.06% (1999 est.)
Nicaragua	R	R		S	S	S	S				✓	0.2% (1999 est.)
Niger	R	R		S			S	M			✓	1.35% (1999 est.)
Nigeria	R	R	S	S	S	S	S	R			✓	5.06% (1999 est.)
Niue	R	R		S			S					NA
Norfolk Island												NA

†The Americas are now polio-free and boosters may be omitted for short-term travellers

Destination	Typhoid	Hepatitis A	Diphtheria	Tuberculosis	Hepatitis B	Rabies	Men. meningitis	Yellow fever	Jap B enceph	Tick-borne encephalitis	Malaria risk	HIV Prevalence (est. 1999)
Northern Mariana Islands	R	R	S		S							NA
Norway										S		less than 100 (1999 est.)
Oman	S	S	S		S	S					✓	0.11% (1999 est.)
Pakistan	R	R	S	S	S	S			S		✓	0.1% (1999 est.)
Palau	R	R	S		S							NA
Panama	R	R	S		S	S		R			✓	1.54% (1999 est.)
Papua New Guinea	R	R	S	S	S				S		✓	0.22% (1999 est.)
Paraguay	R	R	S	S	S	S					✓	0.11% (1999 est.)
Peru	R	R	S	S	S	S		R			✓	0.35% (1999 est.)
Philippines	S	S	S	S	S	S			S		✓	0.07% (1999 est.)
Pitcairn Islands	S	S	S		S							NA
Poland			S		S	S				S		0.07% (1999 est.)
Portugal		S										0.74% (1999 est.)
Puerto Rico	S	S	S	S	S	S						NA
Qatar	S	S	S		S	S						0.09% (1999 est.)
Reunion	R	R	S		S	S						NA
Romania		S	S	S	S	S				S		0.02% (1999 est.)
Russia	S	S	S	S	S	S	S		S	S		0.18% (1999 est.)
Rwanda	R	R	S		S	S		M			✓	11.21% (1999 est.)
Saint Helena	R	R	S		S	S						NA
Saint Kitts and Nevis	S	S	S		S							NA

†The Americas are now polio-free and boosters may be omitted for short-term travellers

Key to immunization recommendations

M = immunization mandatory

R = immunization recommended as risk of infection is substantial

S = immunization sometimes recommended

Vaccines recommended in some circumstances S are for more than three visits in a year, or a stay of more than three months in a rural area, or if the traveller is in a high-risk occupation. Seek specialist advice for complex itineraries.

NB Receiving country outside a yellow fever zone may require a valid yellow fever certificate from travellers going through yellow fever countries.

No vaccines recommended

There are no particular health or vaccine recommendations for the following countries, but travellers to these and all other countries should have their tetanus and polio immunizations up to date.

Australia	Austria❖	Azores	Belgium	Canada	Canary Islands*
Corfu*	Corsica	Crete*	Cyprus	Denmark	Falkland Islands
Finland❖	France	Germany	Gibraltar	Greece*	Hawaii
Hungary❖	Ibiza*	Iceland	Ireland	Italy	Luxembourg
Madeira*	Majorca*	Malta*	Minorca*	Monaco	Netherlands
New Zealand	Norway❖	Portugal*	Sardinia	Spain*	Sweden❖
Switzerland❖	USA				

*Longer-term travellers should also consider hepatitis A immunization.

❖Longer-term travellers should also consider tick-borne encephalitis immunization.

Destination	Typhoid	Hepatitis A	Diphtheria	Tuberculosis	Hepatitis B	Rabies	Men. meningitis	Yellow fever	Jap B enceph	Tick-borne encephalitis	Malaria risk	HIV Prevalence (est. 1999)
Saint Lucia	S	S	S	S	S							NA
Saint Pierre and Miquelon												NA
Saint Vincent and the Grenadines	S	S	S				S					NA
Samoa	R	R	S	S	S							NA
San Marino												NA
Sao Tome and Principe	R	R	S		S	S		M			✓	NA
Sardinia												
Saudi Arabia	S	S	S		S		S				✓	0.01% (1999 est.)
Senegal	R	R	S		S	S	S	R			✓	1.77% (1999 est.)
Seychelles	R	R	S	S	S	S						NA
Sierra Leone	R	R	S		S	S	S	R			✓	2.99% (1999 est.)
Singapore	S	S	S	S	S							0.19% (1999 est.)
Slovakia			S	S	S		S			S		less than 0.01% (1999 est.)
Slovenia			S	S	S		S			S		0.02% (1999 est.)
Solomon Islands	R	R	S	S	S						✓	NA
Somalia	R	R	S		S	S	S	R			✓	NA
South Africa	R	R	S	S	S	S					✓	19.94% (1999 est.)
Spain												0.58% (1999 est.)
Sri Lanka	R	R	S	S	S	S			S		✓	0.07% (1999 est.)

†The Americas are now polio-free and boosters may be omitted for short-term travellers

Key to immunization recommendations

M = immunization mandatory
R = immunization recommended as risk of infection is substantial
S = immunization sometimes recommended

Vaccines recommended in some circumstances S are for more than three visits in a year, or a stay of more than three months in a rural area, or if the traveller is in a high-risk occupation. Seek specialist advice for complex itineraries.

NB Receiving country outside a yellow fever zone may require a valid yellow fever certificate from travellers going through yellow fever countries.

No vaccines recommended

There are no particular health or vaccine recommendations for the following countries, but travellers to these and all other countries should have their tetanus and polio immunizations up to date.

Australia	Austria✣	Azores	Belgium	Canada	Canary Islands*
Corfu*	Corsica	Crete*	Cyprus	Denmark	Falkland Islands
Finland✣	France	Germany	Gibraltar	Greece*	Hawaii
Hungary✣	Ibiza*	Iceland	Ireland	Italy	Luxembourg
Madeira*	Majorca*	Malta*	Minorca*	Monaco	Netherlands
New Zealand	Norway✣	Portugal*	Sardinia	Spain*	Sweden✣
Switzerland✣	USA				

*Longer-term travellers should also consider hepatitis A immunization.
✣Longer-term travellers should also consider tick-borne encephalitis immunization.

Destination	Typhoid	Hepatitis A	Diphtheria	Tuberculosis	Hepatitis B	Rabies	Men. meningitis	Yellow fever	Jap B enceph	Tick-borne encephalitis	Malaria risk	HIV Prevalence (est. 1999)
Sudan	R	R	S		S	S	S	R			✓	0.99% (1999 est.)
Suriname	R	R	S		S	S		R				1.26% (1999 est.)
Svalbard												0% (2001)
Swaziland	R	R	S	S	S	S					✓	25.25% (1999 est.)
Sweden										S		0.08% (1999 est.)
Switzerland										S		0.46% (1999 est.)
Syria	S	S	S		S	S					✓	0.01% (1999 est.)
Tajikistan	S	S	S		S	S				S	✓	less than 0.01% (1999 est.)
Tanzania	R	R	S	S	S	S	S	R			✓	8.09% (1999 est.)
Thailand	S	S	S	S	S	S			S		✓	2.15% (1999 est.)
Togo	R	R	S		S	S	S	M			✓	5.98% (1999 est.)
Tokelau												NA
Tonga	R	R	S			S						NA
Trinidad and Tobago	S	S	S	S	S	S		R				1.05% (1999 est.)
Tunisia	S	S	S		S	S						0.04% (1999 est.)
Turkey	S	S	S	S	S	S					✓	0.01% (1999 est.)
Turkmenistan	S	S	S		S	S				S	✓	0.01% (1999 est.)
Turks and Caicos Islands	S	S	S			S						NA
Tuvalu	R	R	S			S						NA
Uganda	R	R	S	S	S	S	S	R			✓	8.3% (1999 est.)
Ukraine		S	S		S	S				S		0.96% (1999 est.)

†The Americas are now polio-free and boosters may be omitted for short-term travellers

Key to immunization recommendations

M = immunization mandatory

R = immunization recommended as risk of infection is substantial

S = immunization sometimes recommended

Vaccines recommended in some circumstances S are for more than three visits in a year, or a stay of more than three months in a rural area, or if the traveller is in a high-risk occupation. Seek specialist advice for complex itineraries.

NB Receiving country outside a yellow fever zone may require a valid yellow fever certificate from travellers going through yellow fever countries.

No vaccines recommended

There are no particular health or vaccine recommendations for the following countries, but travellers to these and all other countries should have their tetanus and polio immunizations up to date.

Australia	Austria✜	Azores	Belgium	Canada	Canary Islands*
Corfu*	Corsica	Crete*	Cyprus	Denmark	Falkland Islands
Finland✜	France	Germany	Gibraltar	Greece*	Hawaii
Hungary✜	Ibiza*	Iceland	Ireland	Italy	Luxembourg
Madeira*	Majorca*	Malta*	Minorca*	Monaco	Netherlands
New Zealand	Norway✜	Portugal*	Sardinia	Spain*	Sweden✜
Switzerland✜	USA				

*Longer-term travellers should also consider hepatitis A immunization.

✜Longer-term travellers should also consider tick-borne encephalitis immunization.

Destination	Typhoid	Hepatitis A	Diphtheria	Tuberculosis	Hepatitis B	Rabies	Men. meningitis	Yellow fever	Jap B enceph	Tick-borne encephalitis	Malaria risk	HIV Prevalence (est. 1999)
United Arab Emirates	S	S	S		S	S						0.18% (1999 est.)
United Kingdom												0.11% (1999 est.)
United States												0.61% (1999 est.)
Uruguay	S	R	S	S	S	S						0.33% (1999 est.)
Uzbekistan	S	S	S		S	S				S		less than 0.01% (1999 est.)
Vanuata	R	R	S	S	S						✓	NA
Venezuela	R	R	S	S	S	S		R			✓	0.49% (1999 est.)
Vietnam	S	S	S		S	S			S		✓	0.24% (1999 est.)
Virgin Islands	S	S	S		S							NA
West Bank												NA
Western Sahara												NA
World												NA
Yemen	S	S	S		S	S					✓	0.01% (1999 est.)
Yugoslavia		S	S		S	S				S		NA
Zambia	R	R	S	S	S	S	S	R			✓	19.95% (1999 est.)
Zimbabwe	R	R	S	S	S	S					✓	25.06% (1999 est.)

†The Americas are now polio-free and boosters may be omitted for short-term travellers

Key to immunization recommendations

M = immunization mandatory

R = immunization recommended as risk of infection is substantial

S = immunization sometimes recommended

Vaccines recommended in some circumstances S are for more than three visits in a year, or a stay of more than three months in a rural area, or if the traveller is in a high-risk occupation. Seek specialist advice for complex itineraries.

NB Receiving country outside a yellow fever zone may require a valid yellow fever certificate from travellers going through yellow fever countries.

No vaccines recommended

There are no particular health or vaccine recommendations for the following countries, but travellers to these and all other countries should have their tetanus and polio immunizations up to date.

Australia	Austria✤	Azores	Belgium	Canada	Canary Islands*
Corfu*	Corsica	Crete*	Cyprus	Denmark	Falkland Islands
Finland✤	France	Germany	Gibraltar	Greece*	Hawaii
Hungary✤	Ibiza*	Iceland	Ireland	Italy	Luxembourg
Madeira*	Majorca*	Malta*	Minorca*	Monaco	Netherlands
New Zealand	Norway✤	Portugal*	Sardinia	Spain*	Sweden✤
Switzerland✤	USA				

*Longer-term travellers should also consider hepatitis A immunization.

✤Longer-term travellers should also consider tick-borne encephalitis immunization.

Index